Henke's
Med-Math

Dosage Calculation, Preparation & Administration

Eighth Edition

Susan Buchholz, RN, MSN, CNE
Associate Professor
Herzing University
Atlanta, Georgia

. Wolters Kluwer

Philadelphia · Baltimore · New York · London
Buenos Aires · Hong Kong · Sydney · Tokyo

Executive Editor: Sherry Dickinson
Product Development Editor: Matt Hauber
Marketing Manager: Carolyn Fox
Editorial Assistant: Dan Reilly
Production Project Manager: Cynthia Rudy
Design Coordinator: Holly Reid McLaughlin
Illustration Coordinator: Jennifer Clements
Manufacturing Coordinator: Karin Duffield
Prepress Vendor: S4Carlisle Publishing Services

8th edition

9 8 7 6 5 4 3 2

Printed in China

Library of Congress Cataloging-in-Publication Data
Buchholz, Susan, author.
  Henke's med-math : dosage calculation, preparation & administration / Susan Buchholz.—Eighth edition.
     p. ; cm.
  Med-math
  Includes index.
  ISBN 978-1-4963-0284-7
  I. Title. II. Title: Med-math.
  [DNLM: 1. Pharmaceutical Preparations—administration & dosage—Nurses' Instruction. 2. Pharmaceutical Preparations—administration & dosage—Programmed Instruction. 3. Drug Dosage Calculations—Nurses' Instruction. 4. Drug Dosage Calculations—Programmed Instruction. QV 18.2]
  RS57
  615.1'401513—dc23
                                                                          2015012387

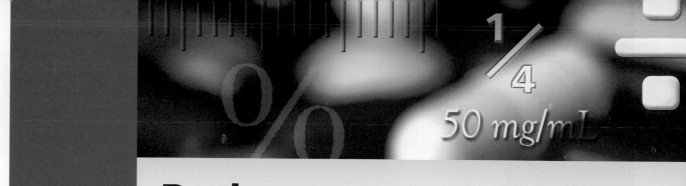

Reviewers

Dana M. Botz, MSN, RN, CNE
Nursing Faculty
North Hennepin Community College
Brooklyn Park, Minnesota

Theresa Buchanan, DNP
Assistant Professor of Nursing
Gordon State College
Barnesville, Georgia

Wendy W. Diment, MSN
Assistant Professor
Piedmont Virginia Community College
Charlottesville, Virginia

Dawn Fucito, MS
Course Coordinator
Middlesex County College
Edison, New Jersey

Sherry Holland, MSN
Instructor
The Community College of Baltimore County
Baltimore, Maryland

Antoinette McCray, RNC, MSN, CNS, CNE
Instructor
Department of Nursing and Allied Health
Norfolk State University
Norfolk, Virginia

Parvaneh Mohammadian, RHP, PhD
Nursing Faculty
California State University Dominguez Hills
Carson, California

Melanie Obispo-Young, RN, APRN
Assistant Professor
Lewis University
Romeoville, Illinois

Joscelyn Richey, MSN, ARNP, CDE
Nursing Faculty
Hillsborough Community College
Tampa, Florida

Ellis Siegel, MSN, BSN, RN
Nursing Professor
Norfolk State University
Norfolk, Virginia

Susan Snyder, MA
Instructor
Antelope Valley College
Lancaster, California

Karen Walton, MSN, RN
Faculty
Wallace State Community College
Hanceville, Alabama

Preface

"It takes a village to raise a child" . . . and revise a book.

This may seem a strange way to start a dosage calculation textbook, but I wanted to acknowledge that there are many students, educators, and nurses who have helped me make this book the best it can be. Despite lengthy proofreading and calculations, I still receive suggestions and solutions from many of you. I wanted to start the book by thanking you for your "eagle eyes" and your feedback.

Key Features of the Text

- Step-by-step approach in solving problems
- Text organization that builds from simpler concepts to more complex concepts
- Demonstration of four methods of calculation and side-by-side solutions
- Joint Commission-approved abbreviations
- *Test Your Clinical Savvy*—"what if" situations that stimulate critical thinking
- Glossary with definitions and common abbreviations
- *Putting It Together*—case studies with application of dosage calculations and critical thinking questions, with suggested answers in Appendix B
- Use of self-tests for pre- or posttesting

New to This Edition

- Updated drug labels and drug names
- Addition of problems to each calculation chapter
- Removal of apothecary measures
  - The U.S. Pharmacopeial (USP) Convention has banned the use of grains and other remnants of the apothecary system. However, medication strengths are still expressed as grains on some labels. The equivalencies for the apothecary system have been removed in this edition, although the definitions may still be found in the glossary.
- Clearer design for problems
- **Calculations in Action** animations to show how problems are solved
  - I have wanted to include a dynamic audio and video supplement to this text for a long time. With this edition, we are introducing a new series of animated calculations, tied to content in the book. Identified by a new icon 🎬, these animations will benefit visual learners—and all learners—by actually showing how the problems are solved in separate steps, with voice-over narration explaining the solutions.

The QSEN (Quality and Safety Education for Nurses) core competency that dosage calculation is most closely related to is the topic of safety. The QSEN definition is "minimizes risk of harm to patients and providers through both system effectiveness and individual performance." As such, correct calculation of drug dosages ensures safety in medication administration.

Because new research often becomes dated quickly, the Research Points boxes have been discontinued. Instead, here are some suggested topic areas for research and evidence-based practice (a reliable research database is recommended):

- Dosage calculations and medication errors
- Pediatric medication errors
- Compliance with "Do Not Use" abbreviations
- Relationship of nursing work environments and the occurrence of medication errors
- Medication errors in mislabeling of medications; medications with similar names or similar packaging; medications not commonly used or prescribed; medications that many patients are allergic to; medications that require drug levels and prescribing
- Nurses' self-reporting of medication safety practices
- Development of dosage calculation skills
- Methods of dosage calculation: which ones are the best and/or most error-free?
- Insulin dosage calculation errors
- Heparin dosage calculation errors
- Categories of nursing medication errors
- Technology and medication errors, including CPOE (computer prescriber order entry) and EHR (electronic health records)
- Use of barcode scanning and medication errors
- Errors in intravenous fluid infusion rates

Student and Instructor Resources

Resources and aids for students and faculty are provided on thePoint at thePoint.lww.com/Buchholz8e.

Student Resources

- New **Calculations in Action** animations provide step-by-step demonstrations of how to solve equations presented in the text.
- **Dosage Calculation Quizzes** provide additional practice in solving drug calculations.
- **Journal Articles** provided for each chapter offer access to current research available in Wolters Kluwer journals.

Instructor Resources

Instructors have access to all the Student Resources, in addition to the following:

- **Test Generator**.
- **Image Bank** of all the images in the text.
- **PowerPoint** presentation for each chapter.

Please continue to send suggestions and comments to me to help make each edition better. I appreciate any feedback and hope to continue to make dosage calculations easier, yet always safe for the consumer.

Susan Buchholz, RN, MSN, CNE
Decatur, Georgia
family@mindspring.com

Acknowledgments

Special thanks to:

- Wolters Kluwer editors: **Sherry Dickinson, Matt Hauber**
- **Sister Grace Henke**
- **Lynn Farmer:** Photography
- **Ginger Pyron:** Editor
- **Pharmaceutical companies** for supplying labels
- **Faith community** at **Oakhurst Baptist Church** for their support and prayers
- **Colleagues at Herzing University**
- **Valerie, Andrew**, and **Chelsea** for their love
- "Unofficial" proofreaders:

  Alina-Sarai Gal-Chis

  Jocylyn Lundy

  Michelle Sugden

  Orpha Gehman

  Milly Rodriquez

  Diane Skwisz

  Maritza Cantarero

  Ose Martinez

Contents

CHAPTER 4 Calculation of Oral Medications—Solids and Liquids   81

CHAPTER 5 Liquids for Injection   139

CHAPTER 6 Calculation of Basic IV Drip Rates   213

CHAPTER 7 Special Types of IV Calculations   255

CHAPTER 8 Dosage Problems for Infants and Children   315

CHAPTER 9 Information Basic to Administering Drugs   367

CHAPTER 10 Administration Procedures   391

Arithmetic Needed for Dosage

TOPICS COVERED

1. Multiplication and division of whole numbers, fractions, and decimals
2. Addition and subtraction of fractions
3. Reading decimals
4. Changing decimals to fractions
5. Addition, subtraction, multiplication, and division of decimals
6. Clearing and rounding of decimals
7. Percents
8. Solving ratio and proportion

When a medication order differs from the fixed amount at which a drug is supplied, you must calculate the dose needed. Calculation requires knowledge of the systems of dosage measurements (see Chapter 2) and the ability to solve arithmetic. This chapter covers the common arithmetic functions needed for the safe administration of drugs.

Examples that use basic arithmetic functions include problems in dosage calculations such as:

45.5 mL water + 34.75 mL juice = total intake

administer 1.5 mg of a drug; if you have 0.75 mg on hand, how much more of the drug do you need?

administer 3 tablets; if each tablet is 1.5 mg, what is the total dose?

administer 7.5 mg of a drug; if you have 1.25 mg tablets on hand, how many tablets need to be given?

on hand are two ophthalmic solutions: 0.05% and 0.02%. Which solution is strongest?

Beginning students invariably express anxiety that they will miscalculate a dose and cause harm. Although everyone is capable of error, no one has to cause an error. The surest way to prevent a mistake is to exercise care in performing basic arithmetic operations and practice basic arithmetic calculations.

For students who believe their arithmetic skills are already satisfactory, this chapter contains self-tests and a proficiency exam. Once you pass the proficiency exam, you can move on to other chapters in the book.

Students with math anxiety and those with deficiencies in performing arithmetic will want to work through this chapter. Examples demonstrate how to perform calculations; the self-tests provide practice and drill. FINE POINTS boxes explain details about the calculation. After you've mastered the content, take the proficiency exam to verify your readiness to move on.

Since calculators are readily available, why go through all the arithmetic? For one thing, using a calculator still requires that you to know what numbers and functions to enter. In clinical situations you may encounter some problems that require a calculator's help, but it's good to know how to make calculations on your own. Solving the arithmetic problems yourself helps you think logically about the amount ordered and the relative dose needed. And when you can mentally calculate dosage, you increase your speed and efficiency in preparing medications. Work out the problems in this chapter with and without a calculator.

 ## Multiplying Whole Numbers

If you need a review, study a multiplication table for the numbers 1 through 12, which can be found in a basic math book or on the internet. (Search for "multiplication table." One site is http://www.mathisfun.com/tables). Then do the self-tests, aiming for 100% accuracy.

SELF-TEST 1	Multiplication

Write the answers to these problems. Answers are given at the end of the chapter; aim for 100%.

1. $2 \times 6 =$ _____
2. $9 \times 7 =$ _____
3. $4 \times 8 =$ _____
4. $5 \times 9 =$ _____
5. $12 \times 9 =$ _____
6. $8 \times 3 =$ _____
7. $11 \times 10 =$ _____
8. $2 \times 7 =$ _____
9. $8 \times 6 =$ _____
10. $8 \times 9 =$ _____
11. $3 \times 5 =$ _____
12. $6 \times 7 =$ _____
13. $4 \times 6 =$ _____
14. $9 \times 6 =$ _____
15. $8 \times 8 =$ _____
16. $7 \times 8 =$ _____
17. $2 \times 9 =$ _____
18. $8 \times 11 =$ _____
19. $4 \times 9 =$ _____
20. $3 \times 8 =$ _____
21. $12 \times 11 =$ _____
22. $9 \times 5 =$ _____
23. $9 \times 9 =$ _____
24. $7 \times 5 =$ _____
25. $12 \times 10 =$ _____

Dividing Whole Numbers

Review division if necessary, using a division table which can be found in a basic math book or on the internet. Again, aim for 100% accuracy on the self-test.

SELF-TEST 2	Division

Write the answers to the following problems. Answers are given at the end of the chapter.

1. $63 \div 7 =$ _____
2. $24 \div 6 =$ _____
3. $36 \div 12 =$ _____
4. $42 \div 6 =$ _____
5. $35 \div 5 =$ _____
6. $96 \div 12 =$ _____
7. $12 \div 3 =$ _____
8. $27 \div 9 =$ _____
9. $49 \div 7 =$ _____
10. $18 \div 3 =$ _____
11. $72 \div 8 =$ _____
12. $48 \div 8 =$ _____
13. $28 \div 7 =$ _____
14. $21 \div 7 =$ _____
15. $24 \div 8 =$ _____
16. $84 \div 12 =$ _____
17. $81 \div 9 =$ _____
18. $32 \div 8 =$ _____
19. $36 \div 6 =$ _____
20. $18 \div 9 =$ _____
21. $21 \div 3 =$ _____
22. $48 \div 4 =$ _____
23. $144 \div 12 =$ _____
24. $56 \div 8 =$ _____
25. $60 \div 5 =$ _____

Fractions

A *fraction* is a portion of a whole number. The top number in a fraction is called the *numerator,* and the bottom number is called the *denominator.* The line between the numerator and the denominator is a division sign. Therefore, you can read the fraction $\frac{1}{4}$ as "one divided by four."

EXAMPLE

$$\frac{1}{4} \quad \begin{array}{l} \rightarrow \text{numerator} \\ \rightarrow \text{denominator} \end{array}$$

Types of Fractions

In a proper fraction, the numerator is smaller than the denominator.

EXAMPLE

$\frac{2}{5}$ (Read as "two fifths.")

In an improper fraction, the numerator is larger than the denominator.

EXAMPLE

$\frac{5}{2}$ (Read as "five halves.")

A *mixed number* has a whole number plus a fraction.

EXAMPLE

$1\frac{2}{3}$ (Read as "one and two thirds.")

In a *complex* or *common* fraction, both the numerator and the denominator are already fractions.

EXAMPLE

$\dfrac{\frac{1}{2}}{\frac{1}{4}}$ (Read as "one half divided by one fourth.")

RULE **REDUCING FRACTIONS**

Find the largest number that can be divided evenly into the numerator and the denominator.

EXAMPLE

EXAMPLE 1:

Reduce $\frac{4}{12}$

$$\frac{\overset{1}{\cancel{\underset{}{4}}}}{\underset{3}{\cancel{12}}} = \frac{1}{3}$$

EXAMPLE 2:

Reduce $\frac{7}{49}$

$$\frac{\overset{1}{\cancel{7}}}{\underset{7}{\cancel{49}}} = \frac{1}{7}$$

 FINE POINTS

Check to see if the denominator is evenly divisible by the numerator. In this example, the number 7 can be evenly divided into 49.

Sometimes fractions are more difficult to reduce because the answer is not obvious.

EXAMPLE

EXAMPLE 1:

Reduce $\frac{56}{96}$

$$\frac{56}{96} = \frac{\overset{1}{\cancel{8}} \times 7}{\underset{1}{\cancel{8}} \times 12} = \frac{7}{12}$$

FINE POINTS

In Example 1, note both the numerator and denominator can be evenly divided by 8. In Example 2 both can be evenly divided by 9.

EXAMPLE 2:

Reduce $\frac{54}{99}$

$$\frac{54}{99} = \frac{\overset{1}{\cancel{9}} \times 6}{\underset{1}{\cancel{9}} \times 11} = \frac{6}{11}$$

When you need to reduce a very large fraction, it may be difficult to determine the largest number that will divide evenly into both the numerator and the denominator. You may have to reduce the fraction several times.

EXAMPLE

EXAMPLE 1:

Reduce $\frac{189}{216}$

Try to divide both by 3 $\quad \dfrac{\overset{63}{\cancel{189}}}{\underset{72}{\cancel{216}}} = \dfrac{63}{72}$

Then use multiples $\quad \dfrac{63}{72} = \dfrac{\overset{1}{\cancel{9}} \times 7}{\underset{1}{\cancel{9}} \times 8} = \dfrac{7}{8}$

FINE POINTS

Prime numbers cannot be reduced any further. Examples are 2, 3, 5, 7, and 11.

When reducing, if the last number is even or a zero, try 2.

If the last number is a zero or 5, try 5.

If the last number is odd, try 3, 7, or 11.

EXAMPLE 2:

Reduce $\frac{27}{135}$

Try to divide both by 3 $\quad \dfrac{\overset{9}{\cancel{27}}}{\underset{45}{\cancel{135}}} = \dfrac{\overset{1}{\cancel{9}}}{\underset{5}{\cancel{45}}} = \dfrac{1}{5}$

Then divide by 9.

SELF-TEST 3   **Reducing Fractions**

Reduce these fractions to their lowest terms. Answers are given at the end of the chapter.

1. $\frac{16}{24}$

2. $\frac{36}{216}$

3. $\frac{18}{96}$

4. $\frac{70}{490}$

5. $\frac{18}{81}$

6. $\frac{8}{48}$

7. $\frac{12}{30}$

8. $\frac{68}{136}$

9. $\frac{55}{121}$

10. $\frac{15}{60}$

Adding Fractions

If you need to add two fractions that have the *same* denominator, first add the two numerators; write that sum over the denominator and, if necessary, reduce.

$$\frac{1}{5} + \frac{3}{5} = \frac{4}{5}$$

If the two fractions have *different* denominators, the process takes two steps. First convert each fraction, multiplying both of its numbers by their lowest common denominator. After you've converted both fractions, add their two numerators together. If necessary, reduce.

$$\frac{3}{5} + \frac{2}{3}$$

$$= \frac{3\,(\times 3)}{5\,(\times 3)} = \frac{9}{15} = \frac{3}{5}$$

$$\frac{2\,(\times 5)}{3\,(\times 5)} = \frac{10}{15} = \frac{2}{3}$$

$$\frac{9}{15} + \frac{10}{15} = \frac{19}{15} \quad \text{or} \quad 1\frac{4}{15}$$

Subtracting Fractions

To subtract two fractions that have the *same* denominator, first subtract their numerators and then write the difference over the denominator. Reduce if necessary.

$$\frac{27}{32} - \frac{18}{32} = \frac{9}{32}$$

If the two fractions have *different* denominators, first convert each fraction using the lowest common denominator (just as you did in the adding example above). Then subtract the numerators, and reduce again if necessary.

$$\frac{7}{8} - \frac{2}{3}$$

$$= \frac{7\,(\times 3)}{8\,(\times 3)} = \frac{21}{24} = \frac{7}{8}$$

$$\frac{2\,(\times 8)}{3\,(\times 8)} = \frac{16}{24} = \frac{2}{3}$$

$$\frac{21}{24} - \frac{16}{24} = \frac{5}{24}$$

SELF-TEST 4 **Adding and Subtracting Fractions**

Add and subtract these fractions. Answers are given at the end of the chapter.

1. $\frac{3}{7} + \frac{2}{7} =$

2. $\frac{3}{5} + \frac{1}{5} =$

3. $\frac{2}{4} + \frac{1}{4} =$

4. $\frac{2}{3} + \frac{1}{6} =$

5. $\frac{1}{2} + \frac{1}{3} =$

6. $\frac{15}{16} - \frac{5}{16} =$

7. $\frac{3}{7} - \frac{2}{7} =$

8. $\frac{3}{5} - \frac{2}{15} =$

9. $\frac{11}{15} - \frac{7}{10} =$

10. $\frac{8}{9} - \frac{5}{12} =$

Multiplying Fractions

There are two ways to multiply fractions. Use whichever method is more comfortable for you.

First Way

Multiply the numerators across. Multiply denominators across. Reduce the answer to its lowest terms.

 EXAMPLE

$$\frac{2}{7} \times \frac{3}{4}$$

$$= \frac{2 \times 3}{7 \times 4}$$

$$= \frac{6}{28}$$

$$= \frac{3 \times \overset{1}{\cancel{2}}}{14 \times \underset{1}{\cancel{2}}}$$

$$= \frac{3}{14}$$

Second Way (When You Are Multiplying Several Fractions)

First, reduce each fraction by dividing its numerator evenly into its denominator. Multiply the remaining numerators across. Multiply the remaining denominators across. Check to see if further reductions are possible. In Example 1, because of several fractions, you can use any numerator to divide into any of the denominators.

EXAMPLE

EXAMPLE 1:

$$\frac{3}{14} \times \frac{7}{10} \times \frac{5}{12}$$

$$= \frac{\overset{1}{\cancel{3}}}{\underset{2}{\cancel{14}}} \times \frac{\overset{1}{\cancel{7}}}{\underset{2}{\cancel{10}}} \times \frac{\overset{1}{\cancel{5}}}{\underset{4}{\cancel{12}}}$$

$$= \frac{1}{16}$$

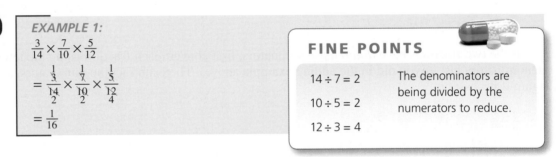

FINE POINTS

$14 \div 7 = 2$

$10 \div 5 = 2$

$12 \div 3 = 4$

The denominators are being divided by the numerators to reduce.

If you're multiplying mixed numbers, you first need to change each of them into an improper fraction. The process: For each fraction, multiply the whole number by the denominator; then add that total to the numerator.

EXAMPLE 2:

$$1\frac{1}{2} \times \frac{4}{6}$$

$$= \frac{\overset{1}{\cancel{3}}}{\underset{1}{\cancel{2}}} \times \frac{\overset{2}{\cancel{4}}}{\underset{2}{\cancel{6}}}$$

$$= \frac{2}{2}$$

$$= 1$$

EXAMPLE 3:

$$\frac{4}{5} \times 6\frac{2}{3}$$

$$= \frac{4}{5} \times \frac{\overset{4}{\cancel{20}}}{\underset{1}{3}}$$

$$= \frac{16}{3}$$

SELF-TEST 5 **Multiplying Fractions**

Multiply these fractions. Reduce if necessary. Answers are given at the end of the chapter.

1. $\frac{1}{6} \times \frac{4}{5} \times \frac{5}{2} =$

2. $\frac{4}{15} \times \frac{3}{2} =$

3. $1\frac{1}{2} \times 4\frac{2}{3} =$

4. $\frac{1}{5} \times \frac{15}{45} =$

5. $3\frac{3}{4} \times 10\frac{2}{3} =$

6. $\frac{7}{20} \times \frac{2}{14} =$

7. $\frac{9}{2} \times \frac{3}{2} =$

8. $6\frac{1}{4} \times 7\frac{1}{9} \times \frac{9}{5} =$

9. $5\frac{1}{8} \times 8\frac{1}{6} \times \frac{1}{7} =$

10. $\frac{11}{12} \times \frac{1}{4} \times \frac{2}{3} =$

Dividing Fractions

To divide two fractions, first invert the fraction that is after the division sign, then change the division sign to a multiplication sign. Reduce to lowest number.

EXAMPLE

EXAMPLE 1:

$\frac{1}{75} \div \frac{1}{150}$

$= \frac{1}{\underset{1}{75}} \times \frac{\overset{2}{150}}{1}$

$= 2$

EXAMPLE 2:

$\frac{\frac{1}{4}}{\frac{3}{8}}$

$= \frac{1}{4} \div \frac{3}{8}$

$= \frac{1}{\underset{1}{4}} \times \frac{\overset{2}{8}}{3}$

$= \frac{2}{3}$

EXAMPLE 3:

$\frac{1\frac{1}{5}}{\frac{2}{3}}$

$= \frac{6}{5} \div \frac{2}{3}$

$= \frac{\overset{3}{6}}{5} \times \frac{3}{\underset{1}{2}}$

$= \frac{9}{5}$ or $1\frac{4}{5}$

FINE POINTS

Complex fractions such as

$\frac{\frac{1}{4}}{\frac{3}{8}}$ are read as $\frac{1}{4} \div \frac{3}{8}$

The vertical arrangement acts just like a division sign.

Divide these fractions. Answers are given at the end of the chapter.

1. $\frac{1}{75} \div \frac{1}{150} =$ 5. $\frac{7}{25} \div \frac{7}{75} =$ 9. $\frac{5}{8} \div \frac{1}{3} =$

2. $\frac{1}{8} \div \frac{1}{4} =$ 6. $\frac{1}{2} \div \frac{1}{4} =$ 10. $5\frac{1}{2} \div \frac{1}{4} =$

3. $2\frac{2}{3} \div \frac{1}{2} =$ 7. $\frac{3}{4} \div \frac{8}{3} =$

4. $75 \div 12\frac{1}{2} =$ 8. $\frac{1}{60} \div \frac{7}{10} =$

Changing Fractions to Decimals

To change a fraction into a decimal, begin by dividing the numerator by the denominator. Remember that the line between the numerator and the denominator is a division sign, so $\frac{1}{4}$ can be read as $1 \div 4$.

In a division problem, each number has a name. The number that's being divided (your fraction's numerator) is the *dividend*; the one that does the dividing (your fraction's denominator) is the *divisor*; and the answer is the *quotient*.

$$\text{divisor} \rightarrow 16\overline{)640.} \leftarrow \text{dividend} \atop \underline{64} \atop 0$$

with $40.$ ← quotient above.

1. Look at the fraction $\frac{1}{4}$

    $\frac{1}{4}$ ← numerator = dividend
       ← denominator = divisor

2. Write

    $4\overline{)1}$

3. Some people find it easier to simply extend the fraction's straight line to the right, then strike out the numerator and place that same number down into the "box."

    $\frac{1}{4} = \dfrac{\cancel{1}}{4\overline{)1}}$

4. Once you've set up the structure for your division problem, place a decimal point immediately after the dividend. Put another decimal point on the quotient line (above), lining up that point exactly with the decimal point below.

    By placing your decimal points carefully, you can avoid serious dosage errors.

    $\dfrac{\cancel{1}}{4\overline{)1.}}$ ← quotient
                 ← dividend

5. Complete the division.

    $\dfrac{\cancel{1}}{4} \dfrac{.25}{\overline{)1.00}} = 0.25$
    $\underline{8}$
    20
    $\underline{20}$
    0

FINE POINTS

If the answer does not have a whole number, place a zero before the decimal point: .25 is incorrect; 0.25 is correct. This is called a leading zero.

The number of places to carry out the decimal will vary depending on the drug and equipment used. For these exercises, when possible, carry answers to the thousandths place (three decimal places).

EXAMPLE

EXAMPLE 1:

$$\frac{5}{16} = \frac{\cancel{5}}{16} \frac{0.312}{)5.000} = 0.312$$

$$\frac{4\ 8}{20}$$
$$\frac{16}{40}$$
$$\frac{32}{8}$$

EXAMPLE 2:

$$\frac{640}{8} = \frac{\cancel{640}}{8} \frac{80.}{)640.} = 80$$

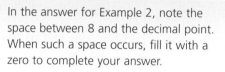

FINE POINTS

In the answer for Example 2, note the space between 8 and the decimal point. When such a space occurs, fill it with a zero to complete your answer.

EXAMPLE 3:

$$\frac{1}{75} = \frac{\cancel{1}}{75} \frac{0.013}{)1.000} = 0.013$$

$$\frac{75}{250}$$
$$\frac{225}{25}$$

SELF-TEST 7   Converting Fractions to Decimals

Divide these fractions to produce decimals. Answers are given at the end of the chapter. Carry decimal point to three decimal places if necessary. (Do not use rounding rules yet!)

1. $\frac{1}{6}$ 5. $\frac{1}{8}$ 9. $\frac{5}{8}$

2. $\frac{6}{8}$ 6. $\frac{1}{7}$ 10. $\frac{1}{5}$

3. $\frac{4}{5}$ 7. $\frac{1}{3}$

4. $\frac{9}{40}$ 8. $\frac{11}{12}$

 # Decimals

Most medication orders are written in the metric system, which uses decimals.

Reading Decimals and Converting Decimals to Fractions

Start by counting how many places come after the decimal point. One space after the decimal point is the *tenths* place. Two spaces is the *hundredths* place. Three places is the *thousandths* place, and so on. When you read the decimal aloud, it sounds like you're reading a fraction:

0.1 is read as "one tenth" $\left(\frac{1}{10}\right)$.

0.01 is read as "one hundredth" $\left(\frac{1}{100}\right)$.

0.001 is read as "one thousandth" $\left(\frac{1}{1000}\right)$.

Always read the number by its name first, then count off the decimal places. If a whole number precedes the decimal, read it just as you normally would.

Since decimals are parts of a whole number, you can write them as fractions:

EXAMPLE

0.56 = "fifty-six hundredths" $\left(\frac{56}{100}\right)$

0.2 = "two tenths" $\left(\frac{2}{10}\right)$

0.194 = "one hundred ninety-four thousandths" $\left(\frac{194}{1000}\right)$

0.31 = "thirty-one hundredths" $\left(\frac{31}{100}\right)$

1.6 = "one and six tenths" $\left(1\frac{6}{10}\right)$

17.354 = "seventeen and three hundred fifty-four thousandths" $\left(17\frac{354}{1000}\right)$.

> **FINE POINTS**
>
> Notice the use of the "leading zero." This is a zero used before a decimal point when writing only a decimal number. This leading zero is used in dosage calculations to reduce errors in writing decimals.

SELF-TEST 8   Reading Decimals

Write these decimals in longhand and as fractions. Do not reduce. Answers are given at the end of the chapter.

1. 0.25 _____

2. 0.004 _____

3. 1.7 _____

4. 0.5 _____

5. 0.334 _____

6. 136.75 _____

7. 0.1 _____

8. 0.15 _____

9. 2.25 _____

10. 10.325 _____

Addition and Subtraction of Decimals

To add decimals, stack them vertically, making sure that all decimal points line up exactly. Starting at the far right of the stack, add each vertical column of numbers. In your answer, be sure your decimal point lines up exactly with the points above it.

EXAMPLE 1:

$$
\begin{array}{r}
0.8 \\
+\,0.6 \\
\hline
1.4
\end{array}
$$

EXAMPLE 2:

$$\begin{array}{r} 10.30 \\ +\ 3.28 \\ \hline 13.58 \end{array}$$

To subtract decimals, stack your two decimals as you did for addition, lining up the decimal points as before. Starting at the far right of the stack, subtract the numbers; again, make sure that the decimal point in your answer aligns with those above it.

EXAMPLE 1:

$$13 - 12.54 = \begin{array}{r} {\scriptstyle 2\ 9\ 10} \\ 13.00 \\ -\ 12.54 \\ \hline 0.46 \end{array}$$

EXAMPLE 2:

$$14.56 - 0.47 = \begin{array}{r} {\scriptstyle 4\ 16} \\ 14.56 \\ -\ 0.47 \\ \hline 14.09 \end{array}$$

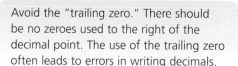

SELF-TEST 9 **Addition and Subtraction of Decimals**

Add and subtract these decimals. Answers are given at the end of the chapter.

1. $0.9 + 0.5 =$
2. $5 + 2.999 =$
3. $10.56 + 357.5 =$
4. $2 + 3.05 + 0.06 =$
5. $15 + 0.19 + 21 =$

6. $98.6 - 66.5 =$
7. $0.45 - 0.38 =$
8. $1.724 - 0.684 =$
9. $7.066 - 0.2 =$
10. $78.56 - 5.77 =$

Multiplying Decimals

Line up the numbers on the right. Do not align the decimal points. Starting on the right, multiply each digit in the top number by each digit in the bottom number, just as you would with whole numbers. Add the products. Place the decimal point in the answer by starting at the right and moving the point the same number of places equal to the sum of the decimal places in both numbers multiplied, count the number of places that you totaled earlier. If you end up with any blank spaces, fill each one with a zero.

EXAMPLE 1:

$2.6 \times 0.03 =$
$$\begin{array}{r} 2.6 \ \text{(1 decimal place)} \\ \times\ 0.03 \ \text{(2 decimal places)} \\ \hline 0.078 \ \text{(3 decimal places from the right)} \end{array}$$

EXAMPLE 2:

$200 \times 0.03 =$
$$\begin{array}{r} 200 \ \text{(no decimal place)} \\ 0.03 \ \text{(2 decimal places)} \\ \hline 6.00 \ \text{(2 decimal places from the right)} \\ \text{or} \\ 6 \end{array}$$

FINE POINTS

Avoid the "trailing zero." There should be no zeroes used to the right of the decimal point. The use of the trailing zero often leads to errors in writing decimals.

FINE POINTS

A quick "double-check" to determine decimal places is to count the number of decimal places in each number that is being multiplied. The answer should have the same number of decimal places.

Dividing Decimals

A reminder: The number being divided is called the *dividend*; the number doing the dividing is called the *divisor*; and the answer is called the *quotient*.

$$\text{divisor} \rightarrow 16\overline{\smash{\big)}\,5.000} \rightarrow \text{dividend}$$
$$0.312 \rightarrow \text{quotient}$$

Note: As soon as you write your dividend, place a decimal point immediately after it. Then place another decimal point directly above it, on the quotient line.

EXAMPLE

$$\frac{13}{16} \quad 16\,\overline{\smash{\big)}\,130}$$

Divide.

EXAMPLE

$$
\begin{array}{r}
0.812 \\
16\,\overline{\smash{\big)}\,13.000} \\
\underline{12\,8} \\
20 \\
\underline{16} \\
40 \\
\underline{32} \\
8
\end{array}
$$

Clearing the Divisor of Decimal Points

Before dividing one decimal by another, clear the divisor of decimal points. To do this, move the decimal point to the far right. Move the decimal point in the dividend *the same number of places* and, directly above it, insert another decimal point in the quotient.

EXAMPLE

EXAMPLE 1:

$$0.2\,\overline{\smash{\big)}\,0.004} = 0.2\,\overline{\smash{\big)}\,0.004}$$

$$\text{Hence, } 2\,\overline{\smash{\big)}\,00.04}$$
$$0.02$$

EXAMPLE 2:

$$
4.3\,\overline{\smash{\big)}\,5.427} \quad \text{becomes} \quad 43.\overline{\smash{\big)}\,54.270}
$$

$$
\begin{array}{r}
1.262 \\
43.\,\overline{\smash{\big)}\,54.270} \\
\underline{43} \\
11\,2 \\
\underline{8\,6} \\
2\,67 \\
\underline{2\,58} \\
90 \\
\underline{86} \\
4
\end{array}
$$

FINE POINTS

When you're dividing, the answer may not come out even. The dosage calculation problems give directions on how many places to carry out your answer. In Example 2, the answer is carried out to three decimal places.

SELF-TEST 10   Multiplication and Division of Decimals

Do these problems in division of decimals. The answers are given at the end of this chapter. If necessary, carry the answer to three places (unless the answer comes out "even"). (Do not use rounding rules yet!)

1. $3.14 \times 0.02 =$

2. $100 \times 0.4 =$

3. $2.76 \times 0.004 =$

4. $6.3 \times 7.6 =$

5. $54 \times 7.41 =$

6. $7.8\overline{)140}$

7. $6\overline{)140}$

8. $0.025\overline{)10}$

9. $1.3\overline{)40}$

10. $7\overline{)18.61}$

Rounding Off Decimals

How do you determine the number of places to carry out division? This question seems to continually confuse students (and teachers sometimes!). The answer depends on the way the drug is dispensed and the equipment needed to administer the drug. Some tablets can be broken into halves or fourths. Some liquids are prepared in units of measurement: tenths, hundredths, or thousandths. Some syringes are marked to the nearest tenth, hundredth, or thousandth place. Intravenous rates are usually rounded to the nearest whole number or sometimes tenth place. Sometimes, determining when to round is dependent on the clinical setting you work in. Pediatric settings often use dosages in tenths, hundredths, and thousandths, while in adult settings, often the answer is rounded to the nearest whole number. As you become familiar with dosage, you'll learn how far to round off your answers. To practice, first review the general rule for rounding off decimals.

RULE   **ROUNDING OFF DECIMALS**

To round off a decimal, you simply drop the final number. Exception: If the final number is 5 or higher, drop it and then increase the adjacent number by 1.

EXAMPLE
> 0.864 becomes 0.86
>
> 1.55 becomes 1.6
>
> 0.33 becomes 0.3
>
> 4.562 becomes 4.56
>
> 2.38 becomes 2.4

To obtain an answer that's rounded off to the nearest tenth, look at the number in the hundredth place and follow the above rule for rounding off.

EXAMPLE
> 0.12 becomes 0.1
>
> 0.667 becomes 0.7
>
> 1.46 becomes 1.5

If you want an answer that's rounded off to the nearest hundredth, look at the number in the thousandth place and follow the above rule for rounding off.

EXAMPLE

0.664 becomes 0.66

0.148 becomes 0.15

2.375 becomes 2.38

And if you want an answer that's rounded off to the nearest thousandth, look at the number in the ten-thousandth place and follow the same rules.

EXAMPLE

1.3758 becomes 1.376

0.0024 becomes 0.002

4.5555 becomes 4.556

SELF-TEST 11   Rounding Decimals

Round off these decimals as indicated. Answers are given at the end of the chapter.

Nearest Tenth	Nearest Hundredth	Nearest Thousandth
1. 0.25 = _____	**6.** 1.268 = _____	**11.** 1.3254 = _____
2. 1.84 = _____	**7.** 0.751 = _____	**12.** 0.0025 = _____
3. 3.27 = _____	**8.** 0.677 = _____	**13.** 0.4521 = _____
4. 0.05 = _____	**9.** 4.539 = _____	**14.** 0.7259 = _____
5. 0.63 = _____	**10.** 1.222 = _____	**15.** 0.3482 = _____

Comparing the Value of Decimals

Understanding which decimal is larger or smaller can help you solve dosage problems. Example: "Will I need more than one tablet or less than one tablet?"

RULE **DETERMINING THE VALUE OF DECIMALS**

The decimal with the higher number in the tenth place has the greater value.

EXAMPLE

Compare 0.25 with 0.5.

Since 5 is higher than 2, the greater of these two decimals is 0.5.

SELF-TEST 12   Value of Decimals

In each pair, underline the decimal with the greater value. Answers are given at the end of the chapter.

1. 0.125 and 0.25

2. 0.04 and 0.1

3. 0.5 and 0.125

4. 0.1 and 0.2

5. 0.825 and 0.44

6. 0.9 and 0.5

7. 0.25 and 0.4

8. 0.7 and 0.35

9. 0.3 and 0.225

10. 0.5 and 0.455

Percents

Percent means "parts per hundred." Percent is a fraction, containing a variable numerator and a denominator that's always 100. You can write a percent as a fraction, a ratio, or a decimal. (To write a ratio, use two numbers separated by a colon. Example: 1:100. Read this ratio as "one is to a hundred.")

Percent written as a fraction: $5\% = \frac{5}{100}$

Percent written as a ratio: $5\% = 5{:}100$

Percent written as a decimal: $5\% = 0.05$

Whole numbers, fractions, and decimals may all be written as percents.

> **FINE POINTS**
>
> These represent the same number:
>
> $5\% = 5{:}100 = 5/100 = 0.05$

EXAMPLE

> Whole number: 4% (four percent)
>
> Decimal: 0.2% (two tenths percent)
>
> Fraction: $\frac{1}{4}\%$ (one fourth percent)

Percents That Are Whole Numbers

EXAMPLE

> *EXAMPLE 1:*
>
> Change to a fraction.
>
> $4\% = \frac{4}{100} = \frac{1}{25}$

> *EXAMPLE 2:*
>
> Change to a decimal.
>
> $4\% = \dfrac{4}{100} \quad \begin{array}{r} .04 \\ 100\overline{)4.00} \end{array} = 0.04$

Percents That Are Decimals

These may be changed in three ways:

By moving the decimal point two places to the left

$0.2\% = \underset{\smile}{00.2} = 0.002$

OR By keeping the decimal, placing the number over 100, and then dividing

$0.2\% = \dfrac{0.2}{100} \quad \begin{array}{r} 0.002 \\ \overline{)0.200} \end{array} = 0.002$

OR By turning it into a complex fraction. If you're using this method, remember to invert the number after the division sign and then multiply. A whole number always has a denominator of 1.

$$0.2\% = \dfrac{\frac{2}{10}}{100}$$

$$= \dfrac{2}{10} \div \dfrac{100}{1}$$

$$= \dfrac{2}{10} \times \dfrac{1}{100} = \dfrac{2}{1000}$$

$$\dfrac{\overset{1}{\cancel{2}}}{\underset{500}{\cancel{1000}}} = \dfrac{1}{500}$$

Percents That Are Fractions

EXAMPLE

EXAMPLE 1:

$$\dfrac{1}{4}\%$$

$$= \dfrac{\frac{1}{4}}{100}$$

$$= \dfrac{1}{4} \div \dfrac{100}{1}$$

$$= \dfrac{1}{4} \times \dfrac{1}{100}$$

$$= \dfrac{1}{400}$$

EXAMPLE 2:

$$\dfrac{1}{2}\%$$

$$= \dfrac{\frac{1}{2}}{100}$$

$$= \dfrac{1}{2} \div \dfrac{100}{1}$$

$$= \dfrac{1}{2} \times \dfrac{1}{100}$$

$$= \dfrac{1}{200}$$

ALTERNATIVE WAY. Because $\frac{1}{2} = 0.5$, $\frac{1}{2}\%$ could also be written as 0.5%. If you follow the rule of clearing a percent by moving the decimal point two places to the left, you get $00.5\% = 0.005$. Note that 0.005 is $\frac{5}{1000} = \frac{1}{200}$. You could also write $\frac{0.5}{100}$

SELF-TEST 13   **Conversion of Percents**

*Change these percents to both a **fraction** and a **decimal**. Reduce if necessary. Answers are given at the end of the chapter.*

1. 10% _____ _____

2. 0.9% _____ _____

3. $\frac{1}{5}\%$ _____ _____

4. 0.01% _____ _____

5. $\frac{2}{3}\%$ _____ _____

6. 0.45% _____ _____

7. 20% _____ _____

8. 0.4% _____ _____

9. $\frac{1}{10}\%$ _____ _____

10. $2\frac{1}{2}\%$ _____ _____

11. 33% _____ _____

12. 50% _____ _____

13. $1\frac{1}{4}\%$ _____ _____

14. 75% _____ _____

15. 25% _____ _____

Fractions, ratios, and decimals also can be converted to percents. Again, remember that percent means "parts of a hundred."

Fractions Converted to Percents

If the denominator is 100, simply write the numerator as a percent:

$\frac{5}{100} = 5\%$

If the denominator is not 100, you must convert the fraction, using 100 as the denominator. In this example, multiply the numerator and denominator, using 20 as the lowest common denominator:

$\frac{3}{5} = \frac{60}{100} = 60\%$

Ratios Converted to Percents

If the second number in the ratio is 100, simply write the first number as a percent:

$1:100 = 1\%$

If the second number in the ratio is not 100, you must convert the ratio, using 100 as the denominator. In this example, multiply the numerator and denominator, using 20 as the lowest common denominator:

$4:5 = 80:100 = 80\%$

Decimals Converted to Percents

Move the decimal point two places to the right and then write the percent sign:

$0.1 = 0.10 = 10\%$

$0.05 = 0.05 = 5\%$

SELF-TEST 14 Fractions, Ratios, and Decimals

Change these percents to a fraction, ratio, and a decimal. Answers are given at the end of the chapter. Do not reduce.

	Fraction	*Ratio*	*Decimal*
1. 32% =	_____	_____	_____
2. 8.5% =	_____	_____	_____
3. 125% =	_____	_____	_____
4. 64% =	_____	_____	_____
5. 11.25% =	_____	_____	_____

Now change these fractions, ratios, and decimals to a percent.

6. $\frac{7}{10}$ =

7. 2:5 =

8. 0.08 =

9. 0.56 =

10. 3 =

Fractions, Ratio, and Proportion

Fractions show how the part (numerator) relates to the whole (denominator). *Ratio* indicates the relationship between two numbers. In this book, ratios are written as two numbers separated by a colon (1:10). Read this ratio as "one is to ten." *Proportion* indicates a relationship between two ratios or two fractions.

EXAMPLE

$\frac{2}{8} = \frac{10}{40}$ (Read the proportion like this: *"two is to eight as ten is to forty."*)

5:30 :: 6:36 (Read as *"five is to thirty as six is to thirty-six."*)

Proportions written with two ratios and the double colon can also be written as fractions. Thus, 5:30 :: 6:36 becomes

$$\frac{5}{30} = \frac{6}{36}$$

Solving Proportions With an Unknown

When one of the numbers in a proportion is unknown, the letter x substitutes for that missing number. By following three steps, you can determine the value of x in a proportion.

Step 1. Cross-multiply.

Step 2. Clear x.

Step 3. Reduce.

Here's how the three steps work.

Proportions Expressed as Two Fractions

Suppose you want to solve this proportion:

$$\frac{1}{0.125} = \frac{x}{0.25}$$

Step 1. Cross-multiply the numerators and denominators.

$$\frac{1}{0.125} \diagdown\diagup \frac{x}{0.25}$$

$$0.125x = 0.25$$

Step 2. Clear x by dividing both sides of the equation with the number that precedes x.

$$x = \frac{0.25}{0.125}$$

Step 3. Reduce the number.

$$0.125\overline{)0.250.}\,\overset{2.}{}$$

$$x = 2$$

EXAMPLE

$$\frac{45}{180} = \frac{3}{x}$$

$$45x = 540$$

$$x = \frac{540}{45}$$

$$x = 12$$

Proportions Expressed as Two Ratios

Suppose you start with this proportion:

$4 : 3.2 :: 7 : x$

Step 1. Cross-multiply the two outside numbers (called *extremes*) and the two inside numbers (called *means*).

$4 : 3.2 :: 7 : x$

$4x = 22.4$

Step 2. Clear x by dividing both sides of the equation with the number that precedes x.

$x = \frac{22.4}{4}$

Step 3. Reduce the number.

$$4\overline{)22.4} \quad 5.6$$

$x = 5.6$

EXAMPLE

$11 : 121 :: 3 : x$

$11x = 363$

$$\begin{array}{r} 33. \\ 11\overline{)363.} \\ \underline{33} \\ 33 \\ \underline{33} \\ \end{array}$$

$x = 33$

SELF-TEST 15 Solving Proportions

Solve these proportions. Answers are given at the end of the chapter.

1. $\frac{120}{4.2} = \frac{16}{x}$

2. $750 : 250 :: x : 5$

3. $\frac{14}{140} = \frac{22}{x}$

4. $2 : 5 :: x : 10$

5. $\frac{81}{3} = \frac{x}{15}$

6. $0.125 : 0.5 :: x : 10$

7. $\frac{1}{50} = \frac{x}{40}$

8. $x : 12 :: 9 : 24$

9. $\frac{0.25}{500} = \frac{x}{1000}$

10. $x : 20 :: 2.5 : 100$

Ratio and Proportion in Dosage: An Introduction

When the amount of drug prescribed by a physician or healthcare provider differs from the supply, you can solve the dosage problem with proportion, using either two ratios or two fractions.

> **EXAMPLE**
>
> Order: 0.5 mg of a drug
>
> Supply: A liquid labeled 0.125 mg per 4 mL

You know that the liquid comes as 0.125 mg in 4 mL. And you know that the amount you want is 0.5 mg. You don't know, however, what amount of liquid is needed to equal 0.5 mg. So, you need one more piece of information: the unknown, or x.

You can set up and solve this arithmetic operation as a proportion, using either two fractions or two ratios. Notice that both methods eventually become the same calculation.

Two Fractions	Two Ratios
$\dfrac{0.5}{0.125} \diagdown \dfrac{x}{4}$ $0.125x = 2$ $\downarrow$ $\dfrac{0.125x}{0.125} = \dfrac{2}{0.125}$ $\downarrow$ $x = \dfrac{2}{0.125}$ $\downarrow$ $x = \dfrac{2}{0.125}$ $0.125\overline{)2.000.}$ $\dfrac{16.}{}$ $1\,25$ 750 $\underline{750}$	$0.5 : 0.125 :: x : 4$ $0.125x = 2$ $\downarrow$ $\dfrac{0.125x}{0.125} = \dfrac{2}{0.125}$ $\downarrow$ $x = \dfrac{2}{0.125}$ $\downarrow$ $x = \dfrac{2}{0.125}$ $0.125\overline{)2.000.}$ $\dfrac{16.}{}$ $1\,25$ 750 $\underline{750}$

$$x = 16$$

So far, you've learned two ways to solve dosage calculation problems: the *ratio method* (i.e., the proportion of two ratios) and the *proportion method* (i.e., the proportion of two fractions). Chapter 4 introduces the simpler *formula method,* which is derived from ratio and proportion. Also, Chapter 4 explains another less complicated way: the *dimensional analysis method.* Throughout the book, self-test and proficiency test problems illustrate solutions reached by all four methods of calculation.

Name: _____

These arithmetic operations are needed to calculate doses. Reduce if necessary. See Appendix A for answers. Your instructor can provide other practice tests if necessary.

A. Multiply

   a) $\begin{array}{r} 647 \\ \times\, 38 \\ \hline \end{array}$
   b) $\frac{8}{9} \times \frac{12}{32}$
   c) $\begin{array}{r} 0.56 \\ \times\, 0.17 \\ \hline \end{array}$

B. Divide. If necessary, round to two decimal places.

   a) $82\overline{)793}$
   b) $5\frac{1}{4} \div \frac{7}{4}$
   c) $0.015\overline{)0.3}$

C. Add and reduce

   a) $\frac{7}{15} + \frac{8}{15}$
   b) $\frac{3}{8} + \frac{2}{5}$
   c) $0.825 + 0.1$

D. Subtract and reduce

   a) $\frac{11}{15} - \frac{7}{10}$
   b) $\frac{8}{15} - \frac{4}{15}$
   c) $1.56 - 0.2$

E. Change to a decimal. If necessary, round to two decimal places (unless the answer comes out "even").

   a) $\frac{1}{18}$
   b) $\frac{3}{8}$

F. Change to a fraction and reduce to lowest terms.

   a) 0.35
   b) 0.08

G. In each set, which number has the greater value?

   a) _____ 0.4 and 0.162

   b) _____ 0.76 and 0.8

   c) _____ 0.5 and 0.83

   d) _____ 0.3 and 0.25

H. Reduce these fractions to their lowest terms as decimals. Round to two decimal places.

   a) $\frac{20}{12}$
   b) $\frac{7}{84}$
   c) $\frac{6}{13}$

I. Round off these decimals as indicated.

   a) nearest tenth   5.349 _____

   b) nearest hundredth   0.6284 _____

   c) nearest thousandth   0.9244 _____

J. Change these percents to a fraction, ratio, and decimal.

   a) $\frac{1}{3}\%$
   b) 0.8%

K. Change these fractions, ratios, and decimals to a percent.

   a) $\frac{7}{100}$
   b) $1 : 10$
   c) 0.008

L. Solve these proportions.

   a) $\frac{32}{128} = \frac{4}{x}$
   b) $8 : 72 :: 5 : x$
   c) $\frac{0.4}{0.12} = \frac{x}{8}$ (nearest whole number)

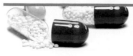

Answers

Self-Test 1 Multiplication

1. 12	**5.** 108	**9.** 48	**13.** 24	**17.** 18	**20.** 24	**23.** 81
2. 63	**6.** 24	**10.** 72	**14.** 54	**18.** 88	**21.** 132	**24.** 35
3. 32	**7.** 110	**11.** 15	**15.** 64	**19.** 36	**22.** 45	**25.** 120
4. 45	**8.** 14	**12.** 42	**16.** 56			

Self-Test 2 Division

1. 9	**5.** 7	**9.** 7	**13.** 4	**17.** 9	**20.** 2	**23.** 12
2. 4	**6.** 8	**10.** 6	**14.** 3	**18.** 4	**21.** 7	**24.** 7
3. 3	**7.** 4	**11.** 9	**15.** 3	**19.** 6	**22.** 12	**25.** 12
4. 7	**8.** 3	**12.** 6	**16.** 7			

Self-Test 3 Reducing Fractions

1. $\frac{16}{24} = \frac{4}{6} = \frac{2}{3}$ (Divide by 4, then 2.)

Alternatively: $\frac{16}{24} = \frac{2}{3}$ (Divide by 8.)

2. $\frac{36}{216} = \frac{6}{36} = \frac{1}{6}$ (Divide by 6, then 6.)

3. $\frac{18}{96} = \frac{9}{48} = \frac{3}{16}$ (Divide by 2, then 3.)

4. $\frac{70}{490} = \frac{7}{49} = \frac{1}{7}$ (Divide by 10, then 7.)

5. $\frac{18}{81} = \frac{2}{9}$ (Divide by 9.)

6. $\frac{8}{48} = \frac{1}{6}$ (Divide by 8.)

7. $\frac{12}{30} = \frac{6}{15} = \frac{2}{5}$ (Divide by 2, then 3.)

Alternatively: $\frac{12}{30} = \frac{2}{5}$ (Divide by 6.)

8. $\frac{68}{136} = \frac{34}{68} = \frac{1}{2}$ (Divide by 2, then 34.)

9. $\frac{55}{121} = \frac{5}{11}$ (Divide by 11.)

10. $\frac{15}{60} = \frac{1}{4}$ (Divide by 15.)

Alternatively: $\frac{15}{60} = \frac{3}{12} = \frac{1}{4}$ (Divide by 5, then 3.)

Self-Test 4 Adding and Subtracting Fractions

1. $\frac{5}{7}$

2. $\frac{4}{5}$

3. $\frac{3}{4}$

4. $\frac{(2 \times 2)}{\underset{6}{\overset{}{3}}} + \frac{1}{6} = \frac{4}{6} + \frac{1}{6} = \frac{5}{6}$

5. $\frac{1}{2} + \frac{1}{3} = \frac{3}{6} + \frac{2}{6} = \frac{5}{6}$

6. $\frac{10}{16}$ or $\frac{5}{8}$

7. $\frac{1}{7}$

8. $\frac{(3 \times 3)}{\underset{15}{\overset{}{5}}} - \frac{2}{15} = \frac{9}{15} - \frac{2}{15} = \frac{7}{15}$

9. $\frac{11}{15} - \frac{7}{10} = \frac{22}{30} - \frac{21}{30} = \frac{1}{30}$

10. $\frac{8}{9} - \frac{5}{12} = \frac{32}{36} - \frac{15}{36} = \frac{17}{36}$

Self-Test 5 Multiplying Fractions (Two Ways to Solve)

First Way

1. $\frac{1}{6} \times \frac{4}{5} \times \frac{5}{2} = \frac{20}{60} = \frac{1}{3}$

2. $\frac{4}{15} \times \frac{3}{2} = \frac{\overset{2}{\cancel{12}}}{\underset{5}{\cancel{30}}} = \frac{2}{5}$

(Divide by 6.)

Second Way

1. $\frac{\overset{}{\cancel{1}}}{\underset{3}{\cancel{6}}} \times \frac{\overset{}{\cancel{4}}}{\underset{1}{\cancel{5}}} \times \frac{\overset{1}{\cancel{5}}}{\underset{1}{\cancel{2}}} = \frac{\overset{1}{\cancel{2}}}{\underset{3}{\cancel{6}}} = \frac{1}{3}$

2. $\frac{\overset{2}{\cancel{4}}}{\underset{5}{\cancel{15}}} \times \frac{\overset{1}{\cancel{3}}}{\underset{1}{\cancel{2}}} = \frac{2}{5}$

(continued)

Answers (Continued)

3. $1\frac{1}{2} \times 4\frac{2}{3} = \frac{3}{2} \times \frac{14}{3} = \frac{\overset{7}{42}}{\underset{1}{6}} = 7$

(Divide by 6.)

4. $\frac{1}{5} \times \frac{15}{45} = \frac{\overset{3}{15}}{\underset{45}{225}} = \frac{3}{45} = \frac{1}{15}$

(Divide by 5.)

5. $3\frac{3}{4} \times 10\frac{2}{3} = \frac{15}{4} \times \frac{32}{3}$

(Too difficult. Use the second way.)

6. $\frac{7}{20} \times \frac{2}{14}$

(Too difficult. Use the second way.)

7. $\frac{9}{2} \times \frac{3}{2} = \frac{27}{4}$ or $6\frac{3}{4}$

8. $6\frac{1}{4} \times 7\frac{1}{9} \times \frac{9}{5} = \frac{25}{4} \times \frac{64}{9} \times \frac{9}{5}$

(Too difficult. Use the second way.)

9. $5\frac{1}{8} \times 8\frac{1}{6} \times \frac{1}{7} = \frac{41}{8} \times \frac{49}{6} \times \frac{1}{7}$

(Too difficult. Use the second way.)

10. $\frac{11}{12} \times \frac{1}{4} \times \frac{2}{3}$

(Too difficult. Use the second way.)

3. $1\frac{1}{2} \times 4\frac{2}{3} = \frac{\overset{1}{3}}{\underset{1}{2}} \times \frac{\overset{7}{14}}{\underset{1}{3}} = 7$

4. $\frac{1}{5} \times \frac{\overset{1}{15}}{\underset{3}{45}} = \frac{1}{15}$

5. $\frac{\overset{5}{15}}{\underset{1}{4}} \times \frac{\overset{8}{32}}{\underset{1}{3}} = 40$

6. $\frac{\overset{1}{\cancel{7}}}{\underset{10}{20}} \times \frac{\overset{1}{\cancel{2}}}{\underset{2}{14}} = \frac{1}{20}$

8. $\frac{\overset{5}{25}}{\underset{1}{4}} \times \frac{\overset{16}{64}}{\underset{1}{9}} \times \frac{\overset{1}{9}}{\underset{1}{5}} = 80$

9. $\frac{41}{8} \times \frac{\overset{7}{49}}{6} \times \frac{1}{\underset{1}{\cancel{7}}} = \frac{287}{48} = 5\frac{47}{48}$

10. $\frac{11}{\underset{6}{12}} \times \frac{1}{4} \times \frac{\overset{1}{2}}{3} = \frac{11}{72}$

Self-Test 6 Dividing Fractions

1. $\frac{1}{75} \div \frac{1}{150} = \frac{1}{\underset{1}{75}} \times \frac{\overset{2}{150}}{1} = 2$

2. $\frac{1}{8} \div \frac{1}{4} = \frac{1}{\underset{2}{8}} \times \frac{\overset{1}{4}}{1} = \frac{1}{2}$

3. $2\frac{2}{3} \div \frac{1}{2} = \frac{8}{3} \times \frac{2}{1} = \frac{16}{3}$ or $5\frac{1}{3}$

4. $75 \div 12\frac{1}{2} = 75 \div \frac{25}{2} = 75 \times \frac{2}{25} = 6$

5. $\frac{7}{25} \div \frac{7}{75} = \frac{\overset{1}{\cancel{7}}}{\underset{1}{25}} \times \frac{\overset{3}{75}}{\underset{1}{\cancel{7}}} = 3$

6. $\frac{1}{2} \div \frac{1}{4} = \frac{1}{\underset{1}{2}} \times \frac{\overset{2}{4}}{1} = 2$

7. $\frac{3}{4} \div \frac{8}{3} = \frac{3}{4} \times \frac{3}{8} = \frac{9}{32}$

8. $\frac{1}{60} \div \frac{7}{10} = \frac{1}{\underset{6}{60}} \times \frac{\overset{1}{10}}{7} = \frac{1}{42}$

9. $\frac{5}{8} \div \frac{1}{3} = \frac{5}{8} \times \frac{3}{1} = \frac{15}{8}$ or $1\frac{7}{8}$

10. $5\frac{1}{2} \div \frac{1}{4} = \frac{11}{\underset{1}{2}} \times \frac{\overset{2}{4}}{1} = 22$

Self-Test 7 Converting Fractions to Decimals

1. $\dfrac{1}{6}$
$$6\overline{)1.000}\;\;.166 = 0.166$$
$$\begin{array}{r}6\\ \hline 40\\ 36\\ \hline 40\\ 36\\ \hline 4\end{array}$$

4. $\dfrac{9}{40}$
$$40\overline{)9.000}\;\;.225 = 0.225$$
$$\begin{array}{r}8\,0\\ \hline 1\,00\\ 80\\ \hline 200\\ 200\\ \hline 0\end{array}$$

7. $\dfrac{1}{3}$
$$3\overline{)1.000}\;\;.333 = 0.333$$
$$\begin{array}{r}9\\ \hline 10\\ 9\\ \hline 10\end{array}$$

2. $\dfrac{\overset{3}{\cancel{6}}}{\underset{4}{\cancel{8}}} = \dfrac{3}{4}$
$$4\overline{)3.00}\;\;.75 = 0.75$$
$$\begin{array}{r}2\,8\\ \hline 20\\ 20\\ \hline 0\end{array}$$

5. $\dfrac{1}{8}$
$$8\overline{)1.000}\;\;.125 = 0.125$$
$$\begin{array}{r}8\\ \hline 20\\ 16\\ \hline 40\\ 40\\ \hline 0\end{array}$$

8. $\dfrac{11}{12}$
$$12\overline{)11.000}\;\;.916 = 0.916$$
$$\begin{array}{r}10\,8\\ \hline 20\\ 12\\ \hline 80\\ 72\end{array}$$

3. $\dfrac{4}{5}$
$$5\overline{)4.0}\;\;.8 = 0.8$$
$$\begin{array}{r}4\,0\\ \hline 0\end{array}$$

6. $\dfrac{1}{7}$
$$7\overline{)1.000}\;\;.142 = 0.142$$
$$\begin{array}{r}7\\ \hline 30\\ 28\\ \hline 20\\ 14\\ \hline 6\end{array}$$

9. $\dfrac{5}{8}$
$$8\overline{)5.000}\;\;.625 = 0.625$$
$$\begin{array}{r}4\,8\\ \hline 20\\ 16\\ \hline 40\\ 40\\ \hline 0\end{array}$$

10. $\dfrac{1}{5}$
$$5\overline{)1.0}\;\;.2 = 0.2$$
$$\begin{array}{r}1\,0\end{array}$$

Self-Test 8 Reading Decimals

1. Twenty-five hundredths $\left(\frac{25}{100}\right)$

2. Four thousandths $\left(\frac{4}{1000}\right)$

3. One and seven tenths $\left(1\frac{7}{10}\right)$

4. Five tenths $\left(\frac{5}{10}\right)$

5. Three hundred thirty-four thousandths $\left(\frac{334}{1000}\right)$

6. One hundred thirty-six and seventy-five hundredths $\left(136\frac{75}{100}\right)$

7. One tenth $\left(\frac{1}{10}\right)$

8. Fifteen hundredths $\left(\frac{15}{100}\right)$

9. Two and twenty-five hundredths $\left(2\frac{25}{100}\right)$

10. Ten and three hundred twenty-five thousandths $\left(10\frac{325}{1000}\right)$

(continued)

Answers (Continued)

Self-Test 9 Addition and Subtraction of Decimals

1.
$$\begin{array}{r} 0.9 \\ +\,0.5 \\ \hline 1.4 \end{array}$$

3.
$$\begin{array}{r} 10.56 \\ +\,357.50 \\ \hline 368.06 \end{array}$$

5.
$$\begin{array}{r} 15.00 \\ 0.19 \\ +\,21.00 \\ \hline 36.19 \end{array}$$

7.
$$\begin{array}{r} 0.\overset{3}{\cancel{4}}5 \\ -\,0.38 \\ \hline 0.07 \end{array}$$

9.
$$\begin{array}{r} \overset{6}{\cancel{7}}.066 \\ -\,0.200 \\ \hline 6.866 \end{array}$$

2.
$$\begin{array}{r} 5.000 \\ +\,2.999 \\ \hline 7.999 \end{array}$$

4.
$$\begin{array}{r} 2.00 \\ 3.05 \\ +\,0.06 \\ \hline 5.11 \end{array}$$

6.
$$\begin{array}{r} 98.6 \\ -\,66.5 \\ \hline 32.1 \end{array}$$

8.
$$\begin{array}{r} 1.\overset{6}{\cancel{7}}24 \\ -\,0.684 \\ \hline 1.040 \text{ or } 1.04 \end{array}$$

10.
$$\begin{array}{r} 7\overset{7}{\cancel{8}}.\overset{4}{\cancel{5}}6 \\ -\,5.77 \\ \hline 72.79 \end{array}$$

Self-Test 10 Multiplication and Division of Decimals

1.
$$\begin{array}{r} 3.14 \\ \times\,0.02 \\ \hline 0.0628 \end{array}$$

2.
$$\begin{array}{r} 100 \\ \times\,0.4 \\ \hline 40.0 \text{ or } 40 \end{array}$$

3.
$$\begin{array}{r} 2.76 \\ \times\,0.004 \\ \hline 0.01104 \end{array}$$

4.
$$\begin{array}{r} 6.3 \\ \times\,7.6 \\ \hline 378 \\ 441 \\ \hline 47.88 \end{array}$$

5.
$$\begin{array}{r} 7.41 \\ \times\,54 \\ \hline 2964 \\ 3705 \\ \hline 400.14 \end{array}$$

6. $7.8\,\overline{)140.0}$ Now it is
$$\begin{array}{r} 17.948 \\ 78\,\overline{)1400.000} \\ \underline{78} \\ 620 \\ \underline{546} \\ 74\,0 \\ \underline{70\,2} \\ 3\,80 \\ \underline{3\,12} \\ 680 \\ \underline{624} \\ 56 \end{array}$$

8. $0.025\,\overline{)10.000}$ Now it is $25\,\overline{)10000.}$ with quotient $400.$

Note that because there are two places between the 4 and the decimal, you had to add two zeros.

9. $1.3\,\overline{)40.0}$ Now it is
$$\begin{array}{r} 30.769 \\ 13\,\overline{)400.0} \\ \underline{39} \\ 10 \\ \underline{0} \\ 100 \\ \underline{91} \\ 90 \\ \underline{78} \\ 120 \\ \underline{117} \\ 3 \end{array}$$

7.
$$\begin{array}{r} 23.333 \\ 6\,\overline{)140.000} \\ \underline{12} \\ 20 \\ \underline{18} \\ 20 \\ \underline{18} \\ 20 \\ \underline{18} \\ 20 \\ \underline{18} \\ 2 \end{array}$$

10.
$$\begin{array}{r} 2.658 \\ 7\,\overline{)18.610} \\ \underline{14} \\ 46 \\ \underline{42} \\ 41 \\ \underline{35} \\ 60 \\ \underline{56} \\ 4 \end{array}$$

Self-Test 11 Rounding Decimals

Nearest Tenth	*Nearest Hundredth*	*Nearest Thousandth*
1. 0.3	**6.** 1.27	**11.** 1.325
2. 1.8	**7.** 0.75	**12.** 0.003
3. 3.3	**8.** 0.68	**13.** 0.452
4. 0.1	**9.** 4.54	**14.** 0.726
5. 0.6	**10.** 1.22	**15.** 0.348

Self-Test 12 Value of Decimals

1. 0.25	**5.** 0.825	**9.** 0.3
2. 0.1	**6.** 0.9	**10.** 0.5
3. 0.5	**7.** 0.4	
4. 0.2	**8.** 0.7	

Self-Test 13 Conversion of Percents

1. Fraction $10\% = \dfrac{\frac{1}{10}}{\frac{100}{10}} = \dfrac{1}{10}$

Decimal $10\% = \dfrac{10}{100} \quad 100\overline{)10.0}^{\,.1} = 0.1$

OR $\quad 10.\% = 0.1$

2. Fraction $0.9\% = \dfrac{\frac{9}{10}}{100} = \dfrac{9}{10} \div 100 = \dfrac{9}{10} \times \dfrac{1}{100} = \dfrac{9}{1000}$

Decimal $0.9\% = \dfrac{0.9}{100} \quad 100\overline{)0.900}^{\,.009} = 0.009$

OR $\quad 00.9\% = 0.009$

3. Fraction $\dfrac{1}{5}\% = \dfrac{\frac{1}{5}}{100} = \dfrac{1}{5} \div 100 = \dfrac{1}{5} \times \dfrac{1}{100} = \dfrac{1}{500}$

Decimal $\dfrac{1}{5}\% = \dfrac{1}{5} \div 100 = \dfrac{1}{500} \quad 500\overline{)1.000}^{\,.002} = 0.002$

OR $\quad \dfrac{1}{5}\% = \dfrac{1}{5} \quad 5\overline{)1.0}^{\,.2} = 0.2\% \quad 00.2 = 0.002$

(continued)

Answers (Continued)

4. Fraction $0.01\% = \dfrac{\frac{1}{100}}{100} = \dfrac{1}{100} \div \dfrac{100}{1} = \dfrac{1}{100} \times \dfrac{1}{100} = \dfrac{1}{10000}$

Decimal $0.01\% = \dfrac{0.01}{100} \overset{0.0001}{\overline{\smash{\big)}\,.0100}} = 0.0001$

OR $00.01 = 0.0001$

5. Fraction $\dfrac{2}{3}\% = \dfrac{\frac{2}{3}}{100} = \dfrac{2}{3} \div \dfrac{100}{1} = \dfrac{2}{3} \times \dfrac{1}{100} = \dfrac{2}{300} = \dfrac{1}{150}$

Decimal $\dfrac{2}{3}\% = \dfrac{2}{3} \div \dfrac{100}{1} = \dfrac{2}{3} \times \dfrac{1}{100} = \dfrac{2}{300} \overset{.0066}{\overline{\smash{\big)}\,2.000}} = 0.0066$ (does not round evenly)

OR $\dfrac{2}{3}\% = \dfrac{2}{3} \overset{.66}{\overline{\smash{\big)}\,2.00}} = 0.66\% = 00.66 = 0.0066$ (does not round evenly)

6. Fraction $0.45\% = \dfrac{\frac{45}{100}}{100} = \dfrac{45}{100} \div \dfrac{100}{1} = \dfrac{45}{100} \times \dfrac{1}{100} = \dfrac{45}{10000} = \dfrac{9}{2000}$

Decimal $0.45\% = \dfrac{.45}{100} \overset{.0045}{\overline{\smash{\big)}\,0.4500}} = 0.0045$

OR $00.45\% = 0.0045$

7. Fraction $\dfrac{\frac{1}{20}}{\underset{5}{100}} = \dfrac{1}{5}$

Decimal $20\% = \dfrac{20}{100} \overset{0.2}{\overline{\smash{\big)}\,20.0}}$

OR $20.\% = 0.2$

8. Fraction $0.4\% = \dfrac{\frac{4}{10}}{100} = \dfrac{4}{10} \div \dfrac{100}{1} = \dfrac{\overset{1}{4}}{10} \times \dfrac{1}{\underset{25}{100}} = \dfrac{1}{250}$

Decimal $0.4\% = \dfrac{0.4}{100} \overset{0.004}{\overline{\smash{\big)}\,0.400}} = 0.004$

OR $00.4\% = 0.004$

9. Fraction $\dfrac{1}{10}\% = \dfrac{\frac{1}{10}}{100} = \dfrac{1}{10} \div \dfrac{100}{1} = \dfrac{1}{10} \times \dfrac{1}{100} = \dfrac{1}{1000}$

Decimal $\dfrac{1}{10}\% = \dfrac{1}{10} \div \dfrac{100}{1} = \dfrac{1}{10} \times \dfrac{1}{100} = \dfrac{1}{1000} \overset{0.001}{\overline{\smash{\big)}\,1.000}} = 0.001$

OR $\dfrac{1}{10}\% = \dfrac{1}{10} \overset{0.1}{\overline{\smash{\big)}\,1.0}} = 0.1\% = 00.1 = 0.001$

10. Fraction $2\frac{1}{2}\% = 2.5\% = \dfrac{\frac{25}{10}}{100} = \dfrac{25}{10} \div \dfrac{100}{1} = \dfrac{25}{10} \times \dfrac{1}{100} = \dfrac{25}{1000} = \dfrac{1}{40}$

Decimal $2.5\% = \dfrac{2.5}{100}$ $100\overline{)2.50}^{\,0.025} = 0.025$

OR $\underset{\smile}{000.}2.5\% = 0.025$

11. Fraction $33\% = \dfrac{33}{100}$

Decimal $33\% = \dfrac{33}{100}$ $100\overline{)33.00}^{\,.33} = 0.33$

OR $\underset{\smile}{33.}\% = 0.33$

12. Fraction $50\% = \dfrac{50}{100} = \dfrac{1}{2}$

Decimal $50\% = \dfrac{50}{100}$ $100\overline{)50.0}^{\,.5} = 0.5$

OR $\underset{\smile}{50.}\% = 0.5$

13. Fraction $1\frac{1}{4}\% = 1.25\% = \dfrac{\frac{125}{100}}{100} = \dfrac{125}{100} \div \dfrac{100}{1} = \dfrac{125}{100} \times \dfrac{1}{100} = \dfrac{125}{10000} = \dfrac{1}{80}$

Decimal $1.25\% = \dfrac{1.25}{100}$ $100\overline{)1.25}^{\,0.0125} = 0.0125$

OR $\underset{\smile}{01.}25\% = 0.0125$

14. Fraction $75\% = \dfrac{75}{100} = \dfrac{3}{4}$

Decimal $75\% = \dfrac{75}{100}$ $100\overline{)75.0}^{\,.75} = 0.75$

OR $\underset{\smile}{75.}\% = 0.75$

15. Fraction $25\% = \dfrac{25}{100} = \dfrac{1}{4}$

Decimal $25\% = \dfrac{25}{100}$ $100\overline{)25.0}^{\,.25} = 0.25$

OR $\underset{\smile}{25.}\% = 0.25$

(continued)

Answers (Continued)

Self-Test 14 Fractions, Ratios, and Decimals

		Fraction	*Ratio*	*Decimal*
1.	32% =	$\dfrac{32}{100}$	32:100	$32\% = 0.32$
2.	8.5% =	$\dfrac{8.5}{100}$ or $\dfrac{85}{1000}$	8.5:100	$08.5\% = 0.085$
3.	125% =	$\dfrac{125}{100}$	125:100	$125\% = 1.25$
4.	64% =	$\dfrac{64}{100}$	64:100	$64\% = 0.64$
5.	11.25% =	$\dfrac{11.25}{100}$ or $\dfrac{1125}{10000}$	11.25:100	$11.25\% = 0.1125$

6. $\dfrac{7}{10} = \dfrac{70}{100} = 70\%$

7. $2:5 = 40:100 = 40\%$

8. $0.08 = 8\%$

9. $0.56 = 56\%$

10. $3.00 = 300\%$

Self-Test 15 Solving Proportions

1. $\dfrac{120}{4.2} = \dfrac{16}{x}$

$120x = 67.2$

$x = 0.56$

$$120\overline{)67.20}$$
$$\underline{60\ 0}$$
$$7\ 20$$
$$\underline{7\ 20}$$

2. $750:250::x:5$

$250x = 750 \times 5$

$x = 15$

$\dfrac{\overset{3}{750} \times 5}{\underset{1}{250}} = 15$

3. $\dfrac{14}{140} = \dfrac{22}{x}$

$14x = 22 \times 140$

$x = 220$

$\dfrac{22 \times \overset{10}{140}}{\underset{1}{14}} = 220$

4. $2:5::x:10$

$5x = 20$

$x = 4$

5. $\dfrac{81}{3} = \dfrac{x}{15}$

$3x = 81 \times 15$

$x = 405$

$\dfrac{81 \times \overset{5}{15}}{\underset{1}{3}} = 405$

6. $0.125:0.5::x:10$

$0.5x = 0.125 \times 10 = \dfrac{\overset{1}{0.125}}{\underset{4}{0.500}} \times 10 = \dfrac{10}{4}$

$x = 2.5$

$$4\overline{)10.0}$$
$$2.5$$

7. $\dfrac{1}{50} = \dfrac{x}{40}$

$50x = 40$

$x = 0.8$

$$50\overline{)40.0}$$
$$\underline{40\ 0}$$
$$0.8$$

8. $x:12::9:24$

$24x = 9 \times 12$

$24x = 108$

$x = 4.5$

9. $\dfrac{0.25}{500} = \dfrac{x}{1000}$

$500\,x = 250$

$x = 0.5$

$$500\overline{)250.0}$$
$$\underline{250\ 0}$$
$$0.5$$

10. $x:20::2.5:100$

$100x = 2.5 \times 20$

$100x = 50$

$x = 0.5$

Metric and Household Systems of Measurement

TOPICS COVERED

1. Metric solid and liquid measures
2. Equivalents within the metric system
3. Liquid household measures
4. Equivalents among metric, liquid, and household systems
5. Temperature conversions
6. Units, milliunits, and milliequivalents

Medication orders are written in metric terms. In this chapter, you will learn solid and liquid measures in the metric system and their equivalents. This will help you in interpreting orders such as:

Administer 30 mL of aluminum hydroxide and magnesium hydroxide (Mylanta) at bedtime.

Administer carvedilol (Coreg) 6.25 mg by mouth four times a day.

When you're preparing liquid doses, a knowledge of household equivalents will help you pour exact amounts. Medications given at home are often prescribed in household measurements. This will help you interpret orders such as:

Administer dextromethorphan (Robitussin) syrup 2 tsp every 4 hours as needed.

Administer sodium polystyrene (Kayexalate) 1 tbsp four times a day.

Medicine cups are marked in metric and household measures; syringes are marked in metric lines. There are many apps available for conversions. Try these key words to find current apps for your handheld device:

metric equivalents

metric converter

temperature conversion

Although the apothecary system was used in the past to write prescriptions, it has gradually been replaced by the metric system. It is rare to see medication orders in the apothecary notation and the Joint Commission wants to place the notation units on the "do not use" list. However, you may see the following terms still used:

Liquid measurements: dram, ounce, drop (gtt), minim (m).

Solid measurement: grain (gr)

Metric System

Measures of Weight

These are the solid measures in the metric system and their abbreviations:

Gram: g

Milligram: mg

Microgram: mcg (µg, which uses the Greek letter mu [µ], is no longer accepted by the Joint Commission for its approved abbreviation list)

Kilogram: kg

Weight Equivalents

These are the basic weight equivalents in the metric system:

1 kg = 1000 g

1 g = 1000 mg

1 mg = 1000 mcg

As you can see, the kilogram is the largest of these.

To equal the weight of a single kilogram, you need 1000 grams.

To equal the weight of a single gram, you need 1000 mg.

To equal the weight of a single milligram, you need 1000 mcg.

The symbol >, which means "greater than," indicates these relationships:

kg > g > mg > mcg

Read this notation as "A kilogram is greater than a gram, which is greater than a milligram, which is greater than a microgram."

Converting Solid Equivalents

If the available supply is not in the same weight measure as the medication order, you will have to calculate how much of a drug to give.

EXAMPLE

Order: 0.25 g

Supply: tablets labeled 125 mg

Since 1 g = 1000 mg, you change 0.25 g to milligrams by multiplying the number of grams by 1000:

$$\begin{array}{r} 0.25 \\ \times\ 1000 \\ \hline 250.00 \end{array}$$

To convert the order, you use 0.25 g = 250 mg (drop the "trailing zero" to the right of the decimal place).

Following this rule, if you are converting grams to milligrams (a larger measurement to a smaller one), multiply the original number by 1000. If you are converting from micrograms to milligrams (a smaller measurement to a larger one), divide the original number by 1000.

[Here's an easy rule to help you remember this type of conversion:

Large to small—multiply by 1000

Small to large—divide by 1000]

[There's another method of conversion as well. In decimals, the thousandth place is three numbers after the decimal point. You can change grams to milligrams by moving the decimal point three places to the *right,* which produces the same answer as multiplying by 1000. You can also change milligrams to grams by moving the decimal point three places to the *left,* which is the same as dividing by 1000. You'll be using this method in some of the calculations to come.]

RULE ➤ **CHANGING GRAMS TO MILLIGRAMS**

To multiply by 1000, move the decimal point three places to the right.

EXAMPLE

EXAMPLE 1:

0.25 g = _____ mg

0.250 = 250

0.25 g = 250 mg

EXAMPLE 2:

0.1 g = _____ mg

0.100 = 100

0.1 g = 100 mg

GRAMS TO MILLIGRAMS QUICK METHOD. Should you move the decimal point to the left or to the right? This Quick Method can help you decide.

1. First, write the order.

2. Write the supply.

3. Show which way the decimal point should move by drawing a "greater than" sign (>).

4. Remember that in the equivalent 1 g = 1000 mg, the gram is the larger measure, with 1000 mg equaling the weight of 1 g.

5. Move the decimal point three places to the right.

EXAMPLE

EXAMPLE 1:

Order: 0.25 g

Supply: 125 mg

You want to convert grams to milligrams.

0.25 g > _____ mg

The "greater than" sign tells you to move the decimal point three places to the *right.*

0.250 = 250

Therefore, 0.25 g = 250 mg.

> *EXAMPLE 2:*
>
> Order: 1.5 g
>
> Supply: 500 mg
>
> You want to convert grams to milligrams.
>
> 1.5 g > _____ mg
>
> The "greater than" sign tells you to move the decimal point three places to the *right*.
>
> 1.500 = 1500
>
> Therefore, 1.5 g = 1500 mg.

SELF-TEST 1 | **Grams to Milligrams**

Convert from grams to milligrams. For correct answers, see the end of the chapter.

1. 0.3 g = _____ mg   **7.** 0.08 g = _____ mg

2. 0.001 g = _____ mg   **8.** 0.275 g = _____ mg

3. 0.02 g = _____ mg   **9.** 0.04 g = _____ mg

4. 1.2 g = _____ mg   **10.** 0.325 g = _____ mg

5. 5 g = _____ mg   **11.** 2 g = _____ mg

6. 0.4 g = _____ mg   **12.** 0.0004 g = _____ mg

RULE   **CHANGING MILLIGRAMS TO GRAMS**

To divide by 1000, move the decimal point three places to the left.

EXAMPLE

> *EXAMPLE 1:*
>
> 100 mg = _____ g
>
> 100. = 0.1
>
> 100 mg = 0.1 g

> *EXAMPLE 2:*
>
> 8 mg = _____ g
>
> 008. = 0.008
>
> 8 mg = 0.008 g

MILLIGRAMS TO GRAMS QUICK METHOD. This method also works to convert milligrams to grams.

1. First, write the order.

2. Write the supply.

3. Show which way the decimal point should move by drawing a "less than" sign (<).

4. Remember that in the equivalent 1 g = 1000 mg, the gram is the larger measure.

5. Move the decimal point three places to the left.

EXAMPLE

EXAMPLE 1:

Order: 15 mg

Supply: 0.03 g

You want to convert milligrams to grams.

15 mg < _____ g

The "less than" sign tells you to move the decimal point three places to the *left*.

015. = 0.015

Therefore, 15 mg = 0.015 g.

EXAMPLE 2:

Order: 500 mg

Supply: 1 g

You want to convert milligrams to grams.

500 mg < _____ g

The "less than" sign tells you to move the decimal point three places to the *left*.

500. = 0.5

Therefore, 500 mg = 0.5 g.

SELF-TEST 2   Milligrams to Grams

Convert from milligrams to grams. For correct answers, see the end of the chapter.

1. 4 mg = _____ g   **7.** 50 mg = _____ g

2. 120 mg = _____ g   **8.** 600 mg = _____ g

3. 40 mg = _____ g   **9.** 5 mg = _____ g

4. 75 mg = _____ g   **10.** 360 mg = _____ g

5. 250 mg = _____ g   **11.** 10 mg = _____ g

6. 1 mg = _____ g   **12.** 0.1 mg = _____ g

RULE ➤ **CHANGING MILLIGRAMS TO MICROGRAMS**

The second major weight equivalent in the metric system is 1 mg = 1000 mcg.

Some medications are so powerful that smaller microgram doses are sufficient to produce a therapeutic effect. Rather than using milligrams written as decimals, it's easier to write orders in micrograms as whole numbers.

To multiply by 1000, move the decimal point three places to the right.

EXAMPLE

> *EXAMPLE 1:*
>
> 0.1 mg = _____ mcg
>
> 0.100 = 100
>
> 0.1 mg = 100 mcg

> *EXAMPLE 2:*
>
> 0.25 mg = _____ mcg
>
> 0.250 = 250
>
> 0.25 mg = 250 mcg

MILLIGRAMS TO MICROGRAMS QUICK METHOD. Should you move the decimal point to the left or to the right? Here are the steps:

1. First, write the order.

2. Write the supply.

3. Show which way the decimal point should move by drawing a "greater than" sign (>).

4. Remember that in the equivalent 1 mg = 1000 mcg, the milligram is the larger measure, with 1000 mcg equaling the weight of 1 mg.

5. Move the decimal point three places to the right.

EXAMPLE

> *EXAMPLE 1:*
>
> Order: 0.1 mg
>
> Supply: 200 mcg
>
> You want to convert milligrams to micrograms.
>
> 0.1 mg > _____ mcg
>
> The "greater than" sign tells you to move the decimal point three places to the *right*.
>
> 0.100 = 100
>
> Therefore, 0.1 mg = 100 mcg.

> *EXAMPLE 2:*
>
> Order: 0.3 mg
>
> Supply: 600 mcg
>
> You want to convert milligrams to micrograms.
>
> 0.3 mg > _____ mcg
>
> The "greater than" sign tells you to move the decimal point three places to the *right*.
>
> 0.300 = 300
>
> Therefore, 0.3 mg = 300 mcg.

SELF-TEST 3   Milligrams to Micrograms

Convert from milligrams to micrograms. For correct answers, see the end of the chapter.

1. 0.3 mg = _____ mcg   **7.** 5 mg = _____ mcg

2. 0.001 mg = _____ mcg   **8.** 0.7 mg = _____ mcg

3. 0.02 mg = _____ mcg   **9.** 0.04 mg = _____ mcg

4. 0.08 mg = _____ mcg   **10.** 10 mg = _____ mcg

5. 1.2 mg = _____ mcg   **11.** 0.9 mg = _____ mcg

6. 0.4 mg = _____ mcg   **12.** 0.01 mg = _____ mcg

RULE ➤   **CHANGING MICROGRAMS TO MILLIGRAMS**

To divide by 1000, move the decimal point three places to the left.

EXAMPLE

EXAMPLE 1:

300 mcg = _____ mg

300. = 0.3

300 mcg = 0.3 mg

EXAMPLE 2:

50 mcg = _____ mg

050. = 0.05

50 mcg = 0.05 mg

MICROGRAMS TO MILLIGRAMS QUICK METHOD. This method also converts micrograms to milligrams.

1. First, write the order.

2. Write the supply.

3. Show which way the decimal point should move by drawing a "less than" sign (<).

4. Remember that in the equivalent 1 mg = 1000 mcg, the milligram is the larger measure.

5. Move the decimal point three places to the left.

EXAMPLE

EXAMPLE 1:

Order: 100 mcg

Supply: 0.1 mg

You want to convert micrograms to milligrams.

100 mcg < _____ mg

The "less than" sign tells you to move the decimal point three places to the *left*.

100. = 0.1

Therefore, 100 mcg = 0.1 mg.

> *EXAMPLE 2:*
>
> Order: 50 mcg
>
> Supply: 0.1 mg
>
> You want to convert micrograms to milligrams.
>
> 50 mcg = _____ mg
>
> mcg < mg
>
> The "less than" sign tells you to move the decimal point three places to the *left*.
>
> 050. = 0.05
>
> Therefore, 50 mcg = 0.05 mg.

SELF-TEST 4   Micrograms to Milligrams

Convert from micrograms to milligrams. For correct answers, see the end of the chapter.

1. 800 mcg = _____ mg
2. 4 mcg = _____ mg
3. 14 mcg = _____ mg
4. 25 mcg = _____ mg
5. 1 mcg = _____ mg
6. 200 mcg = _____ mg
7. 50 mcg = _____ mg
8. 750 mcg = _____ mg
9. 325 mcg = _____ mg
10. 75 mcg = _____ mg
11. 0.1 mcg = _____ mg
12. 150 mcg = _____ mg

SELF-TEST 5   Mixed Conversions

Convert mixed metric weight measures. For correct answers, see the end of the chapter.

1. 0.3 mg = _____ g
2. 0.03 g = _____ mg
3. 15 mcg = _____ mg
4. 0.1 g = _____ mg
5. 100 mcg = _____ mg
6. 50 mg = _____ g
7. 0.014 g = _____ mg
8. 200 mg = _____ g
9. 0.2 mg = _____ mcg
10. 0.65 mg = _____ mcg

SELF-TEST 6   Common Equivalents

Fill in the blanks to convert milligrams to grams or micrograms.

1. 1000 mg = _____ g
2. 600 mg = _____ g
3. 500 mg = _____ g
4. 300 mg = _____ g
5. 200 mg = _____ g
6. 100 mg = _____ g
7. 60 mg = _____ g
8. 30 mg = _____ g
9. 15 mg = _____ g
10. 10 mg = _____ g
11. 0.6 mg = _____ mcg
12. 0.4 mg = _____ mcg
13. 0.3 mg = _____ mcg
14. 0.25 mg = _____ mcg

SELF-TEST 7   Review of Grams to Milligrams

1. What are the methods for converting grams to milligrams? _____

_____

_____

2. 1 g = _____ mg   9. 0.3 g = _____ mg

3. 0.05 g = _____ mg   10. 0.004 g = _____ mg

4. 0.2 g = _____ mg   11. 0.1 g = _____ mg

5. 0.12 g = _____ mg   12. 0.06 g = _____ mg

6. 0.4 g = _____ mg   13. 0.03 g = _____ mg

7. 0.6 g = _____ mg   14. 0.015 g = _____ mg

8. 0.5 g = _____ mg   15. 0.01 g = _____ mg

Household System

Household Measures

Household measures are occasionally used in preparing doses. Equivalents between the metric and household system are also not exact. These are the common ones and their abbreviations:

Teaspoon: tsp

Tablespoon: tbsp

Ounce: oz (or fl oz = fluid ounce)

Pint: pt

Quart: qt

Pound: lb

Household equivalents (approximate conversions):

```
1 tsp = 5 mL
1 tbsp = 15 mL
1 oz (or fl oz) = 30 mL
1 cup = 8 oz = 240–250 mL
1 pt = 500 mL
1 qt = 1 L or 1000 mL
2.2 lb = 1 kg
1 lb = 16 ounces (weight)
1 inch = 2.54 cm (centimeters)
```

Liquid Measures

Metric Liquid Measures

These are the liquid measures in the metric system and their abbreviations:

Liter: L

Milliliter: mL (may be seen as ml)

Cubic centimeter: cc (The use of "cc" is discouraged, however, because of "possible future inclusion in the Official 'Do Not Use' List" by the Joint Commission. See http://www.jointcommission.org for updates.)

Liquid equivalents in the metric system are as follows:

---

1 mL = 1 cc (See previous note regarding use of "cc" as an abbreviation.)

1 L = 1000 mL

Conversions Among Liquid Measures

Figure 2-1 shows a medicine cup with metric and household equivalents. These equivalents are approximate. Figure 2-2 shows syringes marked in mL.

---

1 tsp

15 mL = 1 tbsp = ½ fl oz

30 mL = 2 tbsp = 1 fl oz

1 cup = 8 oz = 240–250 mL

500 mL = 1 pt = 2 cups = 16 oz

1000 mL (1 L) = 1 qt = 2 pt

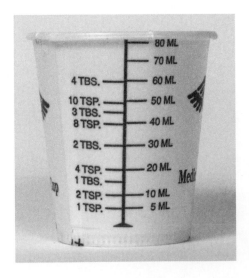

FIGURE 2-1

Medicine cup with metric and household equivalents.

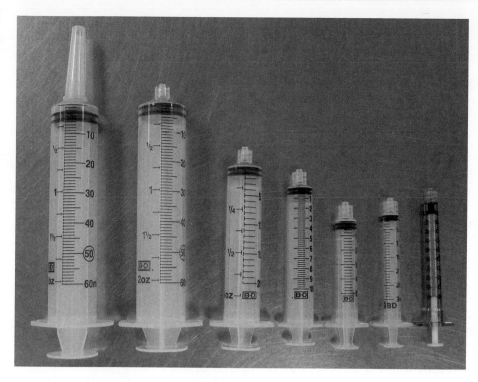

FIGURE 2-2

Syringes showing metric measures.
(Courtesy of Chistopher J. Belisle.)

Other Conversions

Temperature Conversions

Medication orders often use Centigrade temperature (Fig. 2-3). To convert from Fahrenheit to Centigrade, use this formula:

$$°C = (°F - 32) \div 1.8$$

To convert from Centigrade to Fahrenheit, use this formula:

$$°F = (°C \times 1.8) + 32$$

Here is a table of approximate temperature equivalents:

Fahrenheit	Centigrade
212°	100°
105°	40.56°
104°	40°
103°	39.44°
102°	38.89°
101°	38.33°
100°	37.78°
99°	37.22°
98.6°	37°
97°	36.11°
96°	35.56°
32°	0°

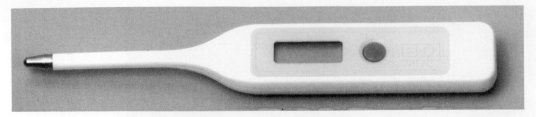

FIGURE 2-3

Digital thermometer that records temperature in Fahrenheit or Centigrade. (Nursing Procedures, 4th Edition. Ambler: Lippincott Williams & Wilkins, 2004.)

Milliunit and Milliequivalent

An unit is a standard of measurement used with drugs such as heparin and penicillin. A milliunit is one thousandth of a unit.

A drug used in obstetrics, oxytocin (Pitocin), is administered in milliunits per minute (see Chapter 7).

United States Pharmacopeia (USP) units are used to measure a vitamin or drug, such as vitamins A and D. USP is a trademark of United States Pharmacopeial Conventions, Inc. (http://www.usp.org). Usually an USP unit is equal to an international unit.

An international unit (IU) is used with vitamins, such as vitamins A, C, and D. Equivalencies of these measurements vary because a unit measures the effect per milligram of this drug. (Websearch "international unit" for more specific information.)

A milliequivalent, abbreviated mEq or meg, is used to measure the amount of solute per liter. It is used when measuring different substances found in biologic fluids, such as the amount of potassium in blood (normal value: 3.5 to 5.0 mEq per liter). Some medications are administered in milliequivalents, such as potassium (Fig. 2-4).

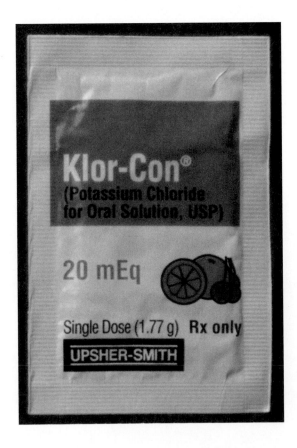

FIGURE 2-4

A medication measured in milliequivalents.

SELF-TEST 8 Liquid Equivalents and Mixed Conversions

Practice exercises in liquid equivalents and mixed conversions. For correct answers, see the end of the chapter. Some equivalencies may be approximate.

1. 1 oz = _____ mL
2. 1 tbsp = _____ mL
3. ½ fl oz = _____ mL
4. 2 fl oz = _____ mL
5. 500 mL = _____ qt
6. 5 mL = _____ tsp
7. 1 tsp = _____ mL
8. 1 fl oz = _____ tbsp
9. ½ tsp = _____ mL
10. 1 L = _____ mL
11. 1000 mL = _____ qt
12. 3 tbsp = _____ mL
13. 1½ fl oz = _____ mL
14. 10 mL = _____ tsp
15. 30 mL = _____ fl oz

16. 30 mL = _____ tbsp
17. 5 tbsp = _____ mL
18. 1 pt = _____ mL
19. 1 qt = _____ mL
20. 500 mL = _____ pt
21. 2 pt = _____ qt
22. 1 qt = _____ L
23. 15 mL = _____ tbsp
24. ½ qt = _____ pt
25. 2 tbsp = _____ fl oz
26. 2.2 lb = _____ kg
27. ½ L = _____ mL
28. 3 tsp = _____ mL
29. 250 mL = _____ pt
30. 1 kg = _____ lb

SELF-TEST 9 Temperature Conversions

Convert from Fahrenheit to Centigrade or from Centigrade to Fahrenheit. For correct answers, see the end of the chapter.

1. 212° F = _____ C
2. 103° F = _____ C
3. 96° F = _____ C
4. 98.6° F = _____ C

5. 38.33° C = _____ F
6. 37.78° C = _____ F
7. 0° C = _____ F
8. 40.56° C = _____ F

| PROFICIENCY TEST 1 | Exercises in Equivalents and Mixed Conversions |

Name:_____

Aim for 100% accuracy on this test. There are 40 items, each worth 2.5 points. See Appendix A for answers. Some equivalencies may be approximate.

1. 100 mg = _____ g

2. 1 fl oz = _____ mL

3. 1 L = _____ mL

4. 1 tsp = _____ mL

5. 0.015 g = _____ mg

6. 10 mg = _____ g

7. 500 mL = _____ L

8. 0.2 g = _____ mg

9. 30 mg = _____ g

10. 500 mg = _____ g

11. 1 fl oz = _____ mL

12. 1 mL = _____ tsp

13. 1 tbsp = _____ mL

14. 1 kg =_____ lb

15. 1 g = _____ mg

16. 60 mg = _____ g

17. 30 mL = _____ fl oz

18. 60 mL = _____ tbsp

19. 3 tbsp = _____ mL

20. 104° F = _____ C

21. 0.1 g = _____ mg

22. 5 mL = _____ tsp

23. 600 mg = _____ g

24. 10 mcg = _____ mg

25. 1000 mL = _____ L

26. 0.5 mcg = _____ mg

27. 0.6 mg = _____ g

28. 250 mcg = _____ mg

29. 1 mg = _____ g

30. 0.125 mg = _____ mcg

31. 0.01 mg = _____ mcg

32. 0.001 mg = _____ mcg

33. 1 qt = _____ mL

34. 6 tsp = _____ fl oz

35. 1 pint = _____ mL

36. ¼ L = _____ mL

37. 110 lb = _____ kg

38. 37.4° = _____ F

39. 100° = _____ C

40. 37° C = _____ F

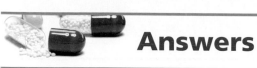

Answers

Self-Test 1 Grams to Milligrams

1. 300	**4.** 1200	**7.** 80	**10.** 325
2. 1	**5.** 5000	**8.** 275	**11.** 2000
3. 20	**6.** 400	**9.** 40	**12.** 0.4

Self-Test 2 Milligrams to Grams

1. 0.004	**4.** 0.075	**7.** 0.05	**10.** 0.36
2. 0.12	**5.** 0.25	**8.** 0.6	**11.** 0.01
3. 0.04	**6.** 0.001	**9.** 0.005	**12.** 0.0001

Self-Test 3 Milligrams to Micrograms

1. 300	**4.** 80	**7.** 5000	**10.** 10000
2. 1	**5.** 1200	**8.** 700	**11.** 900
3. 20	**6.** 400	**9.** 40	**12.** 10

Self-Test 4 Micrograms to Milligrams

1. 0.8	**4.** 0.025	**7.** 0.05	**10.** 0.075
2. 0.004	**5.** 0.001	**8.** 0.75	**11.** 0.0001
3. 0.014	**6.** 0.2	**9.** 0.325	**12.** 0.15

Self-Test 5 Mixed Conversions

1. 0.0003	**4.** 100	**7.** 14	**9.** 200
2. 30	**5.** 0.1	**8.** 0.2	**10.** 650
3. 0.015	**6.** 0.05		

Self-Test 6 Common Equivalents

1. 1	**5.** 0.2	**9.** 0.015	**12.** 400
2. 0.6	**6.** 0.1	**10.** 0.01	**13.** 300
3. 0.5	**7.** 0.06	**11.** 600	**14.** 250
4. 0.3	**8.** 0.03		

Self-Test 7 Review of Grams to Milligrams

1. Multiply grams by 1000 or move decimal point three places to the right or use a "greater than" sign to show movement of decimal point three places to the right.

2. 1000

3. 50

4. 200

5. 120

6. 400

7. 600

8. 500

9. 300

10. 4

11. 100

12. 60

13. 30

14. 15

15. 10

(continued)

Answers (Continued)

Self-Test 8 Liquid Equivalents and Mixed Conversions

1. 30	**9.** 2.5	**17.** 75	**25.** 1
2. 15	**10.** 1000	**18.** 500	**26.** 1
3. 15	**11.** 1	**19.** 1000	**27.** 500
4. 60	**12.** 45	**20.** 1	**28.** 15
5. ½	**13.** 45	**21.** 1	**29.** ½
6. 1	**14.** 2	**22.** 1	**30.** 2.2
7. 5	**15.** 1	**23.** 1	
8. 2	**16.** 2	**24.** 1	

Self-Test 9 Temperature Conversions

1. 100° C	**3.** 35.56° C	**5.** 100.99° F or 101° F	**7.** 32° F
2. 39.44° C	**4.** 37° C	**6.** 100° F	**8.** 105° F

Drug Abbreviations, Labels, and Packaging

TOPICS COVERED

1. Abbreviating times and routes of administration
2. Understanding military time: the 24-hour clock
3. Abbreviating metric, International System of units, and household measures
4. Terms and abbreviations for drug preparations
5. Medication orders and prescriptions
6. Drug labels and drug packaging
7. Equipment to measure doses

 ## Interpreting the Language of Prescriptions

When you're calculating drug dosages, it's important to understand medical abbreviations. Misunderstanding them can lead to medication errors. If you're unsure about what a medical abbreviation stands for, if the handwriting is illegible, or if you have any question about the medication order or prescription, *do not prepare the dose*. Clarify the order, prescription or abbreviation with the healthcare provider who prescribed the medication.

Below are three sample medication orders. They may look confusing now, but after you've worked your way through this chapter, they'll make perfect sense:

Morphine sulfate 15 mg subcutaneously stat and 10 mg q4h prn

Chloromycetin 0.01% Ophth Oint left eye bid

Ampicillin 1 g IVPB q6h

In 2004, the Joint Commission issued a list of "Do Not Use" abbreviations—the ones that were often misread and thus led to medication errors. Some of them (clearly labeled "Do Not Use") appear in this book, either because they are from the minimal required list on the Joint Commission's website or because they supplement that list. To see a complete roster of abbreviations designated "Do Not Use," go to http://www.jointcommission.org or search "prohibited abbreviations." The Institute for Safe Medication Practices also publishes an updated list of "Do Not Use" abbreviations, that include the Joint Commission recommendations in addition to a list of error-prone abbreviations, symbols, and dose designations. Check their website: http://www.ismp.org. Each institution may also have its own "Do Not Use" list. As a nurse, you need to make careful note of abbreviations that are prohibited or dangerous. Search for apps that are available for mobile devices by using key words such as: "medical abbreviations," "military time conversions," "metric and household conversions."

Time of Administration of Drugs

The abbreviations for the times of drug administration appear in the following table. Most of these abbreviations come from Latin words and are given for your reference. Memorize the abbreviations, their meanings, and the sample times that indicate how the abbreviations are interpreted. However, follow your institutional policy for administration times.

Time Abbreviation	Meaning	Explanation		Do Not Use
ac	Before meals	Latin, *ante cibum*		
		SAMPLE TIME	7:30 AM, 11:30 AM, 4:30 PM	
pc	After meals	Latin, *post cibum*		
		SAMPLE TIME	10 AM, 2 PM, 6 PM	
daily	Every day, daily	Latin, *quaque die*		q.d.
		SAMPLE TIME	10 AM	qd
bid	Twice a day	Latin, *bis in die*		
		SAMPLE TIME	10 AM, 6 PM or 9 AM, 9 PM	
tid	Three times a day	Latin, *ter in die*		
		SAMPLE TIME	10 AM, 2 PM, 6 PM or 8 AM, 4 PM, 12	
qid	Four times a day	Latin, *quater in die*		
		SAMPLE TIME	10 AM, 2 PM, 6 PM, 10 PM or 6 AM, 12 PM, 6 PM, 12 AM	
qh	Every hour	Latin, *quaque hora* Because the drug is given every hour, it will be given 24 times in 1 day.		
at bedtime	At bedtime, hour of sleep	Latin, *hora somni*		hs
		SAMPLE TIME	10 PM	h.s.
qn	Every night	Latin, *quaque nocte*		
		SAMPLE TIME	10 PM	
stat	Immediately	Latin, *statim*		
		SAMPLE TIME	Now!	

The time abbreviations in the following table are based on a 24-hour day. To determine the number of times a medication is given in a day, divide 24 by the number given in the abbreviation.

Time Abbreviation	Meaning	Explanation
q2h or q2°	Every 2 hours	The drug will be given 12 times in a 24-hour period (24 ÷ 2).
		SAMPLE TIMES even hours at 2 AM, 4 AM, 6 AM, 8 AM, 10 AM, 12 noon, 2 PM, 4 PM, 6 PM, 8 PM, 10 PM, 12 midnight
q4h or q4°	Every 4 hours	The drug will be given six times in a 24-hour period (24 ÷ 4).
		SAMPLE TIMES 2 AM, 6 AM, 10 AM, 2 PM, 6 PM, 10 PM
q6h or q6°	Every 6 hours	The drug will be given four times in a 24-hour period (24 ÷ 6).
		SAMPLE TIMES 6 AM, 12 noon, 6 PM, 12 midnight
q8h or q8°	Every 8 hours	The drug will be given three times in a 24-hour period (24 ÷ 8).
		SAMPLE TIMES 6 AM, 2 PM, 10 PM
q12h or q12°	Every 12 hours	The drug will be given twice in a 24-hour period (24 ÷ 12).
		SAMPLE TIMES 6 AM, 6 PM

There are four additional time abbreviations that require explanation. They are as follows:

Time Abbreviation	Meaning	Explanation	Do Not Use
every other day	Every other day	Latin, *quaque otra die* This abbreviation is interpreted by the days of the **month**. The nurse writes on the medication record "odd days of the month":	qod q.o.d.
		SAMPLE TIME 10 AM on the first, third, fifth day, and so on	
		The nurse might write "even days of the month":	
		SAMPLE TIME 10 AM on the second, fourth, sixth day, and so on	
prn	As needed	Latin, *pro re nata* **This abbreviation is usually combined with a time abbreviation.**	
		EXAMPLE q4h prn (every 4 hours as needed)	
		This permits the nurse to assess the patient and make a nursing judgment about whether to administer the medication.	
		SAMPLE acetaminophen 650 mg po q4h prn (650 milligrams acetaminophen by mouth, every 4 hours as needed for pain)	

(continued)

Time Abbreviation	Meaning	Explanation	Do Not Use
		The nurse assesses the patient for pain every 4 hours. If the patient has pain, the nurse may administer the drug. This abbreviation has three administration implications: 1. The nurse **must wait** 4 hours before giving the next dose. 2. Once 4 hours have elapsed, the dose may be given any time thereafter. 3. Sample times are not given because the nurse does not know when the patient will need the drug.	
3 times weekly	Three times per week	Latin, *ter in vicis* Time relates to days of the **week.** **SAMPLE TIME** 10 AM on Monday, Wednesday, Friday Do not confuse with tid (three times per **day**).	tiw t.i.w.
biw	Twice per week	Latin, *bis in vicis* Time relates to days of the **week.** **SAMPLE TIME** 10 AM on Monday, Thursday Do not confuse with bid (twice per **day**).	

SELF-TEST 1 Abbreviations

After studying the abbreviations for times of administration, give the meaning of the following terms. Include sample times. Indicate if the abbreviation is "Do Not Use" and which words to substitute for it. The correct answers are given at the end of the chapter.

1. tid _____

2. qn _____

3. pc _____

4. qod _____

5. bid _____

6. hs _____

7. stat _____

8. qid _____

9. q4h _____

10. ac _____

11. qd _____

12. q8h _____

13. qh _____

14. prn _____

15. q4h prn _____

Military Time: The 24-Hour Clock

If a handwritten prescription does not clearly distinguish "AM" from "PM," confusion about times of administration can arise. To prevent error, many institutions have converted from the traditional 12-hour clock to a 24-hour clock, referred to as *military time*. (This text will continue using the normal 12-hour clock.)

The 24-hour clock begins at midnight as 0000. The hours from 1 AM to 12 noon are the same as traditional time; colons and the terms AM and PM are omitted (Fig. 3-1). Examples:

Traditional	Military
12 midnight	0000
1 AM	0100
5 AM	0500
7:30 AM	0730
11:45 AM	1145
12:00 noon	1200

The hours from 1 PM continue numerically; 1 PM becomes 1300. To change traditional time to military time from 1 PM on, add 12. To change military time to traditional time from 1300 on, subtract 12. Examples:

Traditional	Military
1 PM	1300
2:30 PM	1430
5 PM	1700
7:15 PM	1915
10:45 PM	2245
11:59 PM	2359

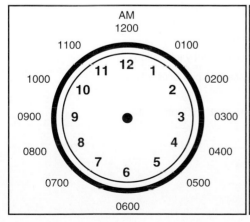 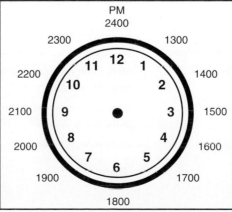

FIGURE 3-1

Example of a military, or 24-hour, clock.

| **SELF-TEST 2** | **Military Time** |

A. Change these traditional times to military time. Answers are given at the end of the chapter.

1. 2 PM _____   **5.** 1:30 AM _____

2. 9 AM _____   **6.** 9:15 PM _____

3. 4 PM _____   **7.** 4:50 AM _____

4. 12 noon _____   **8.** 6:20 PM _____

B. Change these military times to traditional times. Answers are given at the end of the chapter.

1. 0130 _____   **5.** 1910 _____

2. 1745 _____   **6.** 0600 _____

3. 1100 _____   **7.** 0050 _____

4. 2015 _____   **8.** 1000 _____

Routes of Administration

The abbreviations for routes of administration are given in the following table. Latin words are given for reference only. Note the "Do Not Use" abbreviations. Figure 3-2 shows the use of several abbreviations for routes of administration.

Route Abbreviation	Meaning	Origin and Explanation	Do Not Use
Write out	Right ear	Latin, *aures dextra*	AD
Write out	Left ear	Latin, *aures laeva*	AL
Write out	Each ear	Latin, *aures utrae*	AU
HHN	Handheld nebulizer	Medication is placed in a device that produces a fine spray for inhalation.	
IM	Intramuscularly	The injection is given at a 90-degree angle into a muscle.	
IV	Intravenously	The medication or fluid is given into a vein.	
IVP	Intravenous push	Medication is injected directly into a vein.	
IVPB	Intravenous piggyback	Medication prepared in a small volume of fluid is attached to an IV (which is already infusing fluid into a patient's vein) at specified times.	
MDI	Metered-dose inhaler	An aerosol device delivers medication by inhalation.	
NEB	Nebulizer	Medication is placed in a device that produces a fine spray for inhalations.	
NGT or ng	Nasogastric tube	Medication is placed in the stomach through a tube in the nose.	
Write out	In the right eye	Latin, *oculus dextra*	OD

Route Abbreviation	Meaning	Origin and Explanation	Do Not Use
Write out	In the left eye	Latin, *oculus sinister*	OS
Write out	In both eyes	Latin, *oculi utrique*	OU
po or PO	By mouth	Latin, *per os*	
pr or PR	In the rectum	Latin, *per rectum*	
Write out	Subcutaneously, Sub q	The injection is usually given at a 45-degree angle into subcutaneous tissue.	sc sq s.c., s.q.
SL	Sublingual, under the tongue	Latin, *sub lingua*	
S & S	Swish and swallow	By using tongue and cheek muscles, the patient coats his or her mouth with a liquid medication, then swallows.	

SELF-TEST 3	Abbreviations (Routes)

After studying the abbreviations for routes of administration, give the meaning of the following terms. Indicate if the abbreviation is "Do Not Use" and which words substitute for it. The correct answers are given at the end of the chapter.

1. SL _____

2. OU _____

3. NGT _____

4. IV _____

5. po _____

6. OD _____

7. IVPB _____

8. OS _____

9. IM _____

10. pr _____

11. S & S _____

12. sc _____

13. AU _____

14. AL _____

NDC 0517-1130-05
EPINEPHRINE
INJECTION, USP
1:1000 (1 mg/mL)

30 mL
MULTIPLE DOSE VIAL
FOR SC AND IM USE.
FOR IV AND IC USE AFTER
DILUTION.
Rx Only

AMERICAN
REGENT, INC.
SHIRLEY, NY 11967

Each mL contains: Epinephrine 1 mg (as the Hydrochloride), Water for Injection q.s. Sodium Chloride added for isotonicity, Chlorobutanol 0.5% as a preservative and Sodium Metabisulfite not more than 0.15% as an antioxidant. pH adjusted with Sodium Hydroxide and/or Hydrochloric Acid.
PROTECT FROM LIGHT.
Store at controlled room temperature up to 25°C (77°F) (See USP).
Directions for Use: See Package Insert.
Rev. 9/03

Lot / Exp.

FIGURE 3-2

Label states the routes of administration. Epinephrine may be administered intramuscularly (IM) or subcutaneously (SC), or by intravenous (IV) or intracardiac (IC) routes after dilution. (Courtesy of Abbott Laboratories.)

Metric and SI Abbreviations

Metric abbreviations in dosage relate to a drug's weight or volume and are the most common measures in dosage. The International System of Units (Système International d'Unités; SI) was adapted from the metric system in 1960. Most developed countries except the United States have adopted SI nomenclature to provide a standard language of measurement.

Differences between metric and SI systems do not occur in dosage. The meaning and abbreviations for weight and volume are the same. Weight measures are based on the gram; volume measures are based on the liter.

Study the meaning of the abbreviations listed in the following table. In the Explanation column, you'll see one equivalent for each abbreviation to help you understand what kinds of quantities are involved. Equivalents (metric, household) are discussed in Chapter 2. The preferred abbreviation is listed first; variations appear in parentheses.

Metric Abbreviation	Meaning	Explanation	Do Not Use
cc	Cubic centimeter	This is a measure of volume usually reserved for measuring gases. However, you may still find it used as a liquid measure. (One cubic centimeter is approximately equal to 16 drops from a medicine dropper.)	Substitute mL.
g	Gram	This is a solid measure of weight. (One gram is approximately equal to the weight of two paper clips.)	
kg or Kg	Kilogram	This is a weight measure. (One kilogram equals 2.2 pounds.)	
L	Liter	This is a liquid measure. (One liter is a little more than a quart.)	
mcg	Microgram	This is a measure of weight. (1000 micrograms equals 1 milligram.)	μg
mEq or meq	Milliequivalent	No equivalent necessary. Drugs are prepared and ordered in this weight measure.	
mg	Milligram	This is a measure of weight. (1000 milligrams equals 1 gram.)	
mL or ml	Milliliter	This is a liquid measure. The terms *cubic centimeter* (cc) and *milliliter* (mL) are interchangeable in dosage. (One cubic centimeter equals 1 milliliter.)	
unit	Unit	This is a measure of biologic activity. Nurses do not calculate this measure.	U

> **EXAMPLE**   penicillin potassium 300,000 units
>
> *Important:* It is considered safer to write the word unit rather than use the abbreviation because the U could be read as a zero and a medication error might result.

SELF-TEST 4   Abbreviations (Metric)

After studying metric abbreviations, write the meaning of the following terms. Indicate if the abbreviation is not to be used and the words to substitute for it. The correct answers are given at the end of the chapter.

1. 0.3 g _____

2. 150 mcg _____

3. 80 U _____

4. 0.5 mL _____

5. 1.7 cc _____

6. 0.25 mg _____

7. 14 kg _____

8. 20 mEq _____

9. 1.5 L _____

10. 50 μg _____

Household Abbreviations

Physicians and healthcare providers may use these common household measures to order drugs, especially if the drug is to be administered at home. The Explanation column shows metric equivalents.

Household Abbreviation	Meaning	Explanation
pt	Pint	One pint is approximately equal to 500 milliliters: 1 pt ≅ 500 mL. One quart is approximately equal to 1 liter, which is equal to 1000 milliliters; 1 qt ≅ 1 L = 1000 mL.
qt	Quart	One half of a quart is approximately equal to 1 pint; ½ qt ≅ 1 pt = 500 mL.
tbsp	Tablespoon	One tablespoon equals 15 milliliters: 1 tbsp = 15 mL.
tsp	Teaspoon	One teaspoon equals 5 milliliters: 1 tsp = 5 mL.
oz	Ounce	One ounce equals 30 milliliters: 1 oz = 30 mL.

EXAMPLE

6 tsp = 1 oz = 30 mL
3 tsp = ½ oz = 15 mL
2 tbsp = 1 oz = 30 mL = 6 tsp

SELF-TEST 5   Abbreviations (Household)

After studying household measures, write the meaning of the following terms. The correct answers are given at the end of the chapter.

1. 3 tsp _____   **3.** ½ qt _____   **5.** 1 pt _____

2. 1 oz _____   **4.** 1 tsp _____   **6.** 2 tbsp _____

Terms and Abbreviations for Drug Preparations

The following abbreviations and terms are used to describe selected drug preparations. Some of these abbreviations are rarely used yet are included here for reference.

Term Abbreviation	Meaning	Explanation
cap, caps	Capsule	Medication is encased in a gelatin shell.
CR	Controlled release	
LA	Long acting	
SA	Sustained action	These abbreviations indicate that the drug has been prepared in a form that allows extended action. Therefore, the drug is given less frequently.
SR	Slow release or Sustained Release	
DS	Double strength	
EC	Enteric coated	The tablet is coated with a substance that will not dissolve in the acid secretions of the stomach; instead, it dissolves in the more alkaline secretions of the intestines.

(continued)

Term Abbreviation	Meaning	Explanation
el, elix	Elixir	A drug is dissolved in a hydroalcoholic sweetened base.
sol	Solution	The drug is contained in a clear liquid preparation.
sp	Spirit	This is an alcoholic solution of a volatile substance (e.g., spirit of ammonia).
sup, supp	Suppository	This is a solid, cylindrically shaped drug that can be inserted into a body opening (e.g., the rectum or vagina).
susp	Suspension	Small particles of drug are dispersed in a liquid base and must be shaken before being poured; gels and magmas are also suspensions.
syr	Syrup	A sugar is dissolved in a liquid medication and flavored to disguise the taste.
tab, tabs	Tablet	Medication is compressed or molded into a solid form; additional ingredients are used to shape and color the tablet.
tr, tinct.	Tincture	This is a liquid alcoholic or hydroalcoholic solution of a drug.
ung, oint.	Ointment	This is a semisolid drug preparation that is applied to the skin (for external use only).
KVO	Keep vein open	**EXAMPLE ORDER** 1000 mL dextrose 5% in water IV KVO. The nurse is to continue infusing this fluid.
TKO	To keep open	
Discontinue	Discontinue	**EXAMPLE ORDER** Discontinue ampicillin. (Do not use D/C.)
NKA	No known allergies	This is an important assessment that is noted on the medication record of a patient.
NKDA	No known drug allergies	This is an important assessment that is noted on the medication record of a patient.

SELF-TEST 6   **Abbreviations (Drug Preparations)**

After studying the abbreviations for drug preparations, write out the meaning of the following terms. The correct answers are given at the end of the chapter.

1. elix _____
2. DS _____
3. NKA _____
4. caps _____
5. susp _____

6. tab _____
7. SR _____
8. LA _____
9. supp _____
10. tr _____

Now consider the formerly confusing orders that appeared at the beginning of this chapter.

Original: Morphine sulfate 15 mg subcutaneously stat and 10 mg q4h prn

Interpretation: Morphine sulfate 15 mg subcutaneously immediately and 10 mg every 4 hours as needed.

Original: Chloromycetin 0.01% Ophth Oint left eye bid

Interpretation: Chloromycetin 0.01% ophthalmic ointment left eye twice a day.

Original: Ampicillin 1 g IVPB q6h

Interpretation: Ampicillin 1 gram intravenous piggyback every 6 hours.

Drug Labels

An understanding of drug labels and the ways in which drugs are packaged provides a background for dosage and administration.

Labels contain specific facts and appear on drugs intended to be administered as packaged: either in solid form or in liquid form. Occasionally the label does *not* include some details—such as route of administration, usual dose, and storage—because the container is too small. When you need more information than the label provides, consult a professional reference. Figure 3-3 shows a sample drug label.

NDC NUMBER. The National Drug Code (NDC) is a number used by the pharmacist to identify the drug and the method of packaging.

- In Figure 3-3, the NDC is 0165-0022-10. The letters NSN (not shown) mean "national supply number," a code for ordering the drug.

DRUG QUANTITY. This information always appears on the label at the top left, the top right, or the bottom.

- Figure 3-3 indicates 1000 tablets.

TRADE NAME. A drug's trade name (also called brand name or proprietary name) is usually followed by the federal registration symbol ®. Several companies may manufacture the same drug, using different trade names. When a trade name appears on the label, it may be written either in all capital letters or with only the first letter capitalized.

- In Figure 3-3, MagOx400 is the trade name.

GENERIC NAME. The generic name is the official accepted name of a drug, as listed in the United States Pharmacopeia (USP). A drug may have several trade names but only one official generic name. The generic name is not capitalized.

- The generic name given in Figure 3-3 is magnesium oxide.

DRUG STRENGTH. For solid drugs, the label shows metric weights; for liquid drugs, the label states a solution of the drug in a solvent.

- In Figure 3-3, the strength is 400 mg.

DRUG FORM. The label specifies the type of preparation in the container.

- Figure 3-3 indicates that the drug is dispensed in tablets.

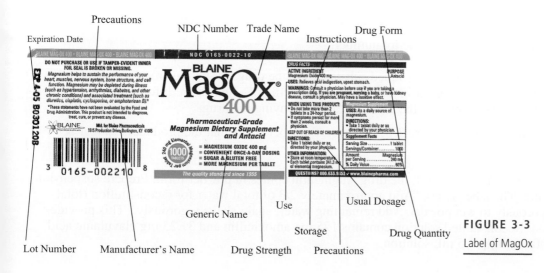

FIGURE 3-3

Label of MagOx

USE. The label may include the indication for the drug.

- Figure 3-3 states "Magnesium helps to sustain the performance of your heart, muscles, nervous system, bone structure and cell function. Magnesium may be depleted during illness (such as hypertension, arrhythmias, diabetes and other chronic conditions) and associated treatment (such as diuretics, cisplatin, cyclosporine or amphoterican B)."

USUAL DOSAGE. The dosage information states how much drug is administered at a single time or during a 24-hour period. It also identifies who should receive the drug.

- Figure 3-3 states, "Usual dosage: take 1 tablet daily or as directed by your physician."

ROUTE OF ADMINISTRATION. The label specifies how the drug is to be given: orally, parenterally (through an injection of some type), or topically (applied to skin or mucous membranes). *If the label does not specify the route, the drug is in an oral form.*

- In Figure 3-3, the route is oral.

STORAGE. Certain conditions are necessary to protect the drug from losing its potency (effectiveness), so this information is crucial. Some drugs come in a dry form and must be dissolved (i.e., reconstituted). The drug may need one kind of storage when it's dry and another kind after reconstitution.

- Figure 3-3 specifies storing the drug at room temperature.

PRECAUTIONS AND WARNINGS. The label may include specific instructions—related to safety, effectiveness, and/or administration—that the nurse must note and follow.

- Figure 3-3 shows these precautions: "Do not purchase or use if tamper-evident inner foil seal is broken or missing. Also, **Warnings:** Consult a physician before use if you are taking a prescription drug. If you are pregnant, nursing a baby, or have kidney disease, consult a physician. May have a laxative effect. The label also states, **When using this product:** Do not take more than 2 tablets in a 24-hour period. If symptoms persist for more than 2 weeks, consult a physician. Keep out of reach of children."

MANUFACTURER'S NAME. If you have any question about the drug, direct them to the manufacturer.

- In Figure 3-3, the manufacturer is Blaine Pharmaceuticals.

EXPIRATION DATE. A drug expires on the last day of the indicated month. After that date, the drug cannot be used.

- Figure 3-3 shows 4-05 as the expiration date.

LOT NUMBER. This number indicates the batch of drug from which the stock came.

- Figure 3-3 shows B030120B as the lot number.

ADDITIVES. The manufacturer may have added substances to the drug, for various reasons: to bind the drug, to make the drug dissolve more easily, to produce a specific pH, and so on. Information about such additives may appear on the label or in the literature accompanying the drug.

- Additives are not shown in Figure 3-3; however, the label states that the product is "sugar & gluten free."

DRUG RECONSTITUTION. In Figure 3-4, the drug Augmentin comes in powder form. Prepare suspension at time of dispensing. The label states, "Add approximately 2/3 of total water for reconstitution (total 90 mL); shake vigorously to wet powder. Add remaining water; again shake vigorously." This provides 100 mL suspension. Reconstituted solution contains 125 mg amoxicillin and 31.25 mg clavulanic acid (as clavulanate potassium) per 5 mL solution.

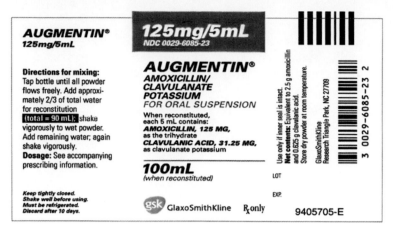

FIGURE 3-4

Label of Augmentin for oral suspension.
(Reproduced with permission of GlaxoSmithKline.)

Combination Medications

Some medication labels indicate more than one drug in the dose form. These combination drugs are ordered according to the number of tablets to give or the amount of liquid to pour.

EXAMPLE

a. Order: Robitussin DM 1 tsp po qid (see Fig. 3-5)

Label: guaifenesin 200 mg/dextromethorphan 30 mg per 10 mL

b. Order: Tylenol #3 tabs ii po q4h prn for pain

Label: acetaminophen 300 mg/codeine 30 mg tablet

c. Order: Talwin Compound 1 tab po q6h

Label: aspirin 325 mg/pentazocine 12.5 mg

d. Order: Phenergan VC Syrup 2 tsp po q6h while awake

Label: phenylephrine 5 mg/promethazine 6.25 mg per 5 mL

 # Drug Packaging

Drugs come in two types of packaging: *unit-dose* and *multidose*. Each type may contain a solid or liquid form of the drug for oral, parenteral, or topical use. Most institutions use a combination of unit-dose and multidose.

Unit-Dose Packaging

In an institutional setting, each dose is individually wrapped and labeled, and a 24-hour supply is prepared by the pharmacy and dispensed. A major value of unit-dose packaging is that two professionals—the pharmacist and the nurse—check the drug and the dose, thereby decreasing the possibility of error.

The medication may be stored in a medication cart, in a locked cabinet at the patient's bedside, or in a locked medication dispensing system, such as the Pyxis.

Unit-dose packaging does not relieve the nurse from responsibility to check the label three times and to calculate the amount of drug needed. Be aware that unit-dose drugs come in different strengths, and when trade names are ordered instead of generic names, there is always a chance of error. A dose may consist of one unit packet, two or more unit packets, or a fraction of one packet. Skilled-care nursing facilities and long-term care facilities often use a system that dispenses the unit-dose medication for 1 month (see Fig. 3-6).

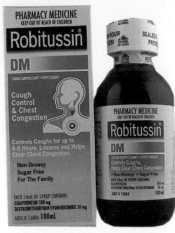

FIGURE 3-5

Robitussin DM, a combination medication

Copyright 2015 L. Farmer Photography

EXAMPLE

A nurse has a unit-dose 100-mg tablet. If an order calls for 50 mg, only half of the tablet should be administered.

If a nurse has an order for 75 mg and each unit packet contains 25-mg tablets, the nurse administers three tablets.

FOR THE ORAL ROUTE. For oral administration, unit-dose packaging comes in a number of forms:

1. Plastic bubble, foil, or paper wrappers containing tablets or capsules (Fig. 3-7A).

2. Plastic or glass containers or sealed packets that hold a single dose of a liquid or powder. The powder is reconstituted to a liquid form by following the directions given on the label (Fig. 3-7B).

3. A sealed medication cup containing a liquid. Once the nurse removes the cover, the medication is ready to administer; the amount administered depends on the correct calculation of the dose (Fig. 3-7C).

FOR THE PARENTERAL ROUTE. These drugs—which may come in a solid or liquid form—are given by injection via the route specified in the medication order (e.g., IV, IM, Subcutaneous, IVPB). Drugs packaged in the containers described below are sterile, and aseptic technique is essential in their preparation and administration.

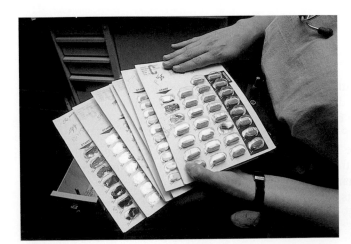

FIGURE 3-6

In long-term care settings, where medication prescriptions remain the same over weeks or months, "bingo" cards are a cost-effective method of dispensing medications. Each bubble contains one dose for the client. (Used with permission from Craven, R. F., & Hirnle, C. J. [2007]. Fundamentals of nursing. Philadelphia, PA: Lippincott Williams & Wilkins, p. 551.)

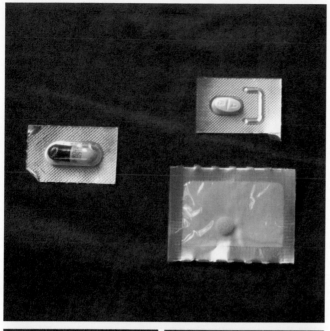

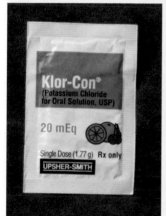

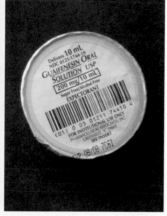

FIGURE 3-7

A. Unit-dose tablets and capsules in foil wrappers.
B. Unit-dose powder in a sealed packet; it is placed in a container and diluted before giving. **C.** Sealed cup containing a liquid medication. (© 2008 Lacey-Bordeaux Photography.)

1. An *ampule* (ampoule) is a glass container that holds a single sterile dose of drug—either a liquid, a powder, or a crystal (Fig. 3-8). The container has a narrow neck that must be broken to reach the drug. Then the nurse uses a sterile syringe to withdraw the medication. Directions tell how to reconstitute the solid forms. Once the glass is broken, the drug cannot be kept sterile, so the nurse must be sure to discard any portion of the drug not immediately used.

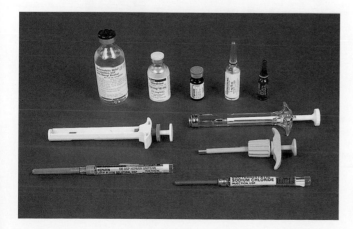

FIGURE 3-8

Parenteral route: **Top row.** Vials and ampules. **Middle/bottom rows.** Prefilled cartridges and holders.

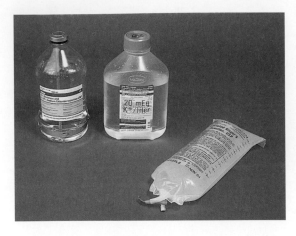

FIGURE 3-9

Flexible plastic bags and glass containers hold medication for IV use.

2. A *vial* is a glass or plastic container with a sealed rubber top (Fig. 3-8). Medication in the container can be kept sterile. The container may have a sterile liquid or a sterile powder that the nurse must reconstitute with a sterile diluent and syringe. Since *single-dose vials* do not contain a preservative or a bacteriostatic agent, the nurse must discard any medication remaining after the dose is prepared.

3. Flexible *plastic bags* or *glass containers* may hold sterile medication for IV use (Fig. 3-9). The nurse administers the fluid via IV tubing connected to a needle or catheter placed in the patient's blood vessel.

4. *Prefilled syringes* contain sterile liquid medication that is ready to administer without further preparation. Although this type of unit-dose packaging is expensive, it can save lives in an emergency when speed is essential (Fig. 3-10).

5. *Prefilled cartridges* are actually small vials with a needle or needleless device attached. They fit into a metal or plastic holder and eject one unit-dose of a sterile drug in liquid form. Brand names include Carpuject and Tubex (Fig. 3-11).

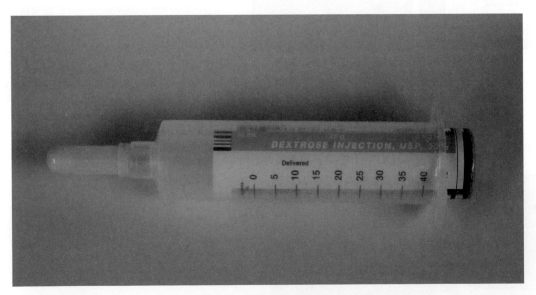

FIGURE 3-10

Prefilled syringe with liquid medication. (© 2010 L. Farmer Photography.)

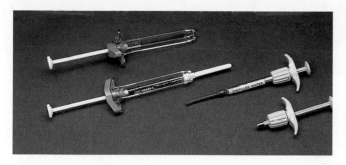

FIGURE 3-11

Prefilled cartridges with injector devices (see http://www.hospira .com/products/CarpujectSyringeSystem.aspx for a visual of putting together a prefilled device and injector).

FOR TOPICAL ADMINISTRATION. Drugs applied to the skin or mucous membranes can achieve a local effect. They can also achieve a systemic effect because they can be absorbed into the circulation.

1. *Transdermal patches* or *pads* are adhesive bandages placed on the skin (Fig. 3-12). They hold a drug form that is slowly absorbed into the circulation over a period ranging from hours to several days.

2. *Lozenges, troches, and pastilles* are disklike solids that slowly dissolve in the mouth (e.g., cough drops). Some drugs are prepared in a gum and are released by chewing (e.g., nicotine).

3. *Suppositories* in foil or plastic wrappers are molded forms that can be inserted into the rectum or vagina (Fig. 3-13). They hold medication in a substance (such as cocoa butter) that melts at body temperature and releases the drug. Suppositories may be used for unconscious patients or those unable to swallow.

4. *Plastic, disposable, squeezable containers* hold either prepared solutions for the vagina (douches) or enema solutions that are administered rectally (Fig. 3-14). To ease insertion, the containers for enemas have a lubricated nozzle. Squeezing the container forces the solution out.

Multidose Packaging

Within an institutional setting, such as a hospital, the nursing floor or unit may receive large stock containers of medications from which doses are poured. Although this type of packaging reduces the pharmacy's workload, it adds to preparation time and increases the possibility of error.

FOR THE ORAL ROUTE. Stock bottles contain a liquid or a solid form such as tablets, capsules, or powders. Large stock bottles hold medication that is dispensed over a period of days. When reconstituting the powders, the nurse must write the date and time of preparation on the container's label and must carefully note storage directions and the expiration date. Caution: Powders, once dissolved, begin losing potency (Fig. 3-15A).

FOR THE PARENTERAL ROUTE. Multidose vials contain either a sterile liquid or a powder to be reconstituted using sterile technique. If reconstituted, the nurse must write the date and time of preparation on the label and must note the expiration date and storage (Fig. 3-15B).

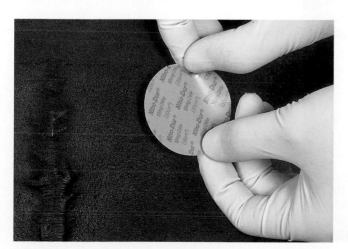

FIGURE 3-12

Transdermal patches or pads are placed on the skin. Drugs prepared in this manner include estrogen, fentanyl, testosterone, and nitroglycerin.

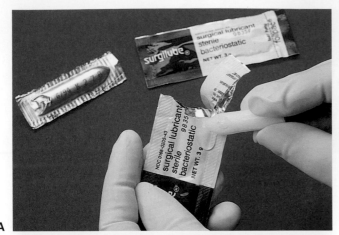

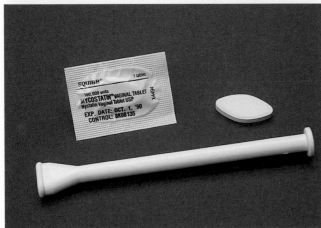

FIGURE 3-13
A. Rectal suppository. **B.** Vaginal suppository and applicator.

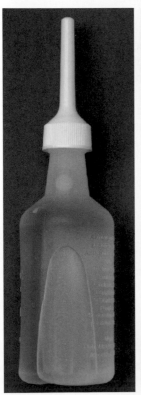

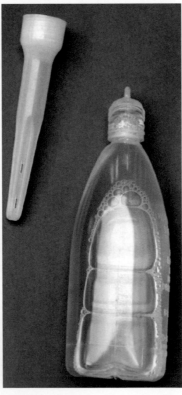

FIGURE 3-14
Unit-dose containers for rectal enema **(A)** and vaginal irrigation **(B)**. (© 2004 Lacey-Bordeaux Photography.)

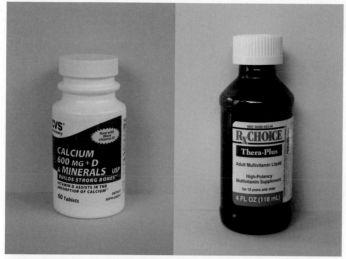

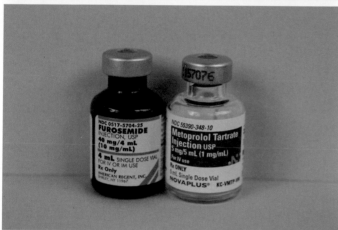

FIGURE 3-15

Multidose packaging. **A.** Oral. **B.** Parenteral. (© 2010 L. Farmer Photography.)

FOR TOPICAL ADMINISTRATION. Since containers for topical medications are used over an extended period of time, it's important to avoid contaminating them. The nurse should label the container with the patient's name and reserve the container's use for only that patient. Here are some guidelines on using containers for topical medication:

1. Metal or plastic tubes often contain ointments or creams for application to the skin or mucous membranes. Squeezing the tubes releases the medication (Fig. 3-16A).

2. To avoid contamination of medicated creams, ointments, and pastes in jars, always use a sterile tongue blade or sterile glove to remove the medication.

3. When using dropper bottles for eye, ear, or nose medications, prevent cross-contamination by labeling each container with the patient's name and using the container only for that patient. The nurse must be careful to avoid touching mucous membranes with the dropper because contamination of the dropper can cause pathogens to grow. Droppers come in two forms: monodrop containers, which are squeezed to release the medication, and containers with removable droppers. Separate, packaged droppers are also available to administer medications; these are sometimes calibrated (i.e., marked in milliliters; Fig. 3-16B, C).

   Eye medications are labeled "ophthalmic" or "for the eye." Ear drugs are labeled "otic" or "auric" or "for the ear." Drugs for nasal administration are labeled "nose drops." Do not interchange these routes.

4. Lozenges and pastilles may be packaged in multidose as well as unit-dose containers.

5. Metered-dose inhalers (MDIs; Fig. 3-17) are aerosol devices with two parts: a canister under pressure and a mouthpiece. The canister contains multiple drug doses in either a liquid form or a microfine

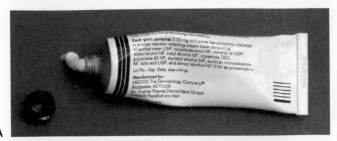

A

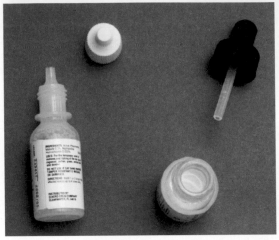

B

C

FIGURE 3-16

Topical multidose containers. **A.** Tubes for creams or ointments. **B.** Monodrop containers—the dropper is attached. **C.** Removable dropper is sometimes calibrated for liquid measures. (© 2004 Lacey-Bordeaux Photography.)

powder or crystal. The mouthpiece fits on the canister, and finger pressure on the mouthpiece opens a valve on the canister that discharges one dose. The physician/healthcare provider's order states the number of inhalations or "puffs" to be taken. Medications for inhalation also may be packaged as liquids in vials or bottles or as capsules containing powder for use with either a handheld nebulizer (HHN) or an intermittent positive-pressure breathing (IPPB) apparatus. Dry powder inhalers (DPIs), such as Advair, contain a set number of doses and are administered in a similar way as MDIs.

Chapter 10 explains specifics of medication administration. Refer also to any nursing fundamentals or pharmacology textbook about medication administration.

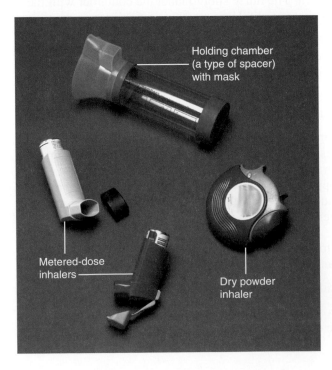

Holding chamber (a type of spacer) with mask

Metered-dose inhalers

Dry powder inhaler

FIGURE 3-17

Examples of MDIs and spacers. (Used with permission from Taylor, C. [2008]. Fundamentals of nursing. Philadelphia, PA: Lippincott Williams & Wilkins, p. 810.)

SELF-TEST 7 Drug Packaging

A. *Match Column A with the letters in Column B to identify the meaning of terms used in drug packaging. Answers are given at the end of the chapter.*

Column A

1. _____ Unit-dose
2. _____ Ampule
3. _____ Parenteral
4. _____ Prefilled cartridge
5. _____ Reconstitution
6. _____ Topical
7. _____ Transdermal patch
8. _____ Vial
9. _____ Lozenge
10. _____ Suppository

Column B

a. Dissolving a powder into solution

b. Glass or plastic container with a sealed rubber top

c. Route of administration to skin or mucous membranes

d. Individually wrapped and labeled drugs

e. Disk-like solid that dissolves in the mouth

f. Molded form of a drug used for insertion in the vagina or rectum

g. General term for an injection route

h. Adhesive bandage applied to the skin that gradually releases a drug

i. Small vial with a needle attached that fits into a syringe holder

j. Glass container that must be broken to obtain the drug

B. *Complete these statements related to drug packaging. Answers are given at the end of the chapter.*

11. The best way to avoid cross-contamination of a multidose tube of ointment is to _____

_____

12. Dropper bottles for eye medications come in two forms: _____

_____

13. The type of drug packaging that decreases the possibility of error is termed _____

_____

14. Drugs administered topically for a local effect may be absorbed and produce another effect

that is called _____

_____

_____

15. The word lozenge describes _____

_____

_____

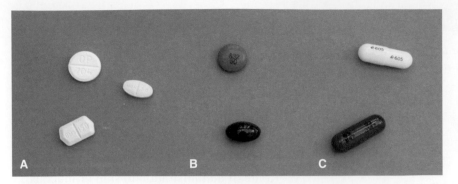

 ## Equipment to Measure Doses

Solids for oral administration come in tablets and capsules. Once you calculate the number to give, you pour the number of tablets or capsules needed into a small container or cup and then discard the container after you've given the medication. Here are a few guidelines about tablets and capsules:

- Tablets may be scored—scored tablets contain a line across the center, so you can easily break them into two halves. Do not break unscored tablets, because you can't be certain that the drug is evenly distributed (Fig. 3-18A).

- Enteric-coated tablets—these tablets have an enteric coating that protects the drug from being inactivated in the stomach. These tablets dissolve in the more alkaline secretions of the intestine rather than in the highly acidic stomach (Fig. 3-18B).

- Prolonged release or extended-release tablets come in three types: XL for extended length, CD for controlled dose, and SR for slow or sustained release. All three disintegrate more slowly and have a longer duration of action than other tablets.

- Capsules are gelatin containers that hold a drug in solid or liquid form (Fig. 3-18C). Avoid opening capsules; this could decrease the drug's potency.

- Enteric-coated, prolonged-release tablets should not be crushed.

Liquids may be prepared as unit doses, ready for you to administer, or they may be stored in stock bottles, thus requiring calculation and measurement. A plastic or paper medicine cup is used to measure liquid. Two practices will help you measure liquids accurately:

1. Pour liquids to a line. Never estimate a dose between two lines.

2. Pour liquids at eye level and on a flat surface (Fig. 3-19). The surface of the liquid has a natural curve called the meniscus. At eye level, the center of the curve should be on the measurement line, while the fluid at the sides of the container will appear to be above the line (Fig. 3-20).

To measure liquids, nurses typically use a medicine cup or a syringe.

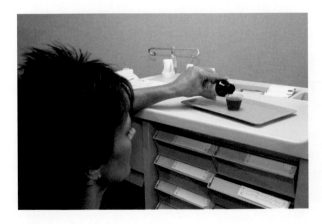

FIGURE 3-19

Liquids are poured at eye level. (Used with permission from Evans-Smith, P. [2005]. Taylor's clinical nursing skills. Philadelphia, PA: Lippincott Williams & Wilkins, p. 117.)

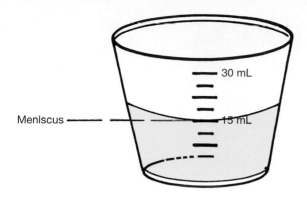

FIGURE 3-20

When viewing the liquid from eye level, the meniscus (lower curve of the fluid) should be on the line.

Syringes

Nurses use several different types of syringes to prepare routine parenteral doses. Each one serves a different purpose (Fig. 3-21).

Here are explanations for four types: the 3-mL syringe, the 1-mL syringe, and two insulin syringes—the 100-unit insulin syringe or low-dose 50-unit insulin syringe.

SYRINGE. The 3-mL syringe shown in Figure 3-22 is routinely used for intramuscular injections. It has a 22-gauge needle, and the needle is 1½ inches long. The term *gauge* indicates the diameter (width) of the needle.

Here's how to use a 3-mL syringe:

- The markings on one side are in mL to the nearest tenth. Each line indicates 0.1 mL.

- When you're preparing a dose, hold the syringe with the needle up, and draw down the medication into the barrel (Fig. 3-23). Suppose you're preparing a dose calculated to be 1.1 mL. Looking at Figure 3-22, count the lines to reach the correct dose.

The 3-mL syringe shows markings for 0.7 mL and 0.8 mL. What would you do if a dosage is 0.75 mL? Although you must not approximate doses between lines, you can handle the problem in two other ways:

First way: Round off 0.75 mL to the nearest tenth. The answer would be 0.8 mL, which can be drawn up to a line. (For details about rounding off numbers, see Chapter 1.)

Second way: Instead, use a *precision syringe,* which shows markings to the nearest hundredth.

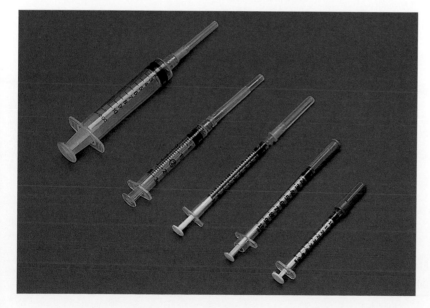

FIGURE 3-21

Various syringe sizes (top to bottom: 12 mL, 3 mL, 1 mL, insulin 100 units, insulin 50 units). (© 2010 L. Farmer Photography.)

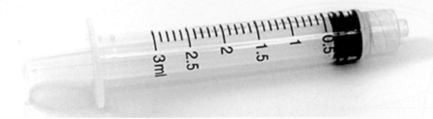

FIGURE 3-22

A 3-mL syringe with metric and apothecary measures. (© 2004 Lacey-Bordeaux Photography.)

PRECISION SYRINGE. The 1-mL precision syringe has a 25-gauge needle that is ⅝-inches long. This syringe is used for subcutaneous and intradermal injections. Of all the syringes nurses use, this one is the most accurate. It is sometimes called a tuberculin syringe. This syringe is marked in hundredths of a milliliter (Fig. 3-24).

Here's how to use a 1-mL precision syringe:

- The markings on the side are in milliliters. There are nine larger lines before 1. Each smaller line is 0.01 mL.

- To prepare an injection, hold the syringe with the needle up, then draw down the medication into the barrel. Suppose you're preparing a dose calculated to be 0.25 mL. Looking at Figure 3-24, count the lines to reach the dose.

ROUNDING WHEN USING A SYRINGE. When rounding injections, current guidelines state to round to the nearest hundredth if the amount is less than 1 mL and to round to the nearest tenth if the amount is greater than 1 mL.

INSULIN SYRINGE. The 1-mL syringe (100 unit) is marked in *units* rather than in milliliters or minims. This syringe usually has a 23- or 25-gauge, ⅝-inch long needle and is used for subcutaneous injection. Use it only to prepare insulin (Fig. 3-25). The physician/healthcare provider orders the type of insulin, the strength of insulin, and the number of units.

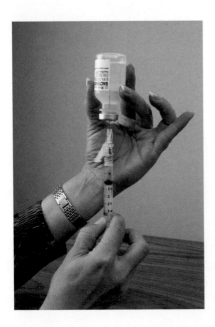

FIGURE 3-23

Drawing liquid medication in a syringe.

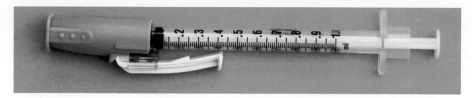

FIGURE 3-24

A 1-mL precision syringe with metric measures. (© 2004 Lacey-Bordeaux Photography.)

EXAMPLE

Order: 20 units NPH insulin every day subcutaneous.

Look at Figure 3-25. Between every 10 units, you'll see four short lines. These markings indicate that each line equals 2 units on this syringe. *Always check the markings on a syringe to be certain you understand what each line equals.*

EXAMPLE

Order: 20 units NPH (unit-100) insulin every day subcutaneous.

To prepare this injection, hold the syringe with the needle up, then draw 20 units of insulin into the barrel.

For odd-numbered insulin doses, do not use the syringe in Figure 3-25. Instead use a low-dose insulin syringe. Make sure the doses are exact, not approximate.

LOW-DOSE INSULIN SYRINGE. The low-dose 50-unit insulin syringe has a 28-gauge needle that is ½-inch long (Fig. 3-26). Notice that between every 5 units, the syringe shows four short lines. These markings indicate that each line equals 1 unit. The syringe is marked for 50 units, so you can use this syringe to draw up any dose of insulin up to 50 units.

More specific information about medication administration is found in Chapter 10. Refer also to any nursing fundamentals pharmacology textbook about medication administration.

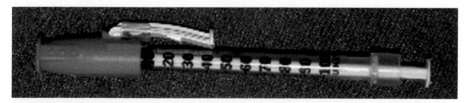

FIGURE 3-25

A 1-mL insulin syringe for 100 units or less. (© 2010 L. Farmer Photography.)

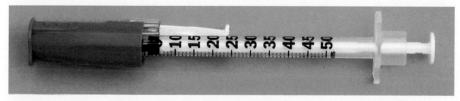

FIGURE 3-26

A ½-mL (low-dose) insulin syringe for 50 units or less. (© 2004 Lacey-Bordeaux Photography.)

| PROFICIENCY TEST 1 | Abbreviations/Military Time |

*Name:*_____

There are 35 items and each is worth 2 points. Indicate if the abbreviation is "Do Not Use" and which words to substitute for it. Change the 12-hour clock time to military time. See Appendix A for answers.

1. bid _____

2. hs _____

3. prn _____

4. OU _____

5. po _____

6. pr _____

7. SL _____

8. S & S _____

9. tiw _____

10. mL _____

11. q4h _____

12. cc _____

13. SC _____

14. AU _____

15. g _____

16. PC _____

17. qd _____

18. stat _____

19. q12h _____

20. tid _____

21. OS _____

22. kg _____

23. qn _____

24. qh _____

25. OD _____

26. mEq _____

27. AC _____

28. qid _____

29. mg _____

30. IM _____

31. 3 PM _____

32. 5:15 PM _____

33. 7 AM _____

34. 10:45 AM _____

35. 8:30 PM _____

Name:_____

A. *Now that you have studied the language of prescriptions, you are ready to interpret medication orders. Write the following orders in longhand. Give sample times. The correct answers are given in Appendix A.*

1. Nembutal 100 mg at bedtime prn po_____

2. Propranolol hydrochloride 40 mg po bid _____

   _____

3. Ampicillin 1 g IVPB q6h _____

   _____

4. Tylenol 325 mg tabs two po stat _____

   _____

5. Pilocarpine drops two OU q3h _____

   _____

6. Scopolamine 0.8 mg subcutaneously stat _____

   _____

7. Digoxin el 0.25 mg po qd _____

   _____

8. Kaochlor 30 mEq po bid _____

   _____

9. Heparin 6000 units subcutaneously q12h _____

   _____

10. Tobramycin 70 mg IM q8h _____

    _____

B. *Below are actual prescriptions written by physicians and other healthcare providers. Interpret each in longhand. In a real-life situation, if the order is not clear, check with the person who wrote the order. Note any Do Not Use abbreviations. The correct answers are given in Appendix A.*

11.	11.
Colace 100 mg po TID	
12.	**12.**
Ativan 1 mg IVP x 1 now	

(continued)

13.	13.
10 meq KCl in 100cc NS over 1h X1	
14.	14.
Tylenol #3 īī tabs po q4h prn Pain	
15.	15.
lopressor 25 mg po BID	

*Name:*_____

A. *Complete these questions. See Appendix A for answers.*

1. Explain the difference between each of these pairs.
   a. Unit-dose _____

      Multidose _____

   b. Ampule _____

      Vial_____

   c. Topical _____

      Parenteral_____

   d. Trade name _____

      Generic name_____

   e. Prefilled _____

      Reconstituted _____

B. 2. *Choose the correct answer.*

    _____ **a.** A major advantage of the unit-dose system of drug administration is that:
        1. the drug supply is always available.
        2. no error is possible.
        3. drugs are less expensive than stock bottles.
        4. the pharmacist provides a second professional check.

    _____ **b.** A major disadvantage of ampules over vials is that ampules:
        1. are only glass.
        2. when opened cannot be kept sterile.
        3. contain only liquids.
        4. cannot be used for injections.

    _____ **c.** Which information is not found on the label for a drug that has been reconstituted?
        1. Date of preparation
        2. Time of preparation
        3. Expiration date
        4. Indications

    _____ **d.** An order reads Valium 5 mg po now. A nurse correctly chooses diazepam. What name does diazepam represent?
        1. Generic
        2. Chemical
        3. Trade
        4. Proprietary

    _____ **e.** Which drug form is safest to administer to an unconscious patient?
        1. Suppository
        2. Lozenge
        3. Liquid in a medication cup
        4. Powder

(continued)

C. 3. *Match the following:*

1. _____ Avoid cross-contamination
2. _____ Removing medication from a jar
3. _____ Eye medication
4. _____ Puffs ordered
5. _____ Date and time label
6. _____ Lozenge
7. _____ Parenteral
8. _____ Combination drugs
9. _____ Transdermal
10. _____ Ear medication

a. Topical applications
b. Auric
c. More than one drug in the dose form
d. Reconstitution
e. Use a tongue blade or clean gloves
f. Cough drop
g. Individual nose, eye, or ear droppers
h. Ophthalmic
i. Inhalation
j. IM, Subcutaneous, IV

D. *Read the label and answer the questions. Use 1 gram as the dosage. See Appendix A for answers.*

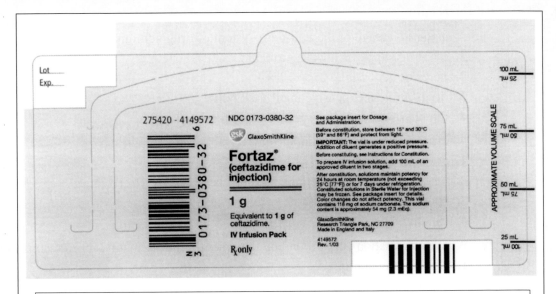

Table 5: Preparation of Fortaz Solutions			
Size	Amount of Diluent to Be Added (mL)	Approximate Available Volume (mL)	Approximate Ceftazidime Concentration (mg/mL)
Intramuscular			
500-mg vial	1.5	1.8	280
1-gram vial	3.0	3.6	280
Intravenous			
500-mg vial	5.0	5.3	100
1-gram vial	10.0	10.6	100
2-gram vial	10.0	11.5	170
Infusion pack			
1-gram vial	100*	100	10
2-gram vial	100*	100	20
Pharmacy bulk package			
6-gram vial	26	30	200

* **Note:** Addition should be in two stages (see Instructions for Constitution).

COMPATIBILITY AND STABILITY:
Intramuscular: Fortaz®, when constituted as directed with sterile water for injection, bacteriostatic water for injection, or 0.5% or 1% lidocaine hydrochloride injection, maintains satisfactory potency for 24 hours at room temperature or for 7 days under refrigeration. Solutions in sterile water for injection that are frozen immediately after constitution in the original container are stable for 3 months when stored at -20°C. Once thawed, solutions should not be refrozen. Thawed solutions may be stored for up to 8 hours at room temperature or for 4 days in a refrigerator.

Preparation of ceftazidime (Fortaz) solutions. (Reproduced with permission of GlaxoSmithKline.)

PROFICIENCY TEST 3 | **Labels and Packaging**

1. Trade name _____

2. Generic name _____

3. Route of administration _____

4. Total volume when reconstituted _____

5. Strength of reconstituted solution _____

6. Directions to reconstitute _____

_____

_____

_____

7. Drug form as dispensed _____

8. Storage _____

_____

_____

9. Expiration date _____

10. Usual dose _____

11. Precautions _____

_____

_____

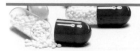 # Answers

Self-Test 1 Abbreviations

1. Three times a day (**sample times:** 10 AM, 2 PM, 6 PM)
2. Every night (**sample time:** 10 PM)
3. After meals (**sample times:** 10 AM, 2 PM, 6 PM)
4. Every other day (**sample times:** odd days of month at 10 AM). Do not use "qod" (write out "every other day").
5. Twice a day (**sample times:** 10 AM, 6 PM or 9 AM, 9 PM)
6. Do not use hs. Use "at bedtime." (**sample time:** 10 PM)
7. Immediately (**sample time:** whatever the time is now)
8. Four times a day (**sample times:** 10 AM, 2 PM, 6 PM, 10 PM or 6 AM, 12 PM, 6 PM, 12 PM)

9. Every 4 hours (sample times: 2 AM, 6 AM, 10 AM, 2 PM, 6 PM, 10 PM)
10. Before meals (**sample times:** 7:30 AM, 11:30 AM, 4:30 PM)
11. Do not use qd; use "every day." (sample time: 10 AM)
12. Every 8 hours (sample times: 6 AM, 2 PM, 10 PM)
13. Every hour
14. Whenever necessary (sample times: No time routine can be written.)
15. Every 4 hours as needed (sample times: No time routine is written because we do not know when the drug will be needed.)

Self-Test 2 Military Time

A.
1. 1400
2. 0900
3. 1600
4. 1200
5. 0130
6. 2115
7. 0450
8. 1820

B.
1. 1:30 AM
2. 5:45 PM
3. 11 AM
4. 8:15 PM
5. 7:10 PM
6. 6 AM
7. 12:50 AM
8. 10 AM

Self-Test 3 Abbreviations (Routes)

1. Sublingual; under the tongue
2. Do not use OU; use "both eyes."
3. Nasogastric tube
4. Intravenously
5. By mouth
6. Do not use OD; use "right eye."
7. Intravenous piggyback
8. Do not use OS; use "left eye."
9. Intramuscularly
10. Rectally
11. Swish and swallow
12. Do not use SC; use "subcutaneously."
13. Do not use au; use "both ears."
14. Do not use al; use "left ear."

Self-Test 4 Abbreviations (Metric)

1. Three tenths of a gram
2. One hundred fifty micrograms
3. Eighty units. Do not use U; use "unit."
4. Five tenths of a milliliter
5. One and seven tenths of a milliliter. Do not use cc; use "milliliter."
6. Twenty-five hundredths of a milligram
7. Fourteen kilograms
8. Twenty milliequivalents
9. One and five tenths of a liter
10. Fifty micrograms. Do not use µg; use "microgram."

(continued)

Answers (Continued)

Self-Test 5 Abbreviations (Household)

1. Three teaspoons
2. One ounce
3. One-half quart
4. One teaspoon
5. One pint
6. Two tablespoons

Self-Test 6 Abbreviations (Drug Preparations)

1. Elixir
2. Double strength
3. No known allergies
4. Capsules
5. Suspension
6. Tablet
7. Slow or sustained release
8. Long acting
9. Suppository
10. Tincture

Self-Test 7 Drug Packaging

A.
1. d
2. j
3. g
4. i
5. a
6. c
7. h
8. b
9. e
10. f

B.
11. Label the tube with one patient's name, and restrict its use to that one patient.
12. Mono drop or containers with removable droppers
13. Unit-dose
14. A systemic effect; the drug reaches the circulation and is carried to other parts of the body.
15. A disklike solid that is slowly dissolved in the mouth (e.g., a cough drop)

Calculation of Oral Medications—Solids and Liquids

TOPICS COVERED

1. Solving oral medication problems:
   a. Using proportion expressed as two ratios
   b. Using proportion expressed as two fractions
   c. Using the formula method
   d. Using dimensional analysis
2. Converting order and supply to the same weight measure
3. Clearing decimal points before solving a problem
4. Interpreting special types of oral solid and liquid orders
5. Oral solid and liquid problems without written calculations

Drugs for oral administration are prepared by pharmaceutical companies as solids (tablets, capsules) and liquids. When the dose ordered by the physician/healthcare provider differs from the supply, you calculate the amount to give to the patient/client. The calculations can be solved in several ways. This chapter shows how to do the math in four different ways: by two fractions, two ratios, the formula method, and the dimensional analysis method.

In dosage calculations, you start with three pieces of information: (we will add the following letters to represent the information)

1. The physician/healthcare provider's order

D = desired dose (order)

2. The quantity or strength of drug on hand

H = on hand or have

3. The solid or liquid form of the supply drug (i.e., the form the drug arrives in)

S = supply

We are solving for x = unknown or answer (amount of drug to give)

With dimensional analysis, you also use conversion factors. These are equivalents necessary to convert between systems of measurement. A conversion factor is a ratio of units that equals 1. For example, a conversion factor of milligrams to grams would be written as 1000 mg/1 g.

Oral Solids

Let's use a real example to illustrate the four different methods of calculation:

EXAMPLE

- Order: carvedilol (Coreg) 6.25 mg po bid
- Read the label.

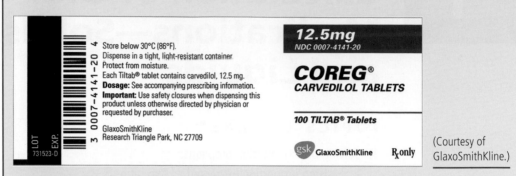

Store below 30°C (86°F).
Dispense in a tight, light-resistant container.
Protect from moisture.
Each Tiltab® tablet contains carvedilol, 12.5 mg.
Dosage: See accompanying prescribing information.
Important: Use safety closures when dispensing this product unless otherwise directed by physician or requested by purchaser.

GlaxoSmithKline
Research Triangle Park, NC 27709

LOT 731523-D   EXP.

0 0007-4141-20 4

3 0007-4141-20 0

12.5mg
NDC 0007-4141-20

COREG®
CARVEDILOL TABLETS

100 TILTAB® Tablets

gsk **GlaxoSmithKline**   R only

(Courtesy of GlaxoSmithKline.)

- Desire: The order. In this example, 6.25 mg is desired.

- Have: The strength of the drug supplied in the container. In the example, the label says that each tablet contains 12.5 mg.

- Supply: The unit form in which the drug comes. Coreg comes in tablet form. Because tablets and capsules are single entities, the supply for oral solid drugs is always 1.

- Amount: How much supply to give. For oral solids, the answer will be the number of tablets or capsules to administer.

So we have:

- Desire: carvedilol (Coreg) 6.25 mg po

- Supply: 1 tablet

- Have: 12.5 mg

> **FINE POINTS**
>
> When you're solving any problem, first check that the order and the supply are in the same weight measure. If they are not, you must convert one or the other amount to its equivalent. With dimensional analysis, you would use a conversion factor. In this example, no equivalent is needed; both the order and the supply are in milligrams.

Proportions Expressed as Two Fractions

Using fractions, set up proportions so that like units are across from each other (the units and the numerator match and the units and denominators match). The first fraction is the known equivalent.

EXAMPLE

To express "One tablet is equal to 12.5 mg," write 1 tablet/12.5 mg.

The second fraction is the unknown, or the desired (ordered) dose.

EXAMPLE

x tablets is equal to 6.25 mg, written as x tablets/6.25 mg.

The completed proportion would be presented as follows:

$$\frac{\text{Supply}}{\text{Have}} = \frac{\text{x}}{\text{Desire}}$$

$$\frac{1 \text{ tablet}}{12.5 \text{ mg}} = \frac{\text{x tablet}}{6.25 \text{ mg}}$$

Next, solve for x. (For a review of how to solve proportions, refer to Chapter 1.)

In our current example, solving for x follows this process:

1. $\dfrac{1 \text{ tablet}}{12.5 \text{ mg}} = \dfrac{\text{x tablet}}{6.25 \text{ mg}}$

$1 \times 6.25 = 12.5\text{x}$

FINE POINTS

$$12.5\overline{)6.25} \;\; .5$$

2. $\dfrac{6.25}{12.5} = \dfrac{\cancel{12.5}\text{x}}{\cancel{12.5}}$

3. $\dfrac{6.25}{12.5} = \dfrac{\cancel{12.5}\text{x}}{\cancel{12.5}}$

$\dfrac{6.25}{12.5} = \text{x}$

Answer: ½ tablet = x

Proportions Expressed as Two Ratios

You can set up a ratio by using colons. Double colons separate the two ratios. The first ratio is the known equivalent; the second ratio is the desired (ordered) dose, or the unknown. The ratio must always follow the same sequence.

The ratio will look like this:

Supply : Have : : x : Desire

1 tablet : 12.5 mg : : x : 6.25 mg

Next, solve for x. (For a review of how to solve ratios, refer to Chapter 1.)

In our current example, solving for x follows this process:

1. 1 tablet : 12.5 mg :: x : 6.25 mg

2. $1 \times 6.25 = 12.5\text{x}$

3. $\dfrac{6.25}{12.5} = \dfrac{\cancel{12.5}\text{x}}{\cancel{12.5}}$

4. $\dfrac{6.25}{12.5} = \dfrac{\cancel{12.5}\text{x}}{\cancel{12.5}}$

5. $\dfrac{6.25}{12.5} = \text{x}$

Answer: ½ tablet = x

FINE POINTS

Note that the ratio and proportion methods end with the same equation—in this case,

$$\frac{6.25}{12.5} = \text{x}$$

When illustrating these two methods, one combined final equation will be shown.

Formula Method

The formula method is simpler than either of the above methods. Using a formula eliminates the need for cross-multiplying, a potential source of error in calculation. When you use this method with oral solids, the supply is typically either 1 tablet or 1 capsule.

Here's how the formula method is set up:

$$\frac{\text{Desire}}{\text{Have}} \times \text{Supply} = x$$

$$\frac{6.25 \text{ mg}}{12.5 \text{ mg}} \times 1 \text{ tablet} = x$$

½ tablet = x

Dimensional Analysis

A fourth method of dosage calculation is called dimensional analysis. This method is used extensively in mathematics and science, especially chemistry calculations. Students often say that once you master dimensional analysis, you tend to use it all the time because it is simpler and more accurate than the other methods.

The dimensional analysis method uses terminology similar to that of other calculation methods. There are several ways to set up the dimensional analysis equation. One way is to set up the equation starting with what unit of measurement you are solving for and how the dose is supplied. A add to this what you have. Then add the desired (ordered) dose. Solve the equation. The equation is set up like a fraction with the appropriate numerators and denominators but looks slightly different.

You can set up the problem using the same terms as above:

$$\frac{\text{Supply}}{\text{Have}} \left| \frac{\text{Desired Dose}}{} \right. = x \text{ or amount}$$

In this example, we are solving for how many tablets of Coreg to administer. Place tablets first in the equation:

tablets

The dose supplied is tablets, and the dose we have is 12.5 mg (per tablet).
So, add to the equation:

$$\frac{1 \text{ tablet}}{12.5 \text{ mg}}$$

Then add the desired dose of 6.25 mg:

$$\frac{1 \text{ tablet}}{12.5 \text{ mg}} \left| 6.25 \text{ mg} \right.$$

According to the basic rules of reducing fractions (review Chapter 1 if necessary), the two "mg" designations cancel each other:

$$\frac{1 \text{ tablet}}{12.5 \text{ mg}} \left| 6.25 \text{ mg} \right.$$

The setup should now look like this:

$$\frac{1 \text{ tablet} \quad | \quad 6.25}{12.5 \quad |}$$

Multiply the numerators, multiply the denominators, and then divide the product of the numerators by the product of the denominators. In this example, the numbers in the numerator are $1 \times 6.25 = 6.25$. The only number in the denominator is 12.5. Divide 6.25 by 12.5 to get ½ tablet. The answer is ½ tablet.

In this example, it would look like this:

$$\frac{1 \text{(tablet)} \quad | \quad 6.25 \text{ mg}}{12.5 \text{ mg} \quad |}$$

Note: When using dimensional analysis, you could also set up the equation starting with the desired dose, then adding the dose supplied and the dose you have. For example, in the problem above, the equation would look like this:

$$\frac{6.25 \text{ mg} \quad | \quad 1 \text{(tablet)}}{| \quad 12.5 \text{ mg}}$$

You would solve the same way, cancelling like units of measurement, reducing if possible, and you will have the same answer:

$$\frac{6.25 \text{ mg} \quad | \quad 1 \text{(tablet)}}{| \quad 12.5 \text{ mg}} = 6.25 \text{ divided by } 12.5 = ½ \text{ tablet}$$

Either way of setting up the dimensional analysis equation will work. This text will use the first way of setting up the problem.

For the purposes of this book, we'll use these four methods—the formula method, the proportion method expressed as two ratios, the proportion method expressed as two fractions, and the dimensional analysis. You just need to see which method makes the most sense to you, then learn it thoroughly and use it. Answers for the self- and proficiency tests in each chapter will include all four methods.

Formula Method	Proportion	Dimensional Analysis
$\dfrac{\text{Desire}}{\text{Have}} \times \text{Supply} = x$	**EXPRESSED AS TWO RATIOS** Supply : Have : : x : Desire **EXPRESSED AS TWO FRACTIONS** $\dfrac{\text{Supply}}{\text{Have}} = \dfrac{x}{\text{Desire}}$	$\dfrac{\text{Supply} \quad | \quad \text{Desire}}{\text{Have} \quad |}$ (add conversion factors as needed)

EXAMPLE

- Order: furosemide (Lasix) 60 mg po every day
- Supply: Read the label.
- No equivalent is needed.

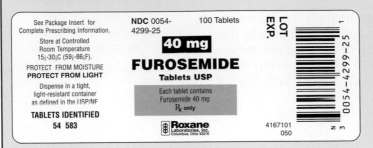

See Package Insert for
Complete Prescribing Information.

Store at Controlled
Room Temperature
15¡-30¡C (59¡-86¡F).

PROTECT FROM MOISTURE
PROTECT FROM LIGHT

Dispense in a tight,
light-resistant container
as defined in the USP/NF

**TABLETS IDENTIFIED
54 583**

NDC 0054-
4299-25   100 Tablets

40 mg

FUROSEMIDE
Tablets USP

Each tablet contains
Furosemide 40 mg
℞ only

Roxane
Laboratories, Inc.
Columbus, Ohio 43216

4167101
050

LOT
EXP.

0054-4299-25

(Courtesy of Boehringer
Ingelheim Roxane.)

So we have:

- Desired dose: 60 mg
- Supply: tablets
- Have: 40 mg (per tablet)

Formula Method	Proportion	Dimensional Analysis
$\dfrac{\overset{1.5}{\cancel{60}} \text{ mg}}{\underset{1}{\cancel{40}} \text{ mg}} \times 1 \text{ tablet}$ $= 1\frac{1}{2} \text{ tablets}$	**EXPRESSED AS TWO RATIOS** $1 \text{ tablet} : 40 \text{ mg} :: x : 60 \text{ mg}$ **EXPRESSED AS TWO FRACTIONS** $\dfrac{1 \text{ tablet}}{40 \text{ mg}} \times \dfrac{x}{60 \text{ mg}}$ **SOLUTION FOR BOTH PROPORTION METHODS** $60 = 40x$ $\dfrac{60}{40} = x$ $1\frac{1}{2} \text{ tablets} = x$	$\dfrac{1 \text{ tablet}}{\underset{2}{\cancel{40}} \text{ mg}} \Bigg| \dfrac{\overset{3}{\cancel{60}} \text{ mg}}{} = \frac{3}{2} = 1\frac{1}{2} \text{ tablets}$

The tablets are scored, so give 1½ tablets.

Let's use another example to show all four methods:

EXAMPLE

- Order: olanzapine (Zyprexa) 7.5 mg po every day
- No equivalent is needed.
- Supply: Read the label.

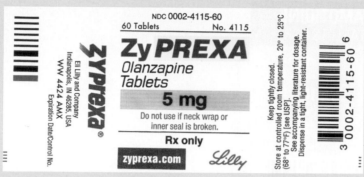

(Courtesy of Lilly Co.)

So we have:

- Desired dose: 7.5 mg
- Supply: tablets
- Have: 5 mg (per tablet)

Formula Method	Proportion	Dimensional Analysis
$\dfrac{\overset{1.5}{\cancel{7.5}}\text{ mg}}{\underset{1}{\cancel{5}}\text{ mg}} \times 1\text{ tablet}$ $= 1\frac{1}{2}\text{ tablets}$	**EXPRESSED AS TWO RATIOS** 1 tablet : 5 mg :: x : 7.5 mg **EXPRESSED AS TWO FRACTIONS** $\dfrac{1\text{ tablet}}{5\text{ mg}} \times \dfrac{x}{7.5\text{ mg}}$ **SOLUTION FOR BOTH PROPORTION METHODS** $7.5 = 5x$ $\dfrac{7.5}{5} = x$ $1\frac{1}{2}\text{ tablets} = x$	$\dfrac{1\,\boxed{\text{tablet}}}{\underset{1}{\cancel{5}}\text{ mg}} \Bigg|\dfrac{\overset{1.5}{\cancel{7.5}}\text{ mg}}{} = 1\frac{1}{2}\text{ tablets}$

Because the supply is scored, you can administer 1½ tablets.

You can also reduce the numbers in the numerator and denominator, using the rules of reducing fractions (see Chapter 1). For this example in the formula and dimensional analysis methods, we could reduce the fraction by dividing 7.5 in the numerator by 5 and then dividing 5 in the denominator by 5.

FINE POINTS

When reducing fractions, first attempt to divide the denominator evenly by the numerator.

EXAMPLE

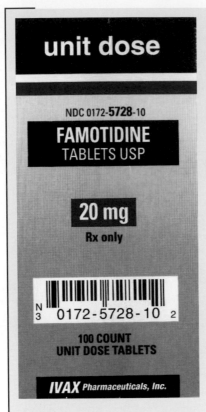

- Desired dose (Order): 40 mg po at bedtime
- Supply: tablets
- Have: 20 mg (per tablet)

Formula Method	Proportion	Dimensional Analysis

Formula Method

$$\frac{\overset{2}{\cancel{40}} \text{ mg}}{\underset{1}{\cancel{20}} \text{ mg}} \times 1 \text{ tablet}$$

$$= 2 \text{ tablets}$$

Proportion

EXPRESSED AS TWO RATIOS

1 tablet : 20 mg : : x : 40 mg

EXPRESSED AS TWO FRACTIONS

$$\frac{1 \text{ tablet}}{20 \text{ mg}} \times \frac{x}{40 \text{ mg}}$$

SOLUTION FOR BOTH PROPORTION METHODS

40 = 20 x

40/20 = x

2 tablets = x

Dimensional Analysis

$$\frac{1 \cancel{\text{tablet}}}{\underset{1}{\cancel{20}} \cancel{\text{mg}}} \left| \frac{\overset{2}{\cancel{40}} \cancel{\text{mg}}}{} \right. = 2 \text{ tablets}$$

EXAMPLE

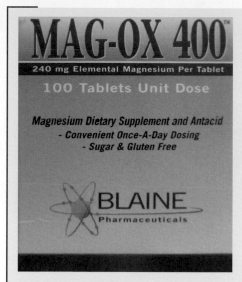

- Desired dose (Order): 200 mg po every day
- Supply: tablets
- Have: 400 mg (per tablet)

Formula Method	Proportion	Dimensional Analysis

Formula Method

$$\frac{\overset{1}{\cancel{200}} \text{ mg}}{\underset{2}{\cancel{400}} \text{ mg}} \times 1 \text{ tablet}$$

$$= \frac{1}{2} \text{ tablet}$$

Proportion

EXPRESSED AS TWO RATIOS

1 tablet : 400 mg :: x : 200 mg

EXPRESSED AS TWO FRACTIONS

$$\frac{1 \text{ tablet}}{400 \text{ mg}} \times \frac{x}{200 \text{ mg}}$$

SOLUTION FOR BOTH PROPORTION METHODS

$$200 = 400\,x$$

$$\frac{200}{400} = x$$

$$\frac{1}{2} \text{ tablet} = x$$

Dimensional Analysis

$$\frac{1 \, \cancel{\text{tablet}}}{\underset{2}{\cancel{400}} \, \cancel{\text{mg}}} \left| \frac{\overset{1}{\cancel{200}} \, \cancel{\text{mg}}}{} \right. = \frac{1}{2} \text{ tablet}$$

Cut the tablet with a pill cutter to obtain ½ tablet.

EXAMPLE

ATENOLOL

| 50 mg | TABLET

N5107968401

Lot 9H328 Exp. 02/11
PKG. BY: UDL, ROCKFORD, IL

- Desired dose (Order): 25 mg po BID
- Supply: tablets
- No equivalent is needed.
- Have: 50 mg (per tablet)

Formula Method	Proportion	Dimensional Analysis

Formula Method

$$\frac{\overset{1}{\cancel{25}} \text{ mg}}{\underset{2}{\cancel{50}} \text{ mg}} \times 1 \text{ tablet}$$

$$= \frac{1}{2} \text{ tablet}$$

Proportion

EXPRESSED AS TWO RATIOS

1 tablet : 50 mg : : x : 25 mg

EXPRESSED AS TWO FRACTIONS

$$\frac{1 \text{ tablet}}{50 \text{ mg}} \times \frac{x}{25 \text{ mg}}$$

**SOLUTION FOR BOTH
PROPORTION METHODS**

$$25 = 50x$$

$$\frac{25}{50} = x$$

$$\frac{1}{2} \text{ tablet} = x$$

Dimensional Analysis

$$\frac{1 \text{ tablet}}{\underset{2}{\cancel{50}} \text{ mg}} \left| \overset{1}{\cancel{25}} \text{ mg} \right. = \frac{1}{2} \text{ tablet}$$

The tablets are scored so give ½ tablet.

Converting Order and Supply to the Same Weight Measure

If the order and supply are in a differing weight measure, then you must convert one or the other amount to its equivalent. For example, if the order states 1 g and the drug is supplied in milligrams, then a conversion is needed from either grams to milligrams or milligrams to grams. Let's take another real-life example to explain this.

EXAMPLE

- Order: amoxicillin (Amoxil) 1 g po q6h
- Supply: Read the label
- Equivalent: 1 g = 1000 mg

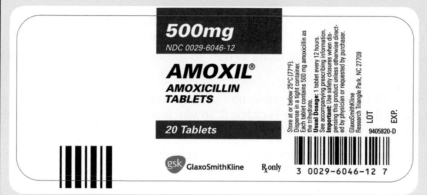

(Courtesy of GlaxoSmithKline.)

So we have:

- Desired dose: 1 g
- Supply: tablets
- Have: 500 mg (per tablet)

Formula Method	Proportion
$$\dfrac{\overset{2}{\cancel{1000}\ \cancel{mg}}}{\underset{1}{\cancel{500}\ \cancel{mg}}} \times 1\ \text{tablet} = 2\ \text{tablets}$$	**EXPRESSED AS TWO RATIOS** 1 tablet : 500 mg : : x : 1000 mg **EXPRESSED AS TWO FRACTIONS** $$\dfrac{1}{500\ \text{mg}} \times \dfrac{x}{1000\ \text{mg}}$$ $$1000 = 500$$ **SOLUTION FOR BOTH PROPORTION METHODS** $$1000 = 500x$$ $$\dfrac{1000}{500} = x$$ $$2\ \text{tablets} = x$$

For dimensional analysis, we include the conversion as an additional step, known as a *conversion factor*. A *conversion factor* is a ratio of units that equals 1. In this example, it will be: $\frac{1000 \text{ mg}}{1 \text{ g}}$.

So the dimensional analysis equation will look like this:

$$\frac{1 \text{ tablet}}{500 \text{ mg}} \left| \frac{1 \text{ g}}{} \right| \frac{1000 \text{ mg}}{1 \text{ g}}$$

Cancel out like units of measurement, in this case, "g" and "mg." Reduce the fraction if possible.

$$\frac{1 \text{ tablet}}{\underset{1}{\cancel{500} \text{ mg}}} \left| \frac{1 \cancel{\text{ g}}}{} \right| \frac{\overset{2}{\cancel{1000} \text{ mg}}}{1 \cancel{\text{ g}}}$$

Solve by multiplying the numerators, $1 \times 1 \times 2 = 2$; multiply the denominators, in this case, it is 1; divide the product of the numerators by the product of the denominators $2 \div 1 = 2$ tablets.

How do you know which conversion factor to use? In the above example, would you use $\frac{1 \text{ g}}{1000 \text{ mg}}$ or $\frac{1000 \text{ mg}}{1 \text{ g}}$?

You use the conversion factor that has the same unit of measurement in the denominator as the ordered unit of measurement. In this example, 1 g is ordered, so you would put 1 g in the denominator and the equivalent, 1000 mg, in the numerator: $\frac{1000 \text{ mg}}{1 \text{ g}}$.

This is so the same units of measurement "cancel" each other out; in this case, the "g's" cancel each other and the "mg's" cancel each other. You are left with "capsules," and that is what you are solving for.

EXAMPLE

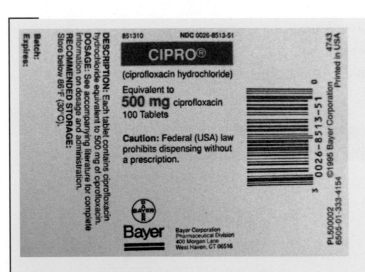

- Desired dose (Order): 0.5 g po every 12 hours
- Supply: tablets
- Equivalent: 0.5 mg = 500 mg
- Have: 500 mg (per tablet)

Formula Method	Proportion	Dimensional Analysis
$\dfrac{\overset{1}{\cancel{500}}\text{ mg}}{\underset{1}{\cancel{500}}\text{ mg}} \times 1 \text{ tablet}$ $= 1 \text{ tablet}$	**EXPRESSED AS TWO RATIOS** 1 tablet : 500 mg : : x : 500 mg **EXPRESSED AS TWO FRACTIONS** $\dfrac{1 \text{ tablet}}{500 \text{ mg}} \times \dfrac{x}{500 \text{ mg}}$ **SOLUTION FOR BOTH PROPORTION METHODS** $500 = 500\,x$ $\dfrac{500}{500} = x$ $1 \text{ tablet} = x$	Use conversion factor 1000 mg/1 g: $\dfrac{1 \text{ tablet}}{\underset{1}{\cancel{500}}\text{ mg}} \left| \, 0.5 \, \cancel{g} \, \right| \dfrac{\overset{2}{\cancel{1000}}\text{ mg}}{1 \, \cancel{g}} = 1 \text{ tablet}$

Clearing Decimals

When the numerator and denominator are decimals, add zeros to make the number of decimal places the same. Then drop the decimal points. This short arithmetic operation replaces long division:

$$\overset{\text{added}}{\underset{\downarrow}{}}$$

$$\frac{0.50\,\text{mg}}{0.25\,\text{mg}} \quad \frac{\text{numerator}}{\text{denominator or divisor}}$$

In division, you must clear the denominator (divisor) of decimal points before you can carry out the arithmetic. Then you move the decimal point in the numerator the same number of places. (For further help in dividing decimals, refer to Chapter 1.)

EXAMPLE

- Order: digoxin (Lanoxin) 0.125 mg po every day

- No equivalent is needed. It is stated on the label as 0.25 mg.

- Supply: Read the label.

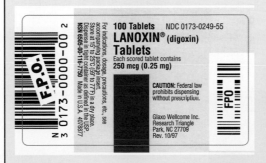

FINE POINTS

Sometimes you will need to add trailing zeros in order to clear the decimal point.

(Used with permission of GlaxoSmithKline.)

So we have:

- Desired dose: 0.125 mg

- Supply: tablets

- Have: 0.25 mg (per tablet)

Formula Method	Proportion	Dimensional Analysis

Formula Method

$$\frac{0.\overset{1}{\cancel{125}}\text{ mg}}{0.\underset{2}{\cancel{250}}\text{ mg}} \times 1 \text{ tablet}$$

$$= \frac{1}{2} \text{ tablet}$$

Proportion

EXPRESSED AS TWO RATIOS

1 tablet : 0.25 mg : : x : 0.125 mg

EXPRESSED AS TWO FRACTIONS

$$\frac{1 \text{ tablet}}{0.25 \text{ mg}} \times \frac{x}{0.125 \text{ mg}}$$

SOLUTION FOR BOTH PROPORTION METHODS

$$0.125 = 0.25x$$

$$\frac{0.\overset{1}{\cancel{125}}\text{ mg}}{0.\underset{2}{\cancel{250}}\text{ mg}} = x$$

$$\frac{1}{2} \text{ tablet} = x$$

Dimensional Analysis

$$\frac{1 \text{ tablet}}{0.\underset{2}{\cancel{250}}\text{ mg}} \mid \frac{0.\overset{1}{\cancel{125}}\text{ mg}}{} = \frac{1}{2} \text{ tablet}$$

EXAMPLE

NDC 0173-0242-56

100 Tablets
(10 blisterpacks of 10 tablets each)

UNIT DOSE PACK

LANOXIN® (digoxin)
Tablets

Each scored tablet contains

125 mcg (0.125 mg)

See package insert for Dosage and Administration.

Store at 25°C (77°F); excursions permitter to 15 to 30°C (59 to 86°F) [see USP Controlled Room Temperature] in a dry place and protect from light.

gsk GlaxoSmithKline

GlaxoSmithKline
Research Triangle Park, NC 27709

- Desired dose (Order): digoxin (Lanoxin) 0.5 mg po daily
- Supply: tablets
- No equivalent is needed.
- Have: 0.125 mg (per tablet)

Formula Method	Proportion	Dimensional Analysis

Formula Method

$$\frac{\overset{4}{\cancel{0.500}} \text{ mg}}{\underset{1}{\cancel{0.125}} \text{ mg}} \times 1 \text{ tablet}$$

$$= 4 \text{ tablets}$$

Proportion

EXPRESSED AS TWO RATIOS

1 tablet : 0.125 mg : : x : 0.5 mg

EXPRESSED AS TWO FRACTIONS

$$\frac{1 \text{ tablet}}{0.125 \text{ mg}} \times \frac{x}{0.5 \text{ mg}}$$

SOLUTION FOR BOTH PROPORTION METHODS

$$0.5 = 0.125x$$

$$\frac{\overset{4}{\cancel{0.500}} \text{ mg}}{\underset{1}{\cancel{0.125}} \text{ mg}} = x$$

$$4 \text{ tablets} = x$$

Dimensional Analysis

$$\frac{1 \text{ tablet}}{\underset{1}{\cancel{0.125}} \text{ mg}} \middle| \frac{\overset{4}{\cancel{0.500}} \text{ mg}}{} = 4 \text{ tablets}$$

SELF-TEST 1 | **Oral Solids**

Solve these practice problems. Answers are given at the end of the chapter. Remember the four methods:

Formula Method	Proportion	Dimensional Analysis

Formula Method

$$\frac{\text{Desire}}{\text{Have}} \times \text{Supply} = x$$

Proportion

EXPRESSED AS TWO RATIOS

Supply : Have : : x : Desire

EXPRESSED AS TWO FRACTIONS

$$\frac{\text{Supply}}{\text{Have}} = \frac{x}{\text{Desire}}$$

Dimensional Analysis

$$\frac{\text{Supply}}{\text{Have}} \middle| \text{Desire} \quad \text{(add conversion factors as needed)}$$

1. Order: dexamethasone (Decadron) 1.5 mg po bid
   Supply: tablets labeled 0.75 mg

2. Order: digoxin (Lanoxin) 0.25 mg po every day
   Supply: scored tablets labeled 0.5 mg

3. Order: ampicillin (Omnipen) 0.5 g po q6h
   Supply: capsules labeled 250 mg

4. Order: prednisone (Deltasone) 10 mg po tid
   Supply: tablets labeled 2.5 mg

5. Order: aspirin 650 mg po stat
   Supply: tablets labeled 325 mg

6. Order: nifedipine (Procardia) 20 mg po bid
   Supply: capsules labeled 10 mg

7. Order: fluphenazine (Prolixin) 10 mg po daily
   Supply: tablets labeled 2.5 mg

(continued)

| SELF-TEST 1 | Oral Solids (Continued) |

8. Order: penicillin G potassium 200,000 units po q8h
   Supply: scored tablets labeled 400,000 units

9. Order: digoxin (Lanoxin) 0.5 mg po every day
   Supply: scored tablets labeled 0.25 mg

10. Order: captopril (Capoten) 18.75 mg po tid
    Supply: scored tablets labeled 12.5 mg

11. Order: quetiapine (Seroquel) 300 mg po bid
    Supply: tablets labeled 200 mg

12. Order: clonidine (Catapres) 0.3 mg po hs
    Supply: tablets labeled 0.1 mg

13. Order: captopril (Capoten) 6.25 mg po bid
    Supply: scored tablets labeled 25 mg

14. Order: clonidine (Catapres) 400 mcg po every day
    Supply: tablets labeled 0.2 mg

15. Order: warfarin (Coumadin) 7.5 mg po every day
    Supply: scored tablets labeled 5 mg

16. Order: glyburide (Micronase) 0.625 mg every day
    Supply: scored tablets labeled 1.25 mg

17. Order: naproxen (Naprosyn) 0.5 g po every day
    Supply: scored tablets labeled 250 mg

18. Order: hydrochlorothiazide (Hydrodiuril) 37.5 mg po every day
    Supply: scored tablets labeled 25 mg

19. Order: cephalexin (Keflex) 1 g po q6h
    Supply: capsules labeled 500 mg

20. Order: baclofen (Lioresal) 25 mg po tid
    Supply: scored tablets labeled 10 mg

Special Types of Oral Solid Orders

Drugs that contain a number of active ingredients are ordered by the number to be administered and do not require calculation. Similarly, over-the-counter (OTC) medications are often ordered by how many are to be administered.

EXAMPLE

EXAMPLE 1:

Vitamin B complex caplets 1 po every day

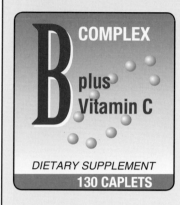

Interpret as "Give 1 vitamin B complex caplet by mouth every day."

EXAMPLE 2:

aspirin/dipyridamole (Aggrenox)

25 mg/200 mg capsules 1 capsule po bid

 FINE POINTS

Notice the label states how much of each drug makes up the drug. This is useful information, especially in medication administration and potential drug allergies.

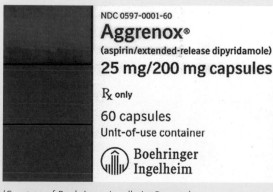

NDC 0597-0001-60

Aggrenox®

(aspirin/extended-release dipyridamole)

25 mg/200 mg capsules

R_x only

60 capsules

Unit-of-use container

Boehringer Ingelheim

Dosage: Read accompanying prescribing information. Store at 25°C (77°F); excursions permitted to 15-30°C (59-86°F). [See USP Controlled Room Temperature.] Protect from excessive moisture.
Mkd. by: Boehringer Ingelheim Pharmaceuticals, Inc. Ridgefield, CT 06877 USA
Mfd. by: Boehringer Ingelheim Pharma GmbH & Co. KG Biberach, Germany
Lic. from: Boehringer Ingelheim International GmbH
U.S. Pat. No. 6,015,577
© Copyright Boehringer Ingelheim International GmbH 2003, ALL RIGHTS RESERVED

Rev 1/30/03
43659/US/3

LOT   EXP

(Courtesy of Boehringer Ingelheim Roxane.)

Interpret as "Give 1 Aggrenox capsule by mouth twice a day."

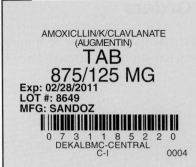

Notice Augmentin contains amoxicillin. Be sure to check if the patient/client is allergic to penicillin before administering.

- Desired dose (Order): Augmentin 1 tablet po BID
- Supply: tablets
- No equivalent is needed
- Interpret as: Give 1 Augmentin by mouth twice a day.

 ## Oral Liquids

For liquids, the three methods are set up just as for oral solids, except the supply will include a liquid measurement, usually milliliters (mL).

Formula Method	Proportion	Dimensional Analysis
$\dfrac{\text{Desire}}{\text{Have}} \times \text{Supply}$ $= \text{Amount (x)}$	**EXPRESSED AS TWO RATIOS** $\text{Supply} : \text{Have} : : x : \text{Desire}$ **EXPRESSED AS TWO FRACTIONS** $\dfrac{\text{Supply}}{\text{Have}} = \dfrac{x}{\text{Desire}}$	$\dfrac{\text{Supply}}{\text{Have}} \left\vert \text{Desire} \right.$ (add conversion factors as needed)

EXAMPLE

- Order: azithromycin (Zithromax) oral susp 400 mg po every day × 4 days
- No equivalent is needed.
- Supply: Read the label.

FOR ORAL USE ONLY.
Store dry powder below 86°F (30°C).
PROTECT FROM FREEZING.
DOSAGE AND USE
See accompanying prescribing information.
MIXING DIRECTIONS:
Tap bottle to loosen powder.
Add 15 mL of water to the bottle.
After mixing, store suspension at
41° to 86°F (5° to 30°C).
Oversized bottle provides extra space
for shaking.
After mixing, use within 10 days. Discard
after full dosing is completed.
SHAKE WELL BEFORE USING.
Contains 1200 mg azithromycin.

NDC 0069-3140-19
30 mL (when mixed)
Zithromax®
(azithromycin for
oral suspension)
CHERRY FLAVORED
200 mg* per 5 mL
Pfizer **Pfizer Labs**
Division of Pfizer Inc, NY, NY 10017

3 N 0069-3140-19   0

6424
MADE IN USA

* When constituted as directed, each teaspoon-
ful (5 mL) contains azithromycin dihydrate
equivalent to 200 mg of azithromycin.

CAUTION: Federal law prohibits
dispensing without prescription.

05-5015-32-0

(Courtesy of Pfizer Labs.)

So we have:

- Desired dose: 400 mg
- Supply: 5 mL
- Have: 200 mg (per 5 mL)

FINE POINTS

Oral liquids may be measured using a medication cup, calibrated dropper, or oral syringe.

Formula Method	Proportion	Dimensional Analysis

Formula Method

$$\frac{\overset{2}{\cancel{400}} \text{ mg}}{\underset{1}{\cancel{200}} \text{ mg}} \times 5 \text{ mL} = 10 \text{ mL}$$

Proportion

EXPRESSED AS TWO RATIOS

5 mL : 200 mg : : x : 400 mg

EXPRESSED AS TWO FRACTIONS

$$\frac{5 \text{ mL}}{200 \text{ mg}} \times \frac{x}{400 \text{ mg}}$$

**SOLUTION FOR BOTH
PROPORTION METHODS**

$$5 \times 400 = 200x$$

$$\frac{2000}{200} = x$$

$$10 \text{ mL} = x$$

Dimensional Analysis

$$\frac{5 \text{ mL}}{\underset{1}{\cancel{200}} \text{ mg}} \; \Big| \; \frac{\overset{2}{\cancel{400}} \text{ mg}}{} = 5 \times 2$$

$$= 10 \text{ mL}$$

FINE POINTS

Before solving each problem, check to be certain that the order and your supply are in the same measure. If they are not, you must convert one or the other to its equivalent. Convert whichever one is easier for you to solve. Dimensional analysis uses a conversion factor in the equation.

30 mL — 2 TBSP
25 mL —
20 mL —
15 mL — 1 TBSP
– 10 mL –
5 mL — 1 TSP

Administer 10 mL of Zithromax po every day for 4 days.

EXAMPLE

- Order: digoxin (Lanoxin) elixir 500 mcg × 1 dose
- Equivalent: 500 mcg = 0.5 mg
- Supply: Read the label.

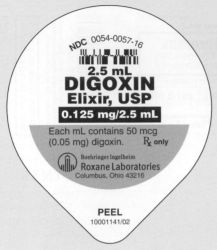

(Courtesy of Boehringer Ingelheim Roxane.)

So we have:

- Desired dose: 500 mcg (0.5 mg)
- Supply: 2.5 mL
- Have: 0.125 mg (per 2.5 mL)

Formula Method	Proportion	Dimensional Analysis

Formula Method

$$\frac{\overset{4}{\cancel{0.5}}\ \text{mg}}{\underset{1}{\cancel{0.125}}\ \text{mg}} \times 2.5\ \text{mL}$$

$$= 10\ \text{mL}$$

Proportion

EXPRESSED AS TWO RATIOS

2.5 mL : 0.125 mg : : x : 0.5 mg

EXPRESSED AS TWO FRACTIONS

$$\frac{2.5\ \text{mL}}{0.125\ \text{mg}} \times \frac{x}{0.5\ \text{mg}}$$

SOLUTION FOR BOTH PROPORTION METHODS

$$2.5 \times 0.5 = 0.125x$$

$$\frac{1.25}{0.125} = x$$

$$10\ \text{mL} = x$$

Dimensional Analysis

Use conversion factor 1 mg/1000 mcg:

$$\frac{\overset{0.5}{\cancel{2.5}}\ \cancel{\text{mL}}}{\underset{0.025}{\cancel{0.125}}\ \text{mg}} \ \Bigg|\ \frac{\overset{1}{\cancel{500}}\ \cancel{\text{mcg}}}{} \ \Bigg|\ \frac{1\ \text{mg}}{\underset{2}{\cancel{1000}}\ \cancel{\text{mcg}}}$$

$$= \frac{0.5}{0.025 \times 2} = 10\ \text{mL}$$

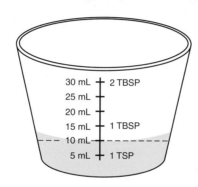

Administer 10 mL of digoxin × 1 dose.

EXAMPLE

- Order: furosemide (Lasix) 34 mg po every day
- No equivalent is needed.
- Supply: Read the label.

FINE POINTS

Because the drug comes with a calibrated dropper, you are alerted that your answer will be a small amount.

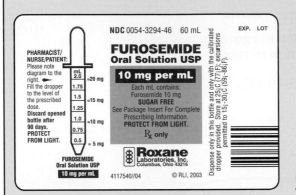

(Courtesy of Boehringer Ingelheim Roxane.)

So we have:

- Desired dose: 34 mg
- Supply: 1 mL
- Have: 10 mg (per mL)

Formula Method	Proportion	Dimensional Analysis
$$\frac{34 \text{ mg}}{10 \text{ mg}} \times 1 \text{ mL} = 3.4 \text{ mL}$$ $$10 \overline{)34.0} \atop \begin{array}{r}3.4\\ \underline{30}\\ 40\end{array}$$	**EXPRESSED AS TWO RATIOS** $$1 \text{ mL} : 10 \text{ mg} :: x : 34 \text{ mg}$$ **EXPRESSED AS TWO FRACTIONS** $$\frac{1 \text{ mL}}{10 \text{ mg}} = \frac{x}{34 \text{ mg}}$$ **SOLUTION FOR BOTH PROPORTION METHODS** $$34 = 10x$$ $$\frac{34}{10} = x$$ $$3.4 \text{ mL} = x$$	$$\frac{1 \text{ mL}}{10 \text{ mg}} \,\bigg|\, \frac{34 \text{ mg}}{} = \frac{34}{10} = x$$ $$3.4 \text{ mL} = x$$

Use the calibrated dropper to administer 3.4 mL.

EXAMPLE

- Order: amoxicillin (Amoxil) oral suspension 500 mg po q8h
- No equivalent is needed.
- Supply: Read the label.

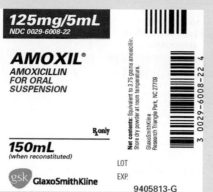

(Courtesy of GlaxoSmithKline.)

So we have:

- Desired dose: 500 mg
- Supply: 5 mL
- Have: 125 mg (per 5 mL)

Formula Method	Proportion	Dimensional Analysis
$\dfrac{\overset{4}{\cancel{500}}\ \text{mg}}{\underset{1}{\cancel{125}}\ \text{mg}} \times 5\ \text{mL} = 4 \times 5$ $= 20\ \text{mL}$	**EXPRESSED AS TWO RATIOS** $5\ \text{mL} : 125\ \text{mg} :: x : 500\ \text{mg}$ **EXPRESSED AS TWO FRACTIONS** $\dfrac{5\ \text{mL}}{125\ \text{mg}} \times \dfrac{x}{500\ \text{mg}}$ **SOLUTION FOR BOTH PROPORTION METHODS** $5 \times 500 = 125x$ $\dfrac{2500}{125} = x$ $20\ \text{mL} = x$	$\dfrac{5\ \cancel{\text{mL}}}{\underset{1}{\cancel{125}}\ \text{mg}} \Big| \dfrac{\overset{4}{\cancel{500}}\ \text{mg}}{} = 5 \times 4$ $= 20\ \text{mL}$

Administer 20 mL of Amoxil po every 8 hours.

EXAMPLE

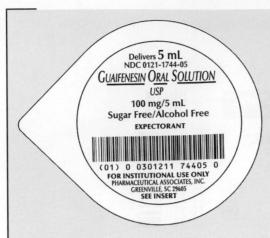

- Desired dose (Order): 250 mg every 4 hours prn cough
- Supply: 10 mL
- Have: 200 mg in 10 mL

Formula Method	Proportion	Dimensional Analysis

Formula Method

$$\frac{\overset{10}{\cancel{250}} \text{ mg}}{\underset{8}{\cancel{200}} \text{ mg}} \times 10 \text{ mL}$$

$$= \frac{10 \times 10}{8} = 12.5 \text{ mL}$$

Proportion

EXPRESSED AS TWO RATIOS

10 mL : 200 mg :: x : 250 mg

EXPRESSED AS TWO FRACTIONS

$$\frac{10 \text{ mL}}{200 \text{ mg}} \times \frac{x}{250 \text{ mg}}$$

SOLUTION FOR BOTH PROPORTION METHODS

$$2500 = 200 \, x$$

$$\frac{2500}{200} = x$$

$$12.5 \text{ mL}$$

Dimensional Analysis

$$\frac{10 \; \cancel{\text{mL}}}{\underset{4}{\cancel{200}} \; \cancel{\text{mg}}} \; \Big| \; \overset{5}{\cancel{\underset{}{250}}} \; \cancel{\text{mg}}$$

$$= \frac{50}{4} = 12.5 \text{ mL}$$

Use an oral syringe to give 12.5 mL.

EXAMPLE

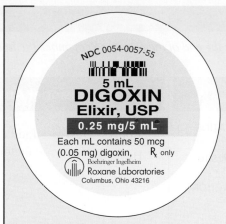

- Equivalent: 250 mcg = 0.25 mg
- Desired dose (Order): Digoxin elixir 250 mcg po daily
- Supply: 5 mL
- Have: 0.25 mg per 5 mL

Formula Method	Proportion	Dimensional Analysis

Formula Method

$$\dfrac{\overset{1}{\cancel{0.25}} \text{ mg}}{\underset{1}{\cancel{0.25}} \text{ mg}} \times 5 \text{ mL}$$

$$= 5 \text{ mL}$$

Proportion

EXPRESSED AS TWO RATIOS

5 mL : 0.25 mg : : x : 0.25 mg

EXPRESSED AS TWO FRACTIONS

$$\frac{5 \text{ mL}}{0.25 \text{ mg}} \times \frac{x}{0.25 \text{ mg}}$$

SOLUTION FOR BOTH PROPORTION METHODS

$$5 \times 0.25 = 0.25\,x$$

$$\frac{1.25}{0.25} = x$$

$$5 \text{ mL} = x$$

Dimensional Analysis

Use conversion factor 1 mg/1000 mcg:

$$\frac{5\,\cancel{\text{mL}} \quad \Big|\quad \overset{1}{\cancel{250}}\ \cancel{\text{mcg}} \quad \Big|\quad 1\ \cancel{\text{mg}}}{0.25\ \cancel{\text{mg}} \quad \Big|\qquad\qquad \Big|\quad \underset{4}{\cancel{1000}}\ \cancel{\text{mcg}}}$$

$$= \frac{5}{0.25 \times 4} = \frac{5}{1} = 5 \text{ mL}$$

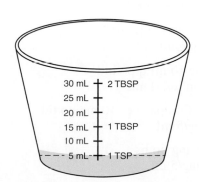

SELF-TEST 2   Oral Liquids

Solve these oral liquid problems. Answers are given at the end of the chapter. Remember the four methods:

Formula Method	Proportion	Dimensional Analysis

$$\frac{\text{Desire}}{\text{Have}} \times \text{Supply} = x$$

EXPRESSED AS TWO RATIOS

Supply : Have : : x : Desire

EXPRESSED AS TWO FRACTIONS

$$\frac{\text{Supply}}{\text{Have}} = \frac{x}{\text{Desire}}$$

Supply	Desire	(add conversion
Have		factors as needed)

1. Order: erythromycin (EES) susp 0.75 g po qid
   Supply: liquid labeled 250 mg/mL

2. Order: ampicillin susp 500 mg po q8h
   Supply: liquid labeled 250 mg/5 mL

3. Order: cephalexin (Keflex) in oral suspension 0.35 g po q6h
   Supply: liquid labeled 125 mg/5 mL

4. Order: cyclosporine (Sandimmune) 150 mg po stat and every day
   Supply: liquid labeled 100 mg/mL in a bottle with a calibrated dropper

5. Order: trifluoperazine (Stelazine) 5 mg po bid
   Supply: liquid labeled 10 mg/mL

6. Order: digoxin (Lanoxin) 0.02 mg po every day
   Supply: pediatric elixir 0.05 mg/mL in a bottle with a dropper marked in tenths of a milliliter

7. Order: potassium chloride 30 mEq po every day
   Supply: liquid labeled 20 mEq/15 mL

8. Order: digoxin (Lanoxin) elixir 0.25 mg via nasogastric tube every day
   Supply: liquid labeled 0.25 mg/mL

9. Order: risperidone (Risperdal) 3 mg po bid
   Supply: liquid labeled 1 mg/mL

10. Order: promethazine (Phenergan) HCl syrup 12.5 mg po tid
    Supply: liquid labeled 6.25 mg/5 mL

11. Order: hydroxyzine (Vistaril) 50 mg po qid
    Supply: syrup labeled 10 mg per 5 mL

12. Order: furosemide (Lasix) 40 mg po q12h
    Supply: liquid labeled 10 mg/mL

13. Order: potassium chloride 10 mEq po bid
    Supply: liquid labeled 20 mEq/30 mL

14. Order: prochlorperazine (Compazine) 10 mg po tid
    Supply: syrup labeled 5 mg/5 mL

15. Order: phenobarbital 100 mg po hs
    Supply: elixir labeled 20 mg/5 mL

SELF-TEST 2	Oral Liquids (Continued)

16. Order: acetaminophen (Tylenol) 650 mg po q4h prn
Supply: elixir labeled 160 mg/5 mL. Round to the nearest whole number

17. Order: diphenhydramine (Benadryl) 25 mg po q4h
Supply: liquid labeled 12.5 mg/5 mL

18. Order: chlorpromazine (Thorazine) 50 mg po tid
Supply: syrup labeled 10 mg/5 mL

19. Order: docusate (Colace) 100 mg po every day
Supply: syrup labeled 50 mg/15 mL

20. Order: codeine 0.06 g po q4–6h prn
Supply: liquid labeled 15 mg/5 mL

Special Types of Oral Liquid Orders

Some liquids, including OTC preparations and multivitamins, are ordered in the amount to be poured and administered. No calculation is required.

EXAMPLE

EXAMPLE 1:

Order: dextromethorphan (Robitussin) syrup 2 tsp q4h prn po

Supply: liquid labeled Robitussin syrup

No calculation is needed. Pour 2 tsp and take every 4 hours by mouth as necessary.

EXAMPLE 2:

Order: milk of magnesia 30 mL tonight po

Supply: liquid labeled milk of magnesia

No calculation is required. Pour 30 mL milk of magnesia and give tonight by mouth.

Oral Solid and Liquid Problems Without Written Calculations/"Common Sense" Calculations

As you develop proficiency in solving problems, you will be able to calculate many answers "in your head" without written work. If you look at a problem that states "1 tablet equals 250 mg" and are asked to solve for 500 mg, you can look at the problem and realize that 250 mg doubled equals 500 mg; therefore, 1 tablet doubled equals 2 tablets, which is the correct dose. Another tip is to "estimate" your answer prior to making calculations. Then, solve the problem. Using "common sense," does the answer "seem" right? One would not administer, say, 20 tablets, or 80 mL of a medication; therefore, the calculation is incorrect and is possibly set up incorrectly. As you continue to practice dosage calculations, try solving problems "in your head" and/or "estimating" your answer and then seeing if the calculated dose "makes sense" (*common sense* loosely defined as "sound, practical judgment").

SELF-TEST 3   Mental Drill Oral Solids and Liquids

Solve the problems "in your head" and write the amount to be given. Answers appear at the end of the chapter.

Order	Supply (scored tablets unless liquid form)	Answer
1. 20 mg	10 mg	_____
2. 0.125 mg	0.25 mg	_____
3. 0.25 mg	0.125 mg	_____
4. 200,000 units	100,000 units	_____
5. 0.5 mg	0.25 mg	_____
6. 0.2 g	400 mg	_____
7. 1 g	1000 mg	_____
8. 0.1 g	100 mg	_____
9. 0.01 g	20 mg	_____
10. 650 mg	325 mg	_____
11. 500 mg	250 mg	_____
12. 0.12 g	60 mg	_____
13. 50 mg	0.1 g	_____
14. 4 mg	2 mg	_____
15. 20 mg	10 mg/5 mL	_____
16. 10 mg	2 mg/5 mL	_____
17. 0.5 g	250 mg/5 mL	_____
18. 0.1 g	200 mg/10 mL	_____
19. 250 mg	0.1 g/6 mL	_____
20. 100 mg	50 mg/10 mL	_____
21. 12 mg	4 mg/5 mL	_____
22. 15 mg	30 mg/10 mL	_____
23. 15 mg	10 mg/4 mL	_____
24. 0.25 mg	0.5 mg/5 mL	_____

Putting it Together

Ms. CM is an 86-year-old women who is being admitted with rapid atrial fibrillation that started about 11:00 PM yesterday. No shortness of breath. Admitted for evaluation.

Past Medical History: Hypertension, intermittent atrial fibrillation 3 to 4 years, chronic aortic insufficiency with dilated left ventricle; previous hospitalization several weeks ago with atrial fibrillation with a rapid ventricular rate. Other medical problems include moderate varicose veins, early dementia, and chronic tobacco use.

No known drug allergies

Current Vital Signs: Blood pressure is 172/58, pulse 120–140/minute, respirations 20/minute, oxygen saturation 96% on 2 L n/c, afebrile

Medication Orders

Warfarin (Coumadin) *anticoagulant* 7.5 mg po daily

Lisinopril (Prinivil) *antihypertensive* 20 mg po q 12

Digoxin (Lanoxin) *antiarrhythmic, increases cardiac contractility*

> **Loading dose:** 0.75 mg po ×1; 0.25 mg po in 6 hours and 12 hours, then
>
> 0.125 mg po daily po hold if HR < 60

Potassium chloride (K-Dur) *potassium supplement* 15 mEq po every day

Alprazolam (Xanax) *antianxiety* 0.25–0.5 mg q 6 hr prn anxiety

Famotidine (Pepcid) *histamine 2 blocker, decreases gastric acid* 40 mg po at bedtime

Acetaminophen (Tylenol) *anti-inflammatory* 650 mg q 4 hour prn mild pain

Calcium carbonate (Tums) *mineral supplement, antacid* 1 g po daily

Calculations

1. Calculate how many tablets of warfarin (Coumadin) to administer. Available supply indicated on the label (scored tablets).

WARFARIN 5 mg.

Lot 628   Exp 2/17

Pkg. by VGS Phil. PA

(continued)

Putting it Together (*Continued*)

2. Calculate how many tablets of lisinopril (Prinivil) to administer. Available supply indicated on the label.

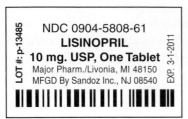

LOT #: p-13485

NDC 0904-5808-61
LISINOPRIL
10 mg. USP, One Tablet
Major Pharm./Livonia, MI 48150
MFGD By Sandoz Inc., NJ 08540

EXP. 3-1-2011

3. Calculate the loading dose of 0.75 mg of digoxin. Available supply indicated on the labels. What are two options of administration?

DIGOXIN
0.25 mg TABLET
NS05281196

Lot 0626   Exp 02/16
Pkg. by: VGS, Atlanta, GA

DIGOXIN
0.5 mg TABLET
NS0105119096

Lot 0726   Exp 02/16
Pkg. by: VGS, Atlanta, GA

4. Calculate the loading dose of 0.25 mg of digoxin. Available supply indicated on the labels under question 3. What are two options of administration?

5. Calculate the maintenance dose of 0.125 mg of digoxin. Available supply read the labels of the two tablets. What are two options of administration?

6. K-Dur 10 mEq is equal to 750 mg of potassium. How many milligrams of potassium would be in 15 mEq?

7. Calculate how many tablets of alprazolam (Xanax) to administer with the range ordered (0.25–0.5 mg). Available supply indicated on the label.

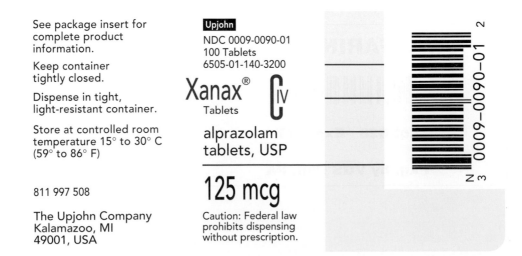

See package insert for complete product information.

Keep container tightly closed.

Dispense in tight, light-resistant container.

Store at controlled room temperature 15° to 30° C (59° to 86° F)

811 997 508

The Upjohn Company
Kalamazoo, MI
49001, USA

Upjohn
NDC 0009-0090-01
100 Tablets
6505-01-140-3200

Xanax® **C**IV
Tablets

alprazolam
tablets, USP

125 mcg

Caution: Federal law prohibits dispensing without prescription.

0009-0090-01

Putting it Together (*Continued*)

8. Calculate how many tablets of famotidine (Pepcid) to administer. Available supply indicated on the label.

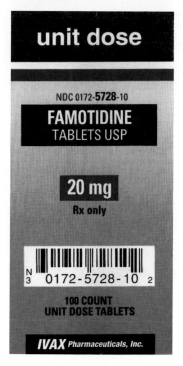

9. Calculate how many milliliters of acetaminophen (Tylenol) to administer. Available supply indicated on the label. Round to the nearest whole number.

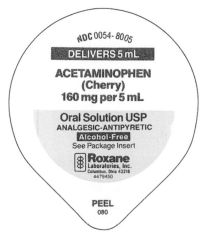

(continued)

Putting it Together (*Continued*)

10. Calculate how many tablets of calcium carbonate (Tums) to administer. Available supply indicated on the label.

CALCIUM

ANTACID TABLETS

200 MG

72 CHEWABLE TABLETS

Critical Thinking Questions

1. What medications would have a higher potential for error in calculation and why?

2. What medications have parameters for administration? Should any of these medications be held given the above scenario?

3. What are some alternatives to giving several tablets of a specific medication (i.e., 4 tablets to equal the ordered dose)?

4. Are there any orders written incorrectly and why? What should you do to correct these?

5. This patient has difficulty with taking medications. What are some alternatives to administration?

Answers in Appendix B.

PROFICIENCY TEST 1 | **Calculation of Oral Doses**

Name: _____

For liquid answers, draw a line on the medicine cup indicating the amount you would pour. Answers are given in Appendix A.

1. Order: KCl elixir 20 mEq po bid
   Supply: liquid labeled 30 mEq/15 mL

   Answer: _____

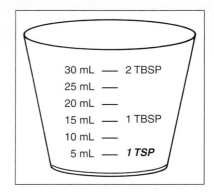

2. Order: phenytoin (Dilantin) susp 150 mg po tid
   Supply: liquid labeled 75 mg/7.5 mL

   Answer: _____

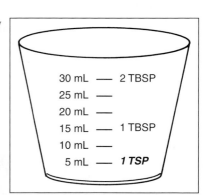

3. Order: digoxin (Lanoxin) elixir 0.125 mg po every day
   Supply: liquid labeled 0.25 mg/10 mL

   Answer: _____

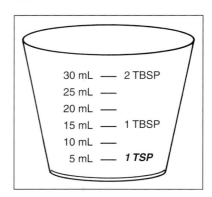

(continued)

Name: _____

4. Order: phenytoin (Dilantin) oral susp 375 mg po tid
   Supply: liquid labeled 125 mg/5 mL

   Answer: _____

30 mL —	2 TBSP
25 mL —	
20 mL —	
15 mL —	1 TBSP
10 mL —	
5 mL —	*1 TSP*

5. Order: cimetidine (Tagamet) 40 mg
   Supply: suspension labeled 20 mg/2.5 mL

   Answer: _____

30 mL —	2 TBSP
25 mL —	
20 mL —	
15 mL —	1 TBSP
10 mL —	
5 mL —	*1 TSP*

6. Order: digoxin (Lanoxin) 0.5 mg po every day
   Supply: tablets labeled 0.25 mg

   Answer: _____

7. Order: digoxin (Lanoxin) 100 mcg every day po
   Supply: 0.1-mg capsules

   Answer: _____

8. Order: allopurinol (Zyloprim) 250 mg po every day
   Supply: scored tablets 100 mg

   Answer: _____

9. Order: ampicillin 0.5 g po q6h
   Supply: capsules labeled 250 mg

   Answer: _____

10. Order: levothyroxine (Synthroid) 0.3 mg po every day
    Supply: tablets labeled 300 mcg scored

    Answer: _____

Name: _____

For liquid answers, draw a line on the medicine cup indicating the amount you would pour.
Answers are given in Appendix A.

1. Order: ibuprofen (Advil) 0.8 g po tid
   Supply: tablets labeled 400 mg

   Answer: _____

2. Order: isoniazid (Niazid) 0.3 g po every day
   Supply: tablets labeled 300 mg

   Answer: _____

3. Order: atenolol (Tenormin) 75 mg po bid
   Supply: 50-mg tablets

   Answer: _____

4. Order: acetaminophen (Tylenol) 0.65 g po q4h
   Supply: tablets labeled 325 mg

   Answer: _____

5. Order: ramipril (Altace) 10 mg po daily

   Supply: tablets labeled 2.5 mg

   Answer: _____

6. Order: nystatin (Mycostatin) oral susp 750,000 units
             po tid
   Supply: liquid labeled 100,000 units/mL

   Answer: _____

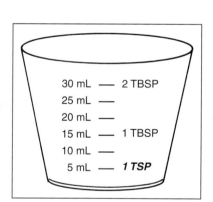

7. Order: oxacillin sodium 0.75 g po q6h
   Supply: liquid labeled 250 mg/5 mL

   Answer: _____

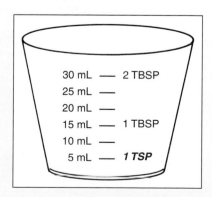

(continued)

Name: _____

8. Order: penicillin V potassium 500 mg po q6h
    Supply: liquid labeled 250 mg/5 mL

    Answer: _____

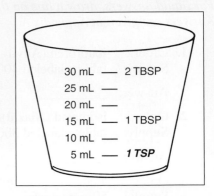

9. Order: aluminum hydroxide/magnesium
    hydroxide/simethicone (Mylanta II)
    30 mL q4h prn
    Supply: liquid labeled aluminum hydroxide/
    magnesium hydroxide/simethicone
    (Mylanta II)

    Answer: _____

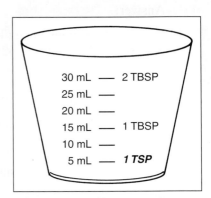

10. Order: theophylline (Theo-Dur) 160 mg po q6h
    Supply: liquid labeled 80 mg/15 mL

    Answer: _____

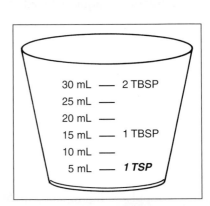

Name: _____

For each question, determine the amount to be given. Answers are given in Appendix A.

1. Order: potassium chloride 20 mEq po in juice bid
   Supply: liquid in a bottle labeled 30 mEq/15 mL

2. Order: syrup of tetracycline (Sumycin) hydrochloride 80 mg po q6h
   Supply: liquid in a dropper bottle labeled 125 mg/5 mL

3. Order: propranolol (Inderal) 0.02 g po bid
   Supply: scored tablets labeled 10 mg

4. Order: ampicillin sodium 0.5 g po q6h
   Supply: capsules of 250 mg

5. Order: digoxin (Lanoxin) 0.5 mg po every day
   Supply: scored tablets of 0.25 mg

6. Order: prednisone (Deltasone) 40 mg po every day
   Supply: liquid in a bottle labeled 5 mg/5 mL

7. Order: hydrochlorothiazide (Hydrodiuril) 75 mg po every day
   Supply: scored tablets 50 mg

8. Order: furosemide (Lasix) 40 mg po every day
   Supply: scored tablets of 80 mg

9. Order: digoxin (Lanoxin) 0.125 mg po
   Supply: liquid in a dropper bottle labeled 500 mcg/10 mL

10. Order: phenytoin (Dilantin) susp 75 mg po tid
    Supply: liquid in a bottle labeled 50 mg/10 mL

11. Order: diazepam (Valium) 5 mg po q4h prn
    Supply: scored tablets 2 mg

12. Order: levothyroxine (Synthroid) 0.15 mg po every day
    Supply: scored tablets 300 mcg

13. Order: disulfiram (Antabuse) 375 mg po today
    Supply: scored tablets 250 mg

14. Order: ibuprofen (Advil) 0.6 g po q4h prn
    Supply: film-coated tablets 300 mg

15. Order: chlorpheniramine maleate (Chlor-Trimeton) syr 1.5 mg po bid
    Supply: liquid in a bottle 1 mg/8 mL

16. Order: diphenhydramine maleate (Benadryl) syrup 25 mg po q4h while awake
    Supply: liquid labeled 12.5 mg/5 mL

17. Order: simethicone (Mylicon) liq 60 mg po in 1/2 glass H_2O
    Supply: liquid in a dropper bottle labeled 40 mg/0.6 mL

18. Order: chlorothiazide (Diuril) oral susp 0.5 g via NGT po every day
    Supply: liquid labeled 250 mg/5 mL

19. Order: meperidine HCl (Demerol) syrup 15 mg po q4h prn
    Supply: liquid labeled 50 mg/5 mL

20. Order: hydroxyzine (Vistaril) susp 50 mg q6h po
    Supply: liquid labeled 25 mg/5 mL

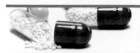

Answers

Self-Test 1 Oral Solids

Formula Method	Proportion	Dimensional Analysis
$\dfrac{\text{Desire}}{\text{Have}} \times \text{Supply} = x$	**EXPRESSED AS TWO RATIOS** Supply : Have : : x : Desire **EXPRESSED AS TWO FRACTIONS** $\dfrac{\text{Supply}}{\text{Have}} = \dfrac{x}{\text{Desire}}$	$\dfrac{\text{Supply} \mid \text{Desire}}{\text{Have} \mid}$ (add conversion factors as needed)

1. No equivalent is needed.

Formula Method	Proportion	Dimensional Analysis
$\dfrac{\overset{2}{\cancel{1.50}} \text{ mg}}{\underset{1}{\cancel{0.75}} \text{ mg}} \times 1 \text{ tablet}$ $= 2 \text{ tablets}$	**EXPRESSED AS TWO RATIOS** 1 tablet : 0.75 mg : : x : 1.5 mg **EXPRESSED AS TWO FRACTIONS** $\dfrac{1 \text{ tablet}}{0.75 \text{ mg}} \times \dfrac{x}{1.5 \text{ mg}}$ **SOLUTION FOR BOTH PROPORTION METHODS** $1.5 = 0.75x$ $\dfrac{1.5}{0.75} = x$ $2 \text{ tablets} = x$	$\dfrac{1 \cancel{\text{tablet}} \mid \overset{0.10}{\cancel{1.5}} \text{ mg}}{\underset{0.05}{\cancel{0.75}} \text{ mg} \mid} = \dfrac{10}{5} = 2 \text{ tablets}$

2. No equivalent is needed.

Formula Method	Proportion	Dimensional Analysis
$\dfrac{\overset{1}{\cancel{0.25}} \text{ mg}}{\underset{2}{\cancel{0.50}} \text{ mg}} \times 1 \text{ tablet}$ $= \frac{1}{2} \text{ tablet}$	**EXPRESSED AS TWO RATIOS** 1 tablet : 0.5 mg : : x : 0.25 mg **EXPRESSED AS TWO FRACTIONS** $\dfrac{1 \text{ tablet}}{0.5 \text{ mg}} \times \dfrac{x}{0.25 \text{ mg}}$ **SOLUTION FOR BOTH PROPORTION METHODS** $0.25 = 0.5x$ $\dfrac{0.25}{0.5} = x$ $0.5 \text{ tablet} = x$ or $\frac{1}{2}$ tablet	$\dfrac{1 \cancel{\text{tablet}} \mid \overset{1}{\cancel{0.25}} \text{ mg}}{\underset{2}{\cancel{0.50}} \text{ mg} \mid} = \frac{1}{2} \text{ tablet}$

(continued)

Answers (Continued)

3. Equivalent 0.5 g = 500 mg

Formula Method	Proportion	Dimensional Analysis
$\dfrac{\overset{2}{\cancel{500}} \text{ mg}}{\underset{1}{\cancel{250}} \text{ mg}} \times 1 \text{ capsule}$ $= 2 \text{ capsules}$	**EXPRESSED AS TWO RATIOS** 1 capsule : 250 mg : : x : 500 mg **EXPRESSED AS TWO FRACTIONS** $\dfrac{1 \text{ capsule}}{250 \text{ mg}} \times \dfrac{x}{500 \text{ mg}}$ **SOLUTION FOR BOTH PROPORTION METHODS** $500 = 250x$ $\dfrac{500}{250} = x$ $2 \text{ capsules} = x$	Use conversion factor 1000 mg/1 g: $\dfrac{1 \text{ capsule}}{\underset{1}{\cancel{250}} \text{ mg}} \left| 0.5 \text{ g} \right| \dfrac{\overset{4}{\cancel{1000}} \text{ mg}}{1 \text{ g}} = 0.5 \times 4$ $= 2 \text{ capsules}$

4. No equivalent is needed.

Formula Method	Proportion	Dimensional Analysis
$\dfrac{\overset{4}{\cancel{10.0}} \text{ mg}}{\underset{1}{\cancel{2.5}} \text{ mg}} \times 1 \text{ tablet}$ $= 4 \text{ tablets}$	**EXPRESSED AS TWO RATIOS** 1 tablet : 2.5 mg : : x : 10 mg **EXPRESSED AS TWO FRACTIONS** $\dfrac{1 \text{ tablet}}{2.5 \text{ mg}} \times \dfrac{x}{10}$ **SOLUTION FOR BOTH PROPORTION METHODS** $10 = 2.5x$ $\dfrac{10}{2.5} = x$ $4 \text{ tablets} = x$	$\dfrac{1 \text{ tablet}}{2.5 \text{ mg}} \left| 10 \text{ mg} \right. = \dfrac{10}{2.5} = 4 \text{ tablets}$

5. No equivalent is needed.

Formula Method	Proportion	Dimensional Analysis
$\dfrac{\overset{2}{\cancel{650}}\ \text{mg}}{\underset{1}{\cancel{325}}\ \text{mg}} \times 1\ \text{tablet}$ $= 2\ \text{tablets}$	**EXPRESSED AS TWO RATIOS** 1 tablet : 325 mg : : x : 650 mg **EXPRESSED AS TWO FRACTIONS** $\dfrac{1\ \text{tablet}}{325\ \text{mg}} \times \dfrac{\text{x}}{650\ \text{mg}}$ **SOLUTION FOR BOTH PROPORTION METHODS** $650 = 325\text{x}$ $\dfrac{650}{325} = \text{x}$ 2 tablets = x	$\dfrac{1\ \cancel{\text{tablet}}}{325\ \cancel{\text{mg}}} \Bigg| \dfrac{650\ \cancel{\text{mg}}}{\ } = \dfrac{650}{325} = 2\ \text{tablets}$

6. No equivalent is needed.

Formula Method	Proportion	Dimensional Analysis
$\dfrac{\cancel{20}\ \text{mg}}{\cancel{10}\ \text{mg}} \times 1\ \text{capsule}$ $= 2\ \text{capsules}$	**EXPRESSED AS TWO RATIOS** 1 capsule : 10 mg : : x : 20 mg **EXPRESSED AS TWO FRACTIONS** $\dfrac{1\ \text{capsule}}{10\ \text{mg}} \times \dfrac{\text{x}}{20\ \text{mg}}$ **SOLUTION FOR BOTH PROPORTION METHODS** $20 = 10\text{x}$ $\dfrac{20}{10} = \text{x}$ 2 capsules = x	$\dfrac{1\ \cancel{\text{capsule}}}{\underset{1}{\cancel{10}}\ \cancel{\text{mg}}} \Bigg| \dfrac{\overset{2}{\cancel{20}}\ \cancel{\text{mg}}}{\ } = 2\ \text{capsules}$

(continued)

Answers (Continued)

7. No equivalent is needed.

Formula Method	Proportion	Dimensional Analysis
$\dfrac{\overset{4}{\cancel{10}}\ \text{mg}}{\underset{1}{\cancel{2.5}}\ \text{mg}} \times 1\ \text{tablet}$ $= 4\ \text{tablets}$	**EXPRESSED AS TWO RATIOS** 1 tablet : 2.5 mg : : x : 10 mg **EXPRESSED AS TWO FRACTIONS** $\dfrac{1\ \text{tablet}}{2.5\ \text{mg}} \times \dfrac{x}{10\ \text{mg}}$ **SOLUTION FOR BOTH PROPORTION METHODS** $10 = 2.5x$ $\dfrac{10}{2.5} = x$ $4\ \text{tablets} = x$	$\dfrac{1\ \text{tablet}}{2.5\ \cancel{\text{mg}}}\ \Bigg|\ 10\ \cancel{\text{mg}} = \dfrac{10}{2.5} = 4\ \text{tablets}$

8. No equivalent is needed.

Formula Method	Proportion	Dimensional Analysis
$\dfrac{\overset{1}{\cancel{200{,}000\ \text{units}}}}{\underset{2}{\cancel{400{,}000\ \text{units}}}} \times 1\ \text{tablet}$ $= \frac{1}{2}\ \text{tablet}$	**EXPRESSED AS TWO RATIOS** 1 tablet : 400,000 units : : x : 200,000 **EXPRESSED AS TWO FRACTIONS** $\dfrac{1\ \text{tablet}}{400{,}000\ \text{units}} \times \dfrac{x}{200{,}000\ \text{units}}$ **SOLUTION FOR BOTH PROPORTION METHODS** $200{,}000 = 400{,}000x$ $\dfrac{200{,}000}{400{,}000} = x$ $0.5\ \text{tablet or } \frac{1}{2}\ \text{tablet} = x$	$\dfrac{1\ \text{tablet}}{\underset{2}{\cancel{400000}}\ \cancel{\text{units}}}\ \Bigg|\ \overset{1}{\cancel{200000}}\ \cancel{\text{units}} = \frac{1}{2}\ \text{tablet}$

9. No equivalent is needed.

Formula Method	Proportion	Dimensional Analysis

Formula Method:

$$\frac{\overset{2}{0.50\ \text{mg}}}{\underset{1}{0.25\ \text{mg}}} \times 1\ \text{tablet}$$

$$= 2\ \text{tablets}$$

Proportion:

EXPRESSED AS TWO RATIOS

1 tablet : 0.25 mg :: x : 0.5 mg

EXPRESSED AS TWO FRACTIONS

$$\frac{1\ \text{tablet}}{0.25\ \text{mg}} \times \frac{x}{0.5\ \text{mg}}$$

SOLUTION FOR BOTH PROPORTION METHODS

$$0.5 = 0.25x$$
$$\frac{0.50}{0.25} = x$$
$$2\ \text{tablets} = x$$

Dimensional Analysis:

$$\frac{1\ \text{tablet}}{0.25\ \text{mg}} \left| \frac{\overset{2}{0.50\ \text{mg}}}{} \right. = 2\ \text{tablets}$$

10. No equivalent is needed.

Formula Method	Proportion	Dimensional Analysis

Formula Method:

$$\frac{\overset{1.5}{18.75\ \text{mg}}}{\underset{1}{12.5\ \text{mg}}} \times 1\ \text{tablet}$$

$$= 1.5\ \text{tablets}$$

or 1½ tablets

Proportion:

EXPRESSED AS TWO RATIOS

1 tablet : 12.5 mg :: x : 18.75 mg

EXPRESSED AS TWO FRACTIONS

$$\frac{1\ \text{tablet}}{12.5\ \text{mg}} \times \frac{x}{18.75\ \text{mg}}$$

SOLUTION FOR BOTH PROPORTION METHODS

$$18.75 = 12.5x$$
$$\frac{18.75}{12.5} = x$$
$$1.5\ \text{tablet or } 1\tfrac{1}{2}\ \text{tablet} = x$$

Dimensional Analysis:

$$\frac{1\ \text{tablet}}{12.5\ \text{mg}} \left| \frac{18.75\ \text{mg}}{} \right. = \frac{18.75}{12.5}$$

$$= 1½\ \text{tablets}$$

(continued)

Answers (Continued)

11. No equivalent is needed.

Formula Method	Proportion	Dimensional Analysis
$$\frac{300 \text{ mg}}{200 \text{ mg}} \times 1 \text{ tablet}$$ $$= 1\frac{1}{2} \text{ tablets}$$	**EXPRESSED AS TWO RATIOS** 1 tablet : 200 mg : : x : 300 mg **EXPRESSED AS TWO FRACTIONS** $$\frac{1 \text{ tablet}}{200 \text{ mg}} \diagdown \frac{x}{300 \text{ mg}}$$ **SOLUTION FOR BOTH PROPORTION METHODS** $$300 = 200x$$ $$\frac{300}{200} = x$$ $$1\frac{1}{2} \text{ tablets} = x$$	$$\frac{1 \text{ tablet}}{200 \text{ mg}} \bigg| \frac{300 \text{ mg}}{} = \frac{3}{2}$$ $$= 1\frac{1}{2} \text{ tablets}$$

12. No equivalent is needed.

Formula Method	Proportion	Dimensional Analysis
$$\frac{0.3 \text{ mg}}{0.1 \text{ mg}} \times 1 \text{ tablet} = 3 \text{ tablets}$$	**EXPRESSED AS TWO RATIOS** 1 tablet : 0.1 mg : : x : 0.3 mg **EXPRESSED AS TWO FRACTIONS** $$\frac{1 \text{ tablet}}{0.1 \text{ mg}} \diagdown \frac{x}{0.3 \text{ mg}}$$ **SOLUTION FOR BOTH PROPORTION METHODS** $$0.3 = 0.1x$$ $$\frac{0.3}{0.1} = x$$ $$3 \text{ tablets} = x$$	$$\frac{1 \text{ tablet}}{0.1 \text{ mg}} \bigg| \frac{0.3 \text{ mg}}{} = \frac{3}{1} = 3 \text{ tablets}$$

13. No equivalent is needed.

Formula Method	Proportion	Dimensional Analysis
$$\dfrac{\overset{0.25}{\cancel{6.25}\text{ mg}}}{\underset{1}{\cancel{25}\text{ mg}}} \times 1 \text{ tablet}$$ $= 0.25$ tablet (tablets can be quartered)	**EXPRESSED AS TWO RATIOS** 1 tablet : 25 mg : : x : 6.25 mg **EXPRESSED AS TWO FRACTIONS** $$\dfrac{1 \text{ tablet}}{25 \text{ mg}} \times \dfrac{x}{6.25 \text{ mg}}$$ **SOLUTION FOR BOTH PROPORTION METHODS** $$6.25 \text{ mg} = 25x$$ $$\dfrac{6.25}{25} = x$$ 0.25 or $\frac{1}{4}$ tablet $= x$	$$\dfrac{1 \text{ tablet}}{25 \text{ mg}} \ \Big|\ \dfrac{6.25 \text{ mg}}{} = \dfrac{6.25}{25} = 0.25$$ or $\frac{1}{4}$ tablet

14. Equivalent: 0.2 mg = 200 mcg

Formula Method	Proportion	Dimensional Analysis
$$\dfrac{\overset{2}{\cancel{400}\text{ mcg}}}{\underset{1}{\cancel{200}\text{ mcg}}} \times 1 \text{ tablet}$$ $= 2$ tablets	**EXPRESSED AS TWO RATIOS** 1 tablet : 200 mcg : : x : 400 mcg **EXPRESSED AS TWO FRACTIONS** $$\dfrac{1 \text{ tablet}}{200 \text{ mcg}} \times \dfrac{x}{400 \text{ mcg}}$$ **SOLUTION FOR BOTH PROPORTION METHODS** $$400 = 200x$$ $$\dfrac{400}{200} = x$$ 2 tablets $= x$	Use conversion factor 1 mg/1000 mcg: $$\dfrac{1 \text{ tablet}}{0.2 \text{ mg}} \ \Big|\ \dfrac{400 \text{ mcg}}{} \ \Big|\ \dfrac{1 \text{ mg}}{1000 \text{ mcg}} = \dfrac{4}{0.2 \times 10}$$ $= 2$ tablets

(continued)

Answers (Continued)

15. No equivalent is needed.

Formula Method	Proportion	Dimensional Analysis
	EXPRESSED AS TWO RATIOS	
$\dfrac{\overset{1.5}{\cancel{7.5}\text{ mg}}}{\cancel{5}\text{ mg}} \times 1 \text{ tablet}$	1 tablet : 5 mg : : x : 7.5 mg	$\dfrac{1 \; \cancel{\text{tablet}}}{5 \; \cancel{\text{mg}}} \Bigg| \; \dfrac{7.5 \; \cancel{\text{mg}}}{} = \dfrac{7.5}{5} = 1\frac{1}{2} \text{ tablet}$
$= 1.5$ tablets	**EXPRESSED AS TWO FRACTIONS**	
or $1\frac{1}{2}$ tablets	$\dfrac{1 \text{ tablet}}{5 \text{ mg}} \bigtimes \dfrac{x}{7.5 \text{ mg}}$	
	SOLUTION FOR BOTH PROPORTION METHODS	
	$7.5 = 5x$	
	$\dfrac{7.5}{5} = x$	
	1.5 or $1\frac{1}{2}$ tablets $= x$	

16. No equivalent is needed.

Formula Method	Proportion	Dimensional Analysis
	EXPRESSED AS TWO RATIOS	
$\dfrac{\overset{0.5}{\cancel{0.625}\text{ mg}}}{\cancel{1.25}\text{ mg}} \times 1 \text{ tablet}$	1 tablet : 1.25 mg : : x : 0.625 mg	$\dfrac{1 \; \cancel{\text{tablet}}}{\underset{2}{\cancel{1.250}}\text{ mg}} \Bigg| \; \dfrac{\overset{1}{\cancel{0.625}}\text{ mg}}{} = \frac{1}{2} \text{ tablet}$
$= 0.5$ tablet	**EXPRESSED AS TWO FRACTIONS**	
or $\frac{1}{2}$ tablet	$\dfrac{1 \text{ tablet}}{1.25 \text{ mg}} \bigtimes \dfrac{x}{0.625 \text{ mg}}$	
	SOLUTION FOR BOTH PROPORTION METHODS	
	$0.625 = 1.25x$	
	$\dfrac{0.625}{1.25} = x$	
	0.5 or $\frac{1}{2}$ tablet $= x$	

17. Equivalent: 0.5 g = 500 mg

Formula Method	Proportion	Dimensional Analysis
$$\dfrac{\overset{2}{500}\ \text{mg}}{\underset{1}{250}\ \text{mg}} \times 1\ \text{tablet}$$ $$= 2\ \text{tablets}$$	**EXPRESSED AS TWO RATIOS** $$1\ \text{tablet} : 250\ \text{mg} :: x : 500\ \text{mg}$$ **EXPRESSED AS TWO FRACTIONS** $$\dfrac{1\ \text{tablet}}{250\ \text{mg}} \times \dfrac{x}{500\ \text{mg}}$$ **SOLUTION FOR BOTH PROPORTION METHODS** $$500 = 250x$$ $$\dfrac{500}{250} = x$$ $$2\ \text{tablets} = x$$	Use conversion factor 1000 mg/1 g: $$\dfrac{1\ \text{tablet}}{\underset{1}{250}\ \text{mg}} \Bigg| \ 0.5\ \text{g} \ \Bigg| \ \dfrac{\overset{4}{1000}\ \text{mg}}{1\ \text{g}} = 0.5 \times 4$$ $$= 2\ \text{tablets}$$

18. No equivalent is needed.

Formula Method	Proportion	Dimensional Analysis
$$\dfrac{\overset{1.5}{37.5}\ \text{mg}}{\underset{1}{25}\ \text{mg}} \times 1\ \text{tablet}$$ $$= 1.5\ \text{tablets}$$ or 1½ tablets	**EXPRESSED AS TWO RATIOS** $$1\ \text{tablet} : 25\ \text{mg} :: x : 37.5\ \text{mg}$$ **EXPRESSED AS TWO FRACTIONS** $$\dfrac{1\ \text{tablet}}{25\ \text{mg}} \times \dfrac{x}{37.5\ \text{mg}}$$ **SOLUTION FOR BOTH PROPORTION METHODS** $$37.5 = 25x$$ $$\dfrac{37.5}{25} = x$$ 1.5 or 1½ tablets = x	$$\dfrac{1\ \text{tablet}}{25\ \text{mg}} \Bigg| \ 37.5\ \text{mg} = \dfrac{37.5}{25} = 1\tfrac{1}{2}\ \text{tablets}$$

(continued)

Answers (Continued)

19. Equivalent: 1 g = 1000 mg

Formula Method	Proportion	Dimensional Analysis
$\dfrac{\overset{2}{\cancel{1000}\text{ mg}}}{\underset{1}{\cancel{500}\text{ mg}}} \times 1\text{ capsule}$ = 2 capsules	**EXPRESSED AS TWO RATIOS** 1 capsule : 500 mg :: x : 1000 mg **EXPRESSED AS TWO FRACTIONS** $\dfrac{1\text{ capsule}}{500\text{ mg}} \times \dfrac{x}{1000\text{ mg}}$ **SOLUTION FOR BOTH** **PROPORTION METHODS** $1000 = 500x$ $\dfrac{1000}{500} = x$ 2 capsules = x	Use conversion factor 1000 mg/1 g: $\dfrac{1\,\cancel{\text{capsule}}}{\cancel{500}\text{ mg}} \,\bigg|\, \dfrac{1\,\cancel{g}}{} \,\bigg|\, \dfrac{\overset{2}{\cancel{1000}}\text{ mg}}{1\,\cancel{g}} = 2\text{ capsules}$

20. No equivalent is needed.

Formula Method	Proportion	Dimensional Analysis
$\dfrac{\overset{2.5}{\cancel{25}\text{ mg}}}{\underset{1}{\cancel{10}\text{ mg}}} \times 1\text{ tablet}$ = 2.5 tablets or 2½ tablets	**EXPRESSED AS TWO RATIOS** 1 tablet : 10 mg :: x : 25 mg **EXPRESSED AS TWO FRACTIONS** $\dfrac{1\text{ tablet}}{10\text{ mg}} \times \dfrac{x}{25\text{ mg}}$ **SOLUTION FOR BOTH** **PROPORTION METHODS** $25 = 10x$ $\dfrac{25}{10} = x$ 2.5 or 2½ tablets = x	$\dfrac{1\,\cancel{\text{tablet}}}{\underset{2}{\cancel{10}}\text{ mg}} \,\bigg|\, \overset{5}{\cancel{25}}\text{ mg} = \dfrac{5}{2} = 2\,½\text{ tablets}$

FINE POINTS

Calculations may be done in different ways. Answers should be the same regardless of the method chosen to solve the problem.

Self-Test 2 Oral Liquids

Formula Method	Proportion	Dimensional Analysis
$\dfrac{\text{Desire}}{\text{Have}} \times \text{Supply} = x$	**EXPRESSED AS TWO RATIOS** Supply : Have : : x : Desire **EXPRESSED AS TWO FRACTIONS** $\dfrac{\text{Supply}}{\text{Have}} = \dfrac{x}{\text{Desire}}$	$\dfrac{\text{Supply} \mid \text{Desire}}{\text{Have} \mid}$ (add conversion factors as needed)

1. Equivalent: 0.75 g = 750 mg

Formula Method	Proportion	Dimensional Analysis
$\dfrac{\overset{3}{\cancel{750}} \text{ mg}}{\underset{1}{\cancel{250}} \text{ mg}} \times 1 \text{ mL} = 3 \text{ mL}$	**EXPRESSED AS TWO RATIOS** 1 mL : 250 mg : : x : 750 mg **EXPRESSED AS TWO FRACTIONS** $\dfrac{1 \text{ mL}}{250 \text{ mg}} \times \dfrac{x}{750 \text{ mg}}$ **SOLUTION FOR BOTH PROPORTION METHODS** $750 = 250x$ $\dfrac{750}{250} = x$ $3 \text{ mL} = x$	Use conversion factor 1000 mg/1 g: $\dfrac{1\,\cancel{\text{mL}}}{\underset{1}{\cancel{250}}\,\cancel{\text{mg}}} \mid \dfrac{0.75\,\cancel{\text{g}}}{} \mid \dfrac{\overset{4}{\cancel{1000}}\,\cancel{\text{mg}}}{1\,\cancel{\text{g}}} = 0.75 \times 4$ $= 3 \text{ mL}$

2. No equivalent is needed.

Formula Method	Proportion	Dimensional Analysis
$\dfrac{\overset{2}{\cancel{500}} \text{ mg}}{\underset{1}{\cancel{250}} \text{ mg}} \times 5 \text{ mL} = 10 \text{ mL}$	**EXPRESSED AS TWO RATIOS** 5 mL : 250 mg : : x : 500 mg **EXPRESSED AS TWO FRACTIONS** $\dfrac{5 \text{ mL}}{250 \text{ mg}} \times \dfrac{x}{500 \text{ mg}}$ **SOLUTION FOR BOTH PROPORTION METHODS** $2500 = 250x$ $\dfrac{2500}{250} = x$ $10 \text{ mL} = x$	$\dfrac{5\,\cancel{\text{mL}}}{\underset{1}{\cancel{250}}\,\cancel{\text{mg}}} \mid \dfrac{\overset{2}{\cancel{500}}\,\cancel{\text{mg}}}{} = 5 \times 2 = 10$

(continued)

Answers (Continued)

3. Equivalent: 0.35 g = 350 mg

Formula Method	Proportion	Dimensional Analysis
$$\frac{\cancel{350}\text{ mg}}{\cancel{125}\text{ mg}} \times \cancel{5}\text{ mL} = 14\text{ mL}$$	**EXPRESSED AS TWO RATIOS** 5 mL : 125 mg : : x : 350 mg **EXPRESSED AS TWO FRACTIONS** $$\frac{5\text{ mL}}{125\text{ mg}} \diagup \frac{x}{350\text{ mg}}$$ **SOLUTION FOR BOTH PROPORTION METHODS** $$1750 = 125x$$ $$\frac{1750}{125} = x$$ $$14\text{ mL} = x$$	Use conversion factor 1000 mg/1 g: $$\frac{5\text{ mL}}{125\text{ mg}} \Big| \frac{0.35\text{ g}}{} \Big| \frac{1000\text{ mg}}{1\text{ g}} = 5 \times 0.35 \times 8$$ $$= 14\text{ mL}$$

4. No equivalent is needed.

Formula Method	Proportion	Dimensional Analysis
$$\frac{\cancel{150}\text{ mg}}{\cancel{100}\text{ mg}} \times 1\text{ mL} = \frac{3}{2}$$ $$= 1.5\text{ mL}$$	**EXPRESSED AS TWO RATIOS** 1 mL : 100 mg : : x : 150 mg **EXPRESSED AS TWO FRACTIONS** $$\frac{1\text{ mL}}{100\text{ mg}} \diagup \frac{x}{150\text{ mg}}$$ **SOLUTION FOR BOTH PROPORTION METHODS** $$150 = 100x$$ $$\frac{150}{100} = x$$ $$1.5\text{ mL} = x$$	$$\frac{1\text{ mL}}{100\text{ mg}} \Big| \frac{150\text{ mg}}{} = \frac{3}{2} = 1.5\text{ mL}$$

5. No equivalent is needed.

Formula Method	Proportion	Dimensional Analysis
$\dfrac{\overset{1}{\cancel{5}}\ \text{mg}}{\underset{2}{\cancel{10}}\ \text{mg}} \times 1\ \text{mL}$ $= \frac{1}{2}$ or 0.5 mL	**EXPRESSED AS TWO RATIOS** 1 mL : 10 mg :: x : 5 mg **EXPRESSED AS TWO FRACTIONS** $\dfrac{1\ \text{mL}}{10\ \text{mg}} \diagdown \dfrac{\text{x}}{5\ \text{mg}}$ **SOLUTION FOR BOTH PROPORTION METHODS** $5 = 10\text{x}$ $\dfrac{5}{10} = \text{x}$ $\frac{1}{2}$ or 0.5 mL = x	$\dfrac{1\,\textcircled{mL}}{\underset{2}{\cancel{10}}\ \text{mg}} \left| \dfrac{\overset{1}{\cancel{5}}\ \text{mg}}{} \right. = \frac{1}{2}$ or 0.5 mL

6. No equivalent is needed.

Formula Method	Proportion	Dimensional Analysis
$\dfrac{0.02\ \text{mg}}{0.05\ \text{mg}} \times 1\ \text{mL} = \dfrac{2}{5}$ $= 0.4\ \text{mL}$	**EXPRESSED AS TWO RATIOS** 1 mL : 0.05 mg :: x : 0.02 mg **EXPRESSED AS TWO FRACTIONS** $\dfrac{1\ \text{mL}}{0.05\ \text{mg}} \diagdown \dfrac{\text{x}}{0.02\ \text{mg}}$ **SOLUTION FOR BOTH PROPORTION METHODS** $0.02 = 0.05\text{x}$ $\dfrac{0.02}{0.05} = \text{x}$ $0.4\ \text{mL} = \text{x}$	$\dfrac{1\,\textcircled{mL}}{0.05\ \text{mg}} \left| \dfrac{0.02\ \text{mg}}{} \right. = \dfrac{2}{5} = 0.4\ \text{mL}$

(continued)

Answers (Continued)

7. No equivalent is needed.

Formula Method	Proportion	Dimensional Analysis
$\dfrac{30\ \text{mEq}}{20\ \text{mEq}} \times 15\ \text{mL} = \dfrac{3 \times 15}{2}$ $= \dfrac{45}{2} = 22.5\ \text{mL}$	**EXPRESSED AS TWO RATIOS** 15 mL : 20 mEq : : x : 30 mEq **EXPRESSED AS TWO FRACTIONS** $\dfrac{15\ \text{mL}}{20\ \text{mEq}} \times \dfrac{x}{30\ \text{mEq}}$ **SOLUTION FOR BOTH PROPORTION METHODS** $15 \times 30 = 20x$ $\dfrac{450}{20} = x$ $22.5\ \text{mL} = x$	$\dfrac{15\ \text{mL}}{20\ \text{mEq}} \ \bigg|\ \dfrac{30\ \text{mEq}}{} = \dfrac{15 \times 3}{2}$ $= 22.5\ \text{mL}$

8. No equivalent is needed.

Formula Method	Proportion	Dimensional Analysis
$\dfrac{0.25\ \text{mg}}{0.25\ \text{mg}} \times 1\ \text{mL} = 1\ \text{mL}$	**EXPRESSED AS TWO RATIOS** 1 mL : 0.25 mg : : x : 0.25 mg **EXPRESSED AS TWO FRACTIONS** $\dfrac{1\ \text{mL}}{0.25\ \text{mg}} \times \dfrac{x}{0.25\ \text{mg}}$ **SOLUTION FOR BOTH PROPORTION METHODS** $0.25 = 0.25x$ $\dfrac{0.25}{0.25} = x$ $1\ \text{mL} = x$	$\dfrac{1\ \text{mL}}{0.25\ \text{mg}} \ \bigg|\ \dfrac{\overset{1}{0.25\ \text{mg}}}{\underset{1}{}} = 1\ \text{mL}$

9. No equivalent is needed.

Formula Method	Proportion	Dimensional Analysis
$\dfrac{3 \text{ mg}}{1 \text{ mg}} \times 1 \text{ mL} = 3 \text{ mL}$	**EXPRESSED AS TWO RATIOS** $1 \text{ mL} : 1 \text{ mg} :: x : 3 \text{ mg}$ **EXPRESSED AS TWO FRACTIONS** $\dfrac{1 \text{ mL}}{1 \text{ mg}} \times \dfrac{x}{3 \text{ mg}}$ **SOLUTION FOR BOTH PROPORTION METHODS** $3 = 1x$ $\dfrac{3}{1} = x$ $3 \text{ mL} = x$	$\dfrac{1 \text{ mL}}{1 \text{ mg}} \left| \dfrac{3 \text{ mg}}{} \right. = 3 \text{ mL}$

10. No equivalent is needed.

Formula Method	Proportion	Dimensional Analysis
$\dfrac{\overset{10}{\cancel{12.5} \text{ mg}}}{\underset{\underset{1}{1.25}}{\cancel{6.25} \text{ mg}}} \times \overset{1}{\cancel{5}} \text{ mL} = 10 \text{ mL}$	**EXPRESSED AS TWO RATIOS** $5 \text{ mL} : 6.25 \text{ mg} :: x : 12.5 \text{ mg}$ **EXPRESSED AS TWO FRACTIONS** $\dfrac{5 \text{ mL}}{6.25 \text{ mg}} \times \dfrac{x}{12.5 \text{ mg}}$ **SOLUTION FOR BOTH PROPORTION METHODS** $62.5 = 6.25x$ $\dfrac{62.5}{6.25} = x$ $10 \text{ mL} = x$	$\dfrac{5 \text{ mL}}{6.25 \text{ mg}} \left| \dfrac{\overset{2}{12.5} \text{ mg}}{} \right. = 5 \times 2 = 10 \text{ mL}$

FINE POINTS

Alternate arithmetic:

$12.5 \times 5 = 62.5$

$$6.25 \overline{)62.50} \overset{10.}{}$$
$$\underline{625}$$
$$0$$

(continued)

Answers (Continued)

11. No equivalent is needed.

Formula Method	Proportion	Dimensional Analysis
$\dfrac{\overset{5}{\cancel{50}} \text{ mg}}{\underset{1}{\cancel{10}} \text{ mg}} \times 5 \text{ mL} = 25 \text{ mL}$	**EXPRESSED AS TWO RATIOS** 5 mL : 10 mg : : x : 50 mg **EXPRESSED AS TWO FRACTIONS** $\dfrac{5 \text{ mL}}{10 \text{ mg}} \times \dfrac{x}{50 \text{ mg}}$ **SOLUTION FOR BOTH PROPORTION METHODS** $5 \times 50 = 10x$ $\dfrac{250}{10} = x$ $25 \text{ mL} = x$	$\dfrac{5\,\cancel{\text{mL}}}{\underset{1}{\cancel{10}} \text{ mg}} \left\vert \dfrac{\overset{5}{\cancel{50}} \text{ mg}}{} \right. = 5 \times 5 = 25 \text{ mL}$

12. No equivalent is needed.

Formula Method	Proportion	Dimensional Analysis
$\dfrac{\overset{4}{\cancel{40}} \text{ mg}}{\underset{1}{\cancel{10}} \text{ mg}} \times 1 \text{ mL} = 4 \text{ mL}$	**EXPRESSED AS TWO RATIOS** 1 mL : 10 mg : : x : 40 mg **EXPRESSED AS TWO FRACTIONS** $\dfrac{1 \text{ mL}}{10 \text{ mg}} \times \dfrac{x}{40 \text{ mg}}$ **SOLUTION FOR BOTH PROPORTION METHODS** $40 = 10x$ $\dfrac{40}{10} = x$ $4 \text{ mL} = x$	$\dfrac{1\,\cancel{\text{mL}}}{\underset{1}{\cancel{10}} \text{ mg}} \left\vert \dfrac{\overset{4}{\cancel{40}} \text{ mg}}{} \right. = 1 \times 4 = 4 \text{ mL}$

13. No equivalent is needed.

Formula Method	Proportion	Dimensional Analysis
$\dfrac{\overset{1}{\cancel{10}}\ \cancel{mEq}}{\underset{2}{\cancel{20}}\ \cancel{mEq}} \times 30\ mL - \dfrac{30}{2}$ $= 15\ mL$	**EXPRESSED AS TWO RATIOS** $30\ mL : 20\ mEq :: x : 10\ mEq$ **EXPRESSED AS TWO FRACTIONS** $\dfrac{30\ mL}{20\ mEq} \times \dfrac{x}{10\ mEq}$ **SOLUTION FOR BOTH** **PROPORTION METHODS** $30 \times 10 = 20x$ $\dfrac{300}{20} = x$ $15\ mL = x$	$\dfrac{\overset{}{\cancel{30}}\ \cancel{mL}}{\underset{2}{\cancel{20}}\ \cancel{mEq}} \left| \dfrac{\overset{1}{\cancel{10}}\ \cancel{mEq}}{} = \dfrac{30}{2} = 15\ mL$

14. No equivalent is needed.

Formula Method	Proportion	Dimensional Analysis
$\dfrac{\overset{2}{\cancel{10}}\ \cancel{mg}}{\underset{1}{\cancel{5}}\ \cancel{mg}} \times 5\ mL = 10\ mL$	**EXPRESSED AS TWO RATIOS** $5\ mL : 5\ mg :: x : 10\ mg$ **EXPRESSED AS TWO FRACTIONS** $\dfrac{5\ mL}{5\ mg} \times \dfrac{x}{10\ mg}$ **SOLUTION FOR BOTH** **PROPORTION METHODS** $10 \times 5 = 5x$ $\dfrac{50}{5} = x$ $10\ mL = x$	$\dfrac{\overset{1}{\cancel{5}}\ \cancel{mL}}{\underset{1}{\cancel{5}}\ mg} \left| \dfrac{10\ \cancel{mg}}{} = 10\ mL$

15. No equivalent is needed.

Formula Method	Proportion	Dimensional Analysis
$\dfrac{\overset{5}{\cancel{100}}\ \cancel{mg}}{\underset{1}{\cancel{20}}\ \cancel{mg}} \times 5\ mL = 25\ mL$	**EXPRESSED AS TWO RATIOS** $5\ mL : 20\ mg :: x : 100\ mg$ **EXPRESSED AS TWO FRACTIONS** $\dfrac{5\ mL}{20\ mg} \times \dfrac{x}{100\ mg}$ **SOLUTION FOR BOTH** **PROPORTION METHODS** $5 \times 100 = 20x$ $\dfrac{500}{20} = x$ $25\ mL = x$	$\dfrac{\overset{}{\cancel{5}}\ \cancel{mL}}{\underset{1}{\cancel{20}}\ \cancel{mg}} \left| \dfrac{\overset{5}{\cancel{100}}\ \cancel{mg}}{} = 5 \times 5 = 25\ mL$

(continued)

Answers (Continued)

16. No equivalent is needed.

Formula Method	Proportion	Dimensional Analysis
$\dfrac{650\ mg}{160\ mg} \times 5\ mL = \dfrac{3250}{160}$ $= 20.31\ or\ 20\ mL$	**EXPRESSED AS TWO RATIOS** $5\ mL : 160\ mg :: x : 650\ mg$ **EXPRESSED AS TWO FRACTIONS** $\dfrac{5\ mL}{160\ mg} \times \dfrac{x}{650\ mg}$ **SOLUTION FOR BOTH PROPORTION METHODS** $650 \times 5 = 160x$ $\dfrac{3250}{160} = x$ $20.31\ or\ 20\ mL = x$	$\dfrac{5\ mL}{160\ mg} \Big| \dfrac{650\ mg}{}$ $= \dfrac{5 \times 650}{160}$ $= 20.31 = 20\ mL$

17. No equivalent is needed.

Formula Method	Proportion	Dimensional Analysis
$\dfrac{\overset{2}{\cancel{25}}\ mg}{\underset{1}{\cancel{12.5}}\ mg} \times 5\ mL = 10\ mL$	**EXPRESSED AS TWO RATIOS** $5\ mL : 12.5\ mg :: x : 25\ mg$ **EXPRESSED AS TWO FRACTIONS** $\dfrac{5\ mL}{12.5\ mg} \times \dfrac{x}{25\ mg}$ **SOLUTION FOR BOTH PROPORTION METHODS** $5 \times 25 = 12.5x$ $\dfrac{125}{12.5} = x$ $10\ mL = x$	$\dfrac{5\ \cancel{mL}}{\underset{1}{\cancel{12.5}}\ \cancel{mg}} \Big| \overset{2}{\cancel{25}}\ \cancel{mg} = 5 \times 2 = 10\ mL$

18. No equivalent is needed.

Formula Method	Proportion	Dimensional Analysis
$\dfrac{\overset{5}{\cancel{50}\ \cancel{mg}}}{\underset{1}{\cancel{10}\ \cancel{mg}}} \times 5\ mL = 25\ mL$	**EXPRESSED AS TWO RATIOS** $5\ mL : 10\ mg :: x : 50\ mg$ **EXPRESSED AS TWO FRACTIONS** $\dfrac{5\ mL}{10\ mg} \times \dfrac{x}{50\ mg}$ **SOLUTION FOR BOTH PROPORTION METHODS** $5 \times 50 = 10x$ $\dfrac{250}{10} = x$ $25\ mL = x$	$\dfrac{5\ \cancel{mL}}{\underset{1}{\cancel{10}\ \cancel{mg}}} \left| \dfrac{\overset{5}{\cancel{50}\ \cancel{mg}}}{} \right. = 5 \times 5 = 25\ mL$

19. No equivalent is needed.

Formula Method	Proportion	Dimensional Analysis
$\dfrac{\overset{2}{\cancel{100}\ \cancel{mg}}}{\underset{1}{\cancel{50}\ \cancel{mg}}} \times 15\ mL = 30\ mL$	**EXPRESSED AS TWO RATIOS** $15\ mL : 50\ mg :: x : 100\ mg$ **EXPRESSED AS TWO FRACTIONS** $\dfrac{15\ mL}{50\ mg} \times \dfrac{x}{100\ mg}$ **SOLUTION FOR BOTH PROPORTION METHODS** $15 \times 100 = 50x$ $\dfrac{1500}{50} = x$ $30\ mL = x$	$\dfrac{15\ \cancel{mL}}{\underset{1}{\cancel{50}\ \cancel{mg}}} \left| \dfrac{\overset{2}{\cancel{100}\ \cancel{mg}}}{} \right. = 15 \times 2 = 30\ mL$

(continued)

Answers (Continued)

20. Equivalent: 0.06 g = 60 mg

Formula Method	Proportion	Dimensional Analysis

Formula Method

$$\frac{\overset{4}{\cancel{60}} \text{ mg}}{\underset{1}{\cancel{15}} \text{ mg}} \times 5 \text{ mL} = 20 \text{ mL}$$

Proportion

EXPRESSED AS TWO RATIOS

$$5 \text{ mL} : 15 \text{ mg} :: x : 60 \text{ mg}$$

EXPRESSED AS TWO FRACTIONS

$$\frac{5 \text{ mL}}{15 \text{ mg}} \times \frac{x}{60 \text{ mg}}$$

SOLUTION FOR BOTH PROPORTION METHODS

$$5 \times 60 = 15x$$

$$\frac{300}{15} = x$$

$$20 \text{ mL} = x$$

Dimensional Analysis

$$\frac{\overset{1}{\cancel{5}} \text{ mL}}{\underset{3}{\cancel{15}} \text{ mg}} \left| \frac{0.06 \cancel{\text{ g}}}{} \right| \frac{1000 \cancel{\text{ mg}}}{1 \cancel{\text{ g}}} = \frac{0.06 \times 1000}{3}$$

$$= 20 \text{ mL}$$

Self-Test 3 Mental Drill Oral Solids and Liquids

1. 2 tablets	**7.** 1 tablet	**13.** ½ tablet	**19.** 15 mL
2. ½ tablet	**8.** 1 tablet	**14.** 2 tablets	**20.** 20 mL
3. 2 tablets	**9.** ½ tablet	**15.** 10 mL	**21.** 15 mL
4. 2 tablets	**10.** 2 tablets	**16.** 25 mL	**22.** 5 mL
5. 2 tablets	**11.** 2 tablets	**17.** 10 mL	**23.** 6 mL
6. ½ tablet	**12.** 2 tablets	**18.** 5 mL	**24.** 2.5 mL

Liquids for Injection

Liquid drugs for injection are prepared by pharmaceutical companies as sterile solutions, powders, or suspensions. Aseptic techniques are used to prepare and administer them. As with oral medications, the nurse may have to calculate the correct dosage. The nurse must also follow correct administration techniques and special considerations (i.e., correct dilution, injection site, size of needle, speed of intravenous injection, etc.). (See Chapter 10 for administration procedures.)

 Syringes and Rounding

These are general acceptable guidelines. Always follow any institution-specific guidelines.

3-mL Syringe

When you're calculating injection answers, the degree of accuracy depends on the syringe you use. Figure 5-1 shows a 3-mL syringe marked in milliliters to the nearest tenth. *To calculate milliliter answers for this 3-mL syringe, carry out the arithmetic to the hundredth place and then round off the answer to the nearest tenth (follow standard rounding rules).*

   1.25 mL becomes 1.3 mL

1-mL Syringe

Figure 5-2 shows a 1-mL syringe (also called a 1-mL precision syringe or a 1-mL tuberculin syringe) marked in milliliters to the nearest hundredth. *To calculate milliliters when the 1-mL syringe is used, carry out the arithmetic to the thousandth place and then round off the answer to the nearest hundredth (follow standard rounding rules).*

   0.978 mL becomes 0.98 mL

   Each of the following examples provides a syringe. (Syringes will be shown without needles.) Calculate milliliters to the degree of accuracy required by the syringe markings.

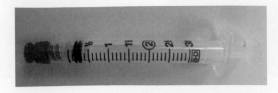

FIGURE 5-1

A 3-mL syringe.

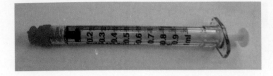

FIGURE 5-2

A 1-mL syringe.

Calculating Liquid Injections

To solve liquid injection problems, use the same rule as for oral solids and liquids.

Formula Method	Proportion	Dimensional Analysis
$\dfrac{\text{Desire}}{\text{Have}} \times \text{Supply} = \text{Amount}$	**EXPRESSED AS TWO RATIOS** Supply : Have :: x : Desire **EXPRESSED AS TWO FRACTIONS** $\dfrac{\text{Supply}}{\text{Have}} = \dfrac{x}{\text{Desire}}$	$\dfrac{\text{Supply}}{\text{Have}} \;\Big|\; \text{Desired Dose}$

EXAMPLE

- Order: trifluoperazine (Stelazine) 1.5 mg IM q6h prn
- Supply: Read the label.

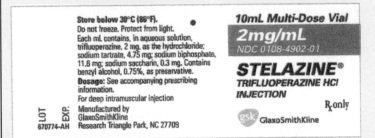

Store below 30°C (86°F). Do not freeze. Protect from light. Each mL contains, in aqueous solution, trifluoperazine, 2 mg. as the hydrochloride; sodium tartrate, 4.75 mg; sodium biphosphate, 11.6 mg; sodium saccharin, 0.3 mg. Contains benzyl alcohol, 0.75%, as preservative. **Dosage:** See accompanying prescribing information. For deep intramuscular injection Manufactured by GlaxoSmithKline Research Triangle Park, NC 27709 LOT EXP: 670774-AH

10mL Multi-Dose Vial
2mg/mL
NDC 0108-4902-01
STELAZINE®
TRIFLUOPERAZINE HCl
INJECTION
R̠only
gsk GlaxoSmithKline

(Courtesy of GlaxoSmithKline.)

- Desire: the amount ordered, here, 1.5 mg
- Have: strength of the drug supplied, here, 2 mg
- Supply: the unit form of the drug, here, 1 mL (for liquid calculations, the supply is usually 1 mL although there are exceptions).
- Amount of liquid to give by injection in milliliters: "x" is used to denote the unknown or answer.

Formula Method	Proportion	Dimensional Analysis
$\dfrac{1.5\ \text{mg}}{2\ \text{mg}} \times 1\ \text{mL} = 0.75\ \text{mL}$	**EXPRESSED AS TWO RATIOS**	$\dfrac{1\ \text{mL}}{2\ \text{mg}} \Bigg|\ \dfrac{1.5\ \text{mg}}{\ } = \dfrac{1.5}{2} = 0.75\ \text{mL}$

Proportion

EXPRESSED AS TWO RATIOS

$$1\ \text{mL} : 2\ \text{mg} :: x : 1.5\ \text{mg}$$

EXPRESSED AS TWO FRACTIONS

$$\frac{1\ \text{mL}}{2\ \text{mg}} \times \frac{x}{1.5\ \text{mg}}$$

SOLUTION FOR BOTH PROPORTION METHODS

$$1.5 = 2x$$
$$\frac{1.5}{2} = x$$
$$0.75\ \text{mL} = x$$

Use a 3-mL syringe. Round to the nearest tenth. Give 0.8 mL IM.

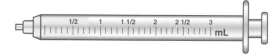

EXAMPLE

- Order: morphine 4 mg IM q4h prn
- Supply: Read the label.

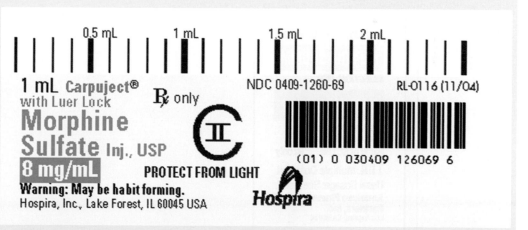

(Courtesy of Abbott Laboratories.)

- Desired dose: 4 mg
- Supply: 1 mL
- Have: 8 mg in 1 mL

Formula Method	Proportion	Dimensional Analysis

Formula Method

$$\frac{\overset{1}{\cancel{4}}\ \cancel{mg}}{\underset{2}{\cancel{8}}\ \cancel{mg}} \times 1\ mL = 0.5\ mL$$

Proportion

EXPRESSED AS TWO RATIOS

$$1\ mL : 8\ mg :: x : 4\ mg$$

EXPRESSED AS TWO FRACTIONS

$$\frac{1\ mL}{8\ mg} \times \frac{x}{4\ mg}$$

SOLUTION FOR BOTH
PROPORTION METHODS

$$4 = 8x$$

$$\frac{4}{8} = x$$

$$0.5\ mL = x$$

Dimensional Analysis

$$\frac{1\ \boxed{mL}}{\underset{2}{\cancel{8}}\ \cancel{mg}} \left|\ \frac{\overset{1}{\cancel{4}}\ \cancel{mg}}{}\right. = 0.5\ mL$$

Give 0.5 mL IM.

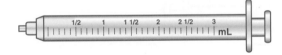

EXAMPLE

- Order: heparin sodium 1500 units subcutaneous bid
- Supply: Read the label.

> NDC 63323-262-01 926201
>
> **HEPARIN SODIUM**
> *INJECTION, USP*
>
> **5,000 USP Units/mL**
> (Derived from Porcine
> Intestinal Mucosa)
> For IV or SC Use   Rx only
> **1 mL** Multiple Dose Vial
> Usual Dosage: See insert.
> **American Pharmaceutical
> Partners, Inc.**
> Los Angeles, CA 90024
>
> **401810A**
>
> LOT 313167
> EXP 09/03

- Desired dose: 1500 units
- Supply: 1 mL
- Have: 5000 units in 1 mL

Formula Method	Proportion	Dimensional Analysis

Formula Method

$$\frac{\overset{3}{\cancel{1500}} \text{ units}}{\underset{10}{\cancel{5000}} \text{ units}} \times 1 \text{ mL}$$

$$= \frac{3}{10} = 0.3 \text{ mL}$$

Proportion

EXPRESSED AS TWO RATIOS

1 mL : 5000 units : : x : 1500 units

EXPRESSED AS TWO FRACTIONS

$$\frac{1 \text{ mL}}{5000 \text{ units}} \times \frac{x}{1500 \text{ units}}$$

SOLUTION FOR BOTH PROPORTION METHODS

$$1500 = 5000x$$

$$\frac{1500}{5000} = x$$

$$0.3 \text{ mL} = x$$

Dimensional Analysis

$$\frac{1 \cancel{\text{ mL}}}{5000 \cancel{\text{ units}}} \bigg| \; 1500 \cancel{\text{ units}} = \frac{15}{50} = 0.3 \text{ mL}$$

Give 0.3 mL.

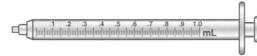

Heparin can also be administered intravenously—this will be covered in Chapter 7.

EXAMPLE

- Order: cyanocobalamin (Vitamin B_{12}) 0.25 mg IM daily × 7 days
- Supply: Read the label.

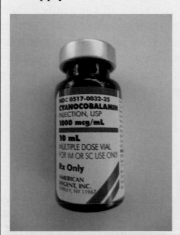

- Conversion: 0.25 mg = 250 mcg
- Desired dose: 250 mcg
- Supply: 1 mL
- Have: 1000 mcg in 1 mL

Formula Method	Proportion	Dimensional Analysis

Formula Method

$$\frac{250 \text{ mcg}}{1000 \text{ mcg}} \times 1 \text{ mL}$$

$$= \frac{250}{1000} = 0.25 \text{ mL}$$

Proportion

EXPRESSED AS TWO RATIOS

$$1 \text{ mL} : 1000 \text{ mcg} :: x : 250 \text{ mcg}$$

EXPRESSED AS TWO FRACTIONS

$$\frac{1 \text{ mL}}{1000 \text{ mcg}} \times \frac{x}{250 \text{ mcg}}$$

SOLUTION FOR BOTH
PROPORTION METHODS

$$250 = 1000x$$

$$\frac{250}{1000} = x$$

$$0.25 \text{ mL} = x$$

Dimensional Analysis

$$\frac{1 \text{ mL}}{1000 \text{ mcg}} \bigg| \frac{0.250 \text{ mg}}{} \bigg| \frac{1000 \text{ mcg}}{1 \text{ mg}}$$

$$= 0.25 \text{ mL}$$

IV Medications

IV push (IVP) medications must be diluted and administered either according to directions in a nursing drug book or according to hospital policy. (Hospital policies often use a greater dilution of certain medications than suggested in drug books. It is safest to follow hospital policy.) First, calculate the correct dose.

EXAMPLE

- Order: digoxin (Lanoxin) loading dose 0.5 mg IV now, then 0.25 mg IV q6h × 2 doses, then maintenance dose of 0.125 mg IV every day.

- A note about maintenance and loading doses: A drug must reach a plateau in the body in order to effectively work. Some drugs have a long half-life, which means it takes longer to reach this plateau and be effective. Digoxin is one of those drugs. Therefore, we administer a higher dose at the start of the drug therapy, also called a loading dose. This may be several higher doses at a closer time interval, or a higher dose one time only. After the plateau is reached, a maintenance dose is ordered, which will be a smaller dose. Work this problem by calculating the two different loading doses. (Consult a nursing pharmacology book for more detailed information on loading and maintenance dosing.)

- Order: digoxin (Lanoxin) 0.5 mg IV now

- Supply: Read the label.

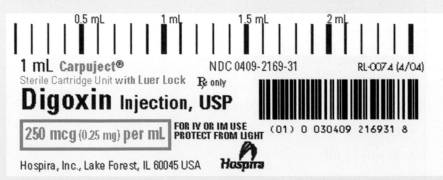

(Used by permission Hospira, Inc.)

- Conversion: 0.5 mg = 500 mcg

- Desired dose: 500 mcg

- Supply: 1 mL

- Have: 250 mcg in 1 mL

Formula Method	Proportion	Dimensional Analysis
$\dfrac{500 \text{ mcg}}{250 \text{ mcg}} \times 1 \text{ mL}$ $= 2 \text{ mL}$	**EXPRESSED AS TWO RATIOS** 1 mL : 250 mcg :: x : 500 mcg **EXPRESSED AS TWO FRACTIONS** $\dfrac{1 \text{ mL}}{250 \text{ mcg}} \times \dfrac{x}{500 \text{ mcg}}$ **SOLUTION FOR BOTH PROPORTION METHODS** $500 = 250x$ $\dfrac{500}{250} = x$ $2 \text{ mL} = x$	$\dfrac{1 \text{ mL}}{250 \text{ mcg}} \ \Big|\ \dfrac{0.5 \text{ mg}}{} \ \Big|\ \dfrac{\overset{4}{1000} \text{ mcg}}{1 \text{ mg}}$ $= 0.5 \times 4$ $= 2 \text{ mL}$

Give 0.25 mL IV either undiluted or dilute in 4 mL of sterile water and give over 5 minutes.

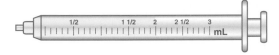

EXAMPLE

- Order: digoxin (Lanoxin) 0.25 mg IV q6h × 2 doses.
- Supply: Read the label.
- Conversion: 0.25 mg = 250 mcg
- Desired dose: 250 mcg
- Supply: 1 mL
- Have: 250 mcg in 1 mL.

Formula Method	Proportion	Dimensional Analysis
$\dfrac{250 \text{ mcg}}{250 \text{ mcg}} \times 1 \text{ mL}$ $= 1 \text{ mL}$	**EXPRESSED AS TWO RATIOS** 1 mL : 250 mcg :: x : 250 mcg **EXPRESSED AS TWO FRACTIONS** $\dfrac{1 \text{ mL}}{250 \text{ mcg}} \times \dfrac{x}{250 \text{ mcg}}$ **SOLUTION FOR BOTH PROPORTION METHODS** $250 = 250x$ $\dfrac{250}{250} = x$ $1 \text{ mL} = x$	$\dfrac{1 \text{ mL}}{250 \text{ mcg}} \ \Big|\ \dfrac{0.25 \text{ mg}}{} \ \Big|\ \dfrac{\overset{4}{1000} \text{ mcg}}{1 \text{ mg}}$ $= 0.25 \times 4$ $= 1 \text{ mL}$

Digoxin IVP is given either undiluted or diluted in 4 mL of sterile water and administered over 5 minutes.

EXAMPLE

- Order: furosemide (Lasix) 20 mg IV q12h
- Supply: Read the label.

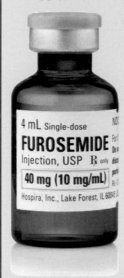

(Used by permission of Hospira, Inc.)

No equivalent is needed.

- Desired dose: 20 mg
- Supply: 1 mL
- Have: 10 mg in 1 mL

Formula Method	Proportion	Dimensional Analysis
$\dfrac{20 \text{ mg}}{10 \text{ mg}} \times 1 \text{ mL} = \dfrac{20}{10} = 2 \text{ mL}$	**EXPRESSED AS TWO RATIOS** 1 mL : 10 mg : : x : 20 mg **EXPRESSED AS TWO FRACTIONS** $\dfrac{1 \text{ mL}}{10 \text{ mg}} \times \dfrac{x}{20 \text{ mg}}$ **SOLUTION FOR BOTH PROPORTION METHODS** $20 = 10x$ $\dfrac{20}{10} = x$ $2 \text{ mL} = x$	$\dfrac{1 \ \textcircled{mL}}{\cancel{10} \text{ mg}} \ \Bigg| \ \dfrac{\cancel{20}^{2} \text{ mg}}{} = 2 \text{ mL}$

Give 2 mL IV.

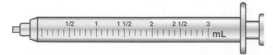

Lasix IVP is given undiluted at a rate of 20 mg over 1 to 2 minutes.

EXAMPLE

• Order: methylprednisolone (A-Methapred) 100 mg IV daily.

• Supply: Read the label.

(This vial is mixed right before administration. Press on the top cap, which pushes the rubber stopper into the vial, mixing the diluent with the powder. Shake gently to mix the two.)

No equivalent needed.

• Desired dose: 100 mg

• Supply: 2 mL

• Have: 125 mg in 2 mL

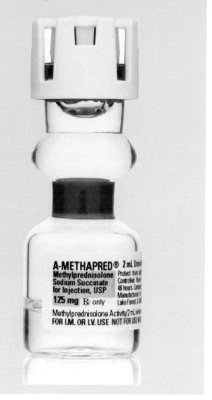

Formula Method	Proportion	Dimensional Analysis

Formula Method

$$\frac{100 \text{ mg}}{125 \text{ mg}} \times 2 \text{ mL} = \frac{200}{125}$$
$$= 1.6 \text{ mL}$$

Proportion

EXPRESSED AS TWO RATIOS

2 mL:125 mg :: x : 100 mg

EXPRESSED AS TWO FRACTIONS

$$\frac{2}{125 \text{ mg}} \times \frac{x}{100 \text{ mg}}$$

SOLUTION FOR BOTH PROPORTION METHODS

$$200 = 125x$$
$$\frac{200}{125} = x$$
$$1.6 \text{ mL} = x$$

Dimensional Analysis

$$\frac{2 \text{ mL}}{125 \text{ mg}} \Bigg| \frac{\overset{20}{100} \text{ mg}}{} = \frac{40}{25} = 1.6 \text{ mL}$$

Administer 1.6 mL over 3-15 minutes IV push

EXAMPLE

- Order: ondansetron (Zofran) 3 mg IV stat
- Supply: Read the label.

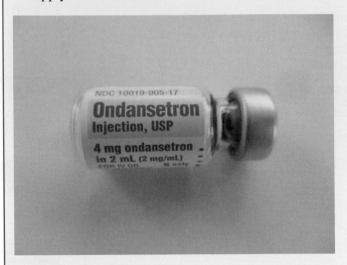

No equivalent is needed.

- Desired dose: 3 mg
- Supply: 2 mL
- Have: 4 mg in 2 mL

Formula Method	Proportion	Dimensional Analysis
$\dfrac{3\,mg}{4\,mg} \times 2\,mL$ $= \dfrac{6}{4} = 1.5\,mL$	**EXPRESSED AS TWO RATIOS** 2 mL : 4 mg :: x : 3 mg **EXPRESSED AS TWO FRACTIONS** $\dfrac{2\ mL}{4\ mg} \times \dfrac{x}{3\ mg}$ **SOLUTION FOR BOTH PROPORTION METHODS** $2 \times 3 = 4x$ $\dfrac{6}{4} = x$ $1.5\ mL = x$	$\dfrac{\overset{1}{2\,mL} \quad\bigg|\quad 3\,mg}{\underset{2}{4\,mg}}$ $= \dfrac{3}{2} = 1.5\,mL$

Administer 1.5 mL over at least 30 seconds or preferably over 2 to 5 minutes.

EXAMPLE

- Order: diphenhydramine (Benadryl) 25 mg IV q4h prn itching
- Supply: Read the label.

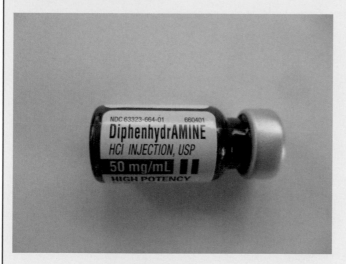

- Desired dose: 25 mg
- Supply: 1 mL
- Have: 50 mg in 1 mL

Formula Method	Proportion	Dimensional Analysis
$\dfrac{25\ \text{mg}}{50\ \text{mg}} \times 1\ \text{mL}$ $= 0.5\ \text{mL}$	**EXPRESSED AS TWO RATIOS** 1 mL : 50 mg :: x : 25 mg **EXPRESSED AS TWO FRACTIONS** $\dfrac{1\ \text{mL}}{50\ \text{mg}} \times \dfrac{x}{25\ \text{mg}}$ **SOLUTION FOR BOTH PROPORTION METHODS** $25 = 50x$ $\dfrac{25}{50} = x$ $0.5\ \text{mL} = x$	$\dfrac{1\ \text{mL} \quad \overset{1}{\cancel{25\ \text{mg}}}}{\underset{2}{\cancel{50\ \text{mg}}}}$ $= 1/2\ \text{or}\ 0.5\ \text{mL}$

May be further diluted in NS. Infuse 0.5 mL at a rate not to exceed 25 mg/minute.

EXAMPLE

- Order: metaclopromide (Reglan) 15 mg IV 30 minutes before meals and at bedtime.
- Supply: Read the label.

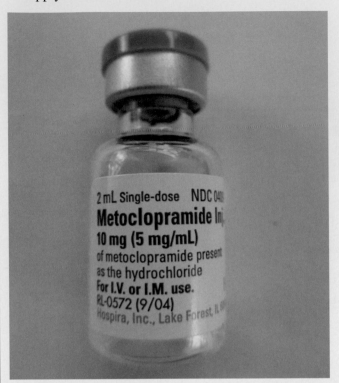

No equivalent is needed.

- Desired dose: 15 mg
- Supply: 1 mL
- Have: 5 mg/mL

Formula Method	Proportion	Dimensional Analysis
$\dfrac{15 \text{ mg}}{5 \text{ mg}} \times 1 \text{ mL}$ $= 3 \text{ mL}$	**EXPRESSED AS TWO RATIOS** $1 \text{ mL} : 5 \text{ mg} :: x : 15 \text{ mg}$ **EXPRESSED AS TWO FRACTIONS** $\dfrac{1 \text{ mL}}{5 \text{ mg}} \times \dfrac{x}{15 \text{ mg}}$ **SOLUTION FOR BOTH PROPORTION METHODS** $15 = 5x$ $\dfrac{15}{5} = x$ $3 \text{ mL} = x$	$\dfrac{1 \text{ mL}}{5 \text{ mg}} \Bigg| \dfrac{\overset{3}{15 \text{ mg}}}{} $ $= 3 \text{ mL}$

Give 3 mL slowly over 1 to 2 minutes.

SELF-TEST 1   Calculation of Liquids for Injection

Practice calculations of injections from a liquid. Report your answer in milliliters; mark the syringe in milliliters. Answers appear at the end of the chapter.

1. Order: clindamycin (Cleocin) 0.3 g IM q6h
   Supply: liquid in a vial labeled 300 mg/2 mL

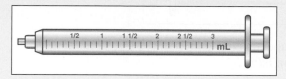

2. Order: morphine 12 mg IV stat
   Supply: vial of liquid labeled 15 mg/mL

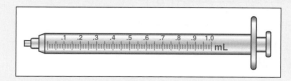

3. Order: vitamin B$_{12}$ 1 mg IM every day
   Supply: vial of liquid labeled 1000 mcg/mL

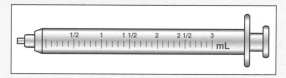

4. Order: gentamicin 9 mg IM q8h
   Supply: pediatric ampule labeled 20 mg/2 mL

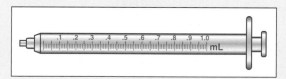

5. Order: gentamicin 50 mg IM q8h
   Supply: vial labeled 40 mg/mL

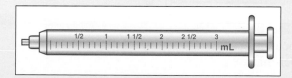

6. Order: phenobarbital 100 mg IM stat
   Supply: ampule labeled 130 mg/mL

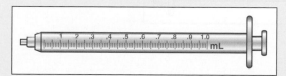

(continued)

7. Order: digoxin (Lanoxin) 0.125 mg IV stat
Supply: ampule labeled 0.5 mg/2 mL

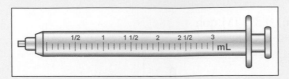

8. Order: heparin 6000 units subcutaneous q4h
Supply: vial labeled 10,000 units/mL

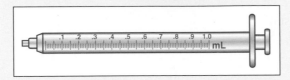

9. Order: terbutaline (Brethine) 0.25 mg subcutaneous
Supply: ampule labeled 1 mg/1 mL

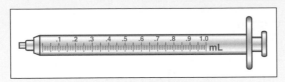

10. Order: labetalol (Normodyne) 20 mg IV stat
Supply: vial labeled 5 mg/mL

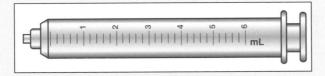

11. Order: haloperidol (Haldol) 2.5 mg IM q4–8h
Supply: vial labeled 5 mg/mL

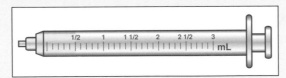

12. Order: methadone 3 mg subcutaneous now
Supply: vial labeled 10 mg per mL

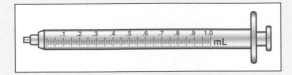

13. Order: amitriptyline (Endep) 0.025 g IM tid
     Supply: vial labeled 10 mg/mL

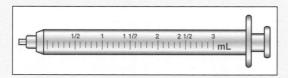

14. Order: chlorpromazine (Thorazine) 50 mg IM now
     Supply: vial labeled 25 mg/mL

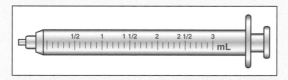

15. Order: dalteparin (Fragmin) 2500 units subcutaneous every day
     Supply: syringe labeled 5000 units in 0.2 mL

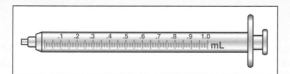

 # Special Types of Problems in Injections From a Liquid

When Supply Is a Ratio

Labels may state the strength of a drug as a ratio.

EXAMPLE

Adrenalin 1:1000

Ratios are always interpreted in the metric system as grams per milliliters. In the example given, 1:1000 means 1 g in 1000 mL. Ratios may be stated in three ways:

    1 g per 1000 mL

    1 g = 1000 mL

    1 g/1000 mL

Write the following ratios in three ways. Answers appear at the end of the chapter.

RATIO	*? g per ? mL*	*? g = ? mL*	*? g/? mL*
1:20			
2:15			

(continued)

SELF-TEST 2	Ratios (Continued)		
1:500	_____	_____	_____
2:2000	_____	_____	_____
1:4	_____	_____	_____
2:25	_____	_____	_____
4:50	_____	_____	_____
1:100	_____	_____	_____
3:75	_____	_____	_____
5:1000	_____	_____	_____

Figure 5-3 shows epinephrine that is labeled 30 mL and is a 1:1000 solution. 1:1000 means 1 g in 1000 mL. 1 g is equivalent to 1000 mg. Therefore, you can interpret the solution as 1000 mg = 1000 mL. If 1000 mL contains 1000 mg, then 1 mL contains 1 mg.

$$\frac{\cancel{1000}\ \text{mg}}{\cancel{1000}\ \text{mL}} = \frac{1\ \text{mg}}{1\ \text{mL}}$$

Since the ampule contains 30 mL, the ampule contains 30 mg of the drug. When reading and writing milligram (mg) and milliliter (mL), remember that milligram is the solid measure; milliliter is the liquid measure.

EXAMPLE

- Order: epinephrine 1 mg subcutaneous stat
- Supply: ampule labeled 1:1000
- Equivalent: 1:1000 means

  1 g in 1000 mL

  1 g = 1000 mg

Therefore, 1000 mL contains 1000 mg and 1 mL contains 1 mg.

- Desired dose: 1 mg
- Supply: 1000 mL
- Have: 1000 mg in 1000 mL

NDC 0517-1130-05
EPINEPHRINE
INJECTION, USP
1:1000 (1 mg/mL)

30 mL
MULTIPLE DOSE VIAL
FOR SC AND IM USE.
FOR IV AND IC USE AFTER
DILUTION.
Rx Only

AMERICAN
REGENT, INC.
SHIRLEY, NY 11967

Each mL contains: Epinephrine 1 mg (as the Hydrochloride), Water for Injection q.s. Sodium Chloride added for isotonicity, Chlorobutanol 0.5% as a preservative and Sodium Metabisulfite not more than 0.15% as an antioxidant. pH adjusted with Sodium Hydroxide and/or Hydrochloric Acid.
PROTECT FROM LIGHT.
Store at controlled room temperature up to 25°C (77°F) (See USP).
Directions for Use: See Package Insert.
Rev. 9/03

Lot / Exp.

FIGURE 5-3

Epinephrine 1:1000. (Courtesy of American Regent Laboratories, Inc.)

Formula Method	Proportion	Dimensional Analysis

Formula Method

$$\frac{1 \text{ mg}}{1000 \text{ mg}} \times \overset{1}{1000} \text{ mL} = 1 \text{ mL}$$

Proportion

EXPRESSED AS TWO RATIOS

1000 mL : 1000 mg : : x : 1 mg

EXPRESSED AS TWO FRACTIONS

$$\frac{1000 \text{ mL}}{1000 \text{ mg}} \times \frac{x}{1 \text{ mg}}$$

SOLUTION FOR BOTH PROPORTION METHODS

$$1000 = 1000x$$

$$\frac{1000}{1000} = x$$

$$1 \text{ mL} = x$$

Dimensional Analysis

$$\frac{\overset{1}{1000} \,\text{mL}}{1 \text{ g}} \left| \frac{1 \text{ mg}}{} \right| \frac{1 \text{ g}}{1000 \text{ mg}} = 1 \text{ mL}$$

Give 1 mL subcutaneously.

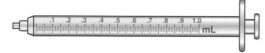

EXAMPLE

- Order: isoproterenol (Isuprel) HCl 0.2 mg IM stat
- Supply: ampule labeled 1:5000
- Equivalent: 1:5000 means

    1 g in 5000 mL
    1 g = 1000 mg

Therefore, 5000 mL contains 1000 mg.

- Desired dose: 0.2 mg
- Supply: 5000 mL
- Have: 1000 mg in 5000 mL

Formula Method	Proportion	Dimensional Analysis

Formula Method

$$\frac{0.2 \text{ mg}}{1000 \text{ mg}} \times \overset{5}{5000} \text{ mL}$$

$$= 0.2 \times 5 = 1 \text{ mL}$$

Proportion

EXPRESSED AS TWO RATIOS

5000 mL : 1000 mg : : x : 0.2 mg

EXPRESSED AS TWO FRACTIONS

$$\frac{5000 \text{ mL}}{1000 \text{ mg}} \times \frac{x}{0.2 \text{ mg}}$$

SOLUTION FOR BOTH PROPORTION METHODS

$$5000 \times 0.2 = 1000x$$

$$\frac{1000}{1000} = x$$

$$1 \text{ mL} = x$$

Dimensional Analysis

$$\frac{\overset{5}{5000} \,\text{mL}}{1 \text{ g}} \left| \frac{0.2 \text{ mg}}{} \right| \frac{1 \text{ g}}{1000 \text{ mg}} = 5 \times 0.2$$

$$= 1 \text{ mL}$$

Give 1 mL IM.

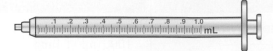

SELF-TEST 3 Using Ratios With Liquids for Injection

Solve these problems involving ratios. Answers appear at the end of the chapter.

1. Order: neostigmine 0.5 mg subcutaneous
Supply: ampule labeled 1:2000

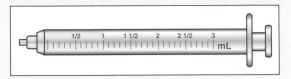

2. Order: isoproterenol (Isuprel) 1 mg: add to IV
Supply: vial labeled 1:5000

A 12-mL syringe is available.

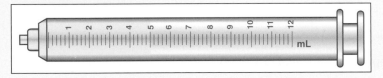

3. Order: neostigmine methylsulfate 0.75 mg subcutaneous
Supply: ampule labeled 1:1000

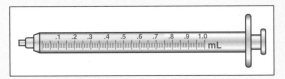

4. Order: epinephrine 0.5 mg subcutaneous stat
Supply: ampule labeled 1:1000

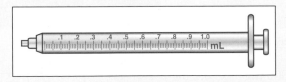

5. Order: neostigmine methylsulfate 1.5 mg IM tid
Supply: ampule labeled 1:2000

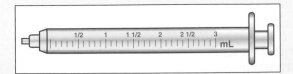

When Supply Is a Percent

Labels may state the strength of a drug as a percent. Percent means parts per hundred. *Percentages are always interpreted in the metric system as grams per 100 mL.*

EXAMPLE

Lidocaine 2% = 2 g in 100 mL

Percents may be stated in three ways:

    2 g per 100 mL

    2 g = 100 mL

    2 g/100 mL

SELF-TEST 4   Percentages

Write the following percentage in three ways. Answers appear at the end of the chapter.

PERCENTAGE	? g per 100 mL	? g = 100 mL	? g/100 mL
0.9%			
10%			
0.45%			
50%			
0.33%			
5%			
30%			
1.5%			
1%			
20%			

To solve percent problems, state the percent as the number of grams per mL. (In the following examples, do not include the total number of mL on the label in the dosage calculation.)

EXAMPLE

- Order: lidocaine 30 mg for injection before suturing wound
- Supply: Read the label.

NDC 0517-0626-25
LIDOCAINE HCl
INJECTION, USP
2%
20 mg/mL

50 mL   MULITPLE DOSE VIAL
FOR INFILTRATION AND NERVE BLOCK
NOT FOR EPIDURAL OR CAUDAL USE
Rx Only
AMERICAN
REGENT, INC.
SHIRLEY, NY 11967

Each mL contains: Lidocaine HCl
20 mg, Sodium Chloride 4.6 mg,
Methylparaben 1 mg, Water for
Injection q.s. pH (range 5.0-7.0)
adjusted with Sodium Hydroxide
and/or Hydrochloric Acid.
**WARNING: CONTAINS A
PRESERVATIVE.**
Store at controlled room
temperature 15°-30°C (59°-86°F)
(See USP). Directions for Use: See
Package Insert.
Rev. 1/03

Lot / Exp.

(Courtesy of American Regent
Laboratories, Inc.)

- Equivalent: 2% means

    2 g in 100 mL

    1 g = 1000 mg

    2 g = 2000 mg

Therefore, 100 mL contains 2000 mg.

- Desired dose: 30 mg
- Supply: 100 mL
- Have: 2000 mg in 100 mL

Formula Method	Proportion	Dimensional Analysis

Formula Method

$$\frac{30 \text{ mg}}{2000 \text{ mg}} \times \overset{1}{100} \text{ mL}$$

$$= \frac{3}{2} \text{ mL} = 1.5 \text{ mL}$$

Proportion

EXPRESSED AS TWO RATIOS

100 mL : 2000 mg : : x : 30 mg

EXPRESSED AS TWO FRACTIONS

$$\frac{100 \text{ mL}}{2000 \text{ mg}} \times \frac{x}{30 \text{ mg}}$$

**SOLUTION FOR BOTH
PROPORTION METHODS**

$$100 \times 30 = 2000x$$

$$\frac{3000}{2000} = x$$

$$1.5 \text{ mL} = x$$

Dimensional Analysis

Use conversion factor 1 g/1000 mg:

$$\frac{\overset{1}{100} \text{ (mL)}}{2 \text{ g}} \left| \frac{\overset{3}{30} \text{ mg}}{} \right| \frac{1 \text{ g}}{\underset{\underset{1}{10}}{1000} \text{ mg}} = \frac{3}{2} = 1.5 \text{ mL}$$

Prepare 1.5 mL or 1½ mL.

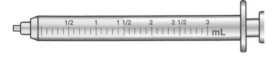

EXAMPLE

- Order: magnesium sulfate 1 g; add to IV stat
- Supply: Read the label.

NDC 0517-2602-25
MAGNESIUM SULFATE
INJECTION, USP
50% (0.5 g/mL)
1 gram/2 mL
(4.06 mEq/mL Magnesium)

2 mL SINGLE DOSE VIAL
FOR IM USE. FOR IV
USE AFTER DILUTION
Rx Only

AMERICAN REGENT, INC.
SHIRLEY, NY 11967

4.06 mOsmol/mL
Contains no more than
12,500 mcg/L of aluminum.
DISCARD UNUSED PORTION.
Store at controlled room temperature
15°-30°C (59°-86°F) (See USP).
Directions for Use: See Package Insert.
Rev. 1/03

Lot / Exp.

(Courtesy of American Regent Laboratories, Inc.)

- Equivalent: 50% means 50 g in 100 mL
- Desired dose: 1 g
- Supply: 100 mL
- Have: 50 g in 100 mL

Formula Method	Proportion	Dimensional Analysis

Formula Method

$$\frac{1 \text{ g}}{\overset{}{\underset{1}{50 \text{ g}}}} \times \overset{2}{100} \text{ mL} = 2 \text{ mL}$$

Proportion

EXPRESSED AS TWO RATIOS

$$100 \text{ mL} : 50 \text{ g} :: x : 1 \text{ g}$$

EXPRESSED AS TWO FRACTIONS

$$\frac{100 \text{ mL}}{50 \text{ g}} \times \frac{x}{1 \text{ g}}$$

SOLUTION FOR BOTH PROPORTION METHODS

$$100 = 50x$$
$$\frac{100}{50} = x$$
$$2 \text{ mL} = x$$

Dimensional Analysis

$$\frac{\overset{2}{100} \text{ mL}}{\underset{1}{50 \text{ g}}} \left| \frac{1 \text{ g}}{} \right. = 2 \text{ mL}$$

Add 2 mL to IV

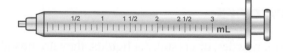

Solve these problems involving percentages. Answers appear at the end of the chapter. Answers are in milliliters (mL).

1. Order: epinephrine 5 mg subcutaneous stat
   Supply: ampule labeled 1%

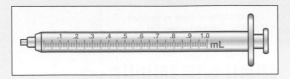

2. Order: lidocaine 15 mg subcutaneous
   Supply: ampule labeled 1%

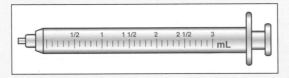

3. Order: phenylephrine HCl (Neo-Synephrine) 3 mg subcutaneous stat
   Supply: ampule labeled 1%

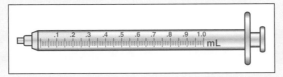

4. Order: Prepare for IV use calcium gluconate 0.3 g
   Supply: ampule labeled 10%

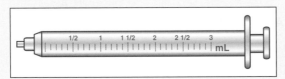

5. Order: dextrose 5 g IV × 1
   Supply: syringe labeled 50%

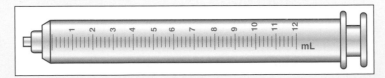

Injections From Powders

Some medications are prepared in a dry form, powder, or crystal. As liquids, they are unstable and lose potency over time. The drug must be reconstituted according to the manufacturer's directions, which will give the type and amount of diluent to use. Most drugs are premixed, and reconstitution is rare. However, in some hospitals and other healthcare settings, the pharmacy is responsible for reconstituting medications. Sometimes, this task becomes your responsibility as a nurse; that's why this book includes these kinds of dosage calculations. Many drugs are reconstituted using a special reconstitution device within an IV bag. (See Chapter 6 for more information.)

To solve injection-from-powder problems, you use the same rule as for oral medications and for injection from a liquid. This is because once the powder is dissolved, the powdered drug takes liquid form.

Formula Method	Proportion	Dimensional Analysis
$\dfrac{\text{Desire}}{\text{Have}} \times \text{Supply} = \text{Amount}$	**EXPRESSED AS TWO RATIOS** Supply : Desire : : x : Have **EXPRESSED AS TWO FRACTIONS** $\dfrac{x}{\text{Desire}} = \dfrac{\text{Supply}}{\text{Have}}$	$\dfrac{\text{Supply}}{\text{Have}} \Big| \text{Desired Dose}$

equivalent to
1gram *cefonicid*
NDC 0007-4353-01

EXP.

MONOCID®
STERILE CEFONICID
SODIUM
(LYOPHILIZED)

LOT

For IV or IM use

NSN 6505-01-189-4698
Before reconstitution protect from light and refrigerate (2° to 8°C). **Usual Adult Dose:** 1 gram every 24 hours as a single dose. See accompanying prescribing information. **For IV Infusion:** See prescribing information. **For IM or IV Direct (Bolus) Injection:** Add 2.5 mL Sterile Water for Injection. Shake Well. Provides an approximate volume of 3.1 mL(325 mg/mL). Properly reconstituted solutions of *Monocid* are stable 24 hours at room temperature or 72 hours if refrigerated (5°C). **Caution:** Federal law prohibits dispensing without prescription.
Glaxo SmithKline Pharmaceuticals
Philadelphia, PA 19101
694021-J

FIGURE 5-4

Label of cefonicid sodium (Monocid). (Courtesy of GlaxoSmithKline Pharmaceuticals.)

EXAMPLE

- Order: cefonicid sodium (Monocid) 0.65 g IM every day (Fig. 5-4).

- Label directions: Add 2.5 mL sterile water for injection. Shake well. Provides an approximate volume of 3.1 mL (325 mg/mL). Stable 24 hours at room temperature or 72 hours if refrigerated (5°C).

- Equivalent: 0.65 g = 650 mg

- Desire: The order in the example is 0.65 g.

- Supply: The fluid portion of the solution made. In this example, it is 1 mL = 325 mg.

- Have: The strength of the drug supplied. The example is 1 g as a dry powder; when reconstituted, it is 325 mg/mL. Remember that the manufacturer gives the strength of the solution; you do not have to determine it.

- Answer: How much liquid to give, stated as mL.

Formula Method	Proportion	Dimensional Analysis

Formula Method

$$\frac{\overset{2}{\cancel{650}} \text{ mg}}{\underset{1}{\cancel{325}} \text{ mg}} \times 1 \text{ mL} = 2 \text{ mL}$$

Proportion

EXPRESSED AS TWO RATIOS

$$1 \text{ mL} : 325 \text{ mg} : : x \text{ mL} : 650 \text{ mg}$$

EXPRESSED AS TWO FRACTIONS

$$\frac{1 \text{ mL}}{325 \text{ mg}} \times \frac{x}{650 \text{ mg}}$$

SOLUTION FOR BOTH PROPORTION METHODS

$$650 = 325x$$
$$\frac{650}{325} = x$$
$$2 \text{ mL} = x$$

Dimensional Analysis

Use conversion factor 1000 mg/1 g:

$$\frac{1 \, \textcircled{mL}}{\underset{65}{\cancel{325} \text{ mg}}} \left| \frac{\overset{0.13}{\cancel{0.65} \text{ g}}}{} \right| \frac{1000 \text{ mg}}{1 \text{ g}} = \frac{0.13 \times 1000}{65}$$

$$= \frac{130}{65} = 2 \text{ mL}$$

Give 2 mL. Store the remaining solution in the refrigerator. Label the vial with the solution made (325 mg/mL), the date and time solution reconstituted, initial of the nurse who dissolve the powder, and the expiration date.

325 mg/mL
10/15/12 1600
SB
Expires 10/18/12

Distinctive Features of Injections From Powders

Aseptic technique is used to prepare and administer the medication, which is given parenterally (usually IM, IV, or intravenous piggyback [IVPB]). The dry drug is supplied in vials of powder or crystals and may come in different strengths. Because powders deteriorate in solution, choose the strength closest to the amount ordered. The powder is usually diluted with one of the following:

Sterile water for injection

Bacteriostatic water for injection with a preservative added

Normal saline for injection (0.9% sodium chloride)

Directions will state which fluids may be used. Read this information carefully, because some fluids may be incompatible (i.e., unsuitable) as diluents. When the powder goes into solution, *displacement* occurs. This means that as the powder dissolves, it increases the volume added to the vial. There is no uniformity in the way powders go into solution.

Refer to the label in Figure 5-4 again. The manufacturer tells the nurse to add 2.5 mL of sterile water to provide an approximate volume of 3.1 mL. In this example, 0.6 mL is the displacement volume. *Injections-from-powder problems are solved by using the solution made, not the displacement volume.* The manufacturer will give the solution.

Where to Find Information About Reconstitution of Powders

Information about reconstitution of powders may be found from the following:

- The label on the vial of powder

- The package insert that comes with the vial of powder

- Nursing drug handbooks

- Other references such as the *Physicians' Desk Reference (PDR)*

STEPS FOR RECONSTITUTING POWDERS WITH DIRECTIONS

1. Read the order.
2. Identify the supply and directions for dilution.
3. Dilute the fluid.
4. Identify the solution and new supply.
5. Calculate the amount to give and prepare the amount.
6. Write on the label the solution made, date, time, your initials, and expiration date.
7. Store according to directions.

EXAMPLE

The package insert information concerning the dilution of cefoperazone (Cefobid) injection is reproduced in Figure 5-5. Examine the directions with the intention of solving the following problem, then read the explanation:

- Order: cefoperazone (Cefobid) 0.5 g IM q12h

- Supply: 1-g vial of powder

Search the directions for three pieces of information to dissolve your supply, which is 1 g:

1. Type of fluid needed to dissolve the powder

2. Amount of fluid to add

3. Solution made

RECONSTITUTION

The following solutions may be used for the initial reconstitution of CEFOBID sterile powder:

Table 1. Solutions for Initial Reconstitution

5% Dextrose Injection (USP)	0.9% Sodium Chloride Injection (USP)
5% Dextrose and 0.9% Sodium Chloride Injection (USP)	Normosol® M and Dextrose Injection
5% Dextrose and 0.2% Sodium Chloride Injection (USP)	Normosol® R
10% Dextrose Injection (USP)	Sterile Water for Injection*
Bacteriostatic Water for Injection [Benzyl Alcohol or Parabens] (USP)*†	

* Not to be used as a vehicle for intravenous infusion.
† Preparation containing Benzyl Alcohol should not be used in neonates.

Preparation for Intramuscular Injection

Any suitable solution listed above may be used to prepare CEFOBID sterile powder for intramuscular injection. When concentrations of 250 mg/ml or more are to be administered, a lidocaine solution should be used. These solutions should be prepared using a combination of Sterile Water for Injection and 2% Lidocaine Hydrochloride Injection (USP) that approximates a 0.5% Lidocaine Hydrochloride Solution. A two-step dilution process as follows is recommended: First, add the required amount of Sterile Water for Injection and agitate until CEFOBID powder is completely dissolved. Second, add the required amount of 2% lidocaine and mix.

	Final Cefoperazone Concentration	Step 1 Volume of Sterile Water	Step 2 Volume of 2% Lidocaine	Withdrawable Volume*†
1 g vial	333 mg/ml	2.0 ml	0.6 ml	3 ml
	250 mg/ml	2.8 ml	1.0 ml	4 ml
2 g vial	333 mg/ml	3.8 ml	1.2 ml	6 ml
	250 mg/ml	5.4 ml	1.8 ml	8 ml

When a diluent other than Lidocaine HCl Injection (USP) is used reconstitute as follows:

	Cefoperazone Concentration	Volume of Diluent to be Added	Withdrawable Volume*
1 g vial	333 mg/ml	2.6 ml	3 ml
	250 mg/ml	3.8 ml	4 ml
2 g vial	333 mg/ml	5.0 ml	6 ml
	250 mg/ml	7.2 ml	8 ml

* There is sufficient excess present to allow for withdrawal of the stated volume.
† Final lidocaine concentration will approximate that obtained if a 0.5% Lidocaine Hydrochloride Solution is used as diluent.

STORAGE AND STABILITY

CEFOBID sterile powder is to be stored at or below 25°C (77°F) and protected from light prior to reconstitution. After reconstitution, protection from light is not necessary.

The following parenteral diluents and approximate concentrations of CEFOBID provide stable solutions under the following conditions for the indicated time periods. (After the indicated time periods, unused portions of solutions should be discarded.)

Controlled Room Temperature (15ϒ–25ϒC/59ϒ–77ϒF)

24 Hours — Approximate

Bacteriostatic Water for Injection [Benzyl Alcohol or Parabens] (USP)	300 mg/ml
5% Dextrose Injection (USP)	2 mg to 50 mg/ml
5% Dextrose and Lactated Ringer's Injection	2 mg to 50 mg/ml
5% Dextrose and 0.9% Sodium Chloride Injection (USP)	2 mg to 50 mg/ml
5% Dextrose and 0.2% Sodium Chloride Injection (USP)	2 mg to 50 mg/ml
10% Dextrose Injection (USP)	2 mg to 50 mg/ml
Lactated Ringer's Injection (USP)	2 mg/ml
0.5% Lidocaine Hydrochloride Injection (USP)	300 mg/ml
0.9% Sodium Chloride Injection (USP)	2 mg to 300 mg/ml
Normosol® M and 5% Dextrose Injection	2 mg to 50 mg/ml
Normosol® R	2 mg to 50 mg/ml
Sterile Water for Injection	300 mg/ml

Reconstituted CEFOBID solutions may be stored in glass or plastic syringes, or in glass or flexible plastic parenteral solution containers.

Refrigerator Temperature (2ϒ–8ϒC/36ϒ–46ϒF)

5 Days — Approximate Concentrations

Bacteriostatic Water for Injection [Benzyl Alcohol or Parabens] (USP)	300 mg/ml
5% Dextrose Injection (USP)	2 mg to 50 mg/ml
5% Dextrose and 0.9% Sodium Chloride Injection (USP)	2 mg to 50 mg/ml
5% Dextrose and 0.2% Sodium Chloride Injection (USP)	2 mg to 50 mg/ml
Lactated Ringer's Injection (USP)	2 mg/ml
0.5% Lidocaine Hydrochloride Injection (USP)	300 mg/ml
0.9% Sodium Chloride Injection (USP)	2 mg to 300 mg/ml
Normosol® M and 5% Dextrose Injection	2 mg to 50 mg/ml
Normosol® R	2 mg to 50 mg/ml
Sterile Water for Injection	300 mg/ml

Reconstituted CEFOBID solutions may be stored in glass or plastic syringes, or in glass or flexible plastic parenteral solution containers.

FIGURE 5-5

Reconstitution directions for cefoperazone (Cefobid). (Courtesy of Pfizer Laboratories.)

Explanation

1. Figure 5-5 gives *Solutions for Initial Reconstitution:* sterile water for injection, bacteriostatic water for injection, and 0.9% sodium chloride injection. Choose one.

2. The heading *Preparation for Intramuscular Injection* states that when a concentration of 250 mg or more is to be administered, a 2% lidocaine solution should be used together with sterile water for injection in a two-step dilution.

3. Two tables are given. The upper table has the two-step dilution; the lower one does not. Because the order requires two steps, use the directions in the top table.

4. Two strengths of powder are listed in the upper table. Look at the extreme left. They are for a 1-g vial and a 2-g vial. Our supply is a 1-g vial. Follow directions for 1 g.

5. The next heading is *Final Cefoperazone Concentration.* Two possibilities are given for the dilution: 333 mg/mL and 250 mg/mL. Because the order calls for 0.5 g, choose 250 mg/mL. Since 0.5 grams = 500 mg, you will need 2 mL of solution.

6. To make the solution of 250 mg/mL, add the following: 2.8 mL sterile water and 1.0 mL 2% lidocaine.

7. The last column on the right, headed *Withdrawable Volume,* lists 4 mL. Ignore this column; it does not affect the answer. When you add 2.8 mL and 1.0 mL, you expect to have 3.8 mL. However, the package insert states that you will end up with 4 mL. The manufacturer is giving the displacement.

8. You now have all of the information needed to prepare the dose ordered. Your solution is 250 mg/mL. Equivalent: 0.5 g = 500 mg.

Formula Method	Proportion	Dimensional Analysis
$$\dfrac{\overset{2}{\cancel{500}}\text{ mg}}{\underset{1}{\cancel{250}}\text{ mg}} \times 1\text{ mL} = 2\text{ mL}$$	**EXPRESSED AS TWO RATIOS** $$1\text{ mL} : 250\text{ mg} :: x : 500\text{ mg}$$ **EXPRESSED AS TWO FRACTIONS** $$\dfrac{1\text{ mL}}{250\text{ mg}} \times \dfrac{x}{500\text{ mg}}$$ **SOLUTION FOR BOTH PROPORTION METHODS** $$500 = 250x$$ $$\dfrac{500}{250} = x$$ $$2\text{ mL} = x$$	Use conversion factor 1000 mg/1 g: $$\dfrac{1\,\cancel{\text{mL}}}{\underset{1}{\cancel{250}}\text{ mg}} \left| 0.5\,\cancel{\text{g}} \right| \dfrac{\overset{4}{\cancel{1000}}\text{ mg}}{1\,\cancel{\text{g}}} = 2\text{ mL}$$

Give 2 mL IM.

9. Write on the label the solution you made, the date, time, your initials, and expiration date.

10. Note the storage directions and stability expiration.

EXAMPLE

- Order: cefazolin (Ancef) 0.3 g IM (Fig. 5-6)

- Supply: 500 mg powder

- Diluting fluid: 2.0 mL sterile water for injection

- Solution and new supply: 225 mg/mL

- Equivalent: 0.3 g = 300 mg

- Desired dose: 300 mg

- Supply: 1 mL

- Have: 225 mg in 1 mL

RECONSTITUTION

Preparation of Parenteral Solution

Parenteral drug products should be SHAKEN WELL when reconstituted, and inspected visually for particulate matter prior to administration. If particulate matter is evident in reconstituted fluids, the drug solutions should be discarded. When reconstituted or diluted according to the instructions below, Ancef (sterile cefazolin sodium, SK&F) is stable for 24 hours at room temperature or for 96 hours if stored under refrigeration. Reconstituted solutions may range in color from pale yellow to yellow without a change in potency.

Single-Dose Vials

For I.M. injection, I.V. direct (bolus) injection, or I.V. infusion, reconstitute with Sterile Water for Injection according to the following table. SHAKE WELL.

Vial Size	Amount of Diluent	Approximate Concentration	Approximate Available Volume
250 mg.	2.0 ml.	125 mg./ml.	2.0 ml.
500 mg.	2.0 ml.	225 mg./ml.	2.2 ml.
1 gram	2.5 ml.	330 mg./ml.	3.0 ml.

FIGURE 5-6

Reconstitution directions for cefazolin (Ancef). (Courtesy of GlaxoSmithKline.)

Formula Method	Proportion	Dimensional Analysis

Formula Method

Equivalent: 0.3 g = 300 mg

$$\frac{\overset{4}{\underset{12}{\cancel{300}}} \text{ mg}}{\underset{9}{\overset{3}{\cancel{225}}} \text{ mg}} \times 1 \text{ mL} = \frac{4}{3} \text{ mL}$$

$$= 1.33 \text{ or } 1.3 \text{ mL}$$

Proportion

EXPRESSED AS TWO RATIOS

$$1 \text{ mL} : 225 \text{ mg} :: x \text{ mL} : 300 \text{ mg}$$

EXPRESSED AS TWO FRACTIONS

$$\frac{1 \text{ mL}}{225 \text{ mg}} \times \frac{x \text{ mL}}{300 \text{ mg}}$$

SOLUTION FOR BOTH PROPORTION METHODS

$$300 = 225x$$

$$\frac{300}{225} = x$$

$$1.33 \text{ or } 1.3 \text{ mL} = x$$

Dimensional Analysis

Use conversion factor 1000 mg/1 g:

$$\frac{1 \;\cancel{\text{mL}}}{\underset{9}{\cancel{225}} \; \cancel{\text{mg}}} \left| 0.3 \; \cancel{\text{g}} \right| \frac{\overset{40}{\cancel{1000}} \; \cancel{\text{mg}}}{1 \; \cancel{\text{g}}} = \frac{40 \times 0.3}{9}$$

$$= \frac{12}{9} = 1.33 \text{ or } 1.3 \text{ mL}$$

Give 1.3 mL IM.

Write on label: 225 mg/mL, date, time, initials, expiration date.

Storage: Refrigerate; stable for 96 hours.

EXAMPLE

- Order: penicillin G potassium 1 million units IM q6h (Fig. 5-7)
- Supply powder: 5 million unit vial
- Diluting fluid and number of milliliters: Use sterile water for injection. See Figure 5-7.
  - Choose 3 mL to dilute the powder, therefore:
  - Solution and new supply: 1 million units/mL.
- Desired dose: 1 million units
- Supply: 1 mL
- Have: 1 million units in 1 mL

PENICILLIN G POTASSIUM for injection
Preparation of Solutions
Use sterile water for injection
    RECONSTITUTION
1,000,000 u vial

Diluent	Desired Concentration
9.6 ml	100,000 u/ml
4.6 ml	200,000 u/ml
3.6 ml	250,000 u/ml

5,000,000 u vial

Diluent	Desired Concentration
23 ml	200,000 u/ml
18 ml	250,000 u/ml
8 ml	500,000 u/ml
3 ml	1,000,000 u/ml

Storage
Prepared solutions may be kept in the refrigerator one week.

FIGURE 5-7

Preparation of solution for the 1,000,000-unit and the 5,000,000-unit vials of penicillin G potassium.

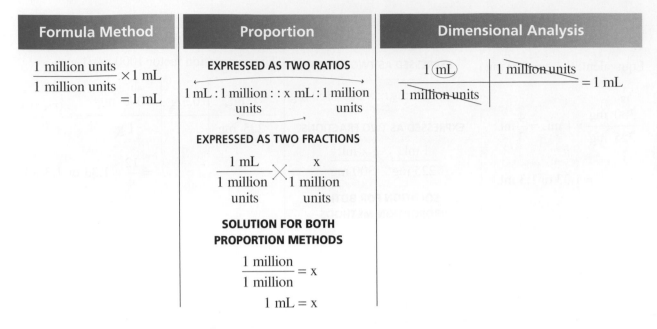

Formula Method	Proportion	Dimensional Analysis

Give 1 mL IM.

Write on label: 1 million units/mL, date, time, initials, expiration date

Storage: Refrigerate; stable for 1 week

Note: This solution (1 million units/mL) may be so concentrated that it is painful when injected. To make a less painful solution, you can dilute the powder with 8 mL to make 500,000 units/mL and give 2 mL to the patient/client.

Here are a few tips before you begin Self-Test 6.

- When reading the directions for reconstitution, look first at the solutions you can make. Think the problem through mentally and choose one dilution so that you will have a focus as you read.

- If your answer is more than 3 mL for an IM injection, consider using two syringes and injecting in two different sites.

- Experience in administering injections will guide you in choosing the solution's concentration. Stronger concentrations, although smaller in volume, may be more painful; a more dilute solution may be more suitable despite its larger volume.

- Each powder problem is unique. Carefully read the directions.

- Choose one diluting fluid for injection: generally, sterile water or 0.9% sodium chloride. You do not need to list all of the fluids in your answer.

- For the following self-tests, assume that the doses ordered and the order are correct. Chapter 9 discusses the nurse's responsibilities in drug knowledge. Dosages for infants and children are discussed in Chapter 8.

SELF-TEST 6	Injections From Powders

Solve the following problems in injections from powders and write your answers using the steps. Answers appear at the end of the chapter. Round to the nearest tenths place.

1. Order: ceftazidime (Ceptaz) 1 g IM q6h (Fig. 5-8)
   Supply: 1 g powder

   a. Diluting fluid and number of milliliters:
   b. Solution and new supply:
   c. Desired dose (and equivalent if necessary):
   d. Answer:
   e. Write on label:
   f. Storage:

CEFTAZIDIME INJECTION

Reconstitution
Single dose vials: Reconstitute with sterile water. Shake well.

Vial Size	Diluent	Approx. Avail. Volume	Approx. Avg. Concentration
IM or IV bolus injection			
1 gram	3.0 mL	3.6 mL	280 mg/mL
IV infusion			
1 gram	10 mL	10.6 mL	95 mg/mL
2 gram	10 mL	11.2 mL	180 mg/mL

Stable for 18 hours at room temperature or seven days if refrigerated.

FIGURE 5-8

Label and reconstitution directions for ceftazidime (Ceptaz).

2. Order: ampicillin sodium (Omnipen) 250 mg IM q6h (Fig. 5-9)
   Supply: 500-mg vial of powder

   a. Diluting fluid and number of milliliters:
   b. Solution and new supply:
   c. Desired dose (and equivalent if necessary):
   d. Answer:
   e. Write on label:
   f. Storage:

AMPICILLIN
Reconstitution
Dissolve contents of a vial with the amount of Sterile Water or Bacteriostatic Water.

Amount Ordered	Recommended Amount of Diluent	Withdraw Volume	Concentration in mg/ml
500 mg	1.8 ml	2.0 ml	250 mg
1.0 Gram	3.4 ml	4.0 ml	250 mg
2.0 gram	6.8 ml	8.0 ml	250 mg

Storage
Use within one hour of reconstitution.

FIGURE 5-9

Reconstitution directions for ampicillin sodium (Omnipen) for IM or IV injection.

(continued)

3. Order: cefazolin sodium (Ancef) 225 mg IM q6h (Fig. 5-10)
    Supply: On the shelf, there are three vial sizes of powder: 250 mg, 500 mg, and 1 g.

   a. Supply chosen:
   b. Diluting fluid and number of milliliters:
   c. Solution and new supply:
   d. Desired dose (and equivalent if necessary):
   e. Answer:
   f. Write on label:
   g. Storage:

RECONSTITUTION

Preparation of Parenteral Solution

Parenteral drug products should be SHAKEN WELL when reconstituted, and inspected visually for particulate matter prior to administration. If particulate matter is evident in reconstituted fluids, the drug solutions should be discarded. When reconstituted or diluted according to the instructions below, Ancef (sterile cefazolin sodium, SK&F) is stable for 24 hours at room temperature or for 96 hours if stored under refrigeration. Reconstituted solutions may range in color from pale yellow to yellow without a change in potency.

Single-Dose Vials

For I.M. injection, I.V. direct (bolus) injection, or I.V. infusion, reconstitute with Sterile Water for Injection according to the following table. SHAKE WELL.

Vial Size	Amount of Diluent	Approximate Concentration	Approximate Available Volume
250 mg.	2.0 ml.	125 mg./ml.	2.0 ml.
500 mg.	2.0 ml.	225 mg./ml.	2.2 ml.
1 gram	2.5 ml.	330 mg./ml.	3.0 ml.

FIGURE 5-10

Reconstitution directions for cefazolin sodium (Ancef). (Courtesy of GlaxoSmithKline.)

4. Order: ceftazidime (Fortaz) 500 mg IM q6h (Fig. 5-11)
   Supply: 1 g powder

  a. Diluting fluid and number of milliliters:
  b. Solution and new supply:
  c. Desired dose (and equivalent if necessary):
  d. Answer:
  e. Write on label:
  f. Storage:

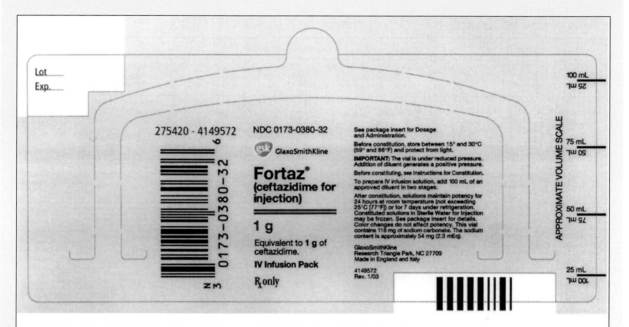

Table 5: Preparation of Fortaz Solutions		
Size	Amount of Diluent to Be Added (mL)	Approximate Available Volume (mL)	Approximate Ceftazidime Concentration (mg/mL)
Intramuscular			
500-mg vial	1.5	1.8	280
1-gram vial	3.0	3.6	280
Intravenous			
500-mg vial	5.0	5.3	100
1-gram vial	10.0	10.6	100
2-gram vial	10.0	11.5	170
Infusion pack			
1-gram vial	100*	100	10
2-gram vial	100*	100	20
Pharmacy bulk package			
6-gram vial	26	30	200

* **Note:** Addition should be in two stages (see Instructions for Constitution).

COMPATIBILITY AND STABILITY:
Intramuscular: Fortaz®, when constituted as directed with sterile water for injection, bacteriostatic water for injection, or 0.5% or 1% lidocaine hydrochloride injection, maintains satisfactory potency for 24 hours at room temperature or for 7 days under refrigeration. Solutions in sterile water for injection that are frozen immediately after constitution in the original container are stable for 3 months when stored at -20°C. Once thawed, solutions should not be refrozen. thawed solutions may be stored for up to 8 hours at room temperature or for 4 days in a refrigerator.

FIGURE 5-11

Preparation of ceftazidime (Fortaz) solutions. (Reproduced with permission of GlaxoSmithKline.)

(continued)

| SELF-TEST 6 | Injections From Powders (Continued) |

5. Order: cefoxitin sodium (Mefoxin) 200 mg IM q4h
Supply: vial of powder labeled 1 g

Refer to Figure 5-12.

a. Diluting fluid and number of milliliters:
b. Solution made and new supply:
c. Desired dose (and equivalent if necessary):
d. Answer:
e. Write on label:
f. Storage:

Table 3 — Preparation of Solution			
Strength	Amount of Diluent to be Added (mL) + +	Approximate Withdrawable Volume (mL)	Approximate Average Concentration (mg/mL)
1 gram Vial	2 (Intramuscular)	2.5	400
2 gram Vial	4 (Intramuscular)	5	400
1 gram Vial	10 (IV)	10.5	95
2 gram Vial	10 or 20 (IV)	11.1 or 21.0	180 or 95
1 gram Infusion Bottle	50 or 100 (IV)	50 or 100	20 or 10
2 gram Infusion Bottle	50 or 100 (IV)	50 or 100	40 or 20
10 gram Bulk	43 or 93 (IV)	49 or 98.5	200 or 100

+ + Shake to dissolve and let stand until clear.

Intramuscular
MEFOXIN, as constituted with Sterile Water for Injection, Bacteriostatic Water for Injection, or 0.5 percent or 1 percent lidocaine hydrochloride solution (without epinephrine), maintains satisfactory potency for 24 hours at room temperature, for one week under refrigeration (below 5°C), and for at least 30 weeks in the frozen state.

FIGURE 5-12

Directions to reconstitute cefoxitin sodium (Mefoxin). (Courtesy of Merck Co. Inc.)

Insulin Injections

Types of Insulin

Insulin is a hormone that regulates glucose metabolism. It is measured in units and is administered by injection. Insulin is supplied in 10-mL vials containing 100 units/mL. Several types of insulin are available: those prepared from animal tissue, or semisynthetically, or synthetically using recombinant DNA.

Insulin cannot be given orally because enzymes in the gastrointestinal tract destroy it. Instead, insulins are administered subcutaneously—except for regular insulin, which can be given either subcutaneously or intravenously. An insulin nasal spray is being developed (search the Internet for the latest news—it is still experimental as of this edition) as well as an insulin patch that will continuously deliver a low dose of insulin through the skin.

Insulins are classified as rapid, intermediate, or long acting. Because onset of action, time of peak activity, and duration of action vary, nurses must be careful to choose and calculate the correct insulin. Table 5-1 summarizes the onset, peak, and duration of various insulins. (Times may vary slightly according to hospital/institutional policies.)

TABLE 5-1 Onset, Peak, and Duration of Different Types of Insulin			
Type	Onset	Peak	Duration
Humalog	5 min	1 h	2–4 h
Regular	1 h	2–4 h	5–7 h
NPH or Lente	1–2.5 h	6–12 h	18–24 h
Ultralente	4–8 h	12–20 h	24–48 h
Mixed insulins	30–60 min, then 1–2 h	2–4 h, then 6–12 h	6–8 h, then 18–24 h
Lantus	1 h	None	24 h

Most hospitals and other institutions require that two licensed nurses double-check the type and amount of insulin prepared. Know the policy of your institution and follow it.

RAPID-ACTING INSULINS. Lispro (Humalog) is the newest human insulin product made by recombinant DNA technology. Like regular insulin, it lowers blood sugar, but much more rapidly.

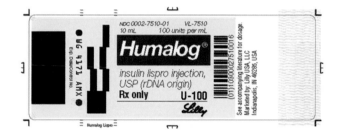

(Courtesy of Eli Lilly Co.)

SHORT-ACTING INSULINS. A large "R" on the label immediately tells you that this is *regular* insulin. Most insulin used clinically is human insulin, Humulin, which is synthesized in the laboratory using recombinant DNA technology. Pork insulin, made from the porcine pancreas, is occasionally used for patients/clients.

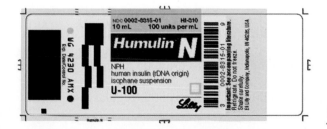

(Courtesy of Eli Lilly Co.)

INTERMEDIATE-ACTING INSULINS. On the label, the letters "N" or "L" or the term *isophane* indicate that regular insulin has been modified, through the addition of zinc and protamine (a basic protein), to delay absorption and prolong the time of action. These intermediate insulins (Humulin N or Humulin L) can be prepared from either pork or Humulin R. The label below may also show the letters "NPH," which denote intermediate action: N means the solution is neutral pH; P indicates the protamine content; and H stands for Hagedorn, the laboratory that first prepared this type of insulin.

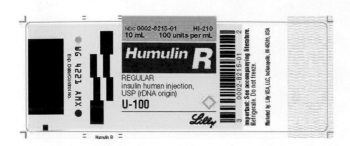

HUMULIN **L**

Lente human insulin (DNA origin)
100 units/mL
10 mL

(Courtesy of Eli Lilly Co.)

LONG-ACTING INSULINS. Lantus insulin is a newer agent that is given subcutaneously and must not be mixed with other insulins. A long duration makes it similar to normal insulin secretion.

Humulin Ultralente is an example of a long-acting insulin. Like the intermediate-acting insulins, long-acting insulins these have been modified with the addition of zinc and protamine. Humulin U or Ultralente is an example of a long-acting insulin.

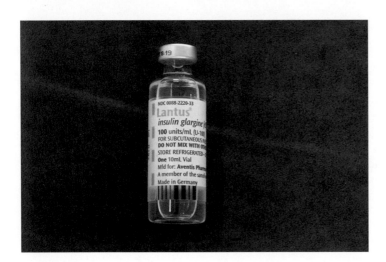

MIXED INSULINS. An order may require that you mix two insulins in one syringe and administer them together. Mixed insulins combine rapid and intermediate insulin. They save nursing time in preparation and are also more convenient for the patient/client, who must learn to draw up and self-administer an injection.

Besides Humulin 70/30 (see illustration), there is also a 50/50 insulin that is 50% regular insulin and 50% NPH.

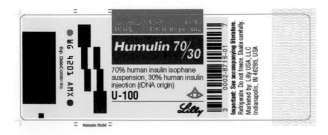

(Courtesy of Eli Lilly Co.)

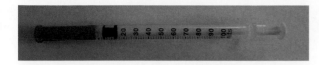

FIGURE 5-13

1-mL syringe marked in units. Each line equals 2 units.

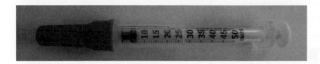

FIGURE 5-14

½-mL low-dose insulin syringe. Each line equals 1 unit.

Regular insulin should appear clear and colorless; it is the only insulin that may be given IV. Other insulins appear cloudy. Gently rotate (don't shake) cloudy insulin vials between your hands to resuspend the particles.

More in-depth information about insulin can be found in pharmacology textbooks or on the Internet.

Types of Insulin Syringes

To administer insulin doses subcutaneously, use an insulin syringe. Two standard syringes measure U 100 insulin. The first measures doses up to 100 units (Fig. 5-13) and the second, called a *low-dose insulin syringe,* measures doses of 50 units or less (Fig. 5-14).

Preparing an Injection Using an Insulin Syringe

The physician or healthcare provider's order for insulin is written as units; the stock comes in 100 units/mL. Both syringes are calibrated (lined) for 100 units/mL. Generally, doses less than 50 units are given with a low-dose insulin syringe. (The insulin syringes are pictured with the needle on the syringe, as they are prepackaged in that manner.)

EXAMPLE

Order: 60 units NPH subcutaneous every day

Supply: Read the label.

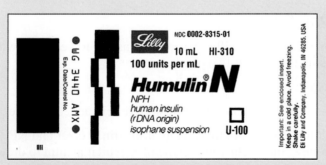

(Courtesy of Eli Lilly Co.)

Ask yourself three questions:

1. What is the order? NPH 60 units
2. What is the supply? NPH U 100/mL
3. Which insulin syringe should I use? The order is 60 units, so use a 1-mL insulin syringe.

Using aseptic technique, draw up the amount required into the syringe.

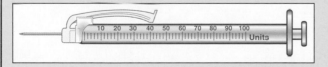

Order: 35 units regular insulin subcutaneous stat

Supply: Read the label.

NDC 0002-8215-01

Lilly

10 mL   HI-210

100 units per mL

Humulin® R

REGULAR
insulin human
injection, USP
(rDNA origin)

◇

U-100

Important: See enclosed insert.
Keep in a cold place. Avoid freezing.
Neutral
Eli Lilly and Company, Indianapolis, IN 46285, USA

(Courtesy of Eli Lilly Co.)

Ask yourself three questions:

1. What is the order? regular insulin 35 units

2. What is the supply? U 100/mL regular insulin

3. What syringe should be used? low-dose insulin syringe since the dose is 35 units

Using aseptic technique, draw up the amount required into the syringe.

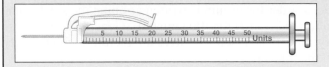

Mixing Two Insulins in One Syringe

Sometimes the physician or healthcare provider will order regular insulin to be mixed with another insulin and injected together at the same site. Remember two points:

1. Always draw up the regular insulin into the syringe first.

2. The total number of units in the syringe equals the two insulin orders added together.

Regular insulin is often ordered with NPH insulin. Since regular insulin is clear and NPH insulin is cloudy, the mnemonic "clear to cloudy" may help you to remember which insulin to draw up first.
   To prepare two insulins with one syringe (Fig. 5-15):

1. Inject into the NPH vial the amount of air equal to the amount of NPH insulin.

2. Inject into the regular vial the amount of air equal to the amount of regular insulin.

3. Withdraw the correct amount of regular insulin ("clear").

4. Withdraw the correct amount of NPH insulin ("cloudy").

5. The total number of units will be the regular insulin amount plus the NPH insulin amount.

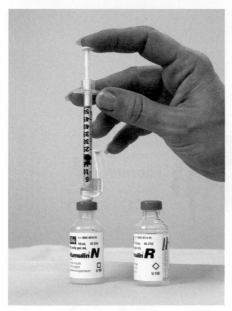

Step 1. Inject air into the NPH vial.

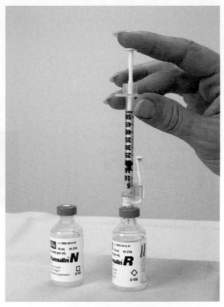

Step 2. Inject air into the regular vial.

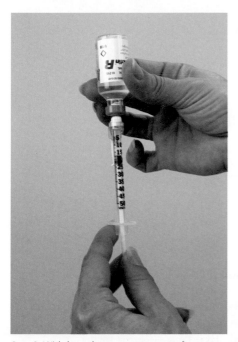

Step 3. Withdraw the correct amount of regular insulin.

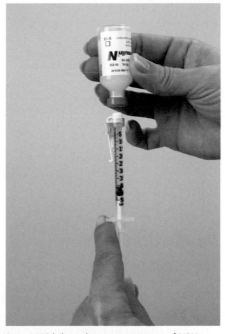

Step 4. Withdraw the correct amount of NPH insulin.

FIGURE 5-15

Mixing two insulins in one syringe. (Used with permission from Evans-Smith, P. [2005]. *Taylor's clinical nursing skills*. Philadelphia, PA: Lippincott Williams & Wilkins, p. 128–129.)

EXAMPLE

Order: regular Humulin insulin 15 units ⎫
                                        ⎬ every day subcutaneously
          NPH Humulin insulin 10 units ⎭

Supply: regular Humulin insulin 100 units/mL

      NPH Humulin insulin 100 units/mL

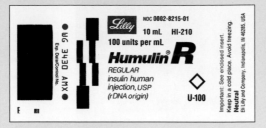 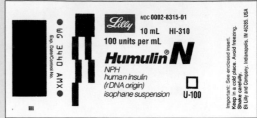

(Courtesy of Eli Lilly Co.)

1. What are the orders? regular (Humulin) insulin 15 units; NPH insulin 10 units (Humulin)

2. What is the supply? regular (Humulin) insulin unit-100/mL; NPH (Humulin) insulin unit-100/mL

3. Which insulin syringe? The total amount is 25 units, so use a low-dose insulin syringe.

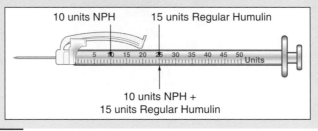

Sliding-Scale Regular Insulin Dosages

Sliding-scale insulin orders refer to a method of insulin administration that is based on the blood glucose result. Sliding-scale orders vary according to institutional policy. The blood glucose result often comes from a finger-stick and uses some type of Accucheck monitor. Another new method is a sensor that the patient/client wears that can monitor the glucose noninvasively. Search for "Glucowatch" on the Internet. The order will read something like this (blood glucose is abbreviated "BG"):

Accuchecks q 4 hours.

For BG 251-300, call physician.

For BG 201-250, give 5 units of regular insulin subcutaneous.

For BG 151-200, give 3 units of regular insulin subcutaneous.

For BG 101-150, give 2 units of regular insulin subcutaneous.

For BG 81-100, give 0 units of regular insulin subcutaneous.

For BG < 80, give 1 amp of D50 and call physician.

In this example, you will test the blood glucose and, according to the results, gives the ordered amount of insulin.

Another type of formula is the calculation, somewhat like this:

Accuchecks q 4 hours.

For BG > 150, give number of units of regular insulin based on: BG−100/40 (blood glucose value minus 100, then divided by 40).

In this formula, the denominator can change depending on the order and how controlled the patient's blood sugar needs to be. A lower number in the denominator, such as BG−100/30, increases the amount of insulin the patient/client receives. This formula also applies when you are giving continuous IV infusion of regular insulin. (See Chapter 7.)

For either type of formula, most hospitals still require that another licensed person double-check both the calculation and the amount of insulin drawn into the syringe.

Order: S/S (sliding scale) insulin. BG−100/40 = number of units of regular insulin.

Blood glucose result: 340

Calculation: 340−100/40

$$= 240/40$$

$$= 6 \text{ units}$$

Administer 6 units.

Since the insulin syringes do not have decimal markings, round the dose to a whole number. Always follow hospital/institutional policy on rounding insulin doses.

Insulin Pens and Prefilled Insulin Devices

Insulin pens and prefilled insulin devices contain insulin in a cartridge. The dose is calculated in the same manner; a needle is attached to the pen or prefilled insulin device and then the number of units is set with a small dial on the insulin pen or prefilled insulin device (Fig. 5-16). The injection is given subcutaneously and held in place for 6 to 10 seconds. Then the needle is removed from the pen or prefilled insulin device and discarded safely. The insulin pen or prefilled insulin device can be used until the insulin cartridge is empty. Usually, the insulin pen or prefilled insulin device is primed with 1 to 2 units before giving the actual dose. There are several advantages, including portability and ease of measuring an accurate dose. However, not all insulins can be supplied, and there is no way to mix insulins with an insulin pen or prefilled insulin device. In a hospital setting, the insulin pen or prefilled insulin device is supplied for only one patient/client, and usually doses must be verified by two licensed nurses.

An insulin pump can administer insulin continuously by the subcutaneous route. A pump is placed near the abdominal area of the patient/client. The pump is preset at a certain rate to deliver the insulin via tubing through a needle inserted in the subcutaneous tissue. Settings can be adjusted to the patient/client's insulin needs. The site is usually changed every 2 to 3 days or as needed (Fig. 5-17). (See the following website: www.minimed.com.)

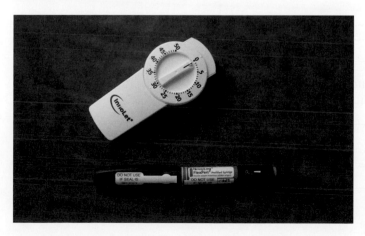

FIGURE 5-16

Insulin pen. (Copyright © 2008 Lacey-Bordeaux Photography.)

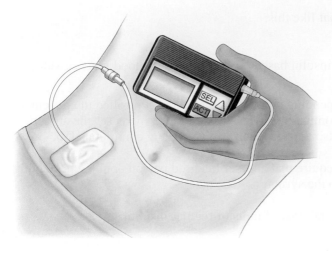

FIGURE 5-17

Insulin pump. (With permission from Taylor, C. [2008]. *Fundamentals of nursing*. Philadelphia, PA: Lippincott Williams & Wilkins, p. 797.)

SELF-TEST 7 | **Insulin Calculations**

Solve these insulin problems. Draw a line on the syringe to indicate the dose you would prepare. Answers appear at the end of the chapter.

1. Order: NPH insulin 56 units subcutaneous every day
   Supply: vial of NPH insulin 100 units/mL

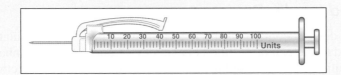

2. Order: 7 units regular insulin and 20 units NPH insulin subcutaneous every day 7 AM
   Supply: vial of regular insulin 100 units/mL and NPH 100 units/mL

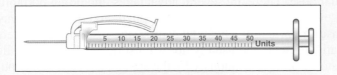

3. Order: regular Humulin insulin 4 units subcutaneous stat
   Supply: vial regular insulin 100 units/mL

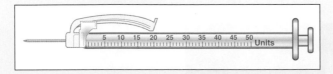

4. Order: NPH insulin 28 units subcutaneous every morning
   Supply: vial of NPH insulin 100 units/mL

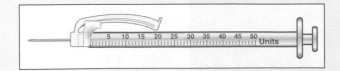

5. Order: 20 units of NPH subcutaneous every day
    Supply: vial of NPH 100 units/mL

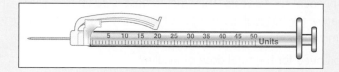

6. Order: regular insulin 16 units with NPH insulin 64 units subcutaneous every day
    Supply: vial of regular insulin 100 units/mL and vial of NPH 100 units/mL

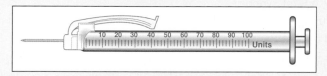

Use the following sliding scale to calculate the insulin dose. Draw a line on the syringe to indicate the dose you would prepare.

Accuchecks q 4 hours.

For BG 251-300, call physician.

For BG 201-250, give 5 units of regular insulin subcutaneous.

For BG 151-200, give 3 units of regular insulin subcutaneous.

For BG 101-150, give 2 units of regular insulin subcutaneous.

For BG 81-100, give 0 units of regular insulin subcutaneous.

For BG < 80, give 1 amp of D50 and call physician.

7. Accucheck 110

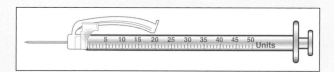

8. Accucheck 175

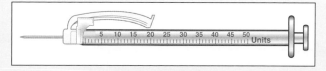

9. Accucheck 251

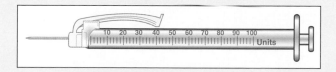

10. Accucheck 75

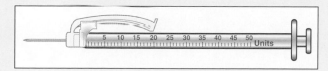

CRITICAL THINKING | TEST YOUR CLINICAL SAVVY

You are a nursing student about to graduate from one of the most prestigious nursing schools in America. On your last day of clinical, you are to give insulin to the last patient/client in your nursing school career. The patient/client has been insulin dependent for 15 years. The ordered dose is 30 units of NPH insulin and 20 units of regular insulin. Unfortunately, the hospital has run out of insulin syringes. Your instructor is going to check your insulin before you administer it.

1. How many milliliters would you need for the total dose of insulin?
2. Could you use a 1-mL syringe to draw up insulin? If so, how would this be done and what would be the precautions?
3. What would be the danger in using a 1-mL syringe?
4. Could you use a 3-mL syringe? A 5-mL syringe?
5. What would be the danger in using a 3-mL or 5-mL syringe?
6. What amount of insulin would be safe to draw up in a 1-mL syringe?

You are working in a medical-surgical unit of a large city hospital. A patient/client is to receive 500,000 units of penicillin G potassium, IV, q 12 hours. Normally, a vial containing 1 million units is considered stock drug (reconstituted: 250,000 units = 1 mL). Because of a nationwide shortage, a vial with 5 million units of penicillin G potassium is supplied (reconstituted 1,000,000 units = 1 mL).

1. What should you do to ensure no mistakes are made for the initial dosing and for subsequent dosing of penicillin?
2. What is the danger in administering too much of any drug?
3. What is the danger in administering too much penicillin and/or potassium?

Putting it Together

Mr. B. is a 54-year-old man with known asthma, recently hospitalized for hematuria and discharged 3 days ago. Since then, he has had dyspnea with wheezing and a dry cough. He has been using nebulized bronchodilators without any relief. Has sinus congestion, no headache, some subjective fevers. No history of pulmonary embolism or DVT. Admitted now for treatment and evaluation of dyspnea.

Past Medical History: renal cell carcinoma, hypertension, asthma, type 2 diabetes, hypercholesterolemia. Previous surgeries: hemorrhoidectomy, hiatal hernia repair, nephrectomy. Obstructive sleep apnea. Social history: lifelong smoker, no alcohol. Lives with his son.

Allergies: Keflex causing rash. Augmentin causing rash. Phenergan causing leg spasm.

Current Vital Signs: Pulse is 96, BP 170/100, RR of 18, sat 96% afebrile.

Medication Orders

Furosemide (Lasix) *diuretic* 40 mg IV q12h

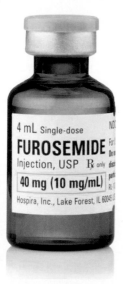

Epoetin (Epogen) *erythropoietin* 8000 units subcutaneous Tuesday/Thursday/Saturday

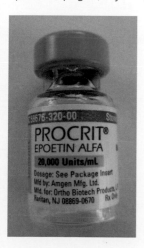

(continued)

Putting it Together (*Continued*)

Heparin *anticoagulant* 2500 units subcutaneous q8h

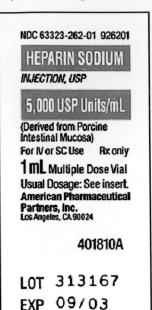

NDC 63323-262-01 926201

HEPARIN SODIUM

INJECTION, USP

5,000 USP Units/mL

(Derived from Porcine Intestinal Mucosa)

For IV or SC Use   Rx only

1 mL Multiple Dose Vial

Usual Dosage: See insert.

American Pharmaceutical Partners, Inc.

Los Angeles, CA 90024

401810A

LOT 313167

EXP 09/03

Theophylline (Theodur) *bronchodilator* 300 mg po q12h

Fluticasone (Flovent) *corticosteroid* 1 puff bid

Amlodipine (Norvasc) antihypertensive 10 mg po daily

Lovastatin (Mevacor) antihyperlipidemic 50 mg po daily

Methylprednisolone (Solu-Medrol) *corticosteroid, glucocorticoid* 100 mg IVP daily

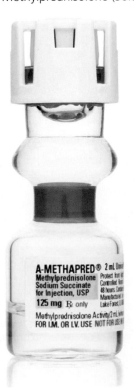

Putting it Together (*Continued*)

Promethazine (Phenergan) *antiemetic* 12.5 mg IV q6h prn nausea

Vancomycin (Vancocin) *anti-infective* 1 g IV q12h

Enalapril (Vasotec) *antihypertensive* 0.625 mg IV q6h over 5 minutes prn SBP >160

ENALAPRIL (Vasotec)

5 MG VIAL   1.25 MG PER ML

39123439

FOR IV USE

Accuchecks ac and hs. For BG >150, Sliding scale: BG −50/20 = units regular insulin subcutaneous

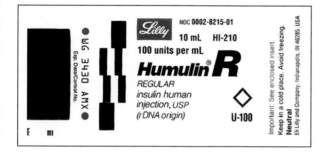

Calculations

1. Calculate how many milliliters of Lasix to administer. Available supply is 10 mg/mL.

2. Calculate how many milliliters of heparin to administer. Available supply is 5000 units/mL.

3. Calculate how many milliliters of Epogen to administer. Available supply is 20,000 units/mL.

4. Calculate how much (if any) insulin to give for blood glucose of 200.

5. Calculate how many mL of Solu-Medrol to administer. Available supply is 125 mg in 2 mL.

6. Calculate how many milliliters of Phenergan to administer. Available supply is 25 mg/mL.

7. What prn medication should be given (if any) for the patient/client's blood pressure? Calculate how many milliliters to administer if the available supply is 1.25 mg/mL.

8. Calculate the amount of Vancocin to add to an IV piggyback for infusion. Available supply is 500 mg/mL after reconstitution.

(continued)

Putting it Together (*Continued*)

Critical Thinking Questions

1. What are precautions that need to be taken with IV push drugs?

2. What are precautions that need to be taken with insulin calculations and administration?

3. What are common mistakes that could happen with insulin dosages?

4. What are common mistakes that could happen with heparin dosages?

5. Why would this patient/client be on insulin coverage if he or she is a type 2 ("non–insulin-dependent") diabetic?

6. What medications should be held and why?

Answers in Appendix B.

PROFICIENCY TEST 1   Calculations of Liquid Injections

*Name:*_____

Solve these injection problems. Draw a line on the syringe indicating the amount you would prepare in milliliters. See Appendix A for answers.

1. Order: sodium amytal 0.1 g IM at 7 AM
   Supply: ampule of liquid labeled 200 mg/3 mL

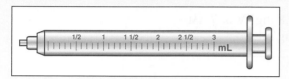

2. Order: morphine sulfate 5 mg IV stat
   Supply: vial of liquid labeled 15 mg/mL

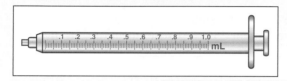

3. Order: diphenhydramine (Benadryl) 25 mg IM q4h prn
   Supply: ampule of liquid labeled 50 mg in 2 mL

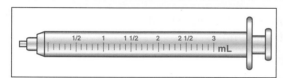

4. Order: NPH insulin 15 units and Humulin insulin 5 units subcutaneous every day 7 AM
   Supply: vials of NPH insulin 100 units/mL and Humulin insulin 100 units/mL

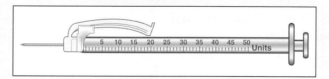

5. Order: add 20 mEq potassium chloride to IV stat
   Supply: vial of liquid labeled 40 mEq per 20 mL

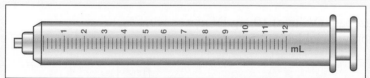

(continued)

6. Order: scopolamine 0.6 mg subcutaneous stat
Supply: vial labeled 0.4 mg/mL

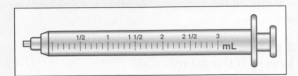

7. Order: atropine sulfate 0.8 mg IV at 7 AM
Supply: vial labeled 0.4 mg/mL

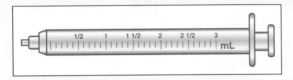

8. Order: add 0.5 g dextrose 25% to IV stat
Supply: vial of liquid labeled infant 25% dextrose injection 250 mg/mL

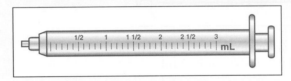

9. Order: ascorbic acid (vitamin C) 200 mg IM bid
Supply: ampule labeled 500 mg/2 mL

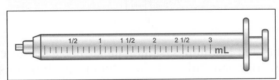

10. Order: epinephrine 7.5 mg subcutaneous stat
Supply: ampule labeled 1:100

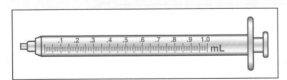

11. Order: diazepam (Valium) 10 mg IV now
Supply: vial labeled 5 mg/mL

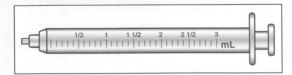

12. Order: chlordiazepoxide (Librium) 25 mg IM bid
     Supply: vial labeled 100 mg per 2 mL

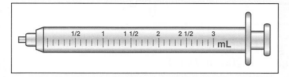

13. Order: hydroxyzine (Vistaril) 50 mg IM bid
     Supply: vial labeled 25 mg/mL

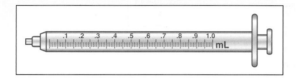

14. Order: lorazepam (Ativan) 0.5 mg IV q4h
     Supply: vial labeled 2 mg/mL

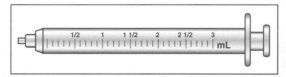

15. Order: phenytoin (Dilantin) 0.2 g IM stat
     Supply: vial labeled 200 mg/2 mL

PROFICIENCY TEST 2 | **Calculations of Liquid Injections and Injections From Powders**

*Name:*_____

Solve these problems for injections from a liquid. Draw a line on the syringe indicating the amount you would prepare in milliliters. See Appendix A for answers. Round to the nearest tenths place.

1. Order: morphine sulfate 10 mg IV stat
   Supply: vial labeled 15 mg/mL (use a 3-mL syringe, round to the nearest tenth)

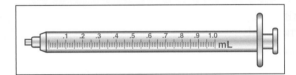

2. Order: phenobarbital 0.1 g IM q6h
   Supply: ampule of liquid labeled 200 mg/3 mL

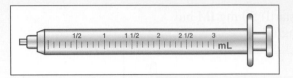

3. Order: vitamin B₁₂ 1000 mcg IM every day
   Supply: vial labeled 5000 mcg/mL

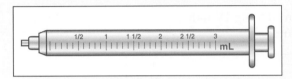

4. Order: prepare 25 mg lidocaine
   Supply: vial of liquid labeled 1%

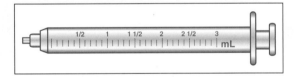

5. Order: scopolamine 0.5 mg subcutaneous stat
   Supply: vial labeled 0.4 mg/mL

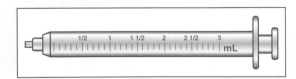

6. Order: NPH insulin 10 units and Humulin insulin 3 units subcutaneous every day 7 AM
   Supply: vials of NPH insulin 100 units/mL and Humulin insulin 100 units/mL

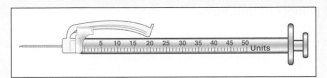

7. Order: add sodium bicarbonate 1.2 mEq to IV stat
   Supply: vial labeled infant 4.2% sodium bicarbonate 5 mEq (0.5 mEq/mL)

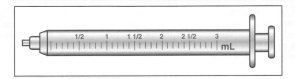

8. Order: epinephrine 500 mcg subcutaneous stat
   Supply: ampule of liquid labeled 1:1000

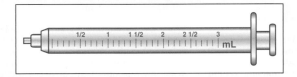

9. Order: ticarcillin disodium (Ticar) 1 g IM
   Supply: vial of powder labeled Ticar 1 g (Fig. 5-18)

   a. Diluting fluid and number of milliliters:
   b. Solution and new stock:
   c. Desired dose (and equivalent if necessary):
   d. Amount to give:
   e. Write on label:
   f. Storage:

DIRECTIONS FOR USE
—1 Gm, 3 Gm and 6 Gm Standard Vials—
INTRAMUSCULAR USE: (Concentration of approximately 385 mg/ml).
For initial reconstitution use Sterile Water for Injection, USP, Sodium Chloride Injection, USP or 1% Lidocaine Hydrochloride solution* (without epinephrine).
Each gram of Ticarcillin should be reconstituted with 2 ml of Sterile Water for Injection, U.S.P., Sodium Chloride Injection, U.S.P. or 1% Lidocaine Hydrochloride solution* (without epinephrine) and **used promptly.** Each 2.6 ml of the resulting solution will then contain 1 Gm of Ticarcillin.
*[For full product information, refer to manufacturer's package insert for Lidocaine Hydrochloride.]
As with all intramuscular preparations, TICAR (Ticarcillin Disodium) should be injected well within the body of a relatively large muscle, using usual techniques and precautions.

FIGURE 5-18

Directions for use of ticarcillin disodium (Ticar). (Courtesy of GlaxoSmithKline.)

(continued)

10. Order: ampicillin sodium 300 mg IM q8h
  Supply: vial of 500 mg powder (Fig. 5-19)

  a. Diluting fluid and number of milliliters:
  b. Solution and new supply:
  c. Desired dose (and equivalent if necessary):
  d. Amount to give:
  e. Write on label:
  f. Storage:

Intramuscular Use: 125 mg vial: Add 1 ml Sterile Water for Injection, USP, or Bacteriostatic Water for Injection, USP (TUBEX® Sterile Cartridge-Needle Unit) to give a final concentration of 125 mg per ml. For fractional doses, withdraw the ampicillin sodium solution as follows:

Dose	Withdraw
25 mg	0.2 ml
50 mg	0.4 ml
75 mg	0.6 ml
100 mg	0.8 ml
125 mg	1 ml

250 mg vial: Add 0.9 ml Sterile Water for Injection, USP, or Bacteriostatic Water for Injection, USP (TUBEX) to give a final concentration of 250 mg/ml. For fractional doses, withdraw the ampicillin sodium solution as follows:

Dose	Withdraw
125 mg	0.5 ml
150 mg	0.6 ml
175 mg	0.7 ml
200 mg	0.8 ml
225 mg	0.9 ml
250 mg	1 ml

For dilution of 500-mg, 1-gram, and 2-gram vials, dissolve contents of a vial with the amount of Sterile water for Injection, USP, or Bacteriostatic Water for Injection, USP, listed in the table below:

Label Claim	Recommended Amount of Diluent	Withdrawable Volume	Concentration in mg/ml
500 mg	1.8 ml	2.0 ml	250 mg
1.0 gram	3.4 ml	4.0 ml	250 mg
2.0 gram	6.8 ml	8.0 ml	250 mg

While the 1-gram and 2-gram vials are primarily for intravenous use, they may be administered intramuscularly when the 250-mg or 500-mg vials are unavailable. In such instances, dissolve in 3.4 or 6.8 ml Sterile Water for Injection, USP, or Bacteriostatic Water for Injection, USP, to give a final concentration of 250 mg/ml

The above solutions must be used within one hour after reconstitution.

FIGURE 5-19

Reconstitution directions for ampicillin sodium for IM or IV injection.

Name:_____

Aim for 90% or better on this test. Assume you have only a 3-mL syringe unless indicated. See Appendix A for answers.

1. Order: digoxin (Lanoxin) 0.25 mg IM every day
   Supply: ampule labeled 0.5 mg/2 mL

2. Order: diphenhydramine hydrochloride (Benadryl) 40 mg IM stat
   Supply: ampule labeled 50 mg in 2 mL

3. Order: morphine sulfate 8 mg IV q4h prn
   Supply: vial labeled 15 mg/mL; round to the nearest tenth

4. Order: meperidine (Demerol) 50 mg IM × 1
   Supply: vial labeled 100 mg/mL (use a 1-mL syringe)

5. Order: ascorbic acid (vitamin C) 200 mg IM every day
   Supply: ampule labeled 500 mg/2 mL

6. Order: vitamin B_{12} 1500 mcg every day IM
   Supply: vial labeled 5000 mcg/mL (use a 1-mL syringe)

7. Order: atropine sulfate 0.6 mg IV at 7:30 AM
   Supply: vial labeled 0.4 mg/mL

8. Order: sodium amytal 0.1 g IM stat
   Supply: ampule 200 mg/3 mL

9. Order: hydromorphone (Dilaudid) 1.5 mg IM q4h prn
   Supply: vial labeled 2 mg/mL (use a 1-mL syringe)

10. Order: penicillin G procaine 600,000 units IM q12h
    Supply: vial labeled 500,000 USP units/mL

11. Order: add nitroglycerin 200 mcg to IV stat
    Supply: vial labeled 0.8 mg/mL (use a 1-mL syringe)

12. Order: neostigmine methylsulfate 500 mcg subcutaneous
    Supply: ampule labeled 1:4000

13. Order: levorphanol tartrate (Levo-Dromoran) 3 mg subcutaneous
    Supply: vial labeled 2 mg/mL

14. Order: epinephrine 0.4 mg subcutaneous stat
    Supply: ampule labeled 1:1000 (2-mL size) (use a 1-mL syringe)

15. Order: magnesium sulfate 500 mg IM
    Supply: ampule labeled 50% (2-mL size)

16. Order: oxymorphone HCl (Numorphan) 0.75 mg subcutaneous
    Supply: vial labeled 1.5 mg/mL (use a 1-mL syringe)

17. Order: add lidocaine 100 mg to IV stat
    Supply: ampule labeled 20% (use a 1-mL syringe)

18. Order: digoxin (Lanoxin) 0.125 mg IV 10 AM
    Supply: ampule labeled 0.25 mg/2 mL

(continued)

PROFICIENCY TEST 3	Calculations of Liquid Injections (Continued)

19. Order: nalbuphine HCl (Nubain) 12 mg IM
        Supply: vial 10 mg/mL

20. Order: add 10 mEq KCl to IV
        Supply: vial 40 mEq/20 mL

PROFICIENCY TEST 4	Mental Drill in Liquids-for-Injection Problems

*Name:*_____

As you develop proficiency in solving problems, you will be able to calculate many answers without written work. This drill combines your knowledge of equivalents and dosages. Solve these problems mentally and write only the amount to give. See Appendix A for answers.

Order	*Supply*	*Give*
1. 0.5 g IM	250 mg/mL	_____
2. 10 mEq IV	40 mEq/20 mL	_____
3. 0.5 mg IM	0.25 mg/mL	_____
4. 100 mg IM	0.2 g/2 mL	_____
5. 50 mg IM	100 mg = 1 mL	_____
6. 0.25 mg IM	0.5 mg/2 mL	_____
7. 0.3 mg subcutaneous	0.4 mg/mL	_____
8. 1 mg subcutaneous	1:1000 solution	_____
9. 1 g IV	5% solution	_____
10. 0.1 g IM	200 mg/5 mL	_____
11. 400,000 units IM	500,000 units/mL	_____
12. 0.5 mg IM	0.5 mg/2 mL	_____
13. 1 g IV	50% solution	_____
14. 75 mg IM	100 mg/2 mL	_____
15. 15 mg IM	1:100 solution	_____
16. 35 mg IM	100 mg/mL	_____
17. 0.6 mg subcutaneous	0.4 mg per mL	_____
18. 0.15 g IM	0.2 g/2 mL	_____

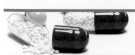

Answers

Self-Test 1 Calculation of Liquids for Injection

1. Equivalent: 0.3 g = 300 mg

Formula Method	Proportion	Dimensional Analysis

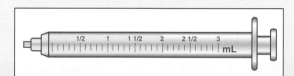

Formula Method:

$$\dfrac{\overset{1}{\cancel{300\ mg}}}{\underset{1}{\cancel{300\ mg}}} \times 2\ mL = 2\ mL$$

Proportion:

EXPRESSED AS TWO RATIOS

2 mL : 300 mg :: x : 300 mg

EXPRESSED AS TWO FRACTIONS

$$\dfrac{2\ mL}{300\ mg} \times \dfrac{x}{300\ mg}$$

SOLUTION FOR BOTH PROPORTION METHODS

$$2 \times 300 = 300x$$

$$\dfrac{600}{300} = x$$

$$2\ mL = x$$

Dimensional Analysis:

Use conversion factor 1000 mg/1 g:

$$\dfrac{2\ \cancel{mL}}{300\ \cancel{mg}} \ \bigg|\ \dfrac{0.3\ \cancel{g}}{} \ \bigg|\ \dfrac{1000\ \cancel{mg}}{1\ \cancel{g}} = \dfrac{2 \times 0.3 \times 10}{3}$$

$$= 2\ mL$$

Give 2 mL IM.

2.

Formula Method	Proportion	Dimensional Analysis

Formula Method:

$$\dfrac{\overset{4}{\cancel{12\ mg}}}{\underset{5}{\cancel{15\ mg}}} \times 1\ mL = \dfrac{4}{5}$$

$$= 0.8\ mL$$

Proportion:

EXPRESSED AS TWO RATIOS

1 mL : 15 mg :: x : 12 mg

EXPRESSED AS TWO FRACTIONS

$$\dfrac{1\ mL}{15\ mg} \times \dfrac{x}{12\ mg}$$

SOLUTION FOR BOTH PROPORTION METHODS

$$12 = 15x$$

$$\dfrac{12}{15} = x$$

$$0.8\ mL = x$$

Dimensional Analysis:

$$\dfrac{1\ \cancel{mL}}{\underset{5}{\cancel{15\ mg}}} \ \bigg|\ \dfrac{\overset{4}{\cancel{12\ mg}}}{} = \dfrac{4}{5} = 0.8\ mL$$

Give 0.8 mL IV. Follow directions for dilution and rate of administration.

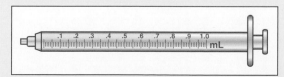

(continued)

Answers (Continued)

3. Equivalent: 1 mg = 1000 mcg

Formula Method	Proportion	Dimensional Analysis
$\dfrac{\overset{1}{\cancel{1000\ \text{mcg}}}}{\underset{1}{\cancel{1000\ \text{mcg}}}} \times 1\ \text{mL} = 1\ \text{mL}$	**EXPRESSED AS TWO RATIOS** 1 mL : 1000 mcg : : x : 1000 mcg **EXPRESSED AS TWO FRACTIONS** $\dfrac{1\ \text{mL}}{1000\ \text{mcg}} \times \dfrac{x}{1000\ \text{mcg}}$ **SOLUTION FOR BOTH PROPORTION METHODS** $1000 = 1000x$ $\dfrac{1000}{1000} = x$ $1\ \text{mL} = x$	Use conversion factor 1000 mcg/1 mg: $\dfrac{1\ \cancel{\text{mL}}}{1000\ \cancel{\text{mcg}}} \Bigg| \dfrac{1\ \cancel{\text{mg}}}{} \Bigg| \dfrac{1000\ \cancel{\text{mcg}}}{1\ \cancel{\text{mg}}} = 1\ \text{mL}$

Give 1 mL IM.

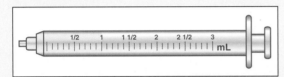

4.

Formula Method	Proportion	Dimensional Analysis
$\dfrac{9\ \text{mg}}{20\ \text{mg}} \times 2\ \text{mL} = \dfrac{18}{20}$ $\qquad\qquad = 0.9\ \text{mL}$	**EXPRESSED AS TWO RATIOS** 2 mL : 20 mg : : x : 9 mg **EXPRESSED AS TWO FRACTIONS** $\dfrac{2\ \text{mL}}{20\ \text{mg}} \times \dfrac{x}{9\ \text{mg}}$ **SOLUTION FOR BOTH PROPORTION METHODS** $2 \times 9 = 20x$ $\dfrac{18}{20} = x$ $0.9\ \text{mL} = x$	$\dfrac{\overset{1}{\cancel{2}}\ \cancel{\text{mL}}}{\underset{10}{\cancel{20}}\ \cancel{\text{mg}}} \Bigg| 9\ \cancel{\text{mg}} = \dfrac{9}{10} = 0.9\ \text{mL}$

Give 0.9 mL IM using a 1-mL precision syringe.

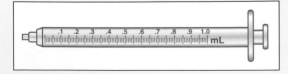

5.

Formula Method	Proportion	Dimensional Analysis

Formula Method

$$\frac{50 \text{ mg}}{40 \text{ mg}} \times 1 \text{ mL} = \frac{5}{4}$$

$$= 1.25 \text{ mL}$$

Proportion

EXPRESSED AS TWO RATIOS

$$1 \text{ mL} : 40 \text{ mg} :: x : 50 \text{ mg}$$

EXPRESSED AS TWO FRACTIONS

$$\frac{1 \text{ mL}}{40 \text{ mg}} \diagup \frac{x}{50 \text{ mg}}$$

SOLUTION FOR BOTH PROPORTION METHODS

$$50 = 40x$$

$$\frac{50}{40} = x$$

$$1.25 \text{ mL} = x$$

Dimensional Analysis

$$\frac{1 \text{ mL}}{40 \text{ mg}} \left| \frac{\overset{5}{\cancel{50}} \text{ mg}}{} \right. = \frac{5}{4} = 1.25 \text{ mL}$$

Give 1.3 mL IM.

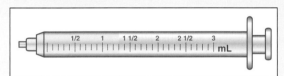

6.

Formula Method	Proportion	Dimensional Analysis

Formula Method

$$\frac{100 \text{ mg}}{130 \text{ mg}} \times 1 \text{ mL} = \frac{10}{13}$$

$$= 0.769 \text{ or } 0.77 \text{ mL}$$

Proportion

EXPRESSED AS TWO RATIOS

$$1 \text{ mL} : 130 \text{ mg} :: x : 100 \text{ mg}$$

EXPRESSED AS TWO FRACTIONS

$$\frac{1 \text{ mL}}{130 \text{ mg}} \diagup \frac{x}{100 \text{ mg}}$$

SOLUTION FOR BOTH PROPORTION METHODS

$$100 = 130x$$

$$\frac{100}{130} = x$$

$$0.769 \text{ or } 0.77 \text{ mL} = x$$

Dimensional Analysis

$$\frac{1 \text{ mL}}{130 \text{ mg}} \left| \frac{\overset{10}{\cancel{100}} \text{ mg}}{13} \right. = \frac{10}{13} = 0.77 \text{ mL}$$

Give 0.77 mL IM using a 1-mL precision syringe (milliliters to the nearest hundredth).

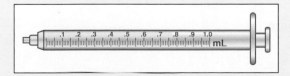

(continued)

Answers (Continued)

7.

Formula Method	Proportion	Dimensional Analysis

Formula Method

$$\frac{0.125 \text{ mg}}{0.5 \text{ mg}} \times 2 \text{ mL}$$

$$= 0.5 \text{ mL}$$

Proportion

EXPRESSED AS TWO RATIOS

2 mL : 0.5 mg :: x : 0.125 mg

EXPRESSED AS TWO FRACTIONS

$$\frac{2 \text{ mL}}{0.5 \text{ mg}} \times \frac{x}{0.125 \text{ mg}}$$

SOLUTION FOR BOTH PROPORTION METHODS

$$0.125 \times 2 = 0.5x$$

$$\frac{0.25}{0.5} = x$$

$$0.5 \text{ mL} = x$$

Dimensional Analysis

$$\frac{\overset{1}{2\,\cancel{mL}}}{\underset{0.25}{0.5\,\cancel{mg}}} \quad \Big| \quad 0.125\,\cancel{mg}$$

$$\frac{0.125 \text{ mg}}{0.25 \text{ mg}} = 0.5 \text{ mL}$$

Give 0.5 mL IV. Follow directions for dilution and rate of medication administration.

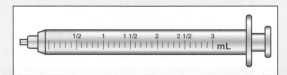

8.

Formula Method	Proportion	Dimensional Analysis

Formula Method

$$\frac{6000 \text{ units}}{10,000 \text{ units}} \times 1 \text{ mL} = \frac{6}{10}$$

$$= 0.6 \text{ mL}$$

Proportion

EXPRESSED AS TWO RATIOS

1 mL : 10,000 :: x : 6000
      units   units

EXPRESSED AS TWO FRACTIONS

$$\frac{1 \text{ mL}}{10,000 \text{ units}} \times \frac{x}{6000 \text{ units}}$$

SOLUTION FOR BOTH PROPORTION METHODS

$$6000 = 10,000x$$

$$\frac{6000}{10,000} = x$$

$$0.6 \text{ mL} = x$$

Dimensional Analysis

$$\frac{1\,\cancel{mL}}{10,000\,\cancel{units}} \quad \Big| \quad 6000\,\cancel{units} = \frac{6}{10} = 0.6 \text{ mL}$$

Give 0.6 mL subcutaneous using a 1-mL precision syringe.

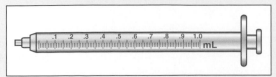

9.

Formula Method	Proportion	Dimensional Analysis

Formula Method

$$\frac{0.25 \text{ mg}}{1 \text{ mg}} \times 1 \text{ mL}$$
$$= 0.25 \text{ mL}$$

Proportion

EXPRESSED AS TWO RATIOS

$1 \text{ mL} : 1 \text{ mg} :: x : 0.25 \text{ mg}$

EXPRESSED AS TWO FRACTIONS

$$\frac{1 \text{ mL}}{1 \text{ mg}} \times \frac{x}{0.25 \text{ mg}}$$

**SOLUTION FOR BOTH
PROPORTION METHODS**

$0.25 = 1x$

$0.25 \text{ mL} = x$

Dimensional Analysis

$$\frac{1 \text{ mL}}{1 \text{ mg}} \left| \frac{0.25 \text{ mg}}{} \right. = 0.25 \text{ mL}$$

Give 0.25 mL subcutaneous using a 1-mL precision syringe.

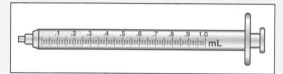

10.

Formula Method	Proportion	Dimensional Analysis

Formula Method

$$\frac{20 \text{ mg}}{5 \text{ mg}} \times 1 \text{ mL} = 4 \text{ mL}$$

Proportion

EXPRESSED AS TWO RATIOS

$1 \text{ mL} : 5 \text{ mg} :: x : 20 \text{ mg}$

EXPRESSED AS TWO FRACTIONS

$$\frac{1 \text{ mL}}{5 \text{ mg}} \times \frac{x}{20 \text{ mg}}$$

**SOLUTION FOR BOTH
PROPORTION METHODS**

$20 = 5x$

$$\frac{20}{5} = x$$

$4 \text{ mL} = x$

Dimensional Analysis

$$\frac{1 \text{ mL}}{\underset{1}{5} \text{ mg}} \left| \frac{\overset{4}{20} \text{ mg}}{} \right. = 4 \text{ mL}$$

Give 4 mL IV. Follow directions for dilution and rate of administration.

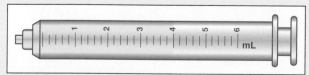

(continued)

Answers (Continued)

11.

Formula Method	Proportion	Dimensional Analysis

Formula Method

$$\frac{2.5 \text{ mg}}{5 \text{ mg}} \times 1 \text{ mL}$$

$$= 0.5 \text{ or } \frac{1}{2} \text{ mL}$$

Proportion

EXPRESSED AS TWO RATIOS

$$1 \text{ mL} : 5 \text{ mg} :: x : 2.5 \text{ mg}$$

EXPRESSED AS TWO FRACTIONS

$$\frac{1 \text{ mL}}{5 \text{ mg}} \times \frac{x}{2.5 \text{ mg}}$$

SOLUTION FOR BOTH PROPORTION METHODS

$$2.5 = 5x$$

$$\frac{2.5}{5} = x$$

$$0.5 \text{ or } \frac{1}{2} \text{ mL} = x$$

Dimensional Analysis

$$\frac{1 \text{ mL}}{5 \text{ mg}} \Bigg| \frac{\overset{0.5}{2.5} \text{ mg}}{1} = 0.5 \text{ mL}$$

Give 0.5 mL IM.

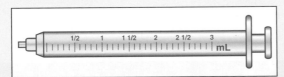

12.

Formula Method	Proportion	Dimensional Analysis

Formula Method

$$\frac{3 \text{ mg}}{10 \text{ mg}} \times 1 \text{ mL} = 0.3 \text{ mL}$$

Proportion

EXPRESSED AS TWO RATIOS

$$1 \text{ mL} : 10 \text{ mg} :: x : 3 \text{ mg}$$

EXPRESSED AS TWO FRACTIONS

$$\frac{1 \text{ mL}}{10 \text{ mg}} \times \frac{x}{3 \text{ mg}}$$

SOLUTION FOR BOTH PROPORTION METHODS

$$3 = 10 x$$

$$\frac{3}{10} = x$$

$$0.3 \text{ mL} = x$$

Dimensional Analysis

$$\frac{1 \text{ mL}}{10 \text{ mg}} \Bigg| 3 \text{ mg} = \frac{3}{10} = 0.3 \text{ mL}$$

Give 0.3 mL subcutaneously using a 1-mL precision syringe.

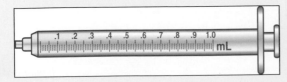

13. 0.025 g = 25 mg

Formula Method	Proportion	Dimensional Analysis
$\dfrac{25\ mg}{10\ mg} \times 1\ mL = 2.5\ mL$	**EXPRESSED AS TWO RATIOS** 1 mL : 10 mg : : x : 25 mg **EXPRESSED AS TWO FRACTIONS** $\dfrac{1\ mL}{10\ mg} \times \dfrac{x}{25\ mg}$ **SOLUTION FOR BOTH PROPORTION METHODS** $25 = 10\ x$ $\dfrac{25}{10} = x$ $2.5\ mL = x$	Use conversion factor 1000 mg/1 g: $\dfrac{1\ mL}{10\ mg} \cdot 0.025\ g \cdot \dfrac{1000\ mg}{1\ g} = 100 \times 0.025$ $= 2.5\ mL$

Give 2.5 mL IM.

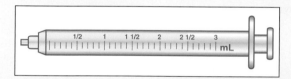

14.

Formula Method	Proportion	Dimensional Analysis
$\dfrac{50\ mg}{25\ mg} \times 1\ mL = 2\ mL$	**EXPRESSED AS TWO RATIOS** 1 mL : 25 mg : : x : 50 mg **EXPRESSED AS TWO FRACTIONS** $\dfrac{1\ mL}{25\ mg} \times \dfrac{x}{50\ mg}$ **SOLUTION FOR BOTH PROPORTION METHODS** $50 = 25x$ $\dfrac{50}{25} = x$ $2\ mL = x$	$\dfrac{1\ mL}{25\ mg} \cdot \dfrac{50\ mg}{1} = 2\ mL$

Give 2 mL IM.

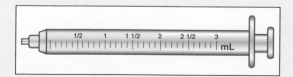

(continued)

Answers (Continued)

15.

Formula Method	Proportion	Dimensional Analysis

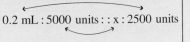

Formula Method

$$\frac{\overset{1}{\cancel{2500}} \text{ units}}{\underset{2}{\cancel{5000}} \text{ units}} \times 0.2 \text{ mL}$$

$$= 0.1 \text{ mL}$$

Proportion

EXPRESSED AS TWO RATIOS

0.2 mL : 5000 units :: x : 2500 units

EXPRESSED AS TWO FRACTIONS

$$\frac{0.2 \text{ mL}}{5000 \text{ units}} \diagdown \frac{x}{2500 \text{ units}}$$

SOLUTION FOR BOTH PROPORTION METHODS

$$0.2 \times 2500 = 5000x$$

$$\frac{500}{5000} = x$$

$$0.1 = x$$

Dimensional Analysis

$$\frac{0.2 \text{ (mL)}}{\underset{2}{\cancel{5000}} \text{ units}} \left| \overset{1}{\cancel{2500}} \text{ units} \right. = \frac{0.2}{2} = 0.1 \text{ mL}$$

Give 0.1 mL subcutaneously using a 1-mL precision syringe.

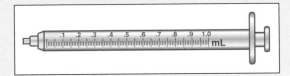

Self-Test 2 Ratios

RATIO	? g per ? mL	? g = ? mL	? g/? mL
1:20	1 g per 20 mL	1 g = 20 mL	1 g/20 mL
2:15	2 g per 15 mL	2 g = 15 mL	2 g/15 mL
1:500	1 g per 500 mL	1 g = 500 mL	1 g/500 mL
2:2000	2 g per 2000 mL	2 g = 2000 mL	2 g/2000 mL
1:4	1 g per 4 mL	1 g = 4 mL	1 g/4 mL
2:25	2 g per 25 mL	2 g = 25 mL	2 g/25 mL
4:50	4 g per 50 mL	4 g = 50 mL	4 g/50 mL
1:100	1 g per 100 mL	1 g = 100 mL	1 g/100 mL
3:75	3 g per 75 mL	3 g = 75 mL	3 g/75 mL
5:1000	5 g per 1000 mL	5 g = 1000 mL	5 g/1000 mL

Self-Test 3 Using Ratios With Liquids for Injection

1. Equivalent: 1:2000 means

1 g in 2000 mL

1 g = 1000 mg

Therefore, the solution is 1000 mg/2000 mL.

Formula Method	**Proportion**	**Dimensional Analysis**
$\dfrac{0.5 \text{ mg}}{1000 \text{ mg}} \times \overset{2}{\cancel{2000}} \text{ mL}$ $= 1 \text{ mL}$	**EXPRESSED AS TWO RATIOS** $2000 \text{ mL} : 1000 \text{ mg} :: x : 0.5 \text{ mg}$ **EXPRESSED AS TWO FRACTIONS** $\dfrac{2000 \text{ mL}}{1000 \text{ mg}} \times \dfrac{x}{0.5 \text{ mg}}$ **SOLUTION FOR BOTH PROPORTION METHODS** $2000 \times 0.5 = 1000x$ $\dfrac{1000}{1000} = x$ $1 \text{ mL} = x$	Use conversion factor 1 g/1000 mg: $\dfrac{\overset{2}{\cancel{2000}} \, \cancel{\text{(mL)}}}{1 \, \cancel{\text{g}}} \Bigg| \dfrac{0.5 \text{ mg}}{} \Bigg| \dfrac{1 \, \cancel{\text{g}}}{\underset{1}{\cancel{1000}} \, \cancel{\text{mg}}} = 2 \times 0.5$ $= 1 \text{ mL}$

Give 1 mL subcutaneous.

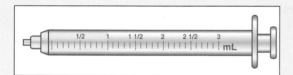

2. Equivalent: 1:5000 means

        1 g in 5000 mL

        1 g = 1000 mg

Therefore, the solution is 1000 mg/5000 mL.

Formula Method	**Proportion**	**Dimensional Analysis**
$\dfrac{1 \text{ mg}}{1000 \text{ mg}} \times \overset{5}{\cancel{5000}} \text{ mL}$ $= 5 \text{ mL}$	**EXPRESSED AS TWO RATIOS** $5000 \text{ mL} : 1000 \text{ mg} :: x : 1 \text{ mg}$ **EXPRESSED AS TWO FRACTIONS** $\dfrac{5000 \text{ mL}}{1000 \text{ mg}} \times \dfrac{x}{1 \text{ mg}}$ **SOLUTION FOR BOTH PROPORTION METHODS** $5000 = 1000x$ $\dfrac{5000}{1000} = x$ $5 \text{ mL} = x$	Use conversion factor 1 g/1000 mg: $\dfrac{\overset{5}{\cancel{5000}} \, \cancel{\text{(mL)}}}{1 \, \cancel{\text{g}}} \Bigg| \dfrac{1 \text{ mg}}{} \Bigg| \dfrac{1 \, \cancel{\text{g}}}{\underset{1}{\cancel{1000}} \, \cancel{\text{mg}}} = 5 \text{ mL}$

Add 5 mL to IV. (This is correct because the route is IV not IM.)

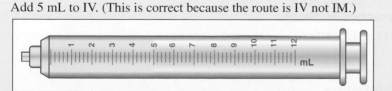

(continued)

Answers (Continued)

3. Equivalent: 1:1000 means

        1 g in 1000 mL

        1 g = 1000 mg

Therefore, the solution is 1000 mg/1000 mL or 1 mg/mL.

Formula Method	Proportion	Dimensional Analysis
$\dfrac{0.75 \text{ mg}}{1 \text{ mg}} \times 1 \text{ mL}$ $= 0.75 \text{ mL}$	**EXPRESSED AS TWO RATIOS** $1 \text{ mL} : 1 \text{ mg} :: x : 0.75 \text{ mg}$ **EXPRESSED AS TWO FRACTIONS** $\dfrac{1 \text{ mL}}{1 \text{ mg}} \times \dfrac{x}{0.75 \text{ mg}}$ **SOLUTION FOR BOTH PROPORTION METHODS** $0.75 = 1x$ $\dfrac{0.75}{1} = x$ $0.75 \text{ mL} = x$	Use conversion factor 1 g/1000 mg: $\dfrac{1000 \text{ (mL)}}{1 \text{ g}} \times \dfrac{0.75 \text{ mg}}{} \times \dfrac{1 \text{ g}}{1000 \text{ mg}} = 0.75 \text{ mL}$

You have a 1-mL syringe marked in hundredths. Draw up 0.75 mL. Do not round.

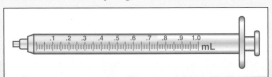

4. Equivalent: 1:1000 means

        1 g in 1000 mL

        1 g = 1000 mg

Therefore, the solution is 1000 mg/1000 mL.

Formula Method	Proportion	Dimensional Analysis
$\dfrac{0.5 \text{ mg}}{1000 \text{ mg}} \times 1000 \text{ mL}$ $= 0.5 \text{ mL}$	**EXPRESSED AS TWO RATIOS** $1000 \text{ mL} : 1000 \text{ mg} :: x : 0.5 \text{ mg}$ **EXPRESSED AS TWO FRACTIONS** $\dfrac{1000 \text{ mL}}{1000 \text{ mg}} \times \dfrac{x}{0.5 \text{ mg}}$ **SOLUTION FOR BOTH PROPORTION METHODS** $1000 \times 0.5 = 1000x$ $\dfrac{500}{1000} = x$ $0.5 \text{ mL} = x$	Use conversion factor 1 g/1000 mg: $\dfrac{1000 \text{ (mL)}}{1 \text{ g}} \times \dfrac{0.5 \text{ mg}}{} \times \dfrac{1 \text{ g}}{1000 \text{ mg}} = 0.5 \text{ mL}$

Give 0.5 mL subcutaneous using a 1-mL precision syringe.

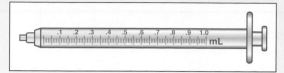

5. Equivalent: 1:2000 means

   1000 mg in 2000 mL

   Therefore, the solution is 1 mg in 2 mL.

Formula Method	Proportion	Dimensional Analysis
$\dfrac{1.5\ \text{mg}}{1\ \text{mg}} \times 2\ \text{mL} = 3\ \text{mL}$	**EXPRESSED AS TWO RATIOS** $2\ \text{mL} : 1\ \text{mg} :: x : 1.5\ \text{mg}$ **EXPRESSED AS TWO FRACTIONS** $\dfrac{2\ \text{mL}}{1\ \text{mg}} \times \dfrac{x}{1.5\ \text{mg}}$ **SOLUTION FOR BOTH PROPORTION METHODS** $2 \times 1.5 = 1x$ $\dfrac{3}{1} = x$ $3\ \text{mL} = x$	Use conversion factor 1 g/1000 mg: $\dfrac{\overset{2}{\cancel{2000}}\ \cancel{\text{mL}}}{\cancel{1\ \text{g}}} \left\lvert\ 1.5\ \cancel{\text{mg}}\ \right\rvert \dfrac{1\ \cancel{\text{g}}}{\underset{1}{\cancel{1000}}\ \cancel{\text{mg}}} = 1.5 \times 2$ $= 3\ \text{mL}$

Give 3 mL IM. May use two syringes of 1.5 mL each.

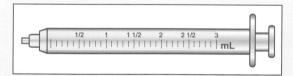

Self-Test 4 Percentages

PERCENTAGE	? g per 100 mL	? g = 100 mL	? g/100 mL
0.9%	0.9 g per 100 mL	0.9 g = 100 mL	0.9 g/100 mL
10%	10 g per 100 mL	10 g = 100 mL	10 g/100 mL
0.45%	0.45 g per 100 mL	0.45 g = 100 mL	0.45 g/100 mL
50%	50 g per 100 mL	50 g = 100 mL	50 g/100 mL
0.33%	0.33 g per 100 mL	0.33 g = 100 mL	0.33 g/100 mL
5%	5 g per 100 mL	5 g = 100 mL	5 g/100 mL
30%	30 g per 100 mL	30 g = 100 mL	30 g/100 mL
1.5%	1.5 g per 100 mL	1.5 g = 100 mL	1.5 g/100 mL
1%	1 g per 100 mL	1 g = 100 mL	1 g/100 mL
20%	20 g per 100 mL	20 g = 100 mL	20 g/100 mL

(continued)

Answers (Continued)

Self-Test 5 Using Percentages With Liquids for Injection

1. Equivalent: 1% 1 g in 100 mL

   1 g = 1000 mg

   Therefore, the solution is 1000 mg/100 mL.

Formula Method	Proportion	Dimensional Analysis
$\dfrac{\overset{1}{\cancel{5}}\text{ mg}}{\underset{\underset{2}{10}}{\cancel{1000}}\text{ mg}} \times \overset{1}{\cancel{100}}\text{ mL}$ $= \dfrac{1}{2}$ mL or 0.5 mL	**EXPRESSED AS TWO RATIOS** 100 mL : 1000 mg :: x : 5 mg **EXPRESSED AS TWO FRACTIONS** $\dfrac{100\text{ mL}}{1000\text{ mg}} \times \dfrac{x}{5\text{ mg}}$ **SOLUTION FOR BOTH PROPORTION METHODS** $100 \times 5 = 1000x$ $\dfrac{500}{1000} = x$ 0.5 mL = x	Use conversion factor 1 g/1000 mg: $\dfrac{\overset{1}{\cancel{100}} \,\cancel{(\text{mL})}}{1\,\cancel{\text{g}}} \left| \dfrac{5\text{ mg}}{} \right| \dfrac{1\,\cancel{\text{g}}}{\underset{10}{\cancel{1000}}\text{ mg}} = \dfrac{5}{10}$ $= \dfrac{1}{2}$ or 0.5 mL

Give 0.5 mL subcutaneous using a 1-mL precision syringe.

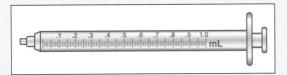

2. Equivalent: 1% 1 g in 100 mL

   1 g = 1000 mg

   Therefore, the solution is 1000 mg/100 mL.

Formula Method	Proportion	Dimensional Analysis
$\dfrac{15\text{ mg}}{\underset{10}{\cancel{1000}}\text{ mg}} \times \overset{1}{\cancel{100}}\text{ mL}$ $= 1.5$ mL or $1\frac{1}{2}$ mL	**EXPRESSED AS TWO RATIOS** 100 mL : 1000 mg :: x : 15 mg **EXPRESSED AS TWO FRACTIONS** $\dfrac{100\text{ mL}}{1000\text{ mg}} \times \dfrac{x}{15\text{ mg}}$ **SOLUTION FOR BOTH PROPORTION METHODS** $100 \times 15 = 1000x$ $\dfrac{1500}{1000} = x$ 1.5 mL = x or $1\frac{1}{2}$ mL	Use conversion factor 1 g/1000 mg: $\dfrac{\overset{1}{\cancel{100}} \,\cancel{(\text{mL})}}{1\,\cancel{\text{g}}} \left| \dfrac{15\text{ mg}}{} \right| \dfrac{1\,\cancel{\text{g}}}{\underset{10}{\cancel{1000}}\text{ mg}} = \dfrac{15}{10} = 1.5$ mL

Give 1.5 mL subcutaneous.

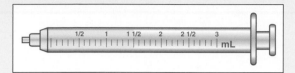

3. Equivalent: 1% 1 g in 100 mL

1 g = 1000 mg

Therefore, the solution is 1000 mg/100 mL.

Formula Method	Proportion	Dimensional Analysis
$\dfrac{3 \text{ mg}}{\underset{10}{1000} \text{ mg}} \times \overset{1}{100} \text{ mL}$ $= 0.3 \text{ mL}$	**EXPRESSED AS TWO RATIOS** 100 mL : 1000 mg :: x : 3 mg **EXPRESSED AS TWO FRACTIONS** $\dfrac{100 \text{ mL}}{1000 \text{ mg}} \times \dfrac{x}{3 \text{ mg}}$ **SOLUTION FOR BOTH PROPORTION METHODS** $100 \times 3 = 1000x$ $\dfrac{300}{1000} = x$ $0.3 \text{ mL} = x$	Use conversion factor 1 g/1000 mg: $\dfrac{\overset{1}{100} \text{ mL}}{1 \text{ g}} \left\vert \dfrac{3 \text{ mg}}{} \right\vert \dfrac{1 \text{ g}}{\underset{10}{1000} \text{ mg}} = \dfrac{3}{10} = 0.3 \text{ mL}$

Give 0.3 mL subcutaneous using a 1-mL precision syringe.

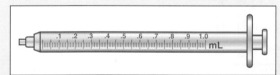

4. Equivalent: 10% means 10 g in 100 mL or 1 g in 10 mL.

Formula Method	Proportion	Dimensional Analysis
$\dfrac{0.3 \text{ g}}{1 \text{ g}} \times 10 \text{ mL} = 3 \text{ mL}$	**EXPRESSED AS TWO RATIOS** 10 mL : 1 g :: x : 0.3 g **EXPRESSED AS TWO FRACTIONS** $\dfrac{10 \text{ mL}}{1 \text{ g}} \times \dfrac{x}{0.3 \text{ g}}$ **SOLUTION FOR BOTH PROPORTION METHODS** $10 \times 0.3 = 1x$ $\dfrac{3}{1} = x$ $3 \text{ mL} = x$	$\dfrac{\overset{10}{100} \text{ mL}}{\underset{1}{10} \text{ g}} \left\vert \dfrac{0.3 \text{ g}}{} \right. = 10 \times 0.3 = 3 \text{ mL}$

(continued)

Answers (Continued)

Prepare the syringe with 3 mL for IV use.

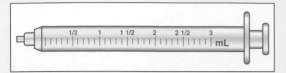

5. Equivalent: 50% means 50 g in 100 mL.

Formula Method	Proportion	Dimensional Analysis
$\dfrac{5\ \cancel{g}^{\,2}}{\cancel{50}\ \cancel{g}_{\,1}} \times \cancel{100}\ \text{mL}$ $= 10\ \text{mL}$	**EXPRESSED AS TWO RATIOS** $100\ \text{mL} : 50\ \text{g} :: x : 5\ \text{g}$ **EXPRESSED AS TWO FRACTIONS** $\dfrac{100\ \text{mL}}{50\ \text{g}} \times \dfrac{x}{5\ \text{g}}$ **SOLUTION FOR BOTH PROPORTION METHODS** $100 \times 5 = 50x$ $\dfrac{500}{50} = x$ $10\ \text{mL} = x$	$\dfrac{\cancel{100}^{\,2}\ \cancel{\text{mL}}}{\cancel{50}\ \cancel{g}_{\,1}} \Bigg| \dfrac{5\ \cancel{g}}{} = 2 \times 5 = 10\ \text{mL}$

Prepare the syringe with 10 mL for IV use.

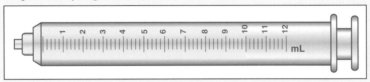

Self-Test 6 Injections From Powders

1. **a.** 3 mL sterile water for injection

   b. 1 g in 3.6 mL; 280 mg/mL

   c. 1 g equivalent: 1 g = 1000 mg

Formula Method	Proportion	Dimensional Analysis
$\dfrac{1000\ \cancel{\text{mg}}}{280\ \cancel{\text{mg}}} \times 1\ \text{mL} = \dfrac{100}{28}$ $= 3.6\ \text{mL}$	**EXPRESSED AS TWO RATIOS** $1\ \text{mL} : 280\ \text{mg} :: x\ \text{mL} : 1000\ \text{mg}$ **EXPRESSED AS TWO FRACTIONS** $\dfrac{1\ \text{mL}}{280\ \text{mg}} \times \dfrac{x}{1000\ \text{mg}}$ **SOLUTION FOR BOTH PROPORTION METHODS** $1000 = 280x$ $\dfrac{1000}{280} = x$ $3.6\ \text{mL} = x$	Use conversion factor 1000 mg/1 g: $\dfrac{1\ \cancel{\text{mL}}}{\cancel{280}\ \cancel{\text{mg}}_{\,28}} \Bigg| \dfrac{1\ \cancel{g}}{} \Bigg| \dfrac{\cancel{1000}^{\,100}\ \cancel{\text{mg}}}{1\ \cancel{g}} = \dfrac{100}{28}$ $= 3.57\ \text{mL or } 3.6\ \text{mL}$ (Round to nearest tenths place) $= 3.6\ \text{mL}$

   d. Give 3.6 mL in two syringes.

   e. Discard the vial; it is empty.

   f. Discard the vial in appropriate receptacle.

2. a. 1.8 mL sterile water for injection

   b. 250 mg/mL

   c. 250 mg

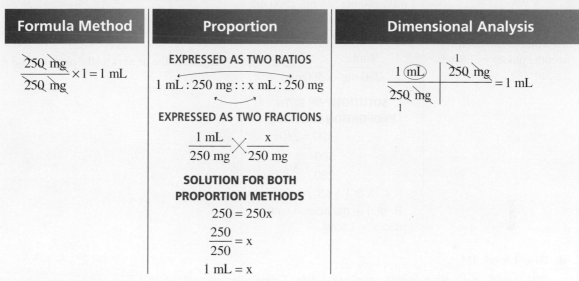

Formula Method	Proportion	Dimensional Analysis

Formula Method

$$\frac{250 \ mg}{250 \ mg} \times 1 = 1 \ mL$$

Proportion

EXPRESSED AS TWO RATIOS

$$1 \ mL : 250 \ mg :: x \ mL : 250 \ mg$$

EXPRESSED AS TWO FRACTIONS

$$\frac{1 \ mL}{250 \ mg} \times \frac{x}{250 \ mg}$$

SOLUTION FOR BOTH PROPORTION METHODS

$$250 = 250x$$

$$\frac{250}{250} = x$$

$$1 \ mL = x$$

Dimensional Analysis

$$\frac{1 \ \textcircled{mL}}{250 \ mg} \ \bigg| \ \frac{\overset{1}{250 \ mg}}{\underset{1}{}} = 1 \ mL$$

   d. Give 1 mL IM.

   e. "The above solutions must be used within 1 hour after reconstitution." You must discard the remaining fluid.

   f. None

3. a. Choose 500 mg powder. (250 mg powder could also work but you would need 1.8 mL to equal 225 mg. Choose the 500 mg powder so that you use only 1 mL for injection)

   b. Add 2 mL sterile water for injection.

   c. 225 mg/mL

   d. 225 mg. NO math needed. 225 mg is in 1 mL.

   e. Give 1 mL IM.

   f. 225 mg/mL, date, time, initials, expiration date: 96 hours after reconstitution

   g. Refrigerate; stable for 96 hours

4. a. 3 mL sterile water for injection

   b. 280 mg/mL

   c. 500 mg

(continued)

Answers (Continued)

Formula Method	Proportion	Dimensional Analysis
$\dfrac{500 \text{ mg}}{280 \text{ mg}} \times 1 \text{ mL} = \dfrac{50}{28}$ $= 1.78$ or 1.8 mL (Round to the nearest tenths place) $= 1.8$ mL	**EXPRESSED AS TWO RATIOS** 1 mL : 280 mg : : x mL : 500 mg **EXPRESSED AS TWO FRACTIONS** $\dfrac{1 \text{ mL}}{280 \text{ mg}} \times \dfrac{\text{x}}{500 \text{ mg}}$ **SOLUTION FOR BOTH PROPORTION METHODS** $500 = 280\text{x}$ $\dfrac{500}{280} = \text{x}$ 1.78 or 1.8 mL $=$ x (Round to the nearest tenths place) $= 1.8$ mL	$\dfrac{1 \text{ mL}}{280 \text{ mg}} \left| \dfrac{\overset{1}{500 \text{ mg}}}{\underset{28}{}} \right. = \dfrac{50}{28}$ mL $= 1.78$ mL or 1.8 mL (Round to the nearest tenths place) $= 1.8$ mL

   d. Give 1.8 mL IM.

   e. 280 mg/mL, date, time, initials, expiration date: 7 days after reconstitution

   f. Refrigerate; stable for 7 days

5. a. Add 2 mL sterile water for injection.

   b. 400 mg/mL

   c. 200 mg

Formula Method	Proportion	Dimensional Analysis
$\dfrac{\overset{1}{200 \text{ mg}}}{\underset{2}{400 \text{ mg}}} \times 1 \text{ mL} = \dfrac{1}{2}$ mL or 0.5 mL	**EXPRESSED AS TWO RATIOS** 1 mL : 400 mg : : x mL : 200 mg **EXPRESSED AS TWO FRACTIONS** $\dfrac{1 \text{ mL}}{400 \text{ mg}} \times \dfrac{\text{x}}{200 \text{ mg}}$ **SOLUTION FOR BOTH PROPORTION METHODS** $200 = 400\text{x}$ $\dfrac{200}{400} = \text{x}$ 0.5 mL $=$ x	$\dfrac{1 \text{ mL}}{\underset{2}{400 \text{ mg}}} \left| \overset{1}{200 \text{ mg}} \right. = \dfrac{1}{2}$ mL or 0.5 mL

   d. Give ½ mL (0.5 mL).

   e. 400 mg/mL, date, time, initials, expiration date: 1 week after reconstitution

   f. Refrigerate; stable for 1 week

Self-Test 7 Insulin Calculations

1.

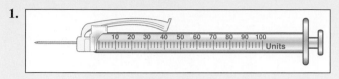

2.

NPH insulin
20 units

Regular insulin
7 units

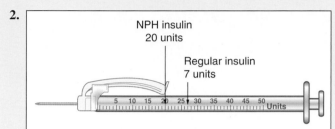

3.

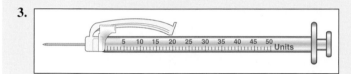

4.

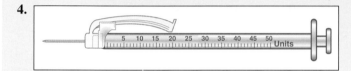

5.

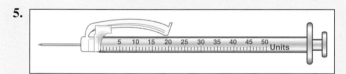

6.

NPH insulin
64 units

Regular insulin
16 units

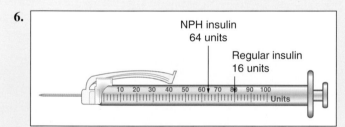

7.

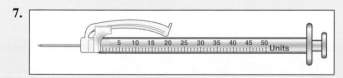

8.

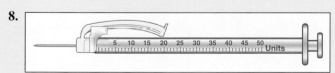

9. Call physician.

10. Give 1 amp D50 and call physician.

Calculation of Basic IV Drip Rates

Administration of parenteral fluids and medications by the IV (intravenous) route is common medical practice and is a specialty within nursing and healthcare. Texts such as *Plumer's Principles and Practice of Intravenous Therapy* (Lippincott Williams & Wilkins, 2006) present detailed and extensive information. This chapter presents basic knowledge—types of fluids, equipment, calculation of drip rates, and recording intake. Chapter 7 presents rules and calculations for special types of IV orders.

Types of IV Fluids

IV fluids are packaged in sterile plastic bags or glass bottles. It is essential to choose the correct IV fluid to avoid serious fluid and electrolyte imbalance that may occur from infusing the wrong solution. Physicians and healthcare providers order IV fluids and the IV flow rate.

If you have any doubt about the correct IV solution, always double-check with another healthcare professional.

Common abbreviations for IV fluids are listed in Table 6-1.

Kinds of IV Drip Factors

IV fluids are administered through infusion sets. These consist of plastic tubing attached at one end to the IV bag and at the other end to a needle or catheter inserted into a blood vessel. The top of the infusion set contains a chamber. Sets with a small needle in the chamber are called *microdrip* because their drops are small. To deliver 1 mL of fluid to the patient/client, 60 drops drip in the drip chamber (60 gtt = 1 mL). All microdrip sets deliver 60 gtt/mL.

TABLE 6-1 Common Abbreviations for IV Fluids	
Abbreviation	**Definition**
D	Dextrose
W	Water
NS	Normal (or isotonic) saline
D5W	5% dextrose in water
0.9% NS	0.9% saline in water (sometimes termed *normal saline*)
0.45% NS	0.45% saline in water (sometimes termed ½ *normal saline*)
0.33% NS	0.33% saline in water (sometimes termed ⅓ *normal saline*)
LR	Lactated Ringer's solution (or Lactated Ringers)

Infusion sets without a small needle in the chamber are called *macrodrip* (Fig. 6-1). Drops per milliliter differ according to the manufacturer. For example, Baxter-Travenol macrodrip sets deliver 10 gtt/mL, so 10 drops drip in the drip chamber (10 gtt = 1 mL); Abbott sets deliver 15 gtt/mL, so 15 drops drip in the drip chamber (15 gtt = 1 mL). The package label states the drops per milliliter (gtt/mL). Sometimes the drop factor is also stated on the top part of the chamber. To calculate IV drip rates, you must know this information (see page 218 on how to choose the correct infusion tubing).

The tubing for these sets includes a roller clamp (Fig. 6-2A) that you can open or close to regulate the drip rate; use a watch or a clock with a second hand to count the number of drops per minute in the chamber (Fig. 6-2B).

The Dial-a-Flow device (sometimes referred to as Dial-a-Flo) is an extension IV tubing that attaches to the primary IV tubing (Fig. 6-3). It is calibrated in milliliters per hour; you "dial" the rate, and the device regulates the flow. The roller clamp must be open all the way. Usually, these devices are not used with an infusion pump. The rate is still an approximate amount, and changes in the patient/client position can affect the flow rate.

Infusion Pumps

Electric infusion pumps also deliver IV fluid. Some are easy to operate; others are more elaborate. You must enter two pieces of information: the total number of milliliters to be infused and the number of milliliters per hour. Pumps used in specialty units also allow you to input the name of the medication, the concentration of the medication, the amount of fluid, and the patient/client's weight. The infusion rate is set in milliliters per hour, and the pump automatically calculates the dose in milligrams, micrograms, etc. There are several manufacturers of IV pumps; some pumps use regular IV tubing, while other pumps use tubing specific to that IV pump. All IV pumps allow you to program the primary IV rate, volume to be infused, secondary IV rate, and total volume that has infused over a period of time. The pump can also calculate the dosage based on weight. Figure 6-4 shows the face of an infusion pump with IV tubing connected.

The tubing factor for an IV infusion pump is 60 gtt/mL; however, the rate is stated and programmed as milliliters per hour.

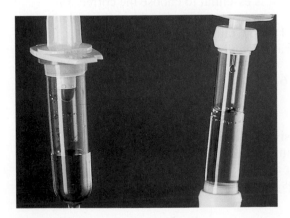

FIGURE 6-1

Drip chambers for macrodrip and microdrip IV tubing.

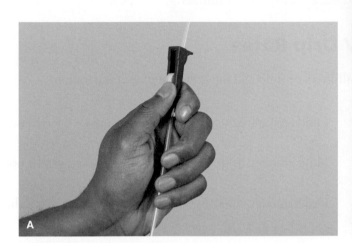
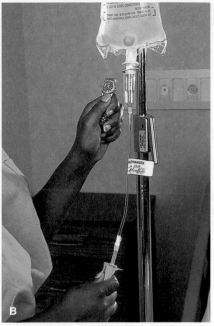

FIGURE 6-2

(A) Roller clamp **(B)** Timing the IV drip rate. (© B. Proud.) (With permission From Taylor, C., Lillis, C., & LeMone, P. [2004]. *Photo atlas of medication administration*. Philadelphia, PA: Lippincott Williams & Wilkins, p. 46.)

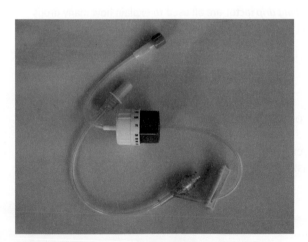

FIGURE 6-3

Dial-a-Flow device. (Copyright 2010 L. Farmer Photography.)

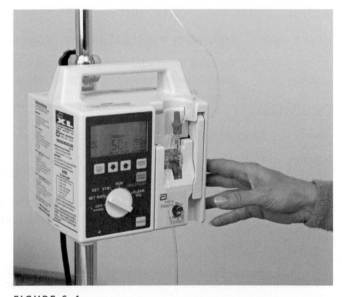

FIGURE 6-4

IV rate is programmed into the infusion pump in milliliters per hour. (With permission from Craven, R. and Himle, C. (2007) *Fundamentals of nursing* (5th ed). Philadelphia, PA: Lippincott Williams and Wilkins, p. 576.)

Labeling IVs

Every IV must be labeled so that any professional can check both the fluid that is infusing and the drip rate. A typical order includes the following information:

- Patient/client name, room, bed number, date, and time
- Order: 500 mL D5W½NS. Rate: 50 mL/hr.

EXAMPLE

LABEL			
Patient/Client	*Andrew Avery*	Room	*1411B*
Date, Time	*6/26, 1000A*	Rate	*50 mL/hr*
Order	*500 mL D5½NS*	Initials	*CB*

Calculating Basic IV Drip Rates

Routine IV orders specify the number of milliliters of fluid and the duration of administration:

EXAMPLE

250 mL D5W IV at 250 mL/hour	Fluid amount: 250 mL	Time: to infuse over 1 hour
1000 mL LR IV 8 AM–8 PM	Fluid amount: 1000 mL	Time: to infuse over 12 hours
500 mL D5½NS with 20 mEq KCl IV to run 75 mL/hr on a pump	Fluid amount: 500 mL	Time: to infuse at 75 mL/hr

As mentioned previously, an infusion pump is set in milliliters per hour, so your dosage calculations are in milliliters per hour as well. IV tubing sets infuse at drops per minute, and the infusion rate depends on the drip rate of the tubing used. Although many institutions only use infusion pumps occasionally you will need to calculate and infuse IV fluid using the drip rate calculation.

RULE ➤ **SOLVING IV CALCULATIONS WITH MICRO- AND MACRODRIP TUBING**

The terms *drop factor, drip factor*, gtt factor, and *tubing drip* factor are all used to explain how many drops per milliliter the tubing delivers. In this text, we will use *drop factor or DF* to mean all of these terms.

Calculation

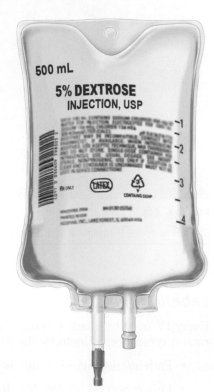

Here's one formula on calculating drip rates:

$$\frac{\text{Number of milliliters to infuse} \times \text{DF}}{\text{Number of minutes to infuse}} = \text{Drops per minute or gtt/minute}$$

For example, the order is to infuse 120 mL of D5W over 60 minutes with a drop factor of 10 drops per milliliter. The calculation is:

$$\frac{120 \times 10}{60} = 20 \text{ gtt/minute}$$

For dimensional analysis, you set up the equation as such:

$$\frac{\text{gtt}}{\text{mL}} \mid \frac{\text{mL to infuse}}{\text{minutes}}$$

In this example:

$$\frac{10 \text{ gtt}}{1 \text{ mL}} \mid \frac{120 \text{ mL}}{60 \text{ minutes}}$$

Cancel "mL." Reduce the fraction. Solve.

$$\frac{10 \text{ gtt}}{1 \text{ mL}} \mid \frac{\overset{2}{120 \text{ mL}}}{\underset{1}{60 \text{ minutes}}} = 10 \times 2 = 20 \text{ gtt/minute}$$

Explanation

DF: the tubing drop factor—either microdrip (60 gtt = 1 mL) or macrodrip. Depending on the manufacturer, macrodrip could be 10 gtt = 1 mL, 15 gtt = 1 mL, or 20 gtt = 1 mL.

Minutes: the number of minutes, specified in every IV order. If the order reads "hour," then you convert to minutes by multiplying by 60 (60 minutes = 1 hour).

gtt/minute: the drip factor, calculated to deliver an even flow of fluid over a specified time. To regulate the drip rate, use a second hand on a watch or a clock. If the drip rate is calculated to be 20 gtt/minute, open the clamp and regulate the drip until you reach that amount. Usually, you break this amount down into seconds rather than counting for a full minute. For this example, 20 gtt/minute becomes approximately 5 gtt every 15 seconds (20 gtt divided by 60 = 0.33 gtt every second. Multiply 0.33 times 15 = approximately 5 gtt every 15 seconds).

The problems requiring calculation in this text will supply the tubing (or drip) factor. When you're working in the clinical area, you must read the package label of the IV tubing to identify the drops per milliliter.

Solving IV Calculations Using an Infusion Pump

Infusion pumps are always calculated in milliliters per hour. Here's how to calculate the example from above, infusing 120 mL of IV fluid over 60 minutes:

$$\frac{\text{Total number of milliliters ordered}}{\text{Number of hours to run}} = \text{mL/hour}$$

The calculation looks like this:

$$\frac{120 \text{ mL}}{1 \text{ hour}} = 120 \text{ mL/hour}$$

Note that 60 minutes was changed to 1 hour (60 minutes = 1 hour).

After calculating, connect the IV fluids to the infusion pump with the appropriate tubing, set the pump at 120 mL/hour, set the volume for infusion—120 mL, and start the infusion.

Explanation

mL: The physician or healthcare provider will indicate the number of milliliters to be infused in the order.

hours: The number of hours to run depends on the way the order is written. For example:

q8h = 8 hours at a time (infuse over 8 hours)

10 AM–4 PM = 6 hours (infuse over 6 hours)

60 minutes = 1 hour (infuse over 1 hour)

90 minutes = 1.5 hours (infuse over 1.5 hour) (to get the number of hours, divide minutes by 60)

Alternate Way

Here's a formula you can use to calculate what rate to set on the infusion pump:

$$\frac{\text{Number of milliliters to infuse} \times \text{DF}}{\text{Number of minutes to infuse}} = \text{Drops per minute or gtt/minute}$$

Since the tubing factor is always 60 gtt/mL with infusion pumps, for the calculation "infuse 120 mL of IV fluid over 60 minutes using an infusion pump," the formula looks like this:

$$\frac{120 \text{ mL} \times 60 \text{ gtt/mL}}{60 \text{ minutes}} = 120 \text{ gtt/minute or } 120 \text{ mL/hour}$$

Drip rates are rounded to the nearest whole number unless using an infusion pump that can infuse in tenths or hundredths (i.e., 8.25 mL/hour). Usually, these infusion pumps are used in a specialty setting such as critical care or pediatrics.

Choosing the Infusion Set

Experience will enable you to judge which IV tubing to use. In clinical settings, the guidelines below will help you make your choice. An electric infusion pump poses no problem, because it will deliver the amount programmed. Specialized pumps in neonatal and intensive care units can deliver 1 mL/hour and even less. Specialized syringe pumps also can deliver less than 1 mL/hour.

When an IV pump is not available, consider these guidelines:

Use microdrip when

- the IV is to be administered over a long period

- a small amount of fluid is to be infused

- the macrodrops per minute are too few (Without an infusion pump, IV fluids flow by gravity. Blood flowing in the vein exerts a pressure. If the IV is too slow, the pressure of the blood in the vein may back up into the tubing, where it may clot and cause the IV to stop infusing.)

Use macrodrip when

- the order specifies a large amount of fluid over a short time

- the microdrips per minute are too many, and counting the drip rate becomes to difficult

---

EXAMPLE

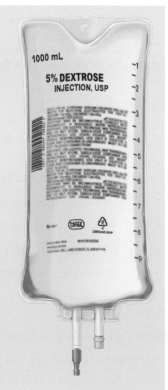

Order: 1000 mL D5W IV 8 AM–8 PM

Available: an infusion pump

8 AM to 8 PM indicates that the IV will run for 12 hours. The infusion pump regulates the rate in milliliters per hour.

$$\frac{\text{Number of mL}}{\text{Number of hours}} = \text{mL/hour}$$

$$\frac{1000 \text{ mL}}{12 \text{ hours}} = 12 \overline{)1000.0} \quad \begin{array}{r} 83.3 \\ \hline 1000.0 \\ 96 \\ \hline 40 \\ 36 \\ \hline 40 \\ 36 \end{array}$$

Label the IV.

Set the pump as follows:

Total volume to infuse: 1000 mL

mL/hour: 83 (Dimensional Analysis: use the same equation, no conversion factor is needed)

EXAMPLE

Order: 500 mL NS IV 12 NOON–4 PM

Available: microdrip at 60 gtt/mL; macrodrip at 20 gtt/mL

The IV will run 4 hours or 240 minutes (4 × 60 minutes). Because no pump is available, the nurse must choose the drip factor. Solve for both drip factors and choose one. Round to the nearest whole number.

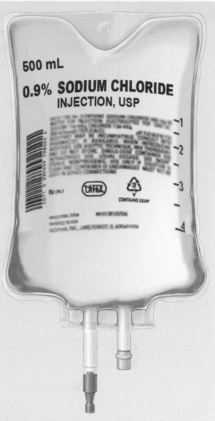

MACRODRIP

$$\frac{500 \text{ mL} \times \overset{1}{\cancel{20}}}{\underset{12}{\cancel{240}}} = \frac{500}{12} = 12\overline{)\begin{array}{l}41.6 \\ 500.0 \\ \underline{48} \\ 20 \\ \underline{12} \\ 80\end{array}}$$

Dimensional Analysis: Use the conversion

factor $\dfrac{1 \text{ hour}}{60 \text{ minutes}}$.

20 gtt	500 mL	1 hour
1 mL	4 hours	60 minutes

Cancel "mL" and "hour." Reduce the fraction. Solve.

$$\frac{\overset{1}{\cancel{\underset{\cancel{5}}{20}}} \text{\cancel{gtt}}}{1 \text{ \cancel{mL}}} \bigg| \frac{500 \text{ \cancel{mL}}}{\underset{1}{\cancel{4}} \text{ \cancel{hours}}} \bigg| \frac{1 \text{ \cancel{hour}}}{\underset{12}{\cancel{60}} \text{ minutes}} = \frac{500}{12} = 41.6 \text{ or } 42 \text{ gtt/minute}$$

Macrodrip at 42 gtt/minute.

MICRODRIP

$$\frac{500 \times \overset{1}{\cancel{60}}}{\underset{4}{\cancel{240}}} = 4\overline{)\begin{array}{l}125 \\ 500 \\ \underline{4} \\ 10 \\ \underline{8} \\ 20\end{array}}$$

Dimensional Analysis:

$$\frac{\overset{1}{\cancel{60}} \text{\cancel{gtt}}}{1 \text{ \cancel{mL}}} \bigg| \frac{\overset{125}{\cancel{500}} \text{ \cancel{mL}}}{\underset{1}{\cancel{4}} \text{ \cancel{hours}}} \bigg| \frac{1 \text{ \cancel{hour}}}{\underset{1}{\cancel{60}} \text{ minutes}} = 125 \text{ gtt/minute}$$

Microdrip at 125 gtt/minute.

Answers are macrodrip at 42 gtt/minute and microdrip at 125 gtt/min. Choose one.

Label the IV.

Set the drip rate.

EXAMPLE

Order: 500 mL D5W IV KVO for 24 hours (KVO stands for "keep vein open." It usually is an IV rate that keeps fluids infusing through a vein. TKO (to keep open) is another abbreviation with the same meaning).

Available: microdrip at 60 gtt/mL; macrodrip 10 gtt/mL

Because no pump is available, choose the IV set. The IV will run 24 hours or 1440 minutes (24 × 60 minutes). Work out the problem for micro- and macrodrip and make a nursing judgment about which tubing to use. Round to the nearest whole number.

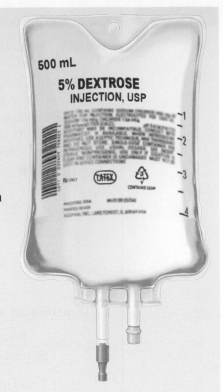

500 mL

5% DEXTROSE
INJECTION, USP

MACRODRIP

$$\frac{500 \text{ mL} \times \overset{1}{\cancel{10}} \text{ gtt}}{\cancel{1440} \text{ minutes}} = \frac{500}{144}$$

$$144 \overline{\smash{)}500.0} \quad \begin{array}{r} 3.4 \\ \underline{432} \\ 680 \\ \underline{576} \\ 104 \end{array}$$

Dimensional Analysis:

$$\frac{\overset{5}{\cancel{10}} \text{ (gtt)}}{1 \text{ mL}} \left| \frac{\overset{100}{\cancel{500}} \text{ mL}}{\underset{12}{\cancel{24}} \text{ hours}} \right| \frac{1 \text{ hour}}{\underset{12}{\cancel{60}} \text{ (minutes)}} = \frac{5 \times 100}{12 \times 12} = \frac{500}{144} = 3.4 \text{ or } 3 \text{ gtt/minute}$$

Macrodrip at 3 gtt/minute.

MICRODRIP

$$\frac{500 \text{ mL} \times \cancel{60} \text{ gtt}}{\cancel{1440} \text{ minutes}} = \frac{3000}{144}$$

$$144 \overline{\smash{)}3000.0} \quad \begin{array}{r} 20.8 \\ \underline{288} \\ 1200 \\ \underline{1152} \\ 48 \end{array}$$

Dimensional Analysis:

$$\frac{\overset{1}{\cancel{60}} \text{ (gtt)}}{1 \text{ mL}} \left| \frac{500 \text{ mL}}{24 \text{ hours}} \right| \frac{1 \text{ hour}}{\underset{1}{\cancel{60}} \text{ (minutes)}} = \frac{500}{24} = 20.8 \text{ or } 21 \text{ gtt/minute}$$

Microdrip at 21 gtt/minute.

A 3-gtt/minute macrodrip is too slow. Choose microdrip. (See the explanation for choosing the infusion set on page 204.)

Label the IV.

Select a microdrip infusion set.

Set the drip rate at 21 gtt/minute.

SELF-TEST 1 Calculation of Drip Rates

Calculate the drip rate for the following IV orders given in milliliters per hour or drops per minute. Answers are given at the end of the chapter. Round to the nearest whole number.

1. Order: 150 mL D5WNS IV q8h
   Available: infusion pump

2. Order: 250 mL D5W; run at 25 mL/hour
   Available: infusion pump

3. Order: 1000 mL D5NS; run 100 mL/hour
   Available: macrodrip (20 gtt/mL); microdrip (60 gtt/mL)

4. Order: 180 mL D5½NS 12 NOON–6 PM
   Available: macrodrip (10 gtt/mL); microdrip (60 gtt/mL)

5. Order: 1000 mL D5W 0.45NS IV 4 PM–12 MIDNIGHT
   Available: macrodrip (15 gtt/mL); microdrip (60 gtt/mL)

6. Order: 250 mL D5W IV q8h
   Available: infusion pump

7. Order: 500 mL NS IV over 2 hours
   Available: infusion pump

8. Order: 1000 mL D5NS IV 4 AM–4 PM
   Available: macrodrip (15 gtt/mL); microdrip (60 gtt/mL)

9. Order: 1000 mL D5W 0.45 NS IV; run 150 mL/hour
   Available: macrodrip (10 gtt/mL); microdrip (60 gtt/mL)

10. Order: 150 mL 0.9 NS IV; over 1 hour
    Available: macrodrip (20 gtt/mL); microdrip (60 gtt/mL)

Determining Hours an IV Will Run

Knowing how to calculate approximately how long an IV will last helps you to know when to prepare the next IV, or to be aware if the IV is infusing too fast or too slow.

$$\frac{\text{Number of milliliters ordered}}{\text{Number of milliliters per hour}} = \text{Number of hours to run}$$

EXAMPLE

Order: 500 mL NS IV; infuse at 75 mL/hour

$$\frac{\text{Number of mL}}{\text{Number of mL/hour}} = \text{Hours}$$

$$\frac{500 \text{ mL}}{75 \text{ mL/hour}} = 75\overline{)\begin{array}{l} 6.67 \\ 500.00 \\ \underline{450} \\ 500 \\ \underline{450} \\ 500 \end{array}}$$

The IV will last approximately 6.7 hours. How many hours and minutes will this be? Since there are 60 minutes in an hour, take 0.7 and multiply by 60, which equals 42 minutes.

What time will the IV be complete? If the IV bag is hung at, say, 8 AM, then add the hours and minutes to calculate when the IV should be complete: 2:42 PM
(6 hours and 42 minutes added to 8 AM).

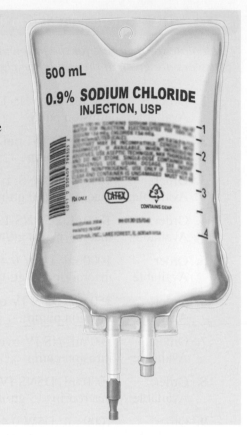

EXAMPLE

Order: 1000 mL ½ NS IV 8 AM–8 PM

No math necessary; 8 AM–8 PM = 12 hours

The IV will last 12 hours.

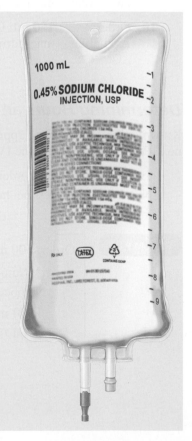

EXAMPLE

Order: D5W IV at 50 mL/hour

$$\frac{\text{Number of mL}}{\text{Number of mL/hour}} = \text{Hours}$$

$$\frac{500 \text{ mL}}{50 \text{ mL}} = 10 \text{ hours}$$

The IV will last 10 hours.

Start the infusion at 10 AM. When will the IV infusion be complete?

10 AM + 10 hours = 8 PM

The infusion will be complete at 8 PM.

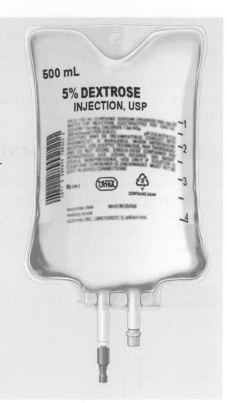

500 mL

5% DEXTROSE
INJECTION, USP

SELF-TEST 2   IV Infusions—Hours

Calculate the hours that the following IV orders will run. Answers are given at the end of this chapter. Convert to hours and minutes if applicable.

1. Order: 250 mL D5½NS IV at 30 mL/hour

2. Order: 500 mL LR IV run at 60 mL/hour

3. Order: 1000 mL D5NS IV 4 PM–2 AM

4. Order: 1000 mL D5W IV KVO 24 hours

5. Order: 500 mL D5½NS at 70 mL/hour

6. Order: 500 mL D5W IV at 50 mL/hour

7. Order: 1000 mL LR IV over 10 hours
Start the IV at 9 AM. When will it be finished?

8. Order: 250 mL NS IV at 100 mL/hour
Start the IV at 1 PM. When will it be finished?

9. Order: 1000 mL NS IV 12 NOON–6 PM

10. Order: 500 mL NS IV over 5 hours

Assessment

Many factors may interfere with the drip rate. When you are not using an infusion pump, gravity will cause the IV to vary from its starting rate; you will need to observe and assess the infusion and IV site frequently. You'll need to monitor other conditions as well. As the amount of fluid decreases in the IV bag, pressure changes occur—and they, too, may affect the rate. The patient/client's movements can kink the tube and shut off the flow; they can change the position of the needle or catheter in the vein.

The needle can become lodged against the side of the blood vessel, thereby altering the flow, or it may be forced out of the vessel, allowing fluid to enter the tissues (infiltration). (Signs of possible infiltration are swelling, pain, coolness, or pallor at the insertion site. If you notice any of these signs, discontinue the IV and start a new one at another insertion site.)

Infusion pumps have an alarm system that beeps to alert you when the rate cannot be maintained or when the infusion is nearly finished. Be sure to check the infusion pump frequently, and know how to troubleshoot the various alarms.

 ## Adding Medications to IVs

When a continuous IV order includes a medication, generally this medication arrives already premixed in the infusion bag or the pharmacist adds it on site. In some institutions, you, the nurse, add the medication to the IV and determine the rate of flow. (Follow the policy at your institution.) If the task falls to you, first calculate how much of the medication to add to the IV fluids and then calculate the drip rate.

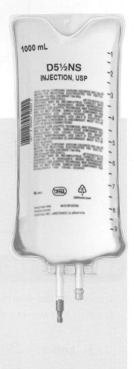

EXAMPLE

Order: 1000 mL D5½NS with 20 mEq KCl IV 10 AM–10 PM

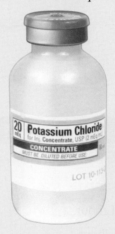

Available: vial of KCl 40 mEq/20 mL, microdrip (60 gtt/minute), macrodrip (20 gtt/minute)

Calculate how many milliliters to add to the IV fluids.

Formula Method	Proportion	Dimensional Analysis

Formula Method

$$\frac{\overset{1}{\cancel{20} \text{ mEq}}}{\underset{2}{\cancel{40} \text{ mEq}}} \times \overset{10}{\cancel{20} \text{ mL}} = 10 \text{ mL}$$

Proportion

EXPRESSED AS TWO RATIOS

$$20 \text{ mL} : 40 \text{ mEq} :: x \text{ mL} : 20 \text{ mEq}$$

EXPRESSED AS TWO FRACTIONS

$$\frac{20 \text{ mL}}{40 \text{ mEq}} \diagup \frac{x}{20 \text{ mEq}}$$

SOLUTION FOR BOTH PROPORTION METHODS

$$20 \times 20 = 40x$$
$$\frac{400}{40} = x$$
$$10 \text{ mL} = x$$

Dimensional Analysis

$$\frac{\overset{1}{\cancel{20} \text{ (mL)}}}{\underset{2}{\cancel{40} \text{ mEq}}} \quad \Big| \quad \frac{20 \text{ mEq}}{} = \frac{20}{2} = 10 \text{ mL}$$

FINE POINTS

Why is the solution not considered to be 1010 mL after adding the KCl? Generally, IV bags are overfilled anyway and we don't need to recalculate when we add the fluid that has the drug in it, unless it is a large amount. For adults, this is usually 25 mL or more; for children we are much more exact and would include the amount of fluid with the drug in it in our total amount of fluid.

Add 10 mL KCl to the IV bag.

Choose the tubing. The IV will run 12 hours.

For macrodrip: $\dfrac{1000 \text{ mL} \times 20 \text{ gtt}}{720 \text{ minutes}} = 28 \text{ gtt/minute}$

For microdrip: $\dfrac{1000 \text{ mL} \times 60 \text{ gtt}}{720 \text{ minutes}} = 83 \text{ gtt/minute}$

Choose either drip rate.

Label the IV.

EXAMPLE

Order: aminophylline 250 mg in 250 mL D5W IV; run at 50 mL/hour for 1 hour.

Available: ampule of aminophylline labeled 1 g in 10 mL; Buretrol that delivers 60 gtt/mL (microdrip). See Figure 6-5.

The ampule of aminophylline has 1 g in 10 mL. This is equivalent to 1000 mg in 10 mL. You want 250 mg.

Calculate how many milliliters to add to the IV fluids.

Formula Method	Proportion	Dimensional Analysis

Formula Method

$\dfrac{\overset{1}{\cancel{250}}}{\underset{4}{\cancel{1000}}} \times 10 = \dfrac{\cancel{10}}{4} \quad 4\overline{)10.0}\;\; 2.5 \text{ mL}$

Proportion

EXPRESSED AS TWO RATIOS

10 mL : 1000 mg :: x mL : 250 mg

EXPRESSED AS TWO FRACTIONS

$\dfrac{10 \text{ mL}}{1000 \text{ mg}} \neq \dfrac{x}{250 \text{ mg}}$

SOLUTION FOR BOTH
PROPORTION METHODS

$10 \times 250 = 1000x$

$\dfrac{2500}{1000} = x$

$2.5 \text{ mL} = x$

Dimensional Analysis

$\dfrac{10 \text{ mL}}{1 \text{ g}} \;\Big|\; \dfrac{\overset{1}{250 \text{ mg}}}{} \;\Big|\; \dfrac{1 \text{ g}}{\underset{4}{1000 \text{ mg}}} = \dfrac{10}{4}$

$= 2.5 \text{ mL}$

Draw up 2.5 mL and inject it into 250 mL D5W. You have 250 mg aminophylline in 250 mL D5W. Label the bag.

You want 50 mL/hour, and you have a Buretrol 60 gtt/mL. Open the Buretrol device, and drip in 50 mL. You will run this amount over 1 hour because that's what the order specified.

$\dfrac{50 \text{ mL} \times \cancel{60} \text{ gtt}}{\cancel{60} \text{ minutes}} = 50 \text{ mL/hour}$

Label the IV: Rate, 50 mL/hour or 50 gtt/minute

FINE POINTS

The Buretrol is microdrip. No calculation is needed:

mL/hour = gtt/minute

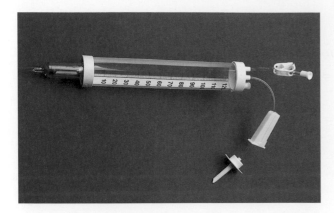

FIGURE 6-5

A Buretrol is an IV delivery system with tubing and a chamber that can hold 150 mL delivered as microdrip (1 mL = 60 drops). (This device is sometimes referred to as a Volutrol.) The top of the Buretrol has a port so that a reservoir of fluid can be added. The Buretrol is a volume control because no more than 150 mL can be infused at one time.

SELF-TEST 3 **IV Infusion Rates**

Calculate how much medication is needed (if applicable) and the infusion rate for the following orders. Answers are given at the end of the chapter. Round to the nearest whole number.

1. Order: 500 mL D5W IV with vitamin C 500 mg at 60 mL/hour
Available: ampule of vitamin C labeled 500 mg/2 mL; microdrip tubing at 60 gtt/mL

2. Order: 250 mg hydrocortisone sodium succinate (Solu-Cortef) in 1000 mL D5W
8 AM–12 MIDNIGHT
Available: vial of hydrocortisone sodium succinate labeled 250 mg with a 2-mL diluent; microdrip tubing

3. Order: aminophylline 250 mg in 250 mL D5W IV; run 50 mL/hour
Available: infusion pump, vial of aminophylline labeled 500 mg/10 mL

4. Order: 250 mL D5½NS with KCl 10 mEq IV 12 NOON–6 PM
Available: microdrip tubing, vial of potassium chloride labeled 20 mEq/10 mL

Medications for Intermittent IV Administration

Some IV medications are administered not continuously but only intermittently, such as every 4, 6, or 8 hours. This route is termed *intravenous piggyback* or (IVPB) (Fig. 6-6). The term admixture refers to the premixed IVPB.

Most of these drugs are prepared in powder form. The manufacturer specifies the type and amount of diluent needed to reconstitute the drug; later, you, the nurse, connect the IVPB (containing the reconstituted drug) by IV tubing to the main IV line. Some IVPB medications come premixed from the manufacturer. For other medications, the institutional pharmacy may reconstitute and prepare IVPB solutions in a sterile environment using a laminar flow hood. This procedure saves nursing time, because when you are ready to administer the drugs, they have already been prepared, labeled, and screened for incompatibilities. Nevertheless, the nurse still bears considerable responsibility: You must check the diluent and volume. You must also check the dose and the expiration date of the reconstituted solution; note whether the IVPB should be refrigerated before use or whether it can remain at room temperature until hung. Finally, you must calculate the drip rate and record this information on the IVPB label before hanging the bag.

The physician or healthcare provider may write a detailed order, such as "Vancomycin 0.5 g IVPB in 100 mL D5W over 1 hour." More often, however, the physician or healthcare provider writes only the drug, route, and time interval, relying on you to research the manufacturer's directions for the amount and type of diluent and the time for the infusion to run (e.g., Order: cefazolin 1 g IVPB q6h).

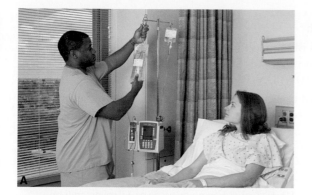
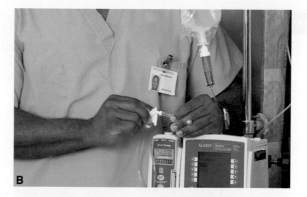
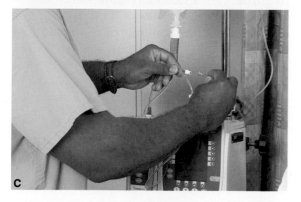
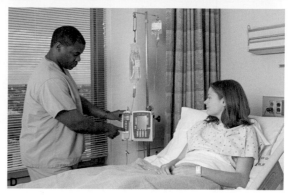
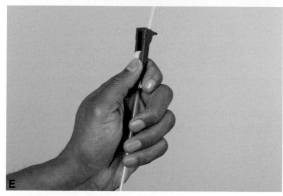

FIGURE 6-6

(A) A primary IV line (left) and an IVPB or secondary line (left). Hang the piggyback higher than the primary line. **(B)** Clean the access port on the primary IV tubing. **(C)** After the piggyback tubing is primed, attach the piggyback setup to the access port. **(D and E).** Set the rate on an infusion pump or use roller clamp on primary infusion tubing to regulate gravity flow. This setup allows the piggyback to flow and the primary infusion is temporarily stopped. After the piggyback has infused, the primary infusion will begin infusing again.

Explanation

To solve IVPB problems, you use a calculation much like the one you used for the IV:

$$\frac{mL \times DF}{minutes} = gtt/minute \quad or \quad \frac{gtt}{mL} \bigg| \frac{mL}{minute}$$

mL: The label or the package insert will state the type and amount of diluent.

DF: The tubing for IVPB is referred to as a secondary administration set and has a macrodrip factor. It is shorter than main line IV tubing. In the clinical setting, check the label for the tubing drip factor.

Minutes: The manufacturer may or may not indicate the number of minutes needed for the IVPB medication to be infused. When the number is not given, follow this general rule for adults: allow 30 minutes for every 50 mL of solution.

EXAMPLE

Order: cefazolin (Ancef) 1 g IVPB q6h

Supply: **package insert** IVPB dilution of cefazolin sodium. Reconstitute with 50 to 100 mL of sodium chloride injection or other solution listed under administration. Other solutions listed include D5W, D10W, D5LR, and D5NS.

Use a 50-mL bag of D5W. It is the most common IVPB diluent. No time for infusion is given in the directions for IVPB; so use 30 minutes for 50 mL. Use an infusion set with a drop factor of 10 gtt/mL.

Here's the calculation:

$$\frac{\text{mL} \times \text{DF}}{\text{minutes}} = \text{gtt/minute}$$

mL = 50 mL D5W
DF = 10 gtt/mL (For a secondary administration, no set time for administration is given. Follow the general adult rule of 30 minutes for every 50 mL.)
minutes = 30

$$\frac{50 \times 10}{30} = 16.6 = 17 \text{ gtt/minute}$$

Dimensional Analysis:

$$\frac{\overset{1}{\cancel{10}} \text{ gtt}}{\cancel{\text{mL}}} \Bigg| \frac{50 \cancel{\text{mL}}}{\underset{3}{\cancel{30}} \text{ minutes}} = \frac{50}{3} = 16.6 \text{ or } 17 \text{ gtt/minute}$$

Before hanging the IVPB, reconstitute the drug. You have a vial of powder labeled 1 g, and you need the whole amount. You have a 50-mL bag of D5W, and you need that whole amount as well. To mix the powder and the diluent, use a reconstitution device—a sterile implement containing two needles or a needleless device that connects the vial and the 50-mL bag. With this device, you can dilute the powder and place it in the IV bag without using a syringe (Fig. 6-7). Some manufacturers now enclose a reconstitution device with the IV bag. Once the powder is reconstituted, label the IV bag.

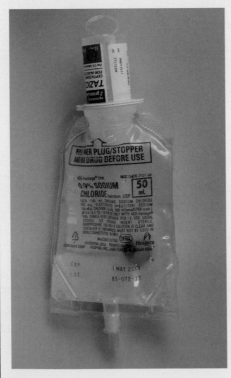

FIGURE 6-7

Reconstitution device: The plug or stopper is removed inside the bag, and the bag is squeezed, forcing the fluid into the powder, which is in the container at the top. Gently shake the bag, diluting and mixing the powder with the fluid. The bag is then hung as a secondary IVPB. (Copyright 2010 L. Farmer Photography.)

The order is q6h, and generally the administration times are 6 AM, 12 NOON, 6 PM, 12 MIDNIGHT. The time of infusion is 30 minutes, and for this label, it will run from 12 NOON to 12:30 PM.

Rather than spending time looking through package inserts for directions, check the concise information in a drug reference such as *Lippincott's Nursing Drug Guide* or a drug information website that your hospital or institution provides.

MEDICATION ADDED

Patient/Client *Chelsea Robertson*	Room *1503*
Medication *cefazolin 1 g*	Flow Rate *17 gtt/minute*
Base Solution *50 mL D5W*	Initials *RT*
	Date, Time *6/14, 12 PM*

EXAMPLE

Order: vancomycin (Vancocin) 1 g in 250 mL D5W IVPB 7 AM

Supply: 500 mg powder reconstitute with 10 mL sterile water to yield 50 mg/mL

DF: 10 gtt/mL

Package insert directions: 250 mL D5W

Run over 2 hours.

$$\frac{mL \times DF}{minutes} = gtt/minute$$

$$\frac{250 \times 10}{120} = \frac{250}{12} \overset{20.8}{\overline{)250.0}} = 21\ gtt/minute$$
$$\phantom{\frac{250 \times 10}{120} = \frac{250}{12}}\ \underline{240}$$
$$\phantom{\frac{250 \times 10}{120} = \frac{250}{12}}\ \ 100$$
$$\phantom{\frac{250 \times 10}{120} = \frac{250}{12}}\ \ \ \underline{96}$$

Dimensional Analysis:

$$\frac{\overset{1}{10}\ gtt}{1\ mL} \left| \frac{\overset{125}{250}\ mL}{\underset{1}{2}\ hours} \right| \frac{1\ hour}{\underset{6}{60}\ minutes} = \frac{125}{6} = 20.8\ or\ 21\ gtt/minute$$

Add 1 g vancomycin (two vials of 500 mg reconstituted) to 250 mL D5W. (Review reconstitution of powders, Chapter 5, if necessary.) Label the IV. Set the rate at 21 gtt/minute. The IVPB will run 2 hours.

When you're using an infusion pump for IVPB, solve the problem by setting 60 gtt as the tubing factor. Most infusion pumps have a special setting for "secondary IV administration." Choose this setting, then program the rate in milliliters per hour. After the IVPB has infused, the pump then either switches back to the primary IV infusion or begins beeping, letting you know that the infusion is complete.

SELF-TEST 4   IVPB Drip Rates

Solve these drip rates for IVPB problems. Answers are given at the end of this chapter. Round your answer to the nearest whole number.

1. Order: acyclovir (Zovirax) 500 mg IVPB q8h
   Supply: 500 mg powder
   Package directions: Reconstitute with 100 mL/D5W. Use a reconstitution device. Infuse over 1 hour/once a day.
   Available: macrodrip tubing at 10 gtt/mL

2. Order: ceftazidime (Ceptaz) 1 g IVPB q12h
   Supply: 1 g powder
   Package directions: Reconstitute with 50 mL D5W. Use a reconstitution device. Infuse over 15–30 minutes.
   Available: macrodrip tubing at 10 gtt/mL

3. Order: cefotaxime (Claforan) 1 g IVPB q6h
   Supply: 1 g powder
   Package directions: Reconstitute with 50 mL D5W. Use a reconstitution device. Infuse over 15–30 minutes.
   Available: macrodrip tubing at 10 gtt/mL

4. Order: ampicillin (Omnipen) 500 mg IV q6h
   Supply: Reconstitute with 4.5 mL sterile water to yield 2 g in 5 mL.
   Package directions: Add to 50 mL D5W. Infuse over 15–30 minutes.
   Available: microdrip tubing at 60 gtt/mL

5. Order: tobramycin (Nebcin) 50 mg IV q8h
   Supply: Reconstitute with 2 mL sterile water to yield 80 mg in 2 mL.
   Package directions: Add to 100 mL/D5W. Infuse over 60 minutes.
   Available: macrodrip tubing at 15 gtt/mL

6. Order: ticarcillin (Timentin) 500 mg IV q6h
   Supply: Reconstitute in 4.5 mL sterile water to yield 1 g in 5 mL.
   Package directions: Add to 50 mL/D5W. Infuse in 30 minutes.
   Available: macrodrip tubing at 15 gtt/mL

Ambulatory Infusion Device

An ambulatory infusion device such as the one pictured in Figure 6-8 is used when a patient/client is receiving long-term antibiotic or other infusion therapy. The device is filled with the medication, and a vacuum within the container infuses the medication over a specific time frame when the device is

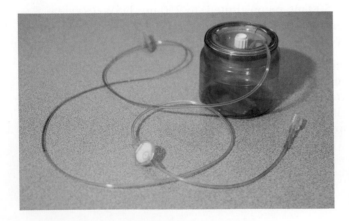

FIGURE 6-8

Ambulatory infusion device.

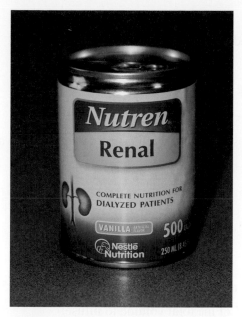

FIGURE 6-9

Commercially prepared tube feeding formula.

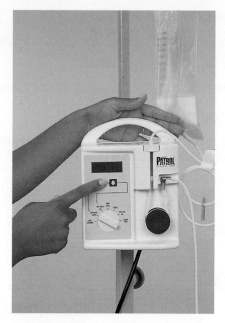

FIGURE 6-10

Feeding pump for infusion of tube feeding. (Used with permission from Craven, R., & Hirnle, C. (2007) *Fundamentals of nursing* (5th ed). Philadelphia, PA: Lippincott Williams & Wilkins, p. 995.)

attached to the patient/client's IV. This is convenient for the patient/client, so that he or she may go home from the hospital on infusion therapy and continue in daily activities. The patient/client may have a peripheral IV site that has to be changed every 3 to 4 days, or he or she may have a long-term indwelling IV catheter, such as a peripherally inserted central catheter (PICC) line.

 Enteral Nutrition

Enteral feeding is used when a patient/client cannot eat or cannot eat enough. A tube is passed through the nasal or oral cavity to the stomach or duodenum, such as with a nasogastric (N/G) tube or orogastric or oral gastric (O/G) tube, or it is placed more permanently, as with a percutaneous endoscopic gastrostomy (PEG) tube, gastrostomy tube (G tube), or jejunostomy tube (J tube). Commercial tube feedings are used as well (Fig. 6-9); these formulas, though varied, usually carry a high-caloric component. They may also include high fiber and high protein and may vary according to a patient/client's disease state.

Tube feedings are administered with a pump that regulates the amount of feeding. The feedings may be *intermittent*, delivering the formula at regular periods of time; *cyclic*, giving the formula over several hours of the day (over 12 to 16 hours); or *continuous*, infusing the formula constantly (Fig. 6-10).

Enteral feedings require careful monitoring to avoid complications and to ensure the patient/client's safety. Full-strength tube feeding is recommended, although diluted tube feedings are still used. The section below discusses common dilutions and the way to calculate the dose. For more information on enteral feedings, consult a basic nursing book such as *Fundamentals of Nursing* by Taylor, Lillis, LeMone, and Lynn (Lippincott Williams & Wilkins, 2013).

Calculation of Tube Feedings

An order for tube feedings will read:

Administer Isocal full strength at 60 mL/hour. Check for residual every 4 hours. Flush tube with 50 mL of water every 4 hours.

This order does not require calculation.

Add Isocal to a tube feeding bag, and set the tube feeding pump at 60 mL/hour.

Complete the other orders per protocol.

Follow hospital protocol for changing of tube feeding bag and tubing.

Dilution Calculations

Diluting tube feeding involves mixing the nutritional supplement with a specific amount of water. The most common dilutions are as follows:

$\frac{1}{4}$ strength (or one-quarter strength)

$\frac{1}{2}$ strength (or one-half strength)

$\frac{3}{4}$ strength (or three-quarter strength)

EXAMPLE

Administer $\frac{1}{4}$ strength Isocal at 60 mL/hour. The total volume will equal 250 mL.

For this problem, begin by taking $\frac{1}{4}$ of the total volume to infuse:

$\frac{1}{4} \times 250$ mL = 62.5 mL

This number tells you how much formula to add to the tube feeding bag.

Next, subtract that number from the total volume:

250 mL − 62.5 mL = 187.5 mL

This new number tells you how much water to add to the tube feeding bag. Now that you have diluted the formula to $\frac{1}{4}$ strength, infuse it at 60 mL/hour.

EXAMPLE

Administer $\frac{1}{2}$ strength Isocal at 60 mL/hour. The total volume will equal 250 mL.

First, take $\frac{1}{2}$ of the total volume:

$\frac{1}{2} \times 250$ mL = 125 mL

Again, this is the volume of formula to add to the tube feeding bag.

Subtract this number from the total volume:

250 mL − 125 mL = 125 mL

This new number tells you how much water to add to the tube feeding bag.

This is the volume of water to dilute. You have diluted the formula to $\frac{1}{2}$ strength; infuse at 60 mL/hour.

EXAMPLE

Administer $\frac{3}{4}$ strength Isocal at 60 mL/hour. The total volume will equal 250 mL.

Take $\frac{3}{4}$ of the total volume:

$\frac{3}{4} \times 250$ mL = 187.5 mL of Isocal

Subtract from the total:

250 mL − 187.5 = 62.5 mL of water to dilute. You have diluted the formula to $\frac{3}{4}$ strength; infuse at 60 mL/hour.

SELF-TEST 5	Calculation of Tube Feedings

Solve these problems stating how much of the feeding and how much water to add. Answers are at the end of the chapter.

1. Prepare ¾ strength Isocal. Total volume is 275 mL. How much Isocal is to be mixed with how much water?

2. Prepare 75 mL of 75% Magnacal. How much Magnacal is to be mixed with how much water?

3. Prepare ½ strength Osmolite. Total volume is 100 mL. How much Osmolite is to be mixed with how much water?

4. Prepare ¼ strength Ensure. Total volume is 85 mL. How much Ensure is to be mixed with how much water?

5. Prepare 25% Renalcal. Total volume is 400 mL. How much Renalcal is to be mixed with how much water?

6. Prepare 50% Suplena. Total volume is 400 mL. How much Suplena is to be mixed with how much water?

Recording Intake

Keep an accurate account of parenteral intake as well as liquids taken orally and/or enterally (e.g., tube feedings). Each institution provides a flow sheet to record fluid input over a specified period of time. Usually, when an IVPB is infusing, the primary IV stops infusing. After the IVPB is completed, the primary IV flow rate begins again. (Refer to Fig. 6-6.)

EXAMPLE

The primary IV is infusing at 50 mL/hour. For 12 hours, the IV intake would be 600 mL (12 hours × 50 mL = 600 mL). If you administer an IVPB of 100 mL once during the 12 hours and infuse the IVPB at 100 mL/hour, then your IV intake would be as follows:

11 hours × 50 mL of primary IV (550 mL) plus 1 hour of 100 mL IVPB, to equal 650 mL IV intake for 12 hours.

An IV infusion pump can keep track of all fluids infused over a specific amount of time. Usually there is a screen titled "volume infused" that shows this value.

SELF-TEST 6	Fluid Intake

Answer the following questions regarding fluid intake. Answers are given at the end of this chapter.

1. A total of 900 mL of an IV solution is to infuse at 100 mL/hour. If it is 9 AM when the infusion starts, at what time will it be completed?

2. A patient/client is receiving an antibiotic IVPB in 75 mL q6h to run over 1 hour plus a maintenance IV of 125 mL/hour. What is the 24-hour intake parenterally?

3. An IV of 1000 mL D5NS is infusing at 10 microdrips/minute. What is the parenteral intake for 8 hours?

4. A doctor orders 500 mL with aminophylline 0.5 g to infuse at 50 mL/hour. How many milligrams will the patient/client receive each hour?

(continued)

SELF-TEST 6   Fluid Intake (Continued)

5. A total of 20,000 units of heparin is added to 500 mL D5W, and the order is to infuse IV at 30 mL/hour. How many hours will the IV run?

6. A patient/client is receiving an antibiotic IVPB in 50 mL q8h to run over 1 hour plus a maintenance IV of 100 mL/hour. What is the 24-hour intake parenterally?

7. A total of 500 mL of an IV solution is to infuse at 50 mL/hour. If it is 6 AM when the infusion starts, at what time is it completed?

8. An IV of D5W 1000 mL is infusing at 125 mL/hour. How many hours will the IV run?

9. A patient/client is receiving an antibiotic IVPB in 250 mL q6h. What is the 24-hour intake parenterally?

10. A physician orders 100 units regular insulin in 100 mL to infuse at 10 mL/hour. How many units will the patient/client receive each hour?

SELF-TEST 7   IV Drip Rates

Solve these problems related to IV and IVPB drip rates. Answers are given at the end of the chapter. Round to the nearest whole number.

1. Order: 1500 mL D5W 8 AM–8 PM
   Available: macrodrip tubing (10 gtt/mL)
   How many drops per minute?

2. Order: 250 mL D5½NS IV KVO (give over 12 hours)
   Available: microdrip tubing
   What is the drip rate?

3. Order: 150 mL D5½NS IV; run 20 mL/hour
   Available: infusion pump

   a. How many drops per minute?
   b. How long will the IV last?

4. Order: 1000 mL D5NS with 15 mEq KCl IV; run 100 mL/hour
   Available: macrotubing (20 gtt/mL) and microdrip

   a. How many hours will this run?
   b. How many milliliters of KCl will you add to the IV if KCl comes in a vial labeled 40 mEq/20 mL?
   c. What tubing will you use?
   d. Calculate drops per minute?

5. Order: aminophylline 1 g in 500 mL D5W IV at 75 mL/hour
   Available: vial of aminophylline 1 g in 10 mL; infusion pump

   a. How many milliliters of aminophylline should be added to the IV?
   b. How will you set the drip rate?

6. Order: amikacin (Amikin) 0.4 g IVPB q8h
   Supply: 2-mL vial labeled 250 mg/mL
   Package directions: 100 mL/D5W 30 minutes
   Available: macrodrip tubing 10 gtt/mL

   a. How many milliliters of amikacin (Amikin) should be added to the IV?
   b. What are the drops per minute?

7. Order: 500 mL D5½NS IV q8h
   Available: microdrip tubing
   What are the drops per minute?

8. Order: 1000 mL D5W IV q24h
   Available: macrodrip tubing (15 gtt/mL)
   What is the drip rate?

9. Order: Heparin 25,000 units in 250 mL NS at 20 mL/hour
   How long will the IV last?

10. Order: 500 mL NS over 4 hours
    Available: macrodrip tubing (20 gtt/mL)
    What is the drip rate?

SELF-TEST 8   **IV Problems**

Solve these problems related to drip rates. Answers are given at the end of this chapter. For drip rates, round to the nearest whole number.

1. Order: aqueous penicillin G 1 milliunit in 100 mL D5W IVPB q6h over 40 minutes (macro-drip tubing at 10 gtt/mL) (milliunits = million units)
   Supply: vial labeled 5 million units of powder. Directions say to inject 18 mL sterile water for injection to yield 20 mL solution. Reconstituted solution is stable for 1 week.

   a. How would you prepare the penicillin?
   b. What solution will you make?
   c. What amount of penicillin solution should be placed into the bag of 100 mL D5W?
   d. What is the drip factor for the IVPB?

2. A total of 1000 mL of an IV solution is to infuse at 100 mL/hour. If the infusion starts at 8 AM, at what time will it be completed?

3. Order: gentamicin (Garamycin) 60 mg IVPB in 50 mL D5W over 30 minutes using macrodrip (20 gtt/mL)
   Supply: vial of gentamicin (Garamycin) 40 mg/mL; 50-mL bag of D5W; order is correct

   a. How many milliliters of gentamicin (Garamycin) will you add to the 50-mL bag of D5W?
   b. What is the drip factor for the IVPB?

4. Calculate the drip factor for 1500 mL D5½NS to run 12 hours by macrodrip (10 gtt/mL).

5. Intralipid, 500 mL q6h, is ordered for a patient/client together with a primary IV that is infusing at 80 mL/hour. Calculate the 24-hour parenteral intake. (Total will be amount of lipids plus primary IV amount.)

6. Order: 1000 mL D5W with 20 mEq KCl and 500 mg of vitamin C at 50 mL/hour. No infusion pump is available.

   a. Approximately how many hours will the IV run?
   b. Which tubing will you choose—macrodrip at 10 gtt/mL or microdrip at 60 gtt/mL?
   c. What are the drops per minute for the tubing that you choose?

Putting it Together

Mrs. Richardson is a 41-year-old woman admitted with nausea, vomiting, and diarrhea. In the emergency room, she had a fever, leukocytosis, and potassium of 5.5.

Past Medical History: end-stage renal disease, diabetes mellitus, hypertension

Post left upper extremity graft placement.

No known drug allergies.

Current Vital Signs: BP 82/50, pulse is 111/minute, respirations 20/minute, oxygen saturation 86% on room air. Temp is 98.6, on admission was 101.7

Medication Orders

gentamicin *anti-infective* 100 mg IV in 100 mL over 1 hour daily

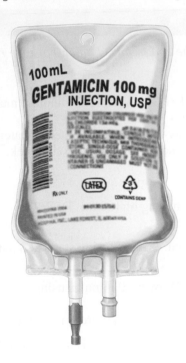

Putting it Together (*Continued*)

daptomycin (Cubicin) *anti-infective* 500 mg in 100 mL NS every 24 hours over 30 minutes

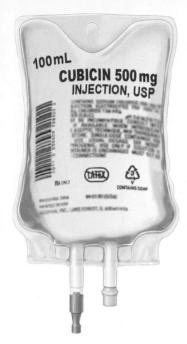

piperacillin and tazobactam (Zosyn) *anti-infective* 3.375 g in 50 mL IV in NS every 6 hours

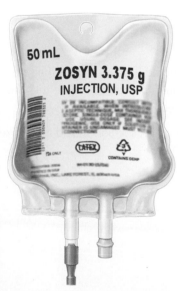

nifedipine (Procardia) XL *antihypertensive* 90 mg po q24h

lisinopril (Prinivil) *antihypertensive* 20 mg po every day

(continued)

Putting it Together (*Continued*)

NS 1000 mL at 40 mL/hour IV

dalteparin (Fragmin) *anticoagulant* 2500 units subcutaneous daily

metoclopramide (Reglan) *antinausea, prokinetic agent* 20 mg IV prn q6h for nausea and vomiting. For doses over 10 mg, must be IVPB.

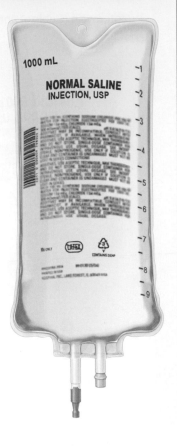

Calculations

1. Calculate the infusion rate for the gentamicin with microdrip and macrodrip (20 gtt/mL) tubing (over 60 minutes).

2. Calculate the infusion rate for the daptomycin (Cubicin) with microdrip and macrodrip (20 gtt/mL) tubing (over 30 minutes).

3. Calculate the infusion rate for piperacillin and tazobactam (Zosyn) with microdrip and macrodrip (15 gtt/mL) tubing (over 30 minutes).

4. Calculate how many hours 1000 mL of NS solution at 40 mL/hour will infuse. Use an infusion pump.

5. Calculate the total intake for 24 hours, including the primary IV and all antibiotics.

Critical Thinking Questions

1. What medications (po or IV) should be held and why?

2. Why would a patient/client receive three antibiotics instead of only one antibiotic?

3. After 6 hours, the NS has only infused 150 mL. How much should have infused? What are some reasons that the IV solution has not infused more? Should the nurse increase the rate of the infusion in order to "catch up" on the total amount needed?

4. Is the metoclopramide (Reglan) to be infused as an IVPB? How much solution should it be mixed with and how long to infuse? (use a drug handbook if needed)

Answers in Appendix B.

*Name:*_____

There are 14 questions related to IV and IVPB and enteral feeding calculations. Answers are given in Appendix A. Round to the nearest whole number.

1. Order: 1000 mL D5NS; run 150 mL/hour IV
   Supply: IV bag of 1000 mL D5NS

   a. Approximately how many hours will the IV run?
   b. Which tubing will you choose—macrodrip (10 gtt/mL) or microdrip (60 gtt/mL)?
   c. How many drops per minute?

2. Order: 100 mL LR 12 NOON–6 PM IV

   a. What size tubing will you use?
   b. What are the drops per minute (macrodrip 10 gtt/mL or microdrip 60 gtt/mL)?

3. Order: 150 mL NS IV over 3 hours
   Supply: bag of 250 mL NS for IV and macrotubing, 15 gtt/mL; microtubing, 60 gtt/mL

   a. What would you do to obtain 150 mL NS?
   b. What IV tubing would you use?
   c. What are the drops per minute?

4. Order: 500 mL D5W IV KVO. Solve for 24 hours. An infusion pump is available. What should be the setting on the infusion pump?

5. Order: doxycycline (Vibramycin) 100 mg IVPB every day
   Supply: 100 mg powder
   Package directions: 250 mL/D5W to infuse over 1 hour; macrodrip tubing 10 gtt/mL

   a. State the amount and type of IV fluid you will use and the time for infusion you will use.
   b. What are the drops per minute?

6. Order: aminophylline 500 mg in 250 mL D5W to run 8 hours IV
   Available: vial of aminophylline labeled 1 g in 10 mL; microdrip tubing

   a. How much aminophylline is needed?
   b. What is the drip rate?

7. A patient/client is receiving a primary IV at the rate of 125 mL/hour. The doctor orders cefoxitin (Mefoxin) 1 g in 75 mL D5W q6h to run over 1 hour. Calculate the 24-hour parenteral intake.

8. Order: 1000 mL D5½NS to run at 90 mL/hour; infusion pump available

   a. What will be the pump setting?
   b. Approximately how long will the IV run?

9. A doctor orders 500 mL aminophylline 0.5 g to infuse at 50 mL/hour. How many milligrams will the patient/client receive each hour?

10. Order: trimethoprim and sulfamethoxazole (Bactrim) 5 mL IVPB q6h
    Supply: vial of 5 mL; one 5-mL vial per 75 mL D5W run over 60 to 90 minutes.
    The main IV line is connected to an infusion pump. What will you do?

    a. State the type and amount of IV fluid you would use and the time for infusion.
    b. How would you program the infusion pump?

(continued)

11. Prepare ¾ strength Isocal. Total volume is 150 mL. How much Isocal is to be mixed with how much water?

12. Prepare ½ strength Vivonex. Total volume is 500 mL. How much Vivonex is to be mixed with how much water?

13. Prepare 25% Osmolite. Total volume is 400 mL. How much Osmolite is to be mixed with how much water?

14. Prepare full strength Isocal. Total volume is 500 mL. How much Isocal is to be mixed with how much water?

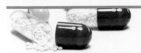

Answers

Self-Test 1 Calculation of Drip Rates

1. This is a continuous IV of 150 mL every 8 hours. There is a pump available.

$$\frac{150 \text{ mL}}{8 \text{ hours}} = 8\overline{)150.0}^{\,18.7}$$
$$\begin{array}{r} 8 \\ \hline 70 \\ 64 \\ \hline 60 \end{array}$$

Label the IV. Set the pump: total volume to infuse = 150 mL; mL/hour = 19.

2. This is a continuous IV. A pump is available. (Dimensional analysis uses the same equation.) The order states mL/hour. There is no calculation needed. Label the IV. Set the pump as follows: total volume to infuse = 250 mL; mL/hour = 25.

3. The order gives 100 mL/hour; mL/hour = gtt/minute microdrip, so you know the microdrip is 100 gtt/minute. Work out the macrodrip factor and choose the tubing.

Macrodrip

$$\frac{\text{mL/hour} \times \text{DF}}{\text{Number of minutes}} = \text{gtt/minute}$$

$$\frac{100 \times \overset{1}{20}}{\underset{3}{60} \text{ minute}} = \frac{100}{3} = 33.3$$

Dimensional Analysis

$$\frac{\overset{1}{20} \text{ gtt}}{1 \text{ mL}} \left| \frac{100 \text{ mL}}{1 \text{ hour}} \right| \frac{1 \text{ hour}}{\underset{3}{60} \text{ minutes}} = \frac{100}{3}$$
$$= 33.3 \text{ or } 33 \text{ gtt/minute}$$

Macrodrip at 33 gtt/minute

Microdrip at 100 gtt/minute (mL/hour = gtt/minute)

Either drip rate could be used. Label the IV.

4. This is a small volume over several hours; use microdrip. Macrodrip would be too slow (5 gtt/minute). Minutes = 6 hours × 60 = 360.

$$\frac{\text{mL/hour} \times \text{DF}}{\text{minutes}} = \text{gtt/minute}$$

$$\frac{180 \text{ mL} \times \overset{1}{60} \text{ gtt}}{\underset{6}{360} \text{ minutes}} = \frac{180}{6} = 6\overline{)180}^{\,30}$$
$$\begin{array}{r} 18 \\ \hline 0 \end{array}$$

Dimensional Analysis

$$\frac{\overset{1}{10} \text{ gtt}}{1 \text{ mL}} \left| \frac{180 \text{ mL}}{6 \text{ hours}} \right| \frac{1 \text{ hour}}{\underset{6}{60} \text{ minutes}} = \frac{180}{6}$$
$$= 30 \text{ gtt/minute}$$

Microdrip is 30 gtt/minute. Label the IV.

5. This is a large volume over several hours. Solve using two steps and decide. Minutes: 8 hours × 60 = 480 minutes

Microdrip

$$\frac{\text{mL/hour} \times \text{DF}}{\text{minutes}} = \text{gtt/minute}$$

$$\frac{1000 \text{ mL} \times \overset{1}{60} \text{ gtt}}{\underset{8}{480} \text{ minutes}} = \frac{1000}{8} = 8\overline{)1000.0}^{\,125.}$$
$$\begin{array}{r} 8 \\ \hline 20 \\ 16 \\ \hline 40 \end{array}$$

Dimensional Analysis

$$\frac{\overset{1}{60} \text{ gtt}}{1 \text{ mL}} \left| \frac{1000 \text{ mL}}{8 \text{ hours}} \right| \frac{1 \text{ hour}}{\underset{1}{60} \text{ minutes}} = \frac{1000}{8}$$
$$= 125 \text{ gtt/minute}$$

Microdrip will be 125 gtt/minute.

Macrodrip

$$\frac{\overset{125}{1000} \times \overset{1}{15}}{\underset{32}{480} \text{ minutes}} = \frac{125}{4} = 4\overline{)125.0}^{\,31.2}$$
$$\begin{array}{r} 12 \\ \hline 5 \\ 4 \\ \hline 10 \\ 8 \end{array}$$

Dimensional Analysis

$$\frac{\overset{1}{15} \text{ gtt}}{1 \text{ mL}} \left| \frac{\overset{250}{1000} \text{ mL}}{8 \text{ hours}} \right| \frac{1 \text{ hour}}{\underset{1}{60} \text{ minutes}} = \frac{250}{8}$$
$$= 31.2 \text{ or } 31 \text{ gtt/minute}$$

Macrodrip at 31 gtt/minute

Microdrip at 125 gtt/minute

Use macrodrip (less fluid per minute).

Label the IV.

(continued)

Answers (Continued)

6. This is a continuous IV of 250 mL every 8 hours. There is a pump available. It will run 8 hours.

$$\frac{250 \text{ mL}}{8} \quad 8\overline{)250.0} \quad \frac{31.2 \text{ mL/hour}}{}$$
$$\underline{24}$$
$$10$$
$$\underline{8}$$
$$2.0$$

Label the IV. Set the pump: total volume to infuse = 250 mL; mL/hour = 31. (Dimensional analysis method uses the same equation.)

7. This is a continuous IV of 500 mL over 2 hours. There is a pump available. It will run 2 hours.

$$\frac{500 \text{ mL}}{2} \quad 2\overline{)500.0} \quad \frac{250.0 \text{ mL/hour}}{}$$
$$\underline{4}$$
$$10$$
$$\underline{10}$$
$$0$$

Label the IV. Set the pump: total volume to infuse = 500 mL; mL/hour = 250. (Dimensional analysis method uses the same equation.)

8. This is a large volume over several hours. Solve using two steps. Minutes: 12 hours × 60 = 720 minutes

$$\frac{\text{mL/hour} \times \text{DF}}{\text{minutes}} = \text{gtt/minute}$$

Macrodrip

$$\frac{1000 \times \overset{1}{\cancel{15}}}{\underset{48}{\cancel{720}} \text{ minutes}} = 48\overline{)1000.0} \quad \frac{20.8}{}$$
$$\underline{96}$$
$$400$$
$$\underline{384}$$
$$6$$

Microdrip

$$\frac{1000 \times \overset{1}{\cancel{60}}}{\underset{12}{\cancel{720}} \text{ minutes}} = 12\overline{)1000} \quad \frac{83}{}$$
$$\underline{96}$$
$$40$$
$$\underline{36}$$
$$4$$

Dimensional Analysis

Macrodrip

$$\frac{\overset{1}{\cancel{15}} \text{ gtt}}{1 \text{ mL}} \left| \frac{\overset{250}{\cancel{1000}} \text{ mL}}{\cancel{12} \text{ hours}} \right| \frac{1 \text{ hour}}{\underset{\underset{1}{4}}{\cancel{60}} \text{ minutes}} = \frac{250}{12}$$

$$= 20.8 \text{ or } 21 \text{ gtt/minute}$$

Microdrip

$$\frac{\overset{1}{\cancel{60}} \text{ gtt}}{1 \text{ mL}} \left| \frac{1000 \text{ mL}}{12 \text{ hours}} \right| \frac{1 \text{ hour}}{\underset{1}{\cancel{60}} \text{ minutes}} = \frac{1000}{12}$$

$$= 83 \text{ gtt/minute}$$

Macrodrip at 21 gtt/minute; microdrip at 83 gtt/minute.

Use macrodrip (less fluid per minute).

Label the IV.

9. This is a large volume at a fast rate. Use macrodrip. Solve using macrodrip factor. Minutes: 1 hour = 60 minutes.

$$\frac{\text{mL/hour} \times \text{DF}}{\text{minutes}} = \text{gtt/minute}$$

$$\frac{150 \times \overset{1}{\cancel{10}}}{\underset{6}{\cancel{60}} \text{ minute}} = \frac{150}{6} \quad 6\overline{)150.0} \quad \frac{25.0 \text{ gtt/minute}}{}$$
$$\underline{12}$$
$$30$$
$$\underline{30}$$
$$0$$

Dimensional Analysis

$$\frac{\overset{1}{\cancel{10}} \text{ gtt}}{1 \text{ mL}} \left| \frac{150 \text{ mL}}{1 \text{ hour}} \right| \frac{1 \text{ hour}}{\underset{6}{\cancel{60}} \text{ minutes}} = \frac{150}{6}$$

$$= 25 \text{ gtt/minute}$$

Macrodrip at 25 gtt/minute; microdrip at 150 gtt/minute.

Use macrodrip (less fluid per minute).

Label the IV.

10. This is a large volume over a short time. Use macrodrip tubing. The rate is 150 mL/hour (150 mL over 1 hour). Solve using macrodrip factor.

$$\frac{\text{mL/hour} \times \text{DF}}{\text{minutes}} = \text{gtt/minute}$$

$$\frac{150 \times \overset{1}{\cancel{20}}}{\underset{3}{\cancel{60}} \text{ minutes}} = \frac{150}{3} \quad 3\overline{)150.0} \quad \frac{50}{}$$
$$\underline{15}$$
$$0$$

Dimensional Analysis

$$\frac{\overset{1}{\cancel{20}} \text{ gtt}}{1 \text{ mL}} \left| \frac{150 \text{ mL}}{1 \text{ hour}} \right| \frac{1 \text{ hour}}{\underset{3}{\cancel{60}} \text{ minutes}} = \frac{150}{3}$$

$$= 50 \text{ gtt/minute}$$

Macrodrip at 50 gtt/minute; microdrip at 150 gtt/minute.

Use macrodrip (less fluid per minute).

Label the IV.

Self-Test 2 IV Infusions—Hours

1. 8.3 hours approximately $\left(\frac{250}{30}=8.3\right)$ or 8 hours 18 minutes

2. 8.3 hours approximately $\left(\frac{500}{60}=8.3\right)$ or 8 hours 18 minutes

3. 10 hours (no math)

4. 24 hours (no math)

5. 7.1 hours approximately $\left(\frac{500}{70}=7.1\right)$ or 7 hours 6 minutes

6. 10 hours $\left(\frac{500}{50}=10\right)$

7. 10 hours (no math) 7 PM

8. 2.5 hours $\left(\frac{250}{100}=2.5\right)$ 3:30 PM or 2 hours 30 minutes

9. 6 hours (no math)

10. 5 hours (no math)

Self-Test 3 IV Infusion Rates

1. You want vitamin C 500 mg, and the supply is 500 mg in 2 mL. Use a syringe to add the 2 mL to 500 mL D5W. Label the IV. You have microdrip available. The IV is to run at 60 mL/hour. No math necessary. Set the microdrip at 60 gtt/minute (mL/hour = gtt/minute for microdrip). Label the IV.

2. You want 250 mg hydrocortisone sodium succinate (Solu Cortef), and it comes in 250 mg with a 2 mL diluent. Use a syringe to reconstitute the hydrocortisone with 2 mL diluent and add it to the IV. 8 AM–12 MIDNIGHT is 16 hours. Minutes: 16 hour × 60 = 960 minutes
mL/hour = gtt/minute for microdrip. No math for microdrip. Microdrip = 63 gtt/minute. Label the IV.
Minutes = 60 × 16 = 960.

$$\frac{1000\ mL \times \overset{1}{\cancel{60}}\ gtt}{\underset{16}{\cancel{960}}\ minutes} = 16\overline{)1000.0}\ \text{or 63 gtt/minute}$$

$$
\begin{array}{r}
62.5 \\
16\overline{)1000.0} \\
96 \\
\hline
40 \\
32 \\
\hline
80 \\
80 \\
\hline
\end{array}
$$

Dimensional Analysis

$$\frac{\overset{1}{\cancel{60}}\ \text{\large(gtt)}}{1\ \cancel{mL}}\ \bigg|\ \frac{1000\ \cancel{mL}}{16\ \cancel{hours}}\ \bigg|\ \frac{1\ \cancel{hour}}{\underset{1}{\cancel{60}}\ \text{\large(minutes)}} = \frac{1000}{16} = 62.5\ \text{or 63 gtt/minute}$$

3. You want 250 mg aminophylline. Supply is 500 mg/10 mL.

Formula Method	Proportion	Dimensional Analysis
$\dfrac{250\ mg}{500\ mg} \times 10\ mL = 5\ mL$	**EXPRESSED AS TWO RATIOS** 10 mL : 500 mg : : x mL : 250 mg **EXPRESSED AS TWO FRACTIONS** $\dfrac{10\ mL}{500\ mg} \times \dfrac{x}{250\ mg}$ **SOLUTION FOR BOTH PROPORTION METHODS** $250 \times 10 = 500x$ $\dfrac{2500}{500} = x$ $5 = x$	$\dfrac{10\ \text{\large(mL)}}{\underset{2}{\cancel{500}}\ mg}\ \bigg|\ \dfrac{\overset{1}{\cancel{250}}\ mg}{}\ = \dfrac{10}{2} = 5\ mL$

Add 5 mL aminophylline to 250 mL D5W. Order is 50 mL/hour. You have an infusion pump. No math. Set the pump as follows: total volume to infuse = 250 mL; mL/hour = 50.

(continued)

Answers (Continued)

4. You want KCl 10 mEq. Supply is 20 mEq/10 mL.

Formula Method	Proportion	Dimensional Analysis

Formula Method

$$\frac{10 \text{ mEq}}{20 \text{ mEq}} \times 10 \text{ mL} = 5 \text{ mL}$$

Proportion

EXPRESSED AS TWO RATIOS

10 mL : 20 mEq :: x mL : 10 mEq

EXPRESSED AS TWO FRACTIONS

$$\frac{10 \text{ mL}}{20 \text{ mEq}} \times \frac{x}{10 \text{ mEq}}$$

SOLUTION FOR BOTH PROPORTION METHODS

$$10 \times 10 = 20x$$

$$\frac{100}{20} = x$$

$$5 \text{ mL} = x$$

Dimensional Analysis

$$\frac{10 \; \cancel{\text{mL}}}{\cancel{20} \; \cancel{\text{mEq}}} \Bigg| \frac{\cancel{10}^{1} \; \cancel{\text{mEq}}}{} = \frac{10}{2} = 5 \text{ mL}$$

Add 5 mL KCl to 250 mL D5W½NS. Label the IV. 12 NOON–6 PM is 6 hours; minutes: 6 hours × 60 = 360 minutes.

$$\frac{250 \text{ mL} \times \cancel{60}^{1} \text{ gtt}}{\cancel{360} \text{ minutes}_{6}} = \frac{250}{6} \quad \begin{array}{r} 41.6 \\ 6\overline{)250.0} \\ \underline{24} \\ 10 \\ \underline{6} \\ 4\,0 \\ \underline{3\,6} \end{array} = 42 \text{ mL/hour}$$

$$\frac{\cancel{60}^{1} \; \cancel{\text{gtt}}}{1 \; \cancel{\text{mL}}} \Bigg| \frac{250 \; \cancel{\text{mL}}}{6 \; \cancel{\text{hours}}} \Bigg| \frac{1 \; \cancel{\text{hour}}}{60 \; \cancel{\text{minutes}}_{1}} = \frac{250}{6}$$

$$= 41.6 \text{ or } 42 \text{ gtt/minutes}$$

mL/hour = gtt/minute microdrip.

Set the microdrip at 42 gtt/minute.

Self-Test 4 IVPB Drip Rates

1. Acyclovir (Zovirax) comes in 500 mg powder. Use a reconstitution device to add the powder to 100 mL D5W; minutes: 1 hour = 60 minutes; DF = 10 gtt/mL for IVPB.

$$\frac{100 \times 10}{60 \text{ minutes}} = \frac{100}{6} \quad \begin{array}{r} 16.6 \\ 6\overline{)100.0} \end{array} = 17 \text{ gtt/minute}$$

Dimensional Analysis

$$\frac{\cancel{10}^{1} \; \cancel{\text{gtt}}}{1 \; \cancel{\text{mL}}} \Bigg| \frac{100 \; \cancel{\text{mL}}}{1 \; \cancel{\text{hour}}} \Bigg| \frac{1 \; \cancel{\text{hour}}}{\cancel{60} \; \cancel{\text{minutes}}_{6}} = \frac{100}{6} = 16.6 \text{ or } 17 \text{ gtt/minute}$$

Label the IVPB.

Set the rate at 17 gtt/minute.

2. Ceftazidime (Ceptaz) comes in a 1-g powder.

Use a reconstitution device to add the powder to 50 mL D5W; use 30 minutes; DF, 10 gtt/mL for IVPB.

$$\frac{50 \times 10}{30 \text{ minutes}} = \frac{50}{3} = 16.6 = 17 \text{ gtt/minute}$$

Dimensional Analysis

$$\frac{\overset{1}{10} \text{ gtt}}{1 \text{ mL}} \left| \frac{50 \text{ mL}}{\underset{3}{30} \text{ minutes}} \right. = \frac{50}{3} = 16.6 \text{ or } 17 \text{ gtt/minute}$$

Label the IVPB.

Set the rate at 17 gtt/minute.

3. Cefotaxime (Claforan) comes as a 1-g powder.

Use a reconstitution device to add the powder to 50 mL D5W; use 30 minutes; DF, 10 gtt/mL for IVPB.

$$\frac{50 \times 10}{30 \text{ minutes}} = 16.6 = 17 \text{ gtt/minute}$$

Dimensional Analysis

$$\frac{\overset{1}{10} \text{ gtt}}{1 \text{ mL}} \left| \frac{50 \text{ mL}}{\underset{3}{30} \text{ minutes}} \right. = \frac{50}{3} = 16.6 \text{ or } 17 \text{ gtt/minute}$$

Label the IVPB.

Set the rate at 17 gtt/minute.

4. Ampicillin (Omnipen) comes as a 2-g powder. Reconstitute in 4.5 mL diluent = total volume 5 mL
   2 g = 2000 mg in 5 mL.

Formula Method	Proportion	Dimensional Analysis
$\frac{500 \text{ mg}}{2000 \text{ mg}} \times 5 \text{ mL}$ $= 1.25 \text{ mL}$	**EXPRESSED AS TWO RATIOS** 5 mL : 2000 mg : : x mL : 500 mg **EXPRESSED AS TWO FRACTIONS** $\frac{5 \text{ mL}}{2000 \text{ mg}} \times \frac{x}{500 \text{ mg}}$ **SOLUTION FOR BOTH** **PROPORTION METHODS** $5 \times 500 = 2000x$ $\frac{2500}{2000} = x$ $1.25 \text{ mL} = x$	Use conversion factor: 1 g/1000 mg $\frac{5 \text{ mL}}{2 \text{ g}} \left| \frac{\overset{1}{500} \text{ mg}}{} \right| \frac{1 \text{ g}}{\underset{2}{1000} \text{ mg}} = \frac{5}{4} = 1.25 \text{ mL}$

Add 1.25 mL to 50 mL D5W. Total minutes = 30; DF = 60 gtt/mL.

$$\frac{50 \times \overset{2}{60}}{\underset{1}{30} \text{ minute}} = 100 \text{ gtt/minute}$$

(continued)

Answers (Continued)

Dimensional Analysis

$$\frac{\overset{1}{\cancel{10}}\ \cancel{gtt}}{1\ \cancel{mL}}\ \bigg|\ \frac{50\ \cancel{mL}}{\underset{3}{\cancel{30}}\ \cancel{minutes}} = \frac{50}{3} = 16.6 \text{ or } 17 \text{ gtt/minute}$$

Label the IVPB.

Set the rate at 100 gtt/minute.

5. Tobramycin (Nebcin) comes as 80 mg in 2 mL after reconstitution.

Formula Method	Proportion	Dimensional Analysis
$\dfrac{50\ mg}{80\ mg} \times 2\ mL = 1.25\ mL$	**EXPRESSED AS TWO RATIOS** 2 mL : 80 mg : : x mL : 50 mg **EXPRESSED AS TWO FRACTIONS** $\dfrac{2\ mL}{80\ mg} \times \dfrac{x}{50\ mg}$ **SOLUTION FOR BOTH PROPORTION METHODS** $2 \times 50 = 80x$ $\dfrac{100}{80} = x$ $1.25\ mL = x$	$\dfrac{2\ \cancel{mL}}{\cancel{80}\ \cancel{mg}}\ \bigg|\ \dfrac{\cancel{50}\ \cancel{mg}}{} = \dfrac{10}{8} = 1.25\ mL$

Add 1.25 mL to 100 mL D5W.

Total minutes = 60; DF = 15 gtt/mL.

$$\frac{mL \times DF}{minutes} = gtt/minute$$

$$\frac{100 \times \overset{1}{\cancel{15}}}{\underset{4}{\cancel{60}}\ minutes} = 25 \text{ gtt/minute}$$

Dimensional Analysis

$$\frac{\overset{1}{\cancel{15}}\ \cancel{gtt}}{1\ \cancel{mL}}\ \bigg|\ \frac{100\ \cancel{mL}}{\underset{4}{\cancel{60}}\ \cancel{minutes}} = \frac{100}{4} = 25 \text{ gtt/minute}$$

Label the IVPB.

Set the rate at 25 gtt/minute.

6. Ticarcillin (Timentin) comes as a 1-g powder. Reconstitute in 4.5 mL of diluent = 5 mL (1 g or 1000 mg = 5 mL)

Formula Method	Proportion	Dimensional Analysis
$\dfrac{500 \text{ mg}}{1000 \text{ mg}} \times 5 \text{ mL}$ $= 2.5 \text{ mL}$	**EXPRESSED AS TWO RATIOS** 5 mL : 1000 mg : : x mL : 500 mg **EXPRESSED AS TWO FRACTIONS** $\dfrac{5 \text{ mL}}{1000 \text{ mg}} \times \dfrac{x}{500 \text{ mg}}$ **SOLUTION FOR BOTH PROPORTION METHODS** $5 \times 500 = 1000x$ $\dfrac{2500}{1000} = x$ $2.5 \text{ mL} = x$	Use conversion factor: 1 g/1000 mg $\dfrac{5 \text{ mL}}{1 \text{ g}} \left| \dfrac{\overset{1}{500 \text{ mg}}}{} \right| \dfrac{1 \text{ g}}{\underset{2}{1000 \text{ mg}}} = \dfrac{5}{2} = 2.5 \text{ mL}$

Add 2.5 mL to 50 mL D5W.

Total minutes, 30; DF, 15 gtt/mL.

$$\frac{\text{mL} \times \text{DF}}{\text{minutes}} = \text{gtt/minute}$$

$$\frac{50 \times \overset{1}{15}}{\underset{2}{30} \text{ minutes}} = 25 \text{ gtt/minute}$$

Dimensional Analysis

$$\frac{\overset{1}{15} \text{ gtt}}{1 \text{ mL}} \left| \frac{50 \text{ mL}}{\underset{2}{30} \text{ minutes}} \right. = \frac{50}{2} = 25 \text{ gtt/minute. Label the IVPB. Set the rate at 25 gtt/minute.}$$

Self-Test 5 Calculation of Tube Feedings

1. 206.25 mL of Isocal. 68.75 mL water.

2. 56.25 mL Magnacal. 18.75 mL water.

3. 50 mL Osmolite. 50 mL water.

4. 21.25 mL Ensure. 63.75 mL water.

5. 100 mL Renalcal. 300 mL water.

6. 200 mL Suplena. 200 mL water.

Self-Test 6 Fluid Intake

1. 900 mL at 100 mL/hour = 9 hours to run. If the IV starts at 9 AM, + 9 hours = 6 PM.

2. IVPB is 75 mL q6h or four times in 24 hours.

75
× 4
300 mL

(continued)

Answers (Continued)

The patient/client is receiving 125 mL for 20 hours (24 hours − 4 hours that the IVPB is running).

$$
\begin{array}{r}
125 \\
\times\ 20 \\
\hline
2500\ \text{mL}
\end{array}
$$

$$
\begin{array}{r}
2500\ \text{mL} \\
+\ 300\ \text{mL} \\
\hline
2800\ \text{mL in 24 hours}
\end{array}
$$

3. IV is infusing at 10 microdrips/minute. (You can also think "10 microdrips/minute = 10 mL/hour. So 8 hours would be $8 \times 10 = 80$ mL/hour") 60 microdrips = 1 mL; every 6 minutes 1 mL infuses ($\frac{60}{10} = 6$ minutes), 10 mL in 60 minutes (1 hour).

$$
\begin{array}{r}
10\ \text{mL in 60 minutes (1 hour)} \\
\times\ 8\ \text{hr} \\
\hline
80\ \text{mL in 8 hours}
\end{array}
$$

4. The IV is 0.5 g or 500 mg in 500 mL. This is equal to 1 mg/mL. The patient/client receives 50 mL/hour, so he or she receives 50 mg each hour.

5. The IV is infusing at 30 mL/hour, and the solution is 500 mL.

$$
\frac{500\ \text{mL}}{30\ \text{mL/hour}} = \frac{50}{3} = 16.6 \text{ hours (approximately) or 16 hours 36 minutes}
$$

6. IVPB is 50 mL q8h or three times in 24 hours.

$$
\begin{array}{r}
50 \\
\times\ 3 \\
\hline
150\ \text{mL}
\end{array}
$$

The patient/client is receiving 100 mL for 21 hours (24 hours − 3 hours that the IVPB is running).

$$
\begin{array}{r}
100 \\
\times\ 21 \\
\hline
2100\ \text{mL}
\end{array}
$$

$$
\begin{array}{r}
2100\ \text{mL} \\
+\ 150\ \text{mL} \\
\hline
2250\ \text{mL in 24 hours}
\end{array}
$$

7. 500 mL at 50 mL/hour = 10 hours to run. If the IV starts at 6 AM, + 10 hours = 4 PM.

8. The IV is infusing at 125 mL/hour and the solution is 1000 mL.

$$
\frac{1000\ \text{mL}}{125\ \text{mL/hour}} = 8 \text{ hours}
$$

9. IVPB is 250 mL q6h or four times in 24 hours.

$$
\begin{array}{r}
250 \\
\times\ 4 \\
\hline
1000\ \text{mL in 24 hours}
\end{array}
$$

10. The IV is 100 units in 100 mL or 1 unit/mL. The patient/client receives 10 mL/hour, so he or she receives 10 units each hour.

Self-Test 7 IV Drip Rates

1. **Macrodrip** $12 \times 60 = 720$ minutes

$$\frac{mL/hour \times DF}{minutes} = gtt/minute \qquad \frac{1500 \; mL \times \overset{1}{\cancel{10}} \; gtt}{\underset{72}{\cancel{720}} \; minutes} = 72\overline{)1500.0}$$

$\begin{array}{r} 20.8 \\ 72\overline{)1500.0} \\ \underline{144} \\ 600 \\ \underline{570} \end{array}$

$= 21 \; gtt/minute$

Dimensional Analysis

$$\frac{\overset{1}{\cancel{10}} \; \text{(gtt)}}{1 \; \cancel{mL}} \; \Bigg| \; \frac{1500 \; \cancel{mL}}{12 \; \cancel{hours}} \; \Bigg| \; \frac{1 \; \cancel{hour}}{\underset{6}{\cancel{60}} \; \text{(minutes)}} = \frac{1500}{72} = 20.8 \; or \; 21 \; gtt/minute$$

Round to 21 gtt/minute.

2. $\dfrac{250 \; mL \times \overset{1}{\cancel{60}} \; gtt}{\underset{12}{\cancel{720}} \; minutes} = \dfrac{250}{12} = 21 \; gtt/minute$

$\begin{array}{r} 20.8 \\ 12\overline{)250.0} \\ \underline{24} \\ 100 \\ \underline{96} \end{array}$

Dimensional Analysis

$$\frac{\overset{1}{\cancel{60}} \; \text{(gtt)}}{1 \; \cancel{mL}} \; \Bigg| \; \frac{250 \; \cancel{mL}}{12 \; \cancel{hour}} \; \Bigg| \; \frac{1 \; \cancel{hour}}{\underset{1}{\cancel{60}} \; \text{(minutes)}} = \frac{250}{12} = 20.8 \; or \; 21 \; gtt/minute$$

You could also say mL/hour = gtt/minute microdrip, so 21 mL/hour = 21 gtt/minute. Round to 21 gtt/minute.

3. $\dfrac{150 \; \cancel{mL}}{20 \; \cancel{mL}/hour} = \dfrac{15}{2} = 2\overline{)15.0}$ hour   or 7 hours 30 minutes

$\begin{array}{r} 7.5 \\ 2\overline{)15.0} \end{array}$

   a. The drip rate is 20 mL/hour. No math is necessary. Set the infusion pump.

   b. The IV will last approximately 7½ hours.

4. a. $\dfrac{\overset{10}{\cancel{1000}} \; mL}{\underset{}{\cancel{100}} \; mL/hour} = 10$ hours

   b.

Formula Method	Proportion	Dimensional Analysis
$\dfrac{15 \; mEq}{\underset{2}{\cancel{40}} \; mEq} \times \overset{1}{\cancel{20}} \; mL = \dfrac{15}{2}$ $= 7.5 \; mL$	**EXPRESSED AS TWO RATIOS** 20 mL : 40 mEq :: x mL : 15 mEq **EXPRESSED AS TWO FRACTIONS** $\dfrac{20 \; mL}{40 \; mEq} \times \dfrac{x}{15 \; mEq}$ **SOLUTION FOR BOTH PROPORTION METHODS** $\dfrac{300}{40} = 7.5 \; mL$	$\dfrac{\overset{1}{\cancel{20}} \; \text{(mL)}}{\underset{2}{\cancel{40}} \; mEq} \; \Bigg| \; \dfrac{15 \; \cancel{mEq}}{} = \dfrac{15}{2} = 7.5 \; mL$

(continued)

Answers (Continued)

c. Microdrip

$$\frac{100 \text{ mL} \times \cancel{60} \text{ gtt}}{\cancel{60} \text{ minutes}} = 100 \text{ gtt/minute}$$

Dimensional Analysis

$$\frac{\cancel{60} \; \cancel{(gtt)}}{1 \; \cancel{mL}} \bigg| \frac{100 \; \cancel{mL}}{1 \; \cancel{hour}} \bigg| \frac{1 \; \cancel{hour}}{\cancel{60} \; \cancel{(minutes)}} = 100 \text{ gtt/minute}$$

Order states to run at 100 mL/hour. mL/hour = gtt/minute microdrip, so microdrip = 100 gtt/minute.

Macrodrip

$$\frac{100 \times \overset{1}{\cancel{20}}}{\underset{3}{\cancel{60}}} = \frac{100}{3} = 33 \text{ gtt/minute}$$

Dimensional Analysis

$$\frac{\overset{1}{\cancel{20}} \; \cancel{(gtt)}}{1 \; \cancel{mL}} \bigg| \frac{100 \; \cancel{mL}}{1 \; \cancel{hour}} \bigg| \frac{1 \; \cancel{hour}}{\underset{3}{\cancel{60}} \; \cancel{(minutes)}} = \frac{100}{3} = 33 \text{ gtt/minute}$$

Choose either tubing.

d. 33 gtt/minute macrodrip: 100 gtt/minute microdrip

5. a. You desire 1 g. Aminophylline comes 1 g in 10 mL. Add 10 mL to the IV of 500 mL D5W and label.

   b. You have an infusion pump; there is no math.

   Set the pump:

   total volume to be infused = 500 mL; mL/hour = 75

6. 0.4 g = 400 mg

   a.

Formula Method	Proportion	Dimensional Analysis
$$\frac{\overset{8}{\cancel{400}} \text{ mg}}{\underset{5}{\cancel{250}} \text{ mg}} \times 1 \text{ mL}$$ $$\frac{8}{5}\overline{)8.0} \quad 1.6 \text{ mL}$$	**EXPRESSED AS TWO RATIOS** 1 mL : 250 mg :: x mL : 400 mg **EXPRESSED AS TWO FRACTIONS** $$\frac{1 \text{ mL}}{250 \text{ mg}} \times \frac{x}{400 \text{ mg}}$$ **SOLUTION FOR BOTH PROPORTION METHODS** $$400 = 250x$$ $$\frac{400}{250} = x$$ $$1.6 \text{ mL} = x$$	Use conversion factor: 1000 mg/1 g $$\frac{1 \; \cancel{(mL)}}{\underset{1}{\cancel{250} \; \cancel{mg}}} \bigg| \frac{0.4 \; \cancel{g}}{} \bigg| \frac{\overset{4}{\cancel{1000} \; \cancel{mg}}}{1 \; \cancel{g}} = 0.4 \times 4 = 1.6 \text{ mL}$$

   b. Add 1.6 mL amikacin (Amikin) to 100 mL D5W.

   DF = 10 gtt/mL for IVPB. Total minutes, 30.

$$\frac{100 \text{ mL} \times 10}{30} = \frac{100}{3} = 33.3 = 33 \text{ gtt/minute}$$

Dimensional Analysis

$$\frac{10 \text{ (gtt)}}{1 \text{ mL}} \Big| \frac{100 \text{ mL}}{30 \text{ (minutes)}} = \frac{100}{3} = 33.3 \text{ or } 33 \text{ gtt/minute}$$

Label the IV.

Round to 33 gtt/minute.

7. Minutes: 8 hours × 60 = 480

$$\frac{500 \text{ mL} \times 60 \text{ gtt}}{480 \text{ minutes}} = \frac{500}{8} \quad 62.5 = 63 \text{ gtt/minute}$$

$$8\overline{)500.0}$$
$$\underline{48}$$
$$20$$
$$\underline{16}$$
$$4\,0$$
$$\underline{4\,0}$$

Dimensional Analysis

$$\frac{60 \text{ (gtt)}}{1 \text{ mL}} \Big| \frac{500 \text{ mL}}{8 \text{ hours}} \Big| \frac{1 \text{ hour}}{60 \text{ (minutes)}} = \frac{500}{8} = 62.5 \text{ or } 63 \text{ gtt/minute}$$

Round to 63 gtt/minute.

You are using microdrip tubing, so mL/hour = gtt/minute. Set the rate at 63 mL/hour.

8. Minutes: 24 hours × 60 = 1440 minutes

$$\frac{1000 \text{ mL} \times 15 \text{ gtt}}{1440 \text{ minutes}} = 96\overline{)1000.0}$$
$$\underline{96}$$
$$40$$
$$\underline{0}$$
$$400$$

10 gtt/minute

Dimensional Analysis

$$\frac{15 \text{ (gtt)}}{1 \text{ mL}} \Big| \frac{1000 \text{ mL}}{24 \text{ hours}} \Big| \frac{1 \text{ hour}}{60 \text{ (minutes)}} = \frac{1000}{96} = 10.4 \text{ or } 10 \text{ gtt/minute}$$

Round to 10 gtt/minute.

9. $$\frac{250 \text{ mL}}{20 \text{ mL/hour}} = \frac{250}{20} \quad 20\overline{)250.0}$$
$$\underline{20}$$
$$50$$
$$\underline{40}$$
$$10\,0$$

The IV will last 12.5 hours or 12 hours 30 minutes.

(continued)

Answers (Continued)

10. Minutes: 4 hours × 60 = 240 minutes

$$\frac{500 \text{ mL} \times \overset{1}{\cancel{20}} \text{ gtt}}{\underset{12}{\cancel{240}} \text{ minute}} = 12\overline{)500.0} \quad \begin{array}{r} 41.6 \\ \underline{48} \\ 20 \\ \underline{12} \\ 80 \end{array}$$

$$= 42 \text{ gtt/minute}$$

Dimensional Analysis

$$\frac{\overset{1}{\cancel{20}} \text{ gtt}}{1 \text{ mL}} \bigg| \frac{500 \text{ mL}}{4 \text{ hours}} \bigg| \frac{1 \text{ hour}}{\underset{3}{\cancel{60}} \text{ minutes}} = \frac{500}{12} = 41.6 \text{ or } 42 \text{ gtt/minute. Round to 42 gtt/minute.}$$

Self-Test 8 IV Problems

1. a. Add 18 mL sterile water for injection to the vial of 5 million units.

b. Solution is 5 milliunits/20 mL (milliunits = million units).

c. You want 1 milliunit.

Formula Method	Proportion	Dimensional Analysis
$\dfrac{1 \text{ milliunit}}{5 \text{ milliunits}} \times \overset{4}{\cancel{20}} \text{ mL}$ $= 4 \text{ mL}$	**EXPRESSED AS TWO RATIOS** 20 mL : 5 milliunits : : x mL : 1 milliunit **EXPRESSED AS TWO FRACTIONS** $\dfrac{20 \text{ mL}}{5 \text{ milliunits}} \diagdown \dfrac{x}{1}$ **SOLUTION FOR BOTH PROPORTION METHODS** $20 = 5x$ $\dfrac{20}{5} = x$ $4 \text{ mL} = x$	$\dfrac{20 \text{ mL}}{5 \text{ milliunits}} \bigg| \dfrac{1 \text{ milliunit}}{} = \dfrac{20}{5} = 4 \text{ mL}$

d.

$$\frac{\overset{25}{\cancel{100}} \text{ mL} \times \cancel{10}}{\underset{1}{\cancel{40}}} = 25 \text{ gtt/minute}$$

Dimensional Analysis

$$\frac{\cancel{10} \text{ gtt}}{1 \text{ mL}} \bigg| \frac{100 \text{ mL}}{40 \text{ minutes}} = \frac{100}{4} = 25 \text{ gtt/minute}$$

2. 1000 mL is infusing at 100 mL/hour, so the IV will take

$$\frac{\overset{10}{\cancel{1000}}}{\underset{1}{\cancel{100}}} = 10 \text{ hours to complete.}$$

If it starts at 8 AM, it should finish 10 hours later at 6 PM.

3. a.

Formula Method	Proportion	Dimensional Analysis
$\dfrac{\overset{3}{\cancel{60} \text{ mg}}}{\underset{2}{\cancel{40} \text{ mg}}} \times 1 \text{ mL} = \dfrac{3}{2}$ $= 1.5 \text{ mL}$	**EXPRESSED AS TWO RATIOS** 1 mL : 40 mg : : x mL : 60 mg **EXPRESSED AS TWO FRACTIONS** $\dfrac{1 \text{ mL}}{40 \text{ mg}} \times \dfrac{x \text{ mL}}{60 \text{ mg}}$ **SOLUTION FOR BOTH PROPORTION METHODS** $60 = 40x$ $\dfrac{60}{40} = x$ $1.5 \text{ mL} = x$	$\dfrac{1 \text{ (mL)}}{\underset{2}{\cancel{40} \text{ mg}}} \left| \overset{3}{\cancel{60} \text{ mg}} \right. = \dfrac{3}{2} = 1.5 \text{ mL}$

Add 1.5 mL gentamicin.

b. $\dfrac{50 \text{ mL} \times \cancel{20}}{\cancel{30} \text{ minutes}} = \dfrac{\cancel{100}}{3}$ $3\overline{)100.00}$ = 33.3 = 33 gtt/minute

Dimensional Analysis

$$\dfrac{\overset{2}{\cancel{20}} \text{ (gtt)}}{1 \text{ mL}} \left| \dfrac{50 \text{ mL}}{\underset{3}{\cancel{30}} \text{ (minutes)}} \right. = \dfrac{100}{3} = 33.3 \text{ or } 33 \text{ gtt/minute. Set the rate at 33 gtt/minute.}$$

4. 12 hours × 60 = 720 minutes

$$\dfrac{1500 \text{ mL} \times \overset{1}{\cancel{10}} \text{ gtt}}{\underset{72}{\cancel{720}} \text{ minute}} = 72\overline{)1500.0} \quad \begin{array}{r} 20.8 \\ \underline{194} \\ 60\ 0 \\ \underline{57\ 6} \end{array}$$

Dimensional Analysis

$$\dfrac{\overset{1}{\cancel{10}} \text{ (gtt)}}{1 \text{ mL}} \left| \dfrac{1500 \text{ mL}}{12 \text{ hours}} \right| \dfrac{1 \text{ hour}}{\underset{6}{\cancel{60}} \text{ (minutes)}} = \dfrac{1500}{72} = 20.8 \text{ or } 21 \text{ gtt/minute. Set the rate at 21 gtt/minute.}$$

(continued)

Answers (Continued)

5. Intralipid 500 mL q6h means the patient/client is receiving 500 mL four times every 24 hours.

$$
\begin{array}{r}
500 \\
\times\ 4 \\
\hline
2000\ \text{mL}
\end{array}
$$

The IV is infusing 80 mL/hour. There are 24 hours in a day, so

$$
\begin{array}{r}
24 \\
\times\ 80 \\
\hline
1920
\end{array}
$$

Adding these, we have
$$
\begin{array}{r}
2000\ \text{mL} \\
+1920\ \text{mL} \\
\hline
3920\ \text{mL}
\end{array}
$$

6. a. You have 1000 mL running at 50 mL/hour, therefore

$$
50\overline{\smash{\big)}\,1000} = 20\ \text{hours}
$$
$$
\underline{100}
$$
$$
0
$$

b. Microdrip 60 gtt/minute

Minutes: 20 hours × 60 = 1200 minutes

$$
\frac{1000\ \text{mL} \times \overset{1}{\cancel{60}}\ \text{gtt}}{\underset{20}{\cancel{1200}}\ \text{minutes}} = \frac{1000}{20} = 50\ \text{gtt/minute}
$$

$$
\frac{\overset{1}{\cancel{60}}\ \text{gtt}}{1\ \text{mL}} \left| \frac{1000\ \cancel{\text{mL}}}{20\ \cancel{\text{hours}}} \right| \frac{1\ \cancel{\text{hour}}}{\underset{1}{\cancel{60}}\ \text{minutes}} = \frac{1000}{20} = 50\ \text{gtt/minute}
$$

Macrodrip tubing 10 gtt/mL

$$
\frac{\cancel{1000}\ \text{mL} \times 10\ \text{gtt}}{\cancel{1200}\ \text{minutes}} = \frac{100}{12} = 8.3\ \text{or 8 gtt/minute}
$$

Dimensional Analysis

$$
\frac{\overset{1}{\cancel{10}}\ \text{gtt}}{1\ \cancel{\text{mL}}} \left| \frac{1000\ \cancel{\text{mL}}}{20\ \cancel{\text{hours}}} \right| \frac{1\ \cancel{\text{hour}}}{\underset{6}{\cancel{60}}\ \text{minutes}} = \frac{1000}{120} = 8.3\ \text{or 8 gtt/minute}
$$

c. The drip factor will be 50 gtt/minute. It is not incorrect to choose the macrodrip at 8 gtt/minute. However, because the IV will run so many hours, a good flow might help to keep the IV running.

Special Types of IV Calculations

TOPICS COVERED

1. Amount of drug in a solution
2. Calculation of rate for special IV orders: units/hour; g/hour; mg/hour, mL/hour, mg/minute, milliunits/minute, mcg/minute, mcg/kg/minute
3. Use of the body surface nomogram and calculation, IV medications based on body surface area
4. Patient-controlled analgesia
5. Special types of calculation: heparin, insulin

In Chapter 6, we studied calculations for microdrip and macrodrip factors, the use of the infusion pump, and IV piggyback (IVPB) orders. In this chapter, we consider calculations for orders written in units, milliunits, milligrams, and micrograms; methods of calculating the safety of doses based on kilograms of body weight and body surface area (BSA); the handling of orders for patient-controlled analgesia (PCA); and special types of calculations in relation to continuous heparin infusion and continuous insulin infusion.

This chapter's dosage calculations are for medications mixed in IV fluids and delivered as continuous infusions. Administering these medications via infusion pumps ensures a correct rate and accuracy of dose (Fig. 7-1). Many infusion pumps can deliver rates less than 1 (e.g., 0.5 mL/hour, 0.25 mL/hour, etc.), and they also can be programmed with the amount of drug, amount of solution, patient/client's weight, and time unit (minutes or hours). Once the pump is set at an infusion rate, the pump calculates how much drug the patient/client is receiving. You, as the nurse, however, still bear the responsibility for double-checking the calculation and entering the correct information on the infusion pump. (Some hospitals require a "double-check" with two licensed staff to verify the pump is set correctly.) (For this chapter, answers will be rounded to the nearest whole number. Follow your institutional policy regarding rounding of IV calculations. Time to run is given in hours and minutes—see Chapter 6 for conversion of hours to minutes.)

Because many of the medications that infuse via continuous infusions are very potent, small changes in the infusion rate can greatly affect the body's physiologic response. In particular, vasopressor drugs

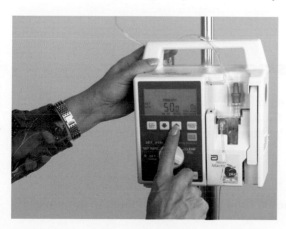

FIGURE 7-1

Infusion pump. (With permission from Evans-Smith, P. [2005]. *Taylor's clinical nursing skills*. Philadelphia, PA: Lippincott Williams & Wilkins.)

such as dopamine, epinephrine, dobutamine, and norepinephrine (Levophed) can affect the patient/client's blood pressure and heart rate, even in small doses. In most hospital settings, the pharmacy prepares medications and IV solutions.

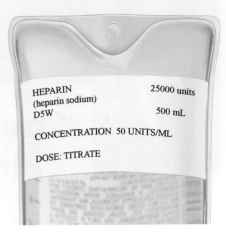

Amount of Drug in a Solution

These calculations can be complicated. One useful technique is reduction: Start with the entire amount of drug mixed in solution and then reduce it to the amount of the drug in only 1 mL of solution.

Here's an example:

Heparin is mixed 25,000 units in 500 mL D5W.

How much heparin is in 1 mL of fluid?

Desired dose: 1 mL

Supply: 25,000 units

Have: 500 mL

To solve:

Formula Method	Proportion	Dimensional Analysis
$\dfrac{25{,}000 \text{ units}}{500 \text{ mL}} \times 1 \text{ mL} = x$ $50 \text{ units} = x$	**EXPRESSED AS TWO RATIOS** $25{,}000 \text{ units} : 500 \text{ mL} :: x : 1 \text{ mL}$ **EXPRESSED AS TWO FRACTIONS** $\dfrac{25{,}000 \text{ units}}{500 \text{ mL}} \times \dfrac{x}{1 \text{ mL}}$ **SOLUTION FOR BOTH PROPORTION METHODS** $25{,}000 = 500x$ $\dfrac{25{,}000}{500} = x$ $50 \text{ units} = x$	Set up the equation. You are solving for units: $\dfrac{25{,}000 \ \text{units}}{500 \text{ mL}} \Big| \dfrac{1 \text{ mL}}{}$ Cancel "mL." Reduce the fraction. Solve. $\dfrac{\overset{50}{\cancel{25{,}000}} \text{ units}}{\underset{1}{\cancel{500}} \ \cancel{\text{mL}}} \Big| \dfrac{1 \ \cancel{\text{mL}}}{} = 50 \text{ units}$

Here's a simple formula you can use for this calculation, instead of the other methods:

$$\frac{\text{Amount of drug}}{\text{Amount of fluid (mL)}} = \text{Amount of drug in 1 mL}$$

Medications Ordered in units/hour or mg/hour

Sometimes patient/client medications are administered as continuous IVs. For these medications, a specific amount of drug is mixed in a specific amount of IV fluid. Check the guidelines (institutional or drug references) to verify dose, dilution, and rate. If any doubts exist, consult with the prescribing physician or healthcare provider.

Units/hour—Calculation of Rate

The order will indicate the amount of drug to be added to the IV fluid and also the amount to administer.

EXAMPLE

Order: heparin, infuse 800 units/hour

Available: heparin 40,000 units in 1000 mL D5W infusion pump

What is the rate?

You know the solution and the amount to administer. Because you'll be using an infusion pump, the answer will be in milliliters per hour.

Desired dose: 800 units/hour

Supply: 40,000 units

Have: 1000 mL

To solve:

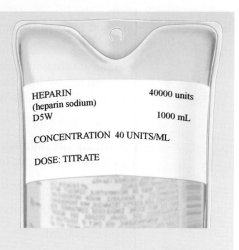

HEPARIN	40000 units
(heparin sodium) D5W	1000 mL

CONCENTRATION 40 UNITS/ML

DOSE: TITRATE

Formula Method	Proportion	Dimensional Analysis

Formula Method

$$\dfrac{\overset{20}{\cancel{800}} \text{ units/hour}}{\underset{\underset{1}{\cancel{40}}}{\cancel{40,000}} \text{ units}} \times \cancel{1000} \text{ mL}$$

= 20 mL/hour on a pump

Note that units cancel out and the answer is milliliters per hour.

Proportion

EXPRESSED AS TWO RATIOS

1000 mL : 40,000 units : : x mL : 800 units

EXPRESSED AS TWO FRACTIONS

$$\dfrac{1000 \text{ mL}}{40,000 \text{ units}} \times \dfrac{x \text{ mL}}{800 \text{ units}}$$

SOLUTION FOR BOTH PROPORTION METHODS

$$800 \times 1000 = 40,000x$$

$$\dfrac{800,000}{40,000} = x$$

$$20 \text{ mL/hour} = x$$

Dimensional Analysis

Set up the equation. You are solving for mL/hour.

$$\dfrac{1000 \, \text{mL}}{40,000 \text{ units}} \quad \dfrac{800 \text{ units}}{\text{hour}}$$

Cancel "units." Reduce the fraction. Solve.

$$\dfrac{1\cancel{000} \, \text{mL}}{\underset{1}{\cancel{40,000}} \text{ units}} \quad \dfrac{\overset{20}{\cancel{800}} \text{ units}}{\text{hour}}$$

= 20 mL/hour

FINE POINTS

Notice that the desired dose, milliliter per hour is set up as a fraction with "mL" in the numerator and "hours" in the denominator.

How many hours will the IV run?

$$\dfrac{\text{Number of milliliters}}{\text{Number of milliliters per hour}}$$

$$\dfrac{1000 \text{ mL}}{20 \text{ mL/hour}} = 50 \text{ hours}$$

Note: Most hospitals require changing the IV fluids every 24 hours.

EXAMPLE

Order: heparin sodium 1100 units/hour IV

Supply: infusion pump, standard solution (premixed by the pharmacy) of 25,000 units in 250 mL D5W

What is the rate?

With an infusion pump, the answer will be in milliliters per hour.

Desired dose: 1100 units/hour

Supply: 25,000 units

Have: 250 mL

To solve:

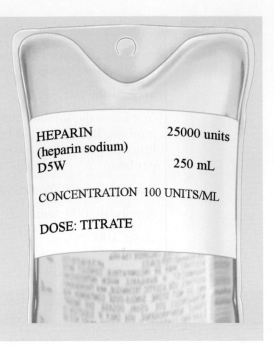

HEPARIN   25000 units
(heparin sodium)
D5W   250 mL

CONCENTRATION 100 UNITS/ML

DOSE: TITRATE

Formula Method	Proportion	Dimensional Analysis

Formula Method

$$\frac{1100 \text{ units/hour}}{25,000 \text{ units}} \times 250 \text{ mL}$$

$$= 11 \text{ mL/hour on a pump}$$

Proportion

EXPRESSED AS TWO RATIOS

250 mL : 25,000 units : : x mL : 1100 units

EXPRESSED AS TWO FRACTIONS

$$\frac{250 \text{ mL}}{25,000 \text{ units}} \times \frac{x \text{ mL}}{1100 \text{ units}}$$

SOLUTION FOR BOTH PROPORTION METHODS

$$250 \times 1100 = 25,000x$$

$$\frac{275,000}{25,000} = x$$

$$11 \text{ mL/hour} = x$$

Dimensional Analysis

Set up the equation. You are solving for milliliters per hour.

$$\frac{250 \text{ mL}}{25,000 \text{ units}} \; \bigg| \; \frac{1100 \text{ units}}{\text{hour}}$$

Cancel "units." Reduce the fraction. Solve.

$$\frac{250 \text{ mL}}{25,000 \text{ units}} \; \bigg| \; \frac{1100 \text{ units}}{\text{hour}} = \frac{11}{1}$$

$$= 11 \text{ mL/hour}$$

How many hours will the IV run?

$$\frac{\text{Number of milliliters}}{\text{Number of milliliters per hour}}$$

$$\frac{250 \text{ mL}}{11 \text{ mL/hour}} = 22.75 \text{ (22 hours 45 minutes) or 23 hours}$$

EXAMPLE

Order: regular insulin 10 units/hour IV

Available: infusion pump, standard solution of 125 units regular insulin in 250 mL NS (normal saline)

What is the rate? Use on infusion pump.

Desired dose: 10 units/hour

Supply: 125 units

Have: 250 mL

To solve:

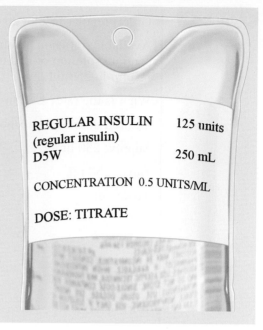

REGULAR INSULIN   125 units
(regular insulin)
D5W   250 mL

CONCENTRATION 0.5 UNITS/ML

DOSE: TITRATE

Formula Method	Proportion	Dimensional Analysis
$\dfrac{10 \text{ units}}{125 \text{ units}} \times \overset{2}{250} \text{ mL}$ $= 20 \text{ mL/hour on a pump}$	**EXPRESSED AS TWO RATIOS** 250 mL : 125 units : : x mL : 10 units **EXPRESSED AS TWO FRACTIONS** $\dfrac{250}{125} \times \dfrac{x \text{ mL}}{10}$ **SOLUTION FOR BOTH PROPORTION METHODS** $250 \times 10 = 125x$ $\dfrac{2500}{125} = x$ $20 \text{ mL/hour} = x$	Set up the equation. You are solving for milliliters per hour. $\dfrac{250 \text{ mL}}{125 \text{ units}} \quad\middle|\quad \dfrac{10 \text{ units}}{\text{hour}}$ Cancel "units." Reduce the fraction. Solve. $\dfrac{\overset{2}{250} \text{ mL}}{\underset{1}{125} \text{ units}} \quad\middle|\quad \dfrac{10 \text{ units}}{\text{hour}} = 10 \times 2$ $= 20 \text{ mL/hour}$

How many hours will the IV run?

$$\frac{\text{Number of milliliters}}{\text{Number of milliliters per hour}}$$

$$\frac{250 \text{ mL}}{20 \text{ mL/hour}} = 12.5 \text{ (12 hours 30 minutes) or approximately 13 hours}$$

EXAMPLE

Order: regular insulin 20 units/hour IV

Available: infusion pump, double concentrate solution of 250 units regular insulin in 250 mL NS

What is the rate? Use an infusion pump.

Desired dose: 20 units/hour

Supply: 250 units

Have: 250 mL

To solve:

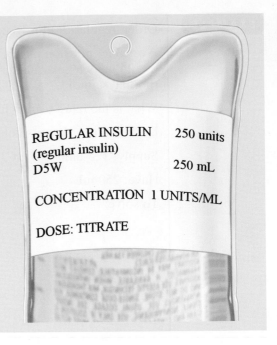

REGULAR INSULIN   250 units
(regular insulin)
D5W   250 mL

CONCENTRATION 1 UNITS/ML

DOSE: TITRATE

Formula Method	Proportion	Dimensional Analysis

Formula Method

$$\frac{20 \text{ units}}{250 \text{ units}} \times \overset{1}{\cancel{250}} \text{ mL}$$

= 20 mL/hour on a pump

Proportion

EXPRESSED AS TWO RATIOS

250 mL : 250 units : : x mL : 20 units

EXPRESSED AS TWO FRACTIONS

$$\frac{250 \text{ mL}}{250 \text{ units}} \times \frac{x}{20 \text{ units}}$$

$$\frac{5000}{250} = x$$

20 mL/hour = x

SOLUTION FOR BOTH PROPORTION METHODS

$$250 \times 20 = 250x$$

$$\frac{5000}{250} = x$$

20 mL/hour = x

Dimensional Analysis

Set up the equation. You are solving for milliliters per hour.

$$\frac{250 \text{ mL}}{250 \text{ units}} \ \Big| \ \frac{20 \text{ units}}{\text{hour}}$$

Cancel "units." Reduce the fraction. Solve.

$$\frac{\overset{1}{\cancel{250}} \text{ mL}}{\cancel{250} \text{ units}} \ \Big| \ \frac{20 \text{ units}}{\text{hour}}$$

= 20 mL/hour

How many hours will the IV run?

$$\frac{\text{Number of milliliters}}{\text{Number of milliliters per hour}}$$

$$\frac{250 \text{ mL}}{20 \text{ mL/hour}} = 12.5 \ (12 \text{ hours } 30 \text{ minutes}) \text{ or approximately } 13 \text{ hours}$$

g/hour; mg/hour—Calculation of Rate

The order will indicate the amount of drug added to the IV fluid and the amount to administer.

EXAMPLE

Order: calcium gluconate 2 g in 100 mL D5W; run 0.25 g/hour IV via infusion pump.

What is the rate?

Because we know the solution and the amount of drug per hour, you can solve the problem and administer the drug in milliliters per hour per infusion pump. Round the final answer to the nearest whole number.

Desired dose: 0.25 g/hour

Supply: 2 g

Have: 100 mL

To solve:

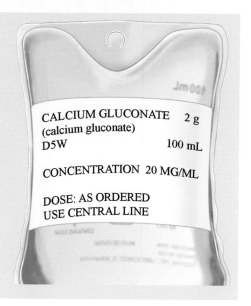

CALCIUM GLUCONATE   2 g
(calcium gluconate)
D5W   100 mL

CONCENTRATION 20 MG/ML

DOSE: AS ORDERED
USE CENTRAL LINE

Formula Method	Proportion	Dimensional Analysis
$\dfrac{0.25\ \cancel{g}\ /\text{hour}}{\cancel{2}\ \cancel{g}} \times \overset{50}{\cancel{100}}\ \text{mL} = 12.5$ $= 13$ mL/hour on a pump	**EXPRESSED AS TWO RATIOS** 100 mL : 2 g : : x mL : 0.25 g **EXPRESSED AS TWO FRACTIONS** $\dfrac{100\ \text{mL}}{2\ \text{g}} \times \dfrac{\text{x mL}}{0.25\ \text{g/hour}}$ **SOLUTION FOR BOTH PROPORTION METHODS** $0.25 \times 100 = 2x$ $\dfrac{25}{2} = x$ 12.5 or 13 mL/hour = x	Set up the equation. You are solving for milliliters per hour. $\dfrac{100\ \text{ⓜ}}{2\ \text{g}}\ \bigg|\ \dfrac{0.25\ \text{g}}{\text{ⓗⓞⓤⓡ}}$ Cancel "g." Reduce the fraction. Solve. $\dfrac{\overset{50}{\cancel{100}}\ \text{ⓜ}}{\underset{1}{\cancel{2}}\ \cancel{g}}\ \bigg|\ \dfrac{0.25\ \cancel{g}}{\text{ⓗⓞⓤⓡ}} = 50 \times 0.25$ $= 12.5$ or 13 mL/hour

How many hours will the IV run?

$$\frac{\text{Number of milliliters}}{\text{Number of milliliters per hour}}$$

$$\frac{100\ \text{mL}}{13\ \text{mL/hour}} = 7.6 \ (7 \text{ hours } 36 \text{ minutes}) \text{ or approximately 8 hours}$$

EXAMPLE

Order: aminophylline 250 mg in 250 mL D5W; run 65 mg/hour IV per infusion pump.

What is the rate? Use an infusion pump.

Desired dose: 65 mg/hour

Supply: 250 mg

Have: 250 mL

To solve:

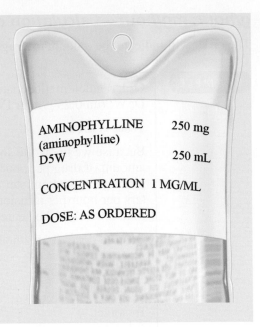

AMINOPHYLLINE   250 mg
(aminophylline)
D5W   250 mL

CONCENTRATION 1 MG/ML

DOSE: AS ORDERED

Formula Method	Proportion	Dimensional Analysis
$$\frac{65 \text{ mg/hour}}{250 \text{ mg}} \times \overset{1}{\cancel{250}} \text{ mL}$$ $$= 65 \text{ mL/hour on a pump}$$	**EXPRESSED AS TWO RATIOS** 250 mL : 250 mg : : x mL : 65 mg **EXPRESSED AS TWO FRACTIONS** $$\frac{250 \text{ mL}}{250 \text{ mg}} \times \frac{x \text{ mL}}{65 \text{ mg}}$$ **SOLUTION FOR BOTH PROPORTION METHODS** $$65 \times 250 = 250x$$ $$\frac{65 \times \cancel{250}}{\cancel{250}} = x$$ $$65 \text{ mL/hour} = x$$	Set up the equation. You are solving for milliliters per hour: $$\frac{250 \text{ mL}}{250 \text{ mg}} \left| \frac{65 \text{ mg}}{\text{hour}} \right.$$ Cancel "mg." Reduce the fraction. Solve. $$\frac{\overset{1}{\cancel{250}} \text{ mL}}{\underset{1}{\cancel{250}} \text{ mg}} \left| \frac{65 \text{ mg}}{\text{hour}} \right. = 65 \text{ mL/hour}$$

How many hours will the IV run?

$$\frac{\text{Number of milliliters}}{\text{Number of milliliters per hour}}$$

$$\frac{250 \text{ mL}}{65 \text{ mL/hour}} = 3.8 \text{ (3 hours 48 minutes) or approximately 4 hours}$$

EXAMPLE

Order: diltiazem (Cardizem) 15 mg/hour

Available: infusion pump, standard solution of 125 mg of diltiazem (Cardizem) in 125 mL NS

What is the rate? Use an infusion pump.

Desired dose: 15 mg/hour

Supply: 125 mg

Have: 125 mL

To solve:

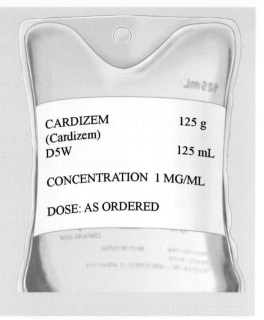

CARDIZEM 125 g
(Cardizem)
D5W 125 mL

CONCENTRATION 1 MG/ML

DOSE: AS ORDERED

Formula Method	Proportion	Dimensional Analysis
$\dfrac{15 \text{ mg/hour}}{125 \text{ mg}} \times 125 \text{ mL}$ = 15 mL/hour on a pump	**EXPRESSED AS TWO RATIOS** 125 mL : 125 mg : : x mL : 15 mg/hour **EXPRESSED AS TWO FRACTIONS** $\dfrac{125 \text{ mL}}{125 \text{ mg}} \times \dfrac{x \text{ mL}}{15 \text{ mg/hour}}$ **SOLUTION FOR BOTH PROPORTION METHODS** $125 \times 15 = 125x$ $\dfrac{1875}{125} = x$ 15 mL/hour = x	Set up the equation. You are solving for milliliters per hour. $\dfrac{125 \text{ mL}}{125 \text{ mg}} \left| \dfrac{15 \text{ mg}}{\text{hour}} \right.$ Cancel "mg." Reduce the fraction. Solve = 15 mL/hour

How many hours will the IV run?

$$\frac{\text{Number of milliliters}}{\text{Number of milliliters per hour}}$$

$$\frac{125 \text{ mL}}{15 \text{ mL/hour}} = 8.3 \text{ (8 hours 18 minutes) or approximately 8 hours}$$

Solve the following problems. Answers appear at the end of this chapter.

1. Order: heparin sodium 800 units/hour IV
   Supply: infusion pump, standard solution of 25,000 units in 250 mL D5W

   a. What is the rate?
   b. How many hours will the IV run?

2. Order: acyclovir (Zovirax) 500 mg in 100 mL D5W IV over 1 hour
   Supply: infusion pump, acyclovir (Zovirax) 500 mg in 100 mL D5W

   What is the rate?

3. Order: aminocaproic acid (Amicar) 24 g over 24 hour IV
   Supply: infusion pump, aminocaproic acid (Amicar) 24 g in 1000 mL D5W

   What is the rate?

4. Order: diltiazem (Cardizem) 10 mg/hour IV
   Supply: infusion pump, diltiazem (Cardizem) 125 mg in 100 mL D5W

   What is the rate?

5. Order: furosemide (Lasix) infuse 4 mg/hour
   Supply: infusion pump, furosemide (Lasix) 100 mg in 100 mL D5W

   What is the rate?

6. Order: regular insulin 15 units/hour IV
   Supply: infusion pump, standard solution of 125 units in 250 mL NS

   a. What is the rate?
   b. How many hours will this IV run?

7. Order: nitroglycerin 50 mg in 250 mL D5W over 24 hour via infusion pump
   What is the rate?

8. Order: heparin 1200 units/hour IV
   Supply: infusion pump, standard solution of 25,000 units in 500 mL D5W

   a. What is the rate?
   b. How many hours will the IV run?

9. Order: regular insulin 23 units/hour IV
   Supply: infusion pump, standard solution of 250 units in 250 mL NS

   a. What is the rate?
   b. How many hours will the IV run?

10. Order: streptokinase (Streptase) 100,000 international units/hour for 24 hour IV
    Supply: infusion pump, standard solution of 750,000 international units in 250 mL NS

    What is the rate?

mg/minute—Calculation of Rate

The order will indicate the amount of drug added to IV fluid and also the amount of drug to administer. These medications are administered through an IV infusion pump in milliliters per hour.

Note: The dimensional analysis method will combine all of the calculation steps into one equation.

EXAMPLE

Order: bretylium (Bretylol) 1 mg/minute IV

Supply: infusion pump, standard solution of 1 g in 500 mL D5W (1000 mg in 500 mL)

The order calls for 1 mg/minute. You need milliliters per hour for the pump.

Convert the order to milligrams per hour by multiplying the drug amount by 60 (60 minutes = 1 hour): 1 mg/minute × 60 minutes = 60 mg in 1 hour.

What is the rate?

Desired dose: 60 mg/hour

Supply: 500 mL

Have: 1 g (1000 mg)

To solve:

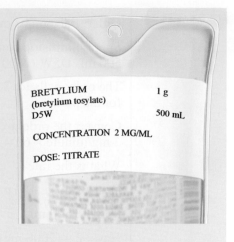

BRETYLIUM   1 g
(bretylium tosylate)
D5W   500 mL

CONCENTRATION 2 MG/ML

DOSE: TITRATE

Formula Method	Proportion	Dimensional Analysis

Formula Method

$$\frac{\overset{30}{\cancel{60} \text{ mg/hour}}}{\underset{\underset{1}{2}}{\cancel{1000} \text{ mg}}} \times \cancel{500} \text{ mL}$$

$$= 30 \text{ mL/hour}$$

Set pump at 30 mL/hour.

Proportion

EXPRESSED AS TWO RATIOS

500 mL : 1000 mg : : x mL : 60 mg

EXPRESSED AS TWO FRACTIONS

$$\frac{500 \text{ mL}}{1000 \text{ mg}} \times \frac{x \text{ mL}}{60 \text{ mg}}$$

SOLUTION FOR BOTH PROPORTION METHODS

$$500 \times 60 = 1000x$$

$$\frac{30,000}{1000} = x$$

$$30 \text{ mL/hour} = x$$

Dimensional Analysis

Set up the equation. You are solving for milliliters per hour. Use the conversion factors:

Use $\dfrac{60 \text{ minutes}}{1 \text{ hour}}$ because the order is in minutes but the answer will be in hours.

Use $\dfrac{1 \text{ g}}{1000 \text{ mg}}$ because the order is in mg but the supply is 1 g in 500 mL.

500 mL	1 mg	1 g	60 minutes
1 g	minutes	1000 mg	1 hour

Cancel "mg," "g," "minutes." Reduce the fraction. Solve.

$$\frac{\overset{1}{\cancel{500} \text{ mL}} \mid 1 \text{ mg} \mid 1 \cancel{g} \mid 60 \cancel{minutes}}{1 \cancel{g} \mid \cancel{minutes} \mid \underset{2}{\cancel{1000} \text{ mg}} \mid 1 \text{ hour}}$$

$$= \frac{60}{2} = 30 \text{ mL/hour}$$

How many hours will the IV run?

$$\frac{\text{Number of milliliters}}{\text{Number of milliliters per hour}}$$

$$\frac{500 \text{ mL}}{30 \text{ mL/hour}} = 16.6 \text{ (16 hours 36 minutes) or approximately 17 hours}$$

FINE POINTS

The conversion factors can be placed anywhere in the equation. All of the "units of measurement" in the conversion factor will be cancelled out in the equation.

EXAMPLE

Order: lidocaine 3 mg/minute IV

Supply: infusion pump, standard solution of 2 g in 500 mL D5W (2000 mg in 500 mL)

The order calls for 3 mg/minute. We need mL/hour for the pump.

Convert the order to milligrams per hour: Multiply 3 mg/minute × 60 = 180 mg/hour

What is the rate?

Desired dose: 180 mg/hour

Supply: 500 mL

Have: 2 g (2000 mg)

To solve:

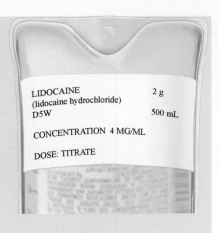

LIDOCAINE   2 g
(lidocaine hydrochloride)
D5W   500 mL

CONCENTRATION 4 MG/ML

DOSE: TITRATE

Formula Method	Proportion	Dimensional Analysis

Formula Method

$$\frac{180 \text{ mg/hour}}{2000 \text{ mg}} \times 500 \text{ mL}$$

$$= \frac{180}{4} = 45 \text{ mL/hour}$$

Proportion

EXPRESSED AS TWO RATIOS

500 mL : 2000 mg :: x mL : 180 mg

EXPRESSED AS TWO FRACTIONS

$$\frac{500 \text{ mL}}{2000 \text{ mg}} \times \frac{x \text{ mL}}{180 \text{ mg}}$$

SOLUTION FOR BOTH PROPORTION METHODS

$$180 \times 500 = 2000x$$

$$\frac{90{,}000}{2000} = x$$

$$45 \text{ mL/hour} = x$$

Dimensional Analysis

Set up the equation. You are solving for milliliters per hour. Use the conversion factors:

Use $\dfrac{60 \text{ minutes}}{1 \text{ hour}}$ because the order is in minutes but the answer will be in hours.

Use $\dfrac{1 \text{ g}}{1000 \text{ mg}}$ because the order is in milligrams but the supply is 2 g in 500 mL.

500 mL	3 mg	1 g	60 minutes
2 g	minutes	1000 mg	1 hour

Cancel "g," "mg," "minutes." Reduce the fraction. Solve.

500 mL	3 mg	1 g	60 minutes
2 g	minutes	1000 mg	1 hour

$$= \frac{3 \times 30}{2} = 45 \text{ mL/hour}$$

Set pump at 45 mL/hour.

How many hours will the IV run?

$$\frac{\text{Number of milliliters}}{\text{Number of milliliters per hour}}$$

$$\frac{500 \text{ mL}}{45 \text{ mL/hour}} = 11.1 \text{ (11 hours 6 minutes) or approximately 11 hours}$$

EXAMPLE

Order: amiodarone 0.5 mg/minute IV

Available: infusion pump, standard solution of 900 mg of amiodarone in 500 mL D5W

The order calls for 0.5 mg/minute. We need mL/hour for the pump.

Convert the order to milligrams per hour: Multiply 0.5 mg/minute × 60 = 30 mg/hour

What is the rate? Use an infusion pump.

Desired dose: 30 mg/hour

Supply: 500 mL

Have: 900 mg

To solve:

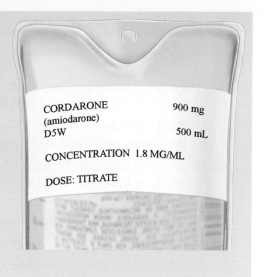

CORDARONE 900 mg
(amiodarone)
D5W 500 mL

CONCENTRATION 1.8 MG/ML

DOSE: TITRATE

Formula Method	Proportion	Dimensional Analysis
$\dfrac{\overset{}{30\ \text{mg/hour}}}{\underset{9}{900\ \text{mg}}} \times \overset{5}{500}\ \text{mL}$ $=\dfrac{30\times 5}{9}$ $=16.6 \text{ or } 17 \text{ mL/hour}$	**EXPRESSED AS TWO RATIOS** 500 mL : 900 mg :: x mL : 30 mg **EXPRESSED AS TWO FRACTIONS** $\dfrac{500\ \text{mL}}{900\ \text{mg}} \times \dfrac{x\ \text{mL}}{30\ \text{mg}}$ $500 \times 30 = 900x$ $500 \times \dfrac{30}{900} = x$ 16.6 or 17 mL/hour = x	Set up the equation. You are solving for milliliters per hour. Use the conversion factors: Use $\dfrac{60 \text{ minutes}}{1 \text{ hour}}$ because the order is in minutes but the answer will be in hour

Dimensional Analysis (continued):

500 mL	0.5 mg	60 minutes
900 mg	minute	hour

Cancel "mg," "minutes."
Reduce the fraction. Solve

$\overset{5}{500}$ mL	0.5 mg	60 minutes
$\underset{9}{900}$ mg	minute	hour

$\dfrac{5 \times 0.5 \times 60}{9} = 17 \text{ mL/hour}$

How many hours will the IV run?

$$\dfrac{\text{Number of milliliters}}{\text{Number of milliliters per hour}}$$

$$\dfrac{500 \text{ mL}}{17 \text{ mL/hour}} = 29.4 \text{ (29 hours 24 minutes) or approximately 29 hours}$$

Most hospitals require changing the IV fluids every 24 hours.

SELF-TEST 2   Infusion Rates for Drugs Ordered in mg/minute

Solve the following problems. Answers appear at the end of the chapter.

1. Order: lidocaine 1 mg/minute IV
   Supply: 2 g in 250 mL D5W, infusion pump

   a. What is the drip rate?
   b. How many hours will the IV run?

2. Order: labetalol (Trandate) 2 mg/minute IV
   Supply: labetalol (Trandate) 300 mg in 300 mL D5W, infusion pump

   a. What is the drip rate?
   b. How many hours will the IV run?

3. Order: bretylium (Bretylol) 2 mg/minute IV
   Supply: bretylium (Bretylol) 1 g in 500 mL D5W, infusion pump

   a. What is the drip rate?
   b. How many hours will the IV run?

4. Order: amiodarone (Cordarone) 1 mg/minute for 6 hours
   Supply: amiodarone (Cordarone) 450 mg in 250 mL D5W, infusion pump

   What is the drip rate?

5. Order: lorazepam (Ativan) 1 mg/minute
   Supply: lorazepam (Ativan) 80 mg in 250 mL NS, infusion pump

   a. What is the drip rate?
   b. How many hours will the IV run?

 # Medications Ordered in mcg/minute, mcg/kg/minute, or milliunits/minute—Calculation of Rate

Intensive care units administer powerful drugs in extremely small amounts called micrograms (1 mg = 1000 mcg). The orders for these drugs often use the patient/client's weight as a determinant, because these drugs are so potent.

EXAMPLE   Order: renal dose dopamine 2 mcg/kg/minute

Order: titrate norepinephrine (Levophed) to maintain arterial mean pressure above 65 mm Hg and below 95 mm Hg

This section shows how to calculate doses in micrograms and in milliunits, and how to use kilograms in determining doses. Most infusion pumps used in hospitals allow you to program these drugs and the pump will calculate the rate for you. However, it is still important to know how to calculate the rate.

mcg/minute—Calculation

Drugs ordered in micrograms per minute are standardized solutions prepared by a pharmacist. They are administered using infusion pumps that deliver medication in milliliters per hour.

   To calculate drugs ordered in micrograms per minute, first determine how much of the drug is in 1 mL of solution (see beginning of this chapter). If the drug is supplied in milligrams, convert it to micrograms; then divide that amount by 60 to get micrograms per minute. The final number tells you how much of the drug is in 1 mL of fluid. You can then use one of the three methods to solve for the infusion rate, on the basis of the ordered dosage. The dimensional analysis method will combine all the steps into one equation.

Solving micrograms per minute requires four steps:

1. Reduce the numbers in the standard solution to milligrams per milliliter.
2. Change milligrams to micrograms.
3. Divide by 60 to get micrograms per minute.
4. Use the formula, ratio, or proportion method to solve for milliliters per hour.

EXAMPLE

Order: dopamine (Intropin) 400 micrograms per minute IV

Supply: infusion pump, standard solution 400 mg in 250 mL D5W

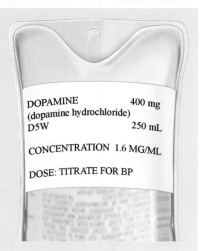

DOPAMINE   400 mg
(dopamine hydrochloride)
D5W   250 mL

CONCENTRATION 1.6 MG/ML

DOSE: TITRATE FOR BP

Step 1. Reduce the numbers in the standard solution.

$$\frac{400 \text{ mg}}{250 \text{ mL}} = 1.6 \text{ mg in 1 mL}$$

Step 2. Change milligrams to micrograms.
$1.6 \text{ mg} \times 1000 = 1600 \text{ mcg}/1 \text{ mL}$

Step 3. Divide by 60 to get micrograms per minute.

$$\frac{1600 \text{ mcg}}{60 \text{ minutes}} = 26.67 \text{ mcg/minute}$$

(Round to hundredths.)

Step 4. Solve for milliliters per hour. (Round to nearest whole number.)

Step 5. Set the infusion pump; program the milliliters per hour and volume to be infused.

Formula Method	Proportion	Dimensional Analysis

Formula Method

$$\frac{400 \text{ mcg/minute}}{26.67 \text{ mcg/minute}} \times 1 \text{ mL}$$

$$= 15 \text{ mL/hour}$$

Proportion

EXPRESSED AS TWO RATIOS

1 mL : 26.67 mcg/minute : : x mL : 400 mcg/minute

EXPRESSED AS TWO FRACTIONS

$$\frac{1 \text{ mL}}{26.67 \text{ mcg/minute}} \times \frac{x \text{ mL}}{400 \text{ mcg/minute}}$$

SOLUTION FOR BOTH PROPORTION METHODS

$$400 = 26.67x$$

$$\frac{400}{26.67} = x$$

$$15 \text{ mL/hour} = x$$

Dimensional Analysis

Set up the equation. You are solving for milliliters per hour. Use the conversion factors:

Use $\dfrac{60 \text{ minutes}}{1 \text{ hour}}$ because the order is in minutes but the answer will be in hours.

Use $\dfrac{1 \text{ mg}}{1000 \text{ mcg}}$ because the order is in mcg, but the supply is 400 mg in 250 mL.

$$\frac{250 \text{ (mL)}}{400 \text{ mg}} \, \Bigg| \, \frac{400 \text{ mcg}}{\text{minutes}} \, \Bigg| \, \frac{60 \text{ minutes}}{1 \text{ (hour)}} \, \Bigg| \, \frac{1 \text{ mg}}{1000 \text{ mcg}}$$

Cancel "mg," "mcg," and "minutes." Reduce the fraction. Solve.

$$\frac{\overset{1}{\cancel{250}} \text{ (mL)}}{\underset{1}{\cancel{400}} \text{ mg}} \, \Bigg| \, \frac{\overset{1}{\cancel{400}} \text{ mcg}}{\cancel{\text{minutes}}} \, \Bigg| \, \frac{60 \cancel{\text{ minutes}}}{1 \text{ (hour)}} \, \Bigg| \, \frac{1 \cancel{\text{ mg}}}{\underset{4}{\cancel{1000}} \text{ mcg}}$$

$$\frac{60}{4} = 15 \text{ mL/hour}$$

> **Step 6.** To set the infusion pump, program the following
> - Total number of milliliters ordered = 250 mL
> - Milliliters per hour to run = 15 mL/hour

EXAMPLE

Order: metaraminol (Aramine) 60 mcg/minute IV

Supply: infusion pump, standard solution 50 mg in 250 mL D5W

> **Step 1.** Reduce the numbers in the standard solution.
> $$\frac{50 \text{ mg}}{250 \text{ mL}} = 0.2 \text{ mg/mL}$$
>
> **Step 2.** Change milligrams to micrograms.
> 0.2 mg = 200 mcg/1 mL
>
> **Step 3.** Divide by 60 to get mcg/minute.
> 3.33 mcg/minute
> Round to hundredths.
>
> **Step 4.** Solve. Round to the nearest whole number.

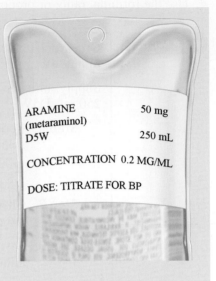

ARAMINE   50 mg
(metaraminol)
D5W   250 mL

CONCENTRATION 0.2 MG/ML

DOSE: TITRATE FOR BP

Formula Method	Proportion	Dimensional Analysis

Formula Method

$$\frac{60 \text{ mcg/minute}}{3.33 \text{ mcg/minute}} \times 1 \text{ mL}$$

$$= 18 \text{ mL/hour}$$

Proportion

EXPRESSED AS TWO RATIOS

1 mL : 3.33 mcg/minute : : x mL : 60 mcg/minute

EXPRESSED AS TWO FRACTIONS

$$\frac{1 \text{ mL}}{3.33 \text{ mcg/minute}} \times \frac{x}{60 \text{ mcg/minute}}$$

SOLUTION FOR BOTH PROPORTION METHODS

$$60 = 3.33x$$
$$\frac{60}{3.33} = x$$
$$18 \text{ mL/hour} = x$$

Dimensional Analysis

Set up the equation. You are solving for milliliters per hour: Use the conversion factors:

Use $\dfrac{60 \text{ minutes}}{1 \text{ hour}}$ because the order is in minutes

but the answer is in hours.

Use $\dfrac{1 \text{ mg}}{1000 \text{ mcg}}$ because the order is in mcg

but the supply is 50 mg in 250 mL.

250 mL	60 mcg	60 minutes	1 mg
50 mg	minutes	1 hour	1000 mcg

Cancel "mg," "mcg," and "minutes." Reduce the fraction. Solve.

¹250 mL	⁶60 mcg	³/₁₅ 60 minutes	1 mg
50 mg	minutes	1 hour	1000 mcg

$$= 6 \times 3 = 18 \text{ mL/hour}$$

> **Step 5.** Set the pump: total number of milliliters = 250 (standard solutions); milliliters per hour = 18.

EXAMPLE

Order: Nitroglycerine, 20 mcg/minute IV

Available: infusion pump, double concentrated solution of 100 mg in 250 mL D5W

Step 1. Reduce the numbers in the solution

100 mg/250 mL = 0.4 mg in 1 mL

Step 2. Change milligrams to micrograms

0.4 mg × 1000 = 400 mcg/1 mL

Step 3. Divide by 60 to get micrograms per minute.

400 mcg/60 minutes = 6.67 mcg/minute (round to hundredths)

Step 4. Solve for milliliters per hour (round to nearest whole number).

Step 5. Set the infusion pump; program the milliliters per hour and volume to be infused.

To solve:

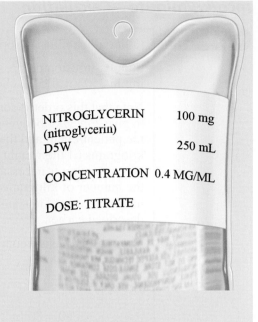

NITROGLYCERIN   100 mg
(nitroglycerin)
D5W   250 mL

CONCENTRATION 0.4 MG/ML

DOSE: TITRATE

Formula Method	Proportion	Dimensional Analysis
$\dfrac{20 \text{ mcg/minute}}{6.67 \text{ mcg/minute}} \times 1 \text{ mL}$ = 3 mL/hr	**EXPRESSED AS TWO RATIOS** 1 mL : 6.67 mcg /minute :: x mL : 20 mcg/minute **EXPRESSED AS TWO FRACTIONS** $\dfrac{1 \text{ mL}}{6.67} \times \dfrac{x}{20 \text{ mcg}}$ **SOLUTION FOR BOTH PROPORTION METHODS** 20 mcg = 6.67x $\dfrac{20}{6.67} = x$ 3 mL/hour = x	Set up the equation. You are solving for milliliters per hour. Use the conversion factors: Use $\dfrac{60 \text{ minutes}}{1 \text{ hour}}$ because the order is in minutes but the answer will be in hours Use $\dfrac{1 \text{ mg}}{1000 \text{ mcg}}$ because the order is in mcg, but the supply is 100mg in 250mL.

For Dimensional Analysis:

$$\frac{250 \text{ mL}}{100 \text{ mg}} \bigg| \frac{20 \text{ mcg}}{\text{minute}} \bigg| \frac{1 \text{ mg}}{1000 \text{ mcg}} \bigg| \frac{60 \text{ minutes}}{\text{hour}}$$

Cancel "mg," "mcg," and "minutes."
Reduce the fraction. Solve

$$\frac{\overset{1}{\cancel{250}} \text{ mL}}{\cancel{100} \text{ mg}} \bigg| \frac{20 \cancel{\text{mcg}}}{\cancel{\text{minute}}} \bigg| \frac{1 \cancel{\text{mg}}}{\underset{4}{\cancel{1000}} \cancel{\text{mcg}}} \bigg| \frac{60 \cancel{\text{minutes}}}{\cancel{\text{hour}}}$$

= 3 mL/hour

mcg/kg/minute—Calculation

EXAMPLE

Order: dopamine (Intropin) 2 mcg/kg/minute

Supply: infusion pump, standard solution 200 mg in 250 mL D5W; client weighs 176 lb

Note that this order is somewhat different. You are to give 2 mcg/kg body weight. First you weigh the patient/client and then convert pounds to kilograms (if the weight is already in kilograms, no conversion is necessary); then multiply the number of kilograms by 2 mcg. Once you have determined this answer, follow the steps described earlier.

The patient/client weighs 176 lb.

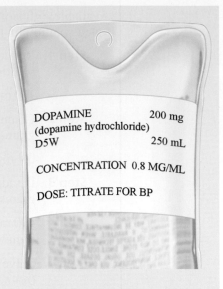

DOPAMINE   200 mg
(dopamine hydrochloride)
D5W   250 mL

CONCENTRATION 0.8 MG/ML

DOSE: TITRATE FOR BP

$$\frac{176 \text{ lb}}{2.2}$$

$$2.2\overline{)176.0} \quad 80 = 80 \text{ kg}$$

$$\begin{array}{r} 80 \text{ kg} \\ \times\ 2 \text{ mcg} \\ \hline 160 \text{ mcg} \end{array}$$ The order now is 160 mcg/minute.

(Dimensional analysis will combine all the steps, including weight conversion, into one equation.)

1. Reduce the numbers in the standard solution.

    $$\frac{200 \text{ mg}}{250 \text{ mL}} = 0.8 \text{ mg/mL}$$

2. Change milligrams to micrograms.

    0.8 = 800 mcg/mL

3. Divide by 60 to get mcg/kg/minute.

    $$\frac{800}{60} = 13.33$$

    Round to hundredths.

4. Solve. Round to the nearest whole number.

Formula Method	Proportion	Dimensional Analysis

Formula Method

$$\frac{160 \text{ mcg/minute}}{13.33 \text{ mcg/minute}} \times 1 \text{ mL}$$

$$= 12 \text{ mL/hour}$$

Proportion

EXPRESSED AS TWO RATIOS

1 mL : 13.33 mcg/minute :: x mL : 160 mcg/minute

EXPRESSED AS TWO FRACTIONS

$$\frac{1 \text{ mL}}{13.33 \text{ mcg/minute}} \diagup \frac{x \text{ mL}}{160 \text{ mg/minute}}$$

SOLUTION FOR BOTH PROPORTION METHODS

$$160 = 13.33x$$

$$\frac{160}{13.33} = x$$

$$12 \text{ mL/hour} = x$$

Dimensional Analysis

Set up the equation. You are solving for milliliters per hour. Use the conversion factors:

Use $\dfrac{60 \text{ minutes}}{1 \text{ hour}}$ because the order is in minutes but the answer will be hours.

Use $\dfrac{1 \text{ mg}}{1000 \text{ mcg}}$ because the order is in mcg, but the supply is 200 mg in 250 mL.

Use $\dfrac{1 \text{ kg}}{2.2 \text{ lb}}$ for the weight conversion.

250 (mL)	2 mcg	60 minutes	1 mg	176 lb	1 kg
200 mg	kg/minute	1 (hour)	1000 mcg		2.2 lb

Cancel "mg," "mcg," "min," "kg," and "lb." Reduce the fraction. Solve.

$$\frac{\overset{1}{250} \text{ (mL)} \mid \overset{1}{\cancel{2}} \text{ mcg} \mid 60 \text{ minutes} \mid 1 \text{ mg} \mid 176 \text{ lb} \mid 1 \text{ kg}}{\underset{100}{200} \text{ mg} \mid \text{kg / minute} \mid 1 \text{ (hour)} \mid \underset{4}{1000} \text{ mcg} \mid \mid 2.2 \text{ lb}}$$

$$= \frac{\overset{15}{60} \times 176}{100 \times \underset{1}{4} \times 2.2} = \frac{15 \times 176}{100 \times 2.2} = \frac{2640}{220} = 12 \text{ mL/hour}$$

FINE POINTS

The order "2 mcg/kg/minute" is written as $\frac{2 \text{mcg}}{\text{kg/minute}}$. The denominator "kg/minute" is a shortened version of the fraction; both "kg" and "minutes" need to be cancelled.

5. Set the pump: total number of milliliters = 250 (standard solution); milliliters per hour = 12.

Milliunits/minute—Calculation

In obstetrics, a oxytocin (Pitocin) drip can initiate labor. The standard solution is 15 units in 250 mL. Because 1 unit = 1000 milliunits, you solve these problems in the same way as micrograms per minute.

EXAMPLE

Order: oxytocin (Pitocin) drip 2 milliunits/minute IV

Supply: infusion pump, standard solution 15 units in NS 250 mL

1. Reduce the numbers in the standard solution

$$\frac{15 \text{ units}}{250 \text{ mL}} = 0.06 \text{ units/mL}$$

2. Change units of pitocin to milliunits

1 unit = 1000 milliunits

$0.06 \times 1000 = 60$ milliunits/mL

3. Divide by 60 to get milliunits per minute

$$\frac{60}{60} = 1 \text{ milliunit/minute}$$

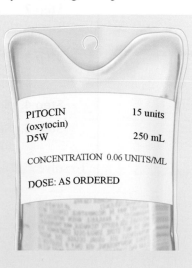

PITOCIN
(oxytocin)
D5W

15 units

250 mL

CONCENTRATION 0.06 UNITS/ML

DOSE: AS ORDERED

4. Solve. Round to the nearest whole number.

Formula Method	Proportion	Dimensional Analysis
$\dfrac{2 \text{ milliunits/minute}}{1 \text{ milliunit/minute}} \times 1 \text{ mL}$ $= 2 \text{ mL/hour}$	**EXPRESSED AS TWO RATIOS** 1 mL : 1 milliunit/minute : : x mL : 2 milliunits/minute **EXPRESSED AS TWO FRACTIONS** $\dfrac{1 \text{ mL}}{1 \text{ milliunit}} \times \dfrac{x}{2 \text{ milliunits}}$ **SOLUTION FOR BOTH PROPORTION METHODS** $2 = 1x$ $\dfrac{2}{1} = x$ $2 \text{ mL/hour} = x$	Set up the equation. You are solving for milliliters per hour. Use the conversion factors: Use $\dfrac{60 \text{ minutes}}{1 \text{ hour}}$ because the order is in minutes but the answer is in hours. Use $\dfrac{1 \text{ unit}}{1000 \text{ milliunits}}$ because the order is in milliunits, but the supply is 15 units in 250 mL.

<table>
<tr><td>250 mL</td><td>2 milliunits</td><td>60 minutes</td><td>1 unit</td></tr>
<tr><td>15 units</td><td>minutes</td><td>1 hour</td><td>1000 milliunits</td></tr>
</table>

Cancel "units," "milliunits," and "minutes." Reduce the fraction. Solve.

<table>
<tr><td>250 mL
(1)</td><td>2 milliunits</td><td>60 minutes
(4)</td><td>1 unit</td></tr>
<tr><td>15 units
(1)</td><td>minutes</td><td>1 hour</td><td>1000 milliunits
(4)</td></tr>
</table>

$= 2 \text{ mL/hour}$

5. Set the pump: total number of milliliters = 250; milliliters per hour = 2.

EXAMPLE

Order: Diprivan 22 mcg/kg/min

Available: infusion pump, standard solution of 1000 mg in 100 mL D5W

The patient weighs 75 kg.

22 mcg × 75 kg = 1650 mcg/minute

(Dimensional analysis will combine all the steps, including weight, into one equation.)

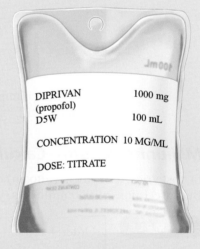

DIPRIVAN	1000 mg
(propofol) D5W	100 mL
CONCENTRATION	10 MG/ML
DOSE: TITRATE	

Step 1. Reduce the numbers in the solution

1000 mg/100 mL = 10 mg/mL

Step 2. Change milligrams to micrograms

10 mg = 10,000 mcg

Step 3. Divide by 60 to get micrograms per minute.

10,000/60 = 166.67 (Round to hundredths.)

Step 4. Solve for milliliters per hour. (Round to nearest whole number.)

Step 5. Set the infusion pump; program the milliliters per hour and volume to be infused.

To solve:

Formula Method	Proportion	Dimensional Analysis

Formula Method

$$\frac{1650}{166.67} \times 1 \text{ mL}$$

$= 9.9$ or 10 mL/hour

Proportion

EXPRESSED AS TWO RATIOS

1 mL:166.67 mcg/minute::x:1650 mcg/minute

EXPRESSED AS TWO FRACTIONS

$$\frac{1 \text{ mL}}{166.67 \text{ mg}} \times \frac{x}{1650 \text{ mcg}}$$

SOLUTION FOR BOTH PROPORTION METHODS

$$1650 = 166.67x$$

$$\frac{1650}{166.67} = x$$

$$9.9 \text{ or } 10 \text{ mL/hour} = x$$

Dimensional Analysis

Set up the equation. You are solving for milliliters per hour. Use the conversion factors:

Use $\dfrac{60 \text{ minutes}}{1 \text{ hour}}$ because the order is in minutes

but answer will be in hours

Use $\dfrac{1 \text{ mg}}{1000 \text{ mcg}}$ because the order is in mcg,

but the supply is 100mg in 250mL.

100 mL	22 mcg	60 minutes	1 mg	75 kg
1000 mg	kg/minute	1 hour	1000 mcg	

Cancel "mg," "mcg," "minutes." Reduce the fraction and Solve.

100 mL	22 mcg	60 minutes	1 mg	75 kg
1000 mg	kg/minute	1 hour	1000 mcg	

$$\frac{22 \times 60 \times 75}{10000} = 10 \text{ mL/hour}$$

Infusion Rates for Drugs Ordered in mcg/minute, mcg/kg/minute, and milliunits/minute

Calculate the number of milliliters to infuse and the rate of infusion. Answers appear at the end of the chapter.

1. Order: dopamine (Intropin) double strength, 800 mcg/minute IV
   Supply: standard solution of 800 mg in 250 mL D5W, infusion pump

2. Order: norepinephrine (Levophed) 12 mcg/minute IV
   Supply: standard solution of 4 mg in 250 mL D5W, infusion pump

3. Order: dobutamine (Dobutrex) 5 mcg/kg/minute IV
   Supply: patient/client weight, 220 lb; standard solution of 1 g in 250 mL D5W, infusion pump

4. Order: dobutamine (Dobutrex) 7 mcg/kg/minute IV
   Supply: patient/client weight, 70 kg; standard solution of 500 mg in 250 mL D5W, infusion pump

5. Order: nitroglycerin 10 mcg/minute IV
   Supply: standard solution of 50 mg in 250 mL D5W, infusion pump

6. Order: oxytocin (Pitocin) 1 milliunit/minute IV
   Supply: standard solution of 15 units in 250 mL NS, infusion pump

7. Order: isoproterenol (Isuprel) titrated at 4 mcg/minute IV
   Supply: solution of 2 mg in 250 mL D5W, infusion pump

8. Order: esmolol (Brevibloc) 50 mcg/kg/minute IV
   Supply: 2.5 g in 250 mL D5W; weight, 58 kg, infusion pump

9. Order: nitroprusside (Nipride) 2 mcg/kg/minute IV
   Supply: patient/client weight, 80 kg; nipride 50 mg in 250 mL D5W, infusion pump

10. Order: amrinone (Inocor) 200 mcg/minute
   Supply: amrinone (Inocor) 0.1 g in 100 mL NS, infusion pump

Body Surface Nomogram

Antineoplastic drugs used in cancer chemotherapy have a narrow therapeutic range. Calculation of these drugs is based on BSA in meters squared—a method considered more precise than mg/kg/body weight. BSA is the measured or calculated area of the body.

There are several mathematical formulas to calculate BSA. The following formula often is used:

$$\sqrt{\frac{weight\,(kg) \times height\,(cm)}{3600}} = BSA$$

You can estimate BSA by using a three-column chart called a nomogram (Fig. 7-2). Mark the patient/client's height in the first column and the weight in the third column. Then draw a line between these two marks. The point at which the line intersects the middle column indicates estimated body surface in meters squared. You'll use a different BSA chart for children because of differences in growth (see Chapter 8).

> **FINE POINTS**
>
> Average BSA:
>
>   "Normal" BSA: 1.7 m²
>
>   Average BSA for men: 1.9 m²
>
>   Average BSA for women: 1.6 m²

The oncologist, a physician who specializes in treating cancer, lists the patient/client's height, weight, and BSA; gives the protocol (drug requirement based on BSA in square meters); and then gives the order.

Figure 7-3 shows a partial order sheet for chemotherapy. Both the pharmacist and you, the nurse, validate the order before preparation.

To determine BSA in square meters, you can use a special calculator obtained from companies manufacturing antineoplastics. Many websites also calculate BSA; see, for example, *www.globalrph.com/bsa2.htm*.

m²—Rule and Calculation

Oncology drugs are prepared by a pharmacist or specially trained technician who is gowned, gloved, and masked and works under a laminar flow hood; these precautions protect the pharmacist or technician and also ensure sterility. When the medication reaches the unit, you, the nurse, bear two responsibilities: checking the doses for accuracy before administration and using an infusion pump for IV orders.

EXAMPLE

Ht, 6′0″; Wt, 175 lb; BSA, 2.0 m²

Order: cisplatin (Platinol) 160 mg (80 mg/m²) IV in 1 L NS with 2 mg magnesium sulfate over 2 hours

1. Check the BSA using the nomogram in Figure 7-2. It is correct. Protocol calls for 80 mg/m²; 160 mg is correct.

2. The IV is prepared by the pharmacy. Determine the rate of infusion.

   1 L = 1000 mL

   $$\frac{Number\ of\ milliliters}{Number\ of\ hours} = Milliliters\ per\ hour \qquad \frac{\overset{500}{\cancel{1000}}}{\underset{1}{\cancel{2}}} = 500\ mL/hour$$

Set the pump: total number of milliliters = 1000; rate in milliliters per hour = 500.

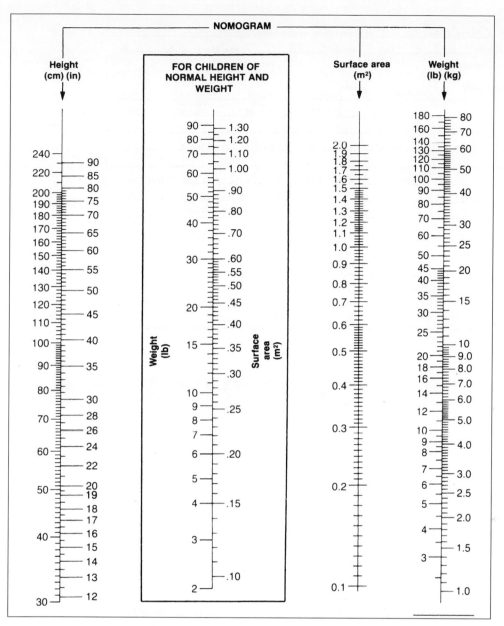

FIGURE 7-2

BSA is critical when calculating dosages for pediatric patients/clients or for drugs that are extremely potent and need to be given in precise amounts. The nomogram shown here lets you plot the patient/client's height and weight to determine the BSA. Here's how it works:

1. Locate the patient/client's height in the left column of the nomogram and the weight in the right column.

2. Use a ruler to draw a straight line connecting the two points. The point where the line intersects the surface area column indicates the patient/client's BSA in meters squared.

3. For an average-sized child, use the simplified nomogram in the box. Just find the child's weight in pounds on the left side of the scale and then read the corresponding BSA on the right side.

	PROTOCOL	PATIENTS	ROUTE AND DILUENT	FREQUENCY AND / OR DOSAGE	# OF
DRUG	DOSAGE	DOSAGE			DAYS
1. MITOMYCIN	12 mg/m²	24 mg	IVP × 1 m 9/08		
2. 5FU	1000 mg/m²	2000 mg	in 1000 mL of NS as a continuous infusion everyday × 4 days on		
3.			9/08, 9/09, 9/10, 9/11		

DIAGNOSIS: COLON CANCER _____ PROTOCOL NAME/NUMBER: _____
PATIENT'S HEIGHT: 6'2 ___ cm   WEIGHT: 186 _____ Kg or BSA: 2.1 ___ m²
VENOUS ACCESS: DEEP ☐   PERIPHERAL ☒
everyday

FIGURE 7-3

Portion of doctor's order form for chemotherapy. The doctor or healthcare provider writes the patient/client's height and weight and calculates the BSA as 2.1 m². The protocol dosage is the guide used to determine the patient/client's dose. For mitomycin, the protocol is 12 mg/m² × 2 m² = 24 mg. For 5FU, the protocol dose is 1000 mg/m² × 2 m² = 2000 mg.

SELF-TEST 4   Use of Nomogram

Solve the following problems. Answers appear at the end of this chapter. Use the nomogram in Figure 7-2 to double-check the BSA.

1. Ht, 6′0″; Wt, 165 lb; BSA, 1.96 m²
   Order: doxorubicin (Doxil) 39 mg (20 mg/m²) in D5W 250 mL to infuse over ½ hour

   a. Is dose correct?
   b. How should the pump be set?

2. Ht, 165 cm; Wt, 70 kg; BSA, 1.77 m²
   Order: CCNU (lomustine) 230 mg po (130 mg/m²) once q6 weeks

   a. Is dose correct?
   b. CCNU (lomustine) comes in tabs of 100 mg and 10 mg. What is the dose?

3. Ht, 6′2″; Wt, 170 lb; BSA, 2.0 m²
   Order: daunorubicin (Cerubidine) 80 mg (40 mg/m²) in D5W over 1 hour IV
   Supply: IV bag labeled 80 mg in 80 mL D5W; infuse in rapidly flowing IV

   a. Is dose correct?
   b. How should the pump be set? (See IVPB administration in Chapter 6.)

4. Ht, 6′5″; Wt, 175 lb; BSA, 2.0 m²
   Order: etoposide (Vepesid) 400 mg po every day × 3 (200 mg/m²)
   Supply: capsules of 50 mg

   a. Is dose correct?
   b. How many capsules should be administered?

5. Ht, 5′3″; Wt, 120 lb; BSA, 1.6 m²
   Order: paclitaxel (Taxol) 216 mg (135 mg/m²) in D5W 500 mL glass bottle over 3 hours

   a. Is dose correct?
   b. How should the pump be set?

Patient-Controlled Analgesia

PCA, an IV method of pain control, allows a patient/client to self-administer a preset dose of pain medication. The physician or healthcare provider prescribes the narcotic dose and concentration, the basal rate, the lockout time, and the total maximum hourly dose (Fig. 7-4).

Basal rate is the amount of medication that is infused continuously each hour. *PCA dose* is the amount of medication infused when the patient/client activates the button control. *Lockout time* or *delay*—a feature that prevents overdosage—is the interval during which the patient/client cannot initiate another dose after giving a self-dose. *Total hourly dose* is the maximum amount of medication the patient/client can receive in an hour. The physician or healthcare provider writes all of this information on an order form.

Figure 7-5 shows a narcotic PCA medication record. Morphine concentration is 1 mg/mL. The pharmacy dispenses a 100-mL NS bag with 100 mL of morphine. The patient/client continuously receives 0.5 mg by infusion pump and can give 1 mg by pressing the PCA button. Eight minutes must elapse before another PCA dose can be delivered. Note that at 12 noon, the nurse charted that the patient/client made three attempts but received only two injections. This indicates that 8 minutes had not elapsed before one of the attempts.

Your responsibility is to assess the patient/client every hour, noting how the patient/client scores his or her pain, the number of PCA attempts, and the total hourly dose received as well as the cumulative dose, the patient/client's level of consciousness, side effects, and respirations. For a pediatric patient/client, a pulse oximeter or apnea/bradycardia monitor is often used.

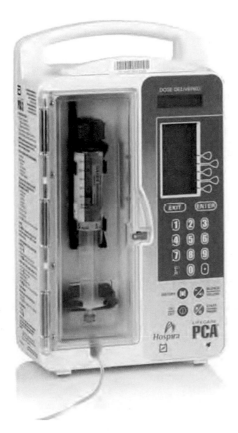

FIGURE 7-4

PCA allows the patient/client to self-administer medication, as necessary, to control pain. (From Roach, S. S. [2004]. *Introductory clinical pharmacology* [7th ed.]. Philadelphia, PA: Lippincott Williams & Wilkins, p. 173.)

AVERY MEDICAL CENTER
Narcotic PCA
Medication Administration Record

Check appropriate order:

Dose: _1_ mg/mL
Lockout: _8_ min
1 hour limit: _8_ mg/mL
Basal _0.5_ mg/hr

_X_ Morphine 1 mg/1 mL:50 mL
___ Fentanyl. Concentration: _____ Volume: _____
___ Demerol 10 mg/1 mL:50 mL
___ Other: _____   Concentration _____ Volume: _____

Infusion started by: _____ RN
    (zero out prior shift volume with each new bag/syringe)
Settings confirmed by: _____ RN
Date/Time discoutinued: _____
Discontinued by: _____ RN
Total Amount Administered: _____
Waste returned to pharmacy: _____

Pharmacist: Witness: Witness:

Date	0600	0800	1000	1200	1400	1600
Number of attempts	3	2	2	3		
Number of injections	3	2	2	2		
Basal dose	0.5	0.5	0.5	0.5		
Total mL	3.5	4.5	4.5	2.5		
Cumulative mL	3.5	8	12.5	15		
Pain score	5	5	5	6		
Level of consciousness	1	1	1	1		
Respiratory rate (per minute)	16	20	16	22		
Nurse's initials	GP	GP	GP	GP		

Level of Consciousness: 1-alert, 2-drowsy, 3-sleeping, 4-confused, 5-difficult to arouse

Nurse's signature _____ Initial _____
Nurse's signature _____ Initial _____
Nurse's signature _____ Initial _____
Nurse's signature _____ Initial _____

FIGURE 7-5

Sample PCA medication record.

Heparin and Insulin Protocols

Many hospitals and other institutions now use protocols to give you more freedom in determining the rate and amount of drug the patient/client is receiving. These protocols are based on a parameter, usually a lab test ordered by the healthcare provider. After receiving the lab test results, you use the protocol to determine the change (if any) in the dosage amount.

Two drugs used in protocols are heparin and insulin. (With insulin, these are sometimes called *sliding scale* protocols.)

Both of these drugs have potential to cause medical problems if the incorrect dose is administered. (Search "heparin errors" or "insulin errors" on the Internet to see how common and serious these errors are.) Most hospitals require another nurse to double-check the dose calculation of heparin and insulin.

Heparin Protocol

Heparin, an anticoagulant, is titrated according to the results of the partial thromboplastin time (PTT) lab test. A weight-based heparin protocol calculates the dose of heparin based on the patient/client's weight.

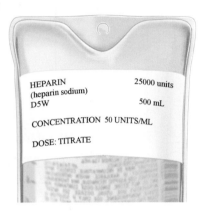

Sample heparin protocol:

Heparin drip: 25,000 units in 500 mL D5W

Bolus or loading dose: 80 units/kg

Starting dose: 18 units/kg/hour

Titrate according to the following chart:

PTT (seconds)	<45 Seconds	45–48 Seconds	49–66 Seconds	67–70 Seconds	71–109 Seconds	110–130 Seconds	>130 Seconds
Bolus or loading dose	Bolus with 40 units/kg	Bolus with 40 units/kg	No bolus	No bolus	No bolus	No bolus	No bolus
Rate adjustment	Increase rate by 3 units/kg/hour	Increase rate by 2 units/kg/hour	Increase rate by 1 unit/kg/hour	No change	No change	Decrease rate by 1 unit/kg/hour	Stop infusion for 1 hour; decrease rate by 2 units/kg/hour
Next lab	PTT in 6 hours	PTT in 6 hours	PTT in 6 hours	PTT next AM	PTT next AM	PTT in 6 hours	PTT in 6 hours

EXAMPLE

Patient/client weight is 70 kg.

1. Calculation for bolus or loading dose: 80 units/kg

    Multiply: 80 units × 70 kg = 5600 units/kg

2. Infusion rate:

    First calculate what the dose will be.

    Starting dose is 18 units/kg/hour.

    Multiply: 18 × 70 kg = 1260 units

    Now use the calculation similar to that on p. 241. (Dimensional analysis will combine all the steps into one equation)

Formula Method	Proportion	Dimensional Analysis
$\dfrac{1260 \text{ units}}{25,000 \text{ units}} \times 500 \text{ mL}$ $= 25.2 \text{ mL/hour}$	**EXPRESSED AS TWO RATIOS** 500 mL : 25,000 units : : x mL : 1260 units **EXPRESSED AS TWO FRACTIONS** $\dfrac{500 \text{ mL}}{25,000 \text{ units}} \times \dfrac{\text{x mL}}{1260 \text{ units}}$ **SOLUTION FOR BOTH PROPORTION METHODS** $500 \times 1260 = 25,000\text{x}$ $\dfrac{500 \times 1260}{25,000} = \text{x}$ $25.2 \text{ mL/hour} = \text{x}$	Set up the equation. You are solving for milliliters per hour: $\dfrac{500 \text{ mL}}{25,000 \text{ units}} \left\| \dfrac{18 \text{ units}}{\text{kg/hour}} \right\| 70 \text{ kg}$ Cancel "units" and "kg." Reduce the fraction. Solve. $\dfrac{\overset{1}{\cancel{500}} \text{ mL}}{\underset{50}{\cancel{25,000}} \text{ units}} \left\| \dfrac{18 \text{ units}}{\text{kg/hour}} \right\| 70 \text{ kg}$ $= \dfrac{18 \times 70}{50} = 25.2 \text{ mL/hour or } 25 \text{ mL/hour}$

Set the pump at 25.2 or 25 mL/hour.

3. The PTT result 6 hours after the infusion started is 50 seconds. According to the table, we increase the drip by 1 unit/kg/hour.

   First, calculate the dose:

   $1 \text{ unit} \times 70 \text{ kg} = 70 \text{ units/kg}$

   Then set up the same formula to solve for the infusion rate change:

Formula Method	Proportion	Dimensional Analysis
$\dfrac{70 \text{ units}}{25,000 \text{ units}} \times 500 \text{ mL}$ $= 1.4 \text{ mL}$	**EXPRESSED AS TWO RATIOS** 500 mL : 25,000 units : : x mL : 70 units **EXPRESSED AS TWO FRACTIONS** $\dfrac{500 \text{ mL}}{25,000 \text{ units}} \times \dfrac{\text{x mL}}{70 \text{ units}}$ **SOLUTION FOR BOTH PROPORTION METHODS** $500 \times 70 = 25,000\text{x}$ $\dfrac{35,000}{25,000} = \text{x}$ $1.4 \text{ mL} = \text{x}$	$\dfrac{\overset{1}{\cancel{500}} \text{ mL}}{\underset{50}{\cancel{25,000}} \text{ units}} \left\| \dfrac{1 \text{ unit}}{\text{kg/hour}} \right\| 70 \text{ kg} = \dfrac{7}{5}$ $= 1.4 \text{ mL}$ Cancel "units" and "kg." Reduce the fraction. Solve.

Increase the infusion rate by 1.4 mL: 25.2 + 1.4 = 26.6 mL/hour. Set the pump at 26.6 or 27 mL/hour.

Recheck the PTT in 6 hours, and titrate according to the result.

SELF-TEST 5 | Heparin Protocol Calculations

Use the chart on page 260 to solve the following problems. Use heparin 25,000 units in 500 mL as your IV solution. The patient/client's weight is 70 kg. Beginning infusion rate for each problem is 25.2 mL/hour. Answers appear at the end of the chapter.

1. The patient/client's PTT is 45 seconds.

   a. Is there a bolus or loading dose? If so, what is the dose?
   b. Is there a change in the infusion rate? Calculate the new infusion rate.

2. The patient/client's PTT is 40 seconds.

   a. Is there a bolus or loading dose? If so, what is the dose?
   b. Is there a change in the infusion rate? Calculate the new infusion rate.

3. The patient/client's PTT is 110 seconds.

   a. Is there a bolus or loading dose? If so, what is the dose?
   b. Is there a change in the infusion rate? Calculate the new infusion rate.

4. The patient/client's PTT is 140 seconds.

   a. Is there a bolus or loading dose? If so, what is the dose?
   b. Is there a change in the infusion rate? Calculate the new infusion rate.

Insulin Protocol

Regular insulin can be given by continuous IV infusion. The rate is titrated according to the blood glucose. Several conditions must be considered before initiating an insulin protocol (also called *hypoglycemic protocol* or *hyperglycemic protocol*); for example, an elevated blood glucose, weight, and renal function. Always follow hospital or institutional policy regarding these variables. This section includes only the calculation of an insulin drip and the titration in infusion rate. (If the blood glucose falls below a certain level, such as 70, the patient/client may need to receive an administration of D50W. Follow hospital policy for hypoglycemia.)

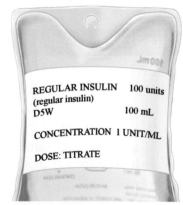

Insulin protocol:

If blood glucose is >150 give IV regular insulin—bolus or loading dose of 0.1 units/kg.

Initiate infusion rate at the calculated dose:

Blood glucose (BG) – 60 × 0.02 = units insulin/hour

(The 0.02 is the "multiplier" or "correction factor." This figure changes according to the blood glucose. See the chart on page 268.)

Regular insulin 100 units in 100 mL of NS.

EXAMPLE

Patient/client weight, 70 kg. Blood glucose, 200.

1. Calculate the bolus or loading dose:

   0.1 units × 70 kg = 7 units of regular insulin IV

2. Calculate the infusion rate:

   (200 – 60) × 0.02 = 2.8 units

3. Now use the calculation similar to that on page 243.

Formula Method	Proportion	Dimensional Analysis
$\dfrac{2.8 \text{ units}}{100 \text{ units}} \times 100 \text{ mL}$ $= 2.8 \text{ mL/hour}$	**EXPRESSED AS TWO RATIOS** $100 \text{ mL} : 100 \text{ units} : : x \text{ mL} : 2.8 \text{ units}$ **EXPRESSED AS TWO FRACTIONS** $\dfrac{100 \text{ mL}}{100 \text{ units}} \times \dfrac{x \text{ mL}}{2.8 \text{ units}}$ **SOLUTION FOR BOTH PROPORTION METHODS** $100 \times 2.8 = 100x$ $\dfrac{100 \times 2.8}{100} = x$ $2.8 \text{ mL/hour} = x$	Set up the equation. You are solving for milliliters per hour: $\dfrac{100 \text{ mL}}{100 \text{ units}} \left| \dfrac{2.8 \text{ units}}{\text{hours}} \right.$ Cancel "units." Reduce the fraction. Solve. $\dfrac{\overset{1}{\cancel{100}} \text{ mL}}{\underset{1}{\cancel{100}} \text{ units}} \left| \dfrac{2.8 \text{ units}}{\text{hours}} \right. = 2.8 \text{ mL/hour}$ or 3 mL/hour

Set the pump at 2.8 mL/hour or 3 mL/hour.

Recheck the blood glucose in 1 hour and titrate.

Sample insulin protocol titration chart:

Blood Glucose Result	Rate/Multiplier Change
80–110	Continue same rate. No change in rate or multiplier.
>110 and <150	Continue same rate. Recheck blood glucose in 1 hour and if >110, increase multiplier by 0.01 and calculate new infusion rate.
>150	Increase multiplier by 0.01 and calculate new infusion rate.

SELF-TEST 6   Insulin Protocol Calculations

Use regular insulin 100 units in 100 mL NS. Patient/client weight of 70 kg. Use initial formula: BG − 60 × 0.02 = units insulin/hour. Use the above chart for changes.

1. Blood glucose is 300.

   a. What is the infusion rate?
   b. Is there a change in the formula? If so, what is the new formula?

2. Blood glucose is 350.

   a. Use the new formula from question 1b. What is the infusion rate?
   b. Is there a change in the formula? If so, what is the new formula?

3. Blood glucose is 140. Rechecked in 1 hour and remains 140.

   a. Use the new formula from question 2b. What is the infusion rate?
   b. Is there a change in the formula? If so, what is the new formula?

4. Blood glucose is 100.

   a. Use the new formula from question 3b. What is the infusion rate?
   b. Is there a change in the formula? If so, what is the new formula?

SELF-TEST 7   Infusion Problems

Solve these problems. Answers are given at the end of the chapter. Answers will be in mL/hour.

1. Order: labetalol (Normadyne) 0.5 mg/minute on pump
   Supply: infusion pump, standard solution of 200 mg in 200 mL D5W

   What is the pump setting?

2. Order: aminophylline at 75 mg/hour IV
   Supply: infusion pump, aminophylline 250 mg in 250 mL D5W

   What is the pump setting?

3. Order: bretylium (Bretylol) 2 g in 500 mL D5W at 4 mg/minute IV
   Supply: infusion pump, standard solution of 2 g in 500 mL D5W

   What is the pump setting?

4. Order: acyclovir (Zovirax) 400 mg in 100 mL D5W over 2 hours
   Supply: infusion pump, acyclovir (Zovirax) 400 mg in 100 mL D5W

   What is the pump setting?

5. Order: urokinase (Abbokinase) 5000 units/hour over 5 hours IV
   Supply: infusion pump, urokinase (Abbokinase) 25,000 units in 250 mL D5W

   What is the pump setting?

6. Order: magnesium sulfate 4 g in 100 mL D5W to infuse over 30 minutes IV
   Supply: infusion pump, magnesium sulfate 4 g in 100 mL D5W

   What is the pump setting?

7. Order: nitroglycerin 80 mcg/minute IV
   Supply: infusion pump, standard solution of 50 mg in 250 mL D5W

   What is the pump setting?

8. Order: dobutamine (Dobutrex) 6 mcg/kg/minute IV
   Supply: infusion pump, solution of 500 mg in 250 mL D5W; weight, 180 lb

   a. Change pounds to kilograms, round to the nearest whole number.
   b. What is the pump setting?

9. Order: oxytocin (Pitocin) 2 milliunits/minute IV
   Supply: infusion pump, solution of 9 units in 150 mL NS

   What is the pump setting?

10. Ht, 6′0″; wt, 110 lb; BSA, 1.55 m²
    Order: cisplatin (Platinol) 124 mg (80 mg/m²) in 1000 mL NS to infuse over 4 hours

    a. Is dose correct?
    b. What is the pump setting?

CRITICAL THINKING   **TEST YOUR CLINICAL SAVVY**

A 65-year-old non–insulin-dependent diabetes mellitus (NIDDM) patient/client with a 10-year history of congestive heart failure is admitted to the intensive care unit with chest pain of more than 24 hours. The patient/client is receiving heparin, insulin, calcium gluconate, and potassium chloride, all intravenously.

A. Why would an infusion pump be needed with these medications?

B. Why would medications that are based on body weight require the use of a pump? Why would medications based on BSA require an infusion pump?

C. Can any of these medications be regulated with standard roller clamp tubing? What would be the advantage? What would be the contraindication?

D. What other information would you need to calculate the drip rates of these medications?

E. Why would it be necessary to calculate how long each infusion will last?

Putting it Together

Mrs. R is a 79-year-old woman with dyspnea without chest pain, fever, chills, or sweats. No evidence for bleeding. Admitted through the ER with BP 82/60, afebrile, sinus tachycardia at 110/minute. She underwent emergency dialysis and developed worsening dyspnea and was transferred to the ICU. BP on admission to ICU was 70/30, tachypneic on 100% nonrebreather mask. No c/o chest discomfort or abdominal pain. Dyspnea worsened and the patient/client became bradycardic and agonal respirations developed. A Code Blue was called and the patient/client was resuscitated after intubation. Spontaneous pulse and atrial fibrillation was noted.

Past Medical History: cardiomegaly, severe cardiomyopathy, chronic atrial fibrillation, unstable angina, hypertension, chronic kidney disease with hemodialysis, TIA in 3/07.

Allergies: calcium channel blockers

Current Vital Signs: pulse 150/minute, blood pressure is 90/40, RR 18 via the ventilator. Afebrile. Weight: 90 kg

Medication Orders

piperacillin/tazobactam (Zosyn) *antibiotic* 0.75 G IV in 50 mL q8h
pantoprazole (Protonix) *antiulcer* 40 mg IV q12h. Dilute in 10 mL NS
and give slow IV push.
phenylephrine (Neo-Synephrine) *vasopressor* drip 30 mg in 500 mL D5W
   100 mcg/minute titrate for SBP >90
norepinephrine (Levophed) *vasopressor* in 4 mg in 500 mL D5W
   Titrate SBP >90 start at 0.5 mcg/minute

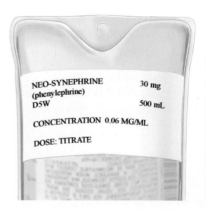

NEO-SYNEPHRINE   30 mg
(phenylephrine)
D5W   500 mL

CONCENTRATION 0.06 MG/ML

DOSE: TITRATE

Putting it Together (*Continued*)

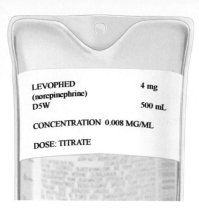

½ NS 1000 mL at 150 mL/hour

Heparin *anticoagulant* 12 units/kg/hour. No loading dose. IV solution 25,000 units in 500 mL D5W. Titrate to keep PTT 49–70.

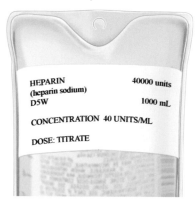

Aspirin *antiplatelet* 81 mg po/N/G daily
digoxin (Lanoxin) *cardiac glycoside* 0.25 mg IV daily
propofol (Diprivan) *sedative* 10 mg/mL
  Titrate 5–50 mcg/kg/min for sedation

Calculations

1. Calculate how many micrograms per milliliter of phenylephrine (Neo-Synephrine).

2. Calculate the rate on the infusion pump of phenylephrine (Neo-Synephrine) 100 mcg/minute.

3. Calculate how many micrograms per milliliter of norepinephrine (Levophed).

4. Calculate the rate on the infusion pump of norepinephrine (Levophed) 0.5 mcg/minute.

5. Calculate the dose of heparin.

6. Calculate the rate on the infusion pump of the heparin dose. When is the next PTT due?

7. Propofol (Diprivan) is mixed in 100 mL. How many milligrams are mixed to equal 10 mg/mL?

8. Calculate the rate on the infusion pump of propofol (Diprivan)—calculate using the range of 5 to 50 mcg/kg/minute.

(continued)

Putting it Together (*Continued*)

Critical Thinking Questions

1. Do any of the patient/client's medical conditions warrant changes in the medication orders?

2. Why would two vasopressors be given together?

3. What is the reason for giving the patient/client propofol (Diprivan)?

4. What medication may help atrial fibrillation yet be contraindicated in this patient/client?

5. What is a possible reason for the sinus tachycardia of 150/minute?

6. What is the reason for giving a drug slow IV push, such as the pantoprazole (Protonix)?

Answers in Appendix B.

PROFICIENCY TEST 1 Special IV Calculations

*Name:*_____

Solve these problems. Answers are given in Appendix A. Answers are in mL/hour.

1. Order: regular insulin 15 units/hour IV
    Supply: infusion pump, standard solution of 125 units in 250 mL NS

    What is the pump setting?

2. Order: heparin sodium 1500 units/hour IV
    Supply: infusion pump, standard solution of 25,000 units in 500 mL D5W IV

    What is the pump setting?

3. Order: bretylium (Bretylol) 2 g in 500 mL D5W at 2 mg/minute IV
    Supply: infusion pump, standard solution of 2 g in 500 mL D5W

    What is the pump setting?

4. Order: diltiazem (Cardizem) at 5 mg/hour IV
    Supply: infusion pump, diltiazem (Cardizem) 125 mg in 100 mL D5W

    What is the pump setting?

5. Order: lidocaine 4 mg/minute IV
    Supply: infusion pump, standard solution of 2 g in 500 mL D5W

    What is the pump setting?

6. Order: KCl 40 mEq/L at 10 mEq/hour IV, in D5W 1000 mL
    Supply: infusion pump, vial of KCl labeled 20 mEq/10 mL

    a. How much KCl should be added?
    b. What is the pump setting?

7. Order: lidocaine 2 mg/minute IV
    Supply: infusion pump, standard solution of 2 g in 500 mL D5W

    What is the pump setting?

8. Order: amphotericin B (Fungizone) 50 mg in 500 mL D5W over 6 hours IV
    Supply: infusion pump, amphotericin B (Fungizone) 50 mg in 500 mL D5W

    What is the pump setting?

9. Order: vasopressin (Pitressin) 18 units/hour IV
    Supply: infusion pump, vasopressin (Pitressin) 200 units in 500 mL D5W

    What is the pump setting?

10. Order: dobutamine (Dobutrex) 250 mcg/minute IV
    Supply: infusion pump, solution of 500 mg in 500 mL D5W

    What is the pump setting?

11. Order: renal dose dopamine (Intropin) 2.5 mcg/kg/minute
    Supply: infusion pump, solution 400 mg in 250 mL D5W; wt, 60 kg

    What is the pump setting?

(continued)

12. Order: oxytocin (Pitocin) 2 milliunits/minute IV
    Supply: infusion pump, solution of 9 units in 150 mL NS

    What is the pump setting?

13. Ht, 5′3″; wt, 143 lb; BSA, 1.7 m²
    Order: Ara-C 170 mg (100 mg/m²) in 1 L D5W over 24 hour

    a. Is dose correct?
    b. How should the pump be set?

14. Order: nitroprusside (Nipride) 5 mcg/kg/minute IV
    Supply: patient/client weight, 90 kg; nitroprusside (Nipride) 50 mg in 250 mL D5W,
                 infusion pump

    What is the pump setting?

15. Order: epinephrine 2 mcg/minute
    Supply: epinephrine 4 mg in 250 mL D5W, infusion pump

    What is the pump setting?

16. Patient/client's PTT is 45 seconds. Use the heparin protocol chart on page 265. Patient/
    client's weight is 90 kg. Heparin 25,000 units in 500 mL. Rate is 32 mL/hour.

    a. Is there a bolus or loading dose? If so, what is the dose?
    b. Is there a change in the infusion rate? Calculate the new infusion rate.

17. Patient/client's PTT is 40 seconds. Use the heparin protocol chart on page 265. Patient/
    client's weight is 90 kg. Heparin 25,000 units in 500 mL. Rate is 32 mL/hour.

    a. Is there a bolus or loading dose? If so, what is the dose?
    b. Is there a change in the infusion rate? Calculate the new infusion rate.

18. Patient/client's PTT is 110 seconds. Use the heparin protocol chart on page 265. Patient/
    client's weight is 90 kg. Heparin 25,000 units in 500 mL. Rate is 32 mL/hour.

    a. Is there a bolus or loading dose? If so, what is the dose?
    b. Is there a change in the infusion rate? Calculate the new infusion rate.

19. Use regular insulin 100 units in 100 mL NS. Patient/client weight of 70 kg. BG – 60 ×
    0.02 = units insulin/hour. Use the insulin protocol chart on page 268 for changes.

    Patient/client's baseline blood glucose is 120. Repeat blood glucose in 1 hour is 125.

    a. What is the infusion rate? (calculate on blood glucose of 125)
    b. Is there a change in the formula? If so, what is the new formula?

20. Use regular insulin 100 units in 100 mL NS. Patient/client weight of 70 kg. Patient's
    blood glucose is 260. BG – 60 × 0.02 = units insulin/hour. Use the chart on page 268 for
    changes.

    a. What is the infusion rate?
    b. Is there a change in the formula? If so, what is the new formula?

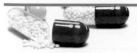

Answers

Self-Test 1 Infusion Rates

1. a.

Formula Method	Proportion	Dimensional Analysis
$\dfrac{\overset{8}{\cancel{800}\ \text{units /hour}}}{\underset{\underset{1}{100}}{\cancel{25,000}\ \text{units}}} \times \overset{1}{\cancel{250}}\ \text{mL}$ $= 8\ \text{mL/hour on a pump}$	**EXPRESSED AS TWO RATIOS** 250 mL : 25,000 units : : x mL : 800 units **EXPRESSED AS TWO FRACTIONS** $\dfrac{250\ \text{mL}}{25,000\ \text{units}} \times \dfrac{\text{x mL}}{800\ \text{units}}$ **SOLUTION FOR BOTH PROPORTION METHODS** $250 \times 800 = 25,000\text{x}$ $\dfrac{200,000}{25,000} = \text{x}$ $8\ \text{mL/hour} = \text{x}$	$\dfrac{\overset{1}{\cancel{250}}\ \text{mL}}{\underset{\underset{1}{100}}{\cancel{25,000}\ \text{units}}} \left| \dfrac{\overset{}{\cancel{800}}\ \text{units}}{\text{hours}} \right. = 8\ \text{mL/hour}$

b.

$$\frac{250\ \text{mL}}{8\ \text{mL/hour}}\ \ 8\overline{)\begin{array}{l}31.2\\250.0\end{array}}$$
$$\begin{array}{r}24\\\hline 10\\8\\\hline 2.0\end{array}$$

= 31 hours 12 minutes or approximately 30 hours; hospital policy states that IV bags be changed after 24 hours

2. Add 500 mg acyclovir to 100 mL D5W using a reconstitution device (see Chapter 6).

$$\frac{\text{Number of milliliters}}{\text{Number of hours}} = \text{Milliliters per hour}$$

$$\frac{100\ \text{mL}}{1\ \text{hour}}\quad \text{No math is necessary. Set the pump at 100 mL/hour.}$$

3. $\dfrac{1000\ \text{mL}}{24\ \text{hour}}\ \ 24\overline{)\begin{array}{l}41.6\\1000.0\end{array}}$

$$\begin{array}{r}96\\\hline 40\\24\\\hline 16.0\\14.4\\\hline\end{array}$$

Set the pump at 42 mL/hour.

(continued)

Answers (Continued)

4.

Formula Method	Proportion	Dimensional Analysis

Formula Method

$$\dfrac{\overset{2}{\cancel{10}} \text{ mg}}{\underset{1}{\cancel{125}} \text{ mg}} \times \overset{4}{\cancel{100}} \text{ mL}$$

$$= 8 \text{ mL/hour}$$

Proportion

EXPRESSED AS TWO RATIOS

$$100 \text{ mL} : 125 \text{ mg} :: x \text{ mL} : 10 \text{ mg}$$

EXPRESSED AS TWO FRACTIONS

$$\dfrac{100 \text{ mL}}{125 \text{ mg}} \diagup\!\!\!\diagdown \dfrac{x \text{ mL}}{10 \text{ mg}}$$

SOLUTION FOR BOTH PROPORTION METHODS

$$100 \times 10 = 125x$$

$$\dfrac{1000}{125} = x$$

$$8 \text{ mL/hour} = x$$

Dimensional Analysis

$$\dfrac{\overset{4}{\cancel{100}} \enspace \cancel{\text{mL}}}{\underset{1}{\cancel{125}} \text{ mg}} \bigg| \dfrac{\overset{2}{\cancel{10}} \text{ mg}}{\cancel{\text{hours}}} = 4 \times 2 = 8 \text{ mL/hour}$$

5.

Formula Method	Proportion	Dimensional Analysis

Formula Method

$$\dfrac{4 \text{ mg /hour}}{\underset{1}{\cancel{100}} \text{ mg}} \times \overset{1}{\cancel{100}} \text{ mL}$$

$$= 4 \text{ mL/hour}$$

Proportion

EXPRESSED AS TWO RATIOS

$$100 \text{ mL} : 100 \text{ mg} :: x \text{ mL} : 4 \text{ mg}$$

EXPRESSED AS TWO FRACTIONS

$$\dfrac{100 \text{ mL}}{100 \text{ mg}} \diagup\!\!\!\diagdown \dfrac{x \text{ mL}}{4 \text{ mg}}$$

SOLUTION FOR BOTH PROPORTION METHODS

$$100 \times 4 = 100x$$

$$\dfrac{400}{100} = x$$

$$4 \text{ mL/hour} = x$$

Dimensional Analysis

$$\dfrac{\overset{1}{\cancel{100}} \enspace \cancel{\text{mL}}}{\underset{1}{\cancel{100}} \text{ mg}} \bigg| \dfrac{4 \text{ mg}}{\cancel{\text{hours}}} = 4 \text{ mL/hour}$$

6. a.

Formula Method	Proportion	Dimensional Analysis
$\dfrac{15 \text{ units}}{125 \text{ units}} \times 250 \text{ mL}$ $= 0.12 \times 250 \text{ mL}$ $= 30 \text{ mL/hour}$	**EXPRESSED AS TWO RATIOS** $250 \text{ mL} : 125 \text{ units} :: x \text{ mL} : 15 \text{ units}$ **EXPRESSED AS TWO FRACTIONS** $\dfrac{250 \text{ mL}}{125 \text{ units}} \diagdown\!\!\!\diagup \dfrac{x \text{ mL}}{15 \text{ units}}$ **SOLUTION FOR BOTH PROPORTION METHODS** $250 \times 15 = 125x$ $\dfrac{3750}{125} = x$ $30 \text{ mL/hour} = x$	$\dfrac{\overset{2}{\cancel{250}} \,\cancel{\text{mL}}}{\underset{1}{\cancel{125}} \,\cancel{\text{units}}} \left| \dfrac{15 \,\cancel{\text{units}}}{\cancel{\text{hours}}} = 15 \times 2 = 30 \text{ mL/hour} \right.$

b. The total volume of medication is 125 units, and the client receives 15 units/hour.

$$\frac{\text{Number of units}}{\text{Number of units per hour}} = \frac{125}{15}$$

$$\begin{array}{r} 8.33 \\ 15\overline{\smash{)}125.00} \\ \underline{120} \\ 5.0 \\ \underline{4.5} \\ 50 \end{array} = 8 \text{ hours } 20 \text{ minutes or approximately } 8 \text{ hours}$$

7. Nitroglycerin is prepared by the pharmacy as a standard solution of 50 mg in 250 mL/24 hours. We only need to calculate milliliters per hour.

$$\frac{250 \text{ mL}}{24 \text{ hours}} \quad \begin{array}{r} 10.4 \\ 24\overline{\smash{)}250.0} \\ \underline{24} \\ 10\,0 \\ \underline{9\,6} \end{array}$$

Set the pump at 10 mL/hour.

(continued)

Answers (Continued)

8. a.

Formula Method	Proportion	Dimensional Analysis
$$\dfrac{\overset{1}{\cancel{1200\ units}}}{\underset{5}{\cancel{25,000\ units}}} \times \overset{}{\cancel{500}}\ mL$$ $$= 24\ mL/hour$$	**EXPRESSED AS TWO RATIOS** 500 mL : 25,000 units : : x mL : 1200 units **EXPRESSED AS TWO FRACTIONS** $$\dfrac{500\ mL}{25,000\ units} \bowtie \dfrac{x\ mL}{1200\ units}$$ **SOLUTION FOR BOTH PROPORTION METHODS** $1200 \times 500 = 25,000x$ $$\dfrac{600,000}{25,000} = x$$ $24\ mL/hour = x$	$$\dfrac{\overset{1}{\cancel{500}}\ \textcircled{mL}}{\underset{50}{\cancel{25,000\ units}}}\ \Bigg|\ \dfrac{1200\ \cancel{units}}{\textcircled{hours}} = \dfrac{1200}{50}$$ $$= 24\ mL/hour$$

b. $\dfrac{500\ mL}{24\ mL/hour} = 20.8$ or approximately 21 hours

9. a.

Formula Method	Proportion	Dimensional Analysis
$$\dfrac{23\ units/hour}{\cancel{250}\ \cancel{units}} \times \cancel{250}\ mL$$ $$= 23\ mL/hour$$	**EXPRESSED AS TWO RATIOS** 250 mL : 250 units : : x mL : 23 units **EXPRESSED AS TWO FRACTIONS** $$\dfrac{250\ mL}{250\ units} \bowtie \dfrac{x\ mL}{23\ units}$$ **SOLUTION FOR BOTH PROPORTION METHODS** $250 \times 23 = 250x$ $$\dfrac{5750}{250} = x$$ $23\ mL/hour = x$	$$\dfrac{\overset{1}{\cancel{250}}\ \textcircled{mL}}{\underset{1}{\cancel{250}\ \cancel{units}}}\ \Bigg|\ \dfrac{23\ \cancel{units}}{\textcircled{hours}} = 23\ mL/hour$$

b. $\dfrac{250\ mL}{23\ mL/hour} = 10.8$ (10 hours 48 minutes) or approximately 11 hours

10.

Formula Method	Proportion	Dimensional Analysis
$\dfrac{100,000 \text{ units}}{750,000 \text{ units}} \times 250 \text{ mL}$ $= 33 \text{ mL/hour}$	**EXPRESSED AS TWO RATIOS** 250 mL : 750,000 units : : x mL : 100,000 units **EXPRESSED AS TWO FRACTIONS** $\dfrac{250 \text{ mL}}{750,000 \text{ units}} \times \dfrac{x \text{ mL}}{100,000 \text{ units}}$ **SOLUTION FOR BOTH PROPORTION METHODS** $100,000 \times 250 = 750,000x$ $\dfrac{100,000 \times 250}{750,000} = x$ $33 \text{ mL/hour} = x$	$\dfrac{250 \text{ mL}}{750,000 \text{ units}} \left\lvert \dfrac{100,000 \text{ units}}{\text{hour}} \right. = \dfrac{2500}{75}$ $= 33 \text{ mL/hours}$

Self-Test 2 Infusion Rates for Drugs Ordered in mg/minute

1. a. Order: 1 mg/minute = 60 mg/hour (1 mg/minute × 60 minutes)

Solution: 2 g in 250 mL

2 g = 2000 mg

Formula Method	Proportion	Dimensional Analysis
$\dfrac{60 \text{ mg/hour}}{\underset{8}{2000 \text{ mg}}} \times \overset{1}{250} \text{ mL}$ $= 7.5 \text{ mL/hour or } 8 \text{ mL/hour}$	**EXPRESSED AS TWO RATIOS** 250 mL : 2000 mg : : x mL : 60 mg **EXPRESSED AS TWO FRACTIONS** $\dfrac{250 \text{ mL}}{2000 \text{ mg}} \times \dfrac{x \text{ mL}}{60 \text{ mg}}$ **SOLUTION FOR BOTH PROPORTION METHODS** $250 \times 60 = 2000x$ $\dfrac{75,000}{2000} = x$ $7.5 \text{ mL/hour} = x$	Use conversion factors: 60 minutes/1 hour 1 g/1000 mg $\dfrac{\overset{1}{250} \text{ mL}}{2 \text{ g}} \left\lvert \dfrac{1 \text{ mg}}{\text{minute}} \right\lvert \dfrac{\overset{15}{60} \text{ minutes}}{1 \text{ hour}} \left\lvert \dfrac{1 \text{ g}}{\underset{\underset{1}{4}}{1000} \text{ mg}} \right.$ $= \dfrac{15}{2} = 7.5 \text{ or } 8 \text{ mL/hour}$

Set the pump at 8 mL/hour.

b. $\dfrac{250 \text{ mL}}{8 \text{ mL/hour}} = 31.25$ (31 hours 15 minutes) or approximately 31 hours; hospital policy requires that IV bags be changed every 24 hours

(continued)

Answers (Continued)

2. a. Order: 2 mg/minute = 120 mg/hour (2 mg/minute × 60 minutes)

Solution: 300 mg in 300 mL D5W

Formula Method	Proportion	Dimensional Analysis
$\dfrac{120 \text{ mg /hour}}{300 \text{ mg}} \times 300 \text{ mL}$ $= 120$ mL/hour	**EXPRESSED AS TWO RATIOS** 300 mL : 300 mg : : x mL : 120 mg **EXPRESSED AS TWO FRACTIONS** $\dfrac{300 \text{ mL}}{300 \text{ mg}} \times \dfrac{x \text{ mL}}{120 \text{ mg}}$ **SOLUTION FOR BOTH PROPORTION METHODS** $300 \times 120 = 300x$ $\dfrac{36{,}000}{300} = x$ 120 mL/hour = x	Use conversion factor 60 minutes/1 hour: $\dfrac{300 \text{ mL}}{300 \text{ mg}} \cdot \dfrac{2 \text{ mg}}{\text{minutes}} \cdot \dfrac{60 \text{ minutes}}{1 \text{ hours}} = 2 \times 60$ $= 120$ mL/hour

b. 300 mL/120 mL/hour = 2.5 or $2\frac{1}{2}$ hours

3. a. Order: 2 mg/minute = 120 mg/hour (2 mg/minute × 60 minutes)

Solution: 1 g in 500 mL

1 g = 1000 mg

Formula Method	Proportion	Dimensional Analysis
$\dfrac{120 \text{ mg /hour}}{1000 \text{ mg}} \times 500 \text{ mL}$ $= 60$ mL/hour	**EXPRESSED AS TWO RATIOS** 500 mL : 1000 mg : : x mL : 120 mg **EXPRESSED AS TWO FRACTIONS** $\dfrac{500 \text{ mL}}{1000 \text{ mg}} \times \dfrac{x \text{ mL}}{120 \text{ mg}}$ **SOLUTION FOR BOTH PROPORTION METHODS** $500 \times 120 = 1000x$ $\dfrac{60{,}000}{1000} = x$ 60 mL/hour = x	Use conversion factors: 60 minutes/1 hour 1 g/1000 mg $\dfrac{500 \text{ mL}}{1 \text{ g}} \cdot \dfrac{2 \text{ mg}}{\text{minutes}} \cdot \dfrac{60 \text{ minutes}}{1 \text{ hour}} \cdot \dfrac{1 \text{ g}}{1000 \text{ mg}}$ $= 60$ mL/hour

Set the pump at 60 mL/hour.

b. $\dfrac{500 \text{ mL}}{60 \text{ mL/hour}} = 8.3$ or approximately 8 hours 18 minutes

4. Order: 1 mg/minute = 60 mg/hour (1 mg/minute × 60 minutes)

Solution: 450 mg in 250 mL

Formula Method	Proportion	Dimensional Analysis
$\dfrac{\cancel{60}\text{ mg /hour}}{\cancel{450}\text{ mg}}\times \overset{5}{\cancel{250}}\text{ mL}$ $= 33.33 \text{ or } 33 \text{ mL/hour}$	**EXPRESSED AS TWO RATIOS** 250 mL : 450 mg : : x mL : 60 mg **EXPRESSED AS TWO FRACTIONS** $\dfrac{250 \text{ mL}}{450 \text{ mg}} \times \dfrac{\text{x mL}}{60 \text{ mg}}$ **SOLUTION FOR BOTH PROPORTION METHODS** $250 \times 60 = 450\text{x}$ $\dfrac{15{,}000}{450} = \text{x}$ 33.33 mL/hour = x	Use conversion factor 60 minutes/1 hour: $\dfrac{\overset{5}{\cancel{250}}\ \cancel{\text{mL}}}{\underset{9}{\cancel{450}}\ \cancel{\text{mg}}}\ \bigg|\ \dfrac{1\ \cancel{\text{mg}}}{\cancel{\text{minute}}}\ \bigg|\ \dfrac{60\ \cancel{\text{minutes}}}{1\ \cancel{\text{hour}}} = \dfrac{5 \times 60}{9}$ $= 33.33 \text{ or } 33 \text{ mL/hour}$

Set the pump at 33 mL/hour. Run for 6 hours.

5. a. Order: 1 mg/minute = 60 mg/hour (1 mg/minute × 60 minutes)

Solution: 80 mg in 250 mL

Formula Method	Proportion	Dimensional Analysis
$\dfrac{\cancel{60}\text{ mg /hour}}{\cancel{80}\text{ mg}}\times 250 \text{ mL}$ $= \dfrac{1500}{8}$ $= 187.5 \text{ or } 188 \text{ mL/hour}$	**EXPRESSED AS TWO RATIOS** 250 mL : 80 mg : : x mL : 60 mg **EXPRESSED AS TWO FRACTIONS** $\dfrac{250 \text{ mL}}{80 \text{ mg}} \times \dfrac{\text{x mL}}{60 \text{ mg}}$ **SOLUTION FOR BOTH PROPORTION METHODS** $250 \times 60 = 80\text{x}$ $\dfrac{15{,}000}{80} = \text{x}$ 187.5 or 188 mL/hour = x	Use conversion factor 60 minutes/1 hour: $\dfrac{250\ \cancel{\text{mL}}}{\underset{10}{\cancel{80}}\ \cancel{\text{mg}}}\ \bigg|\ \dfrac{1\ \cancel{\text{mg}}}{\cancel{\text{minutes}}}\ \bigg|\ \dfrac{\overset{30}{\cancel{60}}\ \cancel{\text{minutes}}}{1\ \cancel{\text{hour}}} = \dfrac{250 \times 3}{4}$ $= 187.5 \text{ or } 188 \text{ mL/hour}$

b. $\dfrac{250 \text{ mL}}{188 \text{ mL/hour}} = 1.33 \text{ hours or } 1 \text{ hour } 20 \text{ minutes}$

(continued)

Answers (Continued)

Self-Test 3 Infusion Rates for Drugs Ordered in mcg/minute, mcg/kg/minute, and milliunits/minute

1. Order: 800 mcg/minute

Standard solution: 800 mg in 250 mL D5W

Step 1. $\dfrac{800 \text{ mg}}{250 \text{ mL}} = 3.2 \text{ mg/mL}$

Step 2. $3.2 \text{ mg} = 3200 \text{ mcg/mL}$

Step 3. $\dfrac{3200}{60} = 53.33 \text{ mcg/minute}$

Step 4. Solve for milliliters per hour:

Formula Method	Proportion	Dimensional Analysis
$\dfrac{800 \text{ mcg/minute}}{53.33 \text{ mcg/minute}} \times 1 \text{ mL}$ $= 15 \text{ mL/hour}$	**EXPRESSED AS TWO RATIOS** $1 \text{ mL} : 53.33 \text{ mcg/minute} :: x \text{ mL} : 800 \text{ mcg/minute}$ **EXPRESSED AS TWO FRACTIONS** $\dfrac{1 \text{ mL}}{53.33} \diagdown \dfrac{x \text{ mL}}{800 \text{ mcg/minute}}$ **SOLUTION FOR BOTH PROPORTION METHODS** $800 = 53.33x$ $\dfrac{800}{53.33} = x$ $15 \text{ mL/hour} = x$	Use conversion factors: 1 mg/1000 mg 60 minutes/1 hour 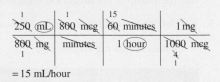 $= 15 \text{ mL/hour}$

Set the pump: total number of milliliters = 250 (standard solution); milliliters per hour = 15.

2. Order: 12 mcg/minute

Standard solution: 4 mg in 250 mL D5W

Step 1. $\dfrac{4 \text{ mg}}{250 \text{ mL}} = 0.016 \text{ mg/mL}$

Step 2. $0.016 \text{ mg} = 16 \text{ mcg/mL}$

Step 3. $\dfrac{16 \text{ mcg}}{60 \text{ minute}} = 0.27 \text{ mcg/minute}$

Step 4. Solve for milliliters per hour:

Formula Method	Proportion	Dimensional Analysis

Formula Method

$$\frac{12 \text{ mcg/minute}}{0.27 \text{ mcg/minute}} \times 1 \text{ mL}$$

$$= 44 \text{ mL/hour}$$

Proportion

EXPRESSED AS TWO RATIOS

1 mL : 0.27 mcg/minute : : x mL : 12 mcg/minute

EXPRESSED AS TWO FRACTIONS

$$\frac{1 \text{ mL}}{0.27} \diagdown \frac{x \text{ mL}}{12 \text{ mcg/minute}}$$

SOLUTION FOR BOTH PROPORTION METHODS

$$12 = 0.27x$$

$$\frac{12}{0.27} = x$$

$$44 \text{ mL/hour} = x$$

Dimensional Analysis

Use conversion factors:
60 minutes/1 hour
1 mg/1000 mcg

$$\frac{\overset{1}{250} \text{ mL}}{4 \text{ mg}} \,\bigg|\, \frac{12 \text{ mcg}}{\text{minutes}} \,\bigg|\, \frac{60 \text{ minutes}}{1 \text{ hour}} \,\bigg|\, \frac{1 \text{ mg}}{\underset{4}{1000} \text{ mcg}}$$

$$= \frac{720}{16} = 45 \text{ mL/hour}$$

(*Note:* Notice the difference in answers. If using a calculator, do not round until the final answer.)

Set the pump: total number of milliliters = 250; milliliters per hour = 44 or 45 (see note above).

3. Order: 5 mcg/kg/minute

Weight: 220 lb

Standard solution: 1 g in 250 mL

Convert pounds to kilograms.

$$\frac{220 \text{ lb}}{2.2 \text{ kg}} \,\bigg)\, \frac{100.0}{220.0} = 100 \text{ kg}$$

To obtain the order in micrograms, multiply 100 kg × 5 mcg/kg/minute:

100 kg
× 5 mcg/kg/minute
500 mcg/minute (order)

Step 1. 1 g = 1000 mg

$$\frac{1000 \text{ mg}}{250 \text{ mL}} = 4 \text{ mg/mL}$$

Step 2. 4 mg = 4000 mcg/mL

Step 3. $\dfrac{4000}{60} = 66.67 \text{ mcg/minute}$

(continued)

Answers (Continued)

Step 4. Solve for milliliters per hour:

Formula Method	Proportion	Dimensional Analysis
$\dfrac{500\text{ mcg/minute}}{66.67\text{ mcg/minute}} \times 1\text{ mL}$ $= 7.49 \text{ or } 8 \text{ mL/hour}$	**EXPRESSED AS TWO RATIOS** 1 mL : 66.67 mcg/minute : : x mL : 500 mcg/minute **EXPRESSED AS TWO FRACTIONS** $\dfrac{1\text{ mL}}{66.67} \times \dfrac{x\text{ mL}}{500\text{ mcg/minute}}$ **SOLUTION FOR BOTH PROPORTION METHODS** $500 = 66.67x$ $\dfrac{500}{66.67} = x$ $7.5 \text{ or } 8 = x$	Use conversion factors: 60 minutes/1 hour 1 g/1000 mg 1 mg/1000 mcg 1 kg/2.2 lb

Dimensional Analysis calculation:

$$\dfrac{1}{250}\ \dfrac{\text{mL}}{1\ \text{g}} \left| \dfrac{1}{5}\ \dfrac{\text{mcg}}{\text{kg/minute}} \right| \dfrac{60\ \text{minutes}}{1\ \text{hour}} \left| \dfrac{1\ \text{g}}{1000\ \text{mg}} \right|_{4} \dfrac{1\ \text{mg}}{1000\ \text{mcg}}_{2}^{200} \left| \dfrac{1}{220}\ \dfrac{\text{lb}}{2.2\ \text{lb}} \right|_{1} \dfrac{1\ \text{kg}}{}$$

$$= \dfrac{60}{4 \times 2} = \dfrac{60}{8} = 7.5 \text{ or } 8 \text{ mL/hour}$$

Set the pump: total number of milliliters = 250 (standard solution); milliliters per hour = 7.5 or 8.

4. Order: 7 mcg/kg/minute

Standard solution: 500 mg in 250 mL D5W

Patient/client's weight: 70 kg

The patient/client weighs
$$\begin{array}{r} 70\text{ kg} \\ \times\,7\text{ mcg/kg/minute} \\ \hline 490\text{ mcg/minute} \end{array}$$

Step 1. $\dfrac{500\text{ mg}}{250\text{ mL}} = 2\text{ mg/mL}$

Step 2. $2 \times 1000 = 2000\text{ mcg/mL}$

Step 3. $\dfrac{2000}{60} = 33.33\text{ mcg/min}$

Step 4. Solve for milliliters per hour:

Formula Method	Proportion	Dimensional Analysis
$\dfrac{490\text{ mcg/minute}}{33.33\text{ mcg/mL/minute}} \times 1\text{ mL} = x$ $x = 14.7 \text{ or } 15 \text{ mL/hour}$	**EXPRESSED AS TWO RATIOS** 1 mL : 33.33 mcg/minute : : x mL : 490 mcg/minute **EXPRESSED AS TWO FRACTIONS** $\dfrac{1\text{ mL}}{33.33} \times \dfrac{x\text{ mL}}{490\text{ mcg/minute}}$ **SOLUTION FOR BOTH PROPORTION METHODS** $490 = 33.33x$ $\dfrac{490}{33.33} = x$ $14.7 \text{ or } 15 \text{ mL/hour} = x$	Use conversion factors: 1 mg/1000 mcg 60 minutes/1 hour

Dimensional Analysis calculation:

$$\dfrac{1}{250}\ \dfrac{\text{mL}}{500\ \text{mg}} \left| \dfrac{7\ \text{mcg}}{\text{kg/minute}} \right| \dfrac{60\ \text{minutes}}{1\ \text{hour}} \left| \dfrac{1\ \text{mg}}{1000\ \text{mcg}}_{4} \right| \dfrac{70\ \text{kg}}{}$$

$$= \dfrac{7 \times 6 \times 7}{20} = \dfrac{294}{20} = 14.7 \text{ or } 15 \text{ mL/hour}$$

Set the pump: total number of milliliters = 250 (standard solution); milliliters per hour = 15.

5. Order: 10 mcg/minute

Standard solution: 50 mg in 250 mL

Step 1. $\dfrac{50 \text{ mg}}{250 \text{ mL}} = 0.2 \text{ mg/mL}$

Step 2. $0.2 \times 1000 = 200 \text{ mcg/mL}$

Step 3. $\dfrac{200 \text{ mcg}}{60 \text{ mL}} = 3.33 \text{ mcg/minute}$

Step 4. Solve for milliliters per hour:

Formula Method	Proportion	Dimensional Analysis

Formula Method

$\dfrac{10 \text{ mcg /minute}}{3.33 \text{ mcg /minute}} \times 1 \text{ mL} = x$

$x = 3 \text{ mL/hour}$

Proportion

EXPRESSED AS TWO RATIOS

$1 \text{ mL} : 3.33 \text{ mcg/minute} :: x \text{ mL} : 10 \text{ mcg/minute}$

EXPRESSED AS TWO FRACTIONS

$\dfrac{1 \text{ mL}}{3.33} \times \dfrac{x \text{ mL}}{10 \text{ mcg/minute}}$

SOLUTION FOR BOTH PROPORTION METHODS

$10 = 3.33x$

$\dfrac{10}{3.33} = 3.33$

$3 \text{ mL/hour} = x$

Dimensional Analysis

Use conversion factors:
1 mg/1000 mcg
60 minutes/1 hour

$$\dfrac{\overset{1}{250} \text{ mL}}{\underset{5}{50} \text{ mg}} \bigg| \dfrac{\overset{1}{10} \text{ mcg}}{\text{minutes}} \bigg| \dfrac{60 \text{ minutes}}{1 \text{ hour}} \bigg| \dfrac{1 \text{ mg}}{\underset{4}{1000} \text{ mcg}}$$

$$= \dfrac{60}{5 \times 4} = \dfrac{60}{20} = 3 \text{ mL/hour}$$

Set the pump: total number of milliliters = 250; milliliters per hour = 3.

6. Order: 1 milliunit/minute

Standard solution: 15 units in 250 mL NS

Step 1. $\dfrac{15 \text{ units}}{250 \text{ mL}} = 0.06 \text{ units/mL}$

Step 2. 1 unit = 1000 milliunits

0.06 units = 60 milliunits

Step 3. $\dfrac{60}{60} = 1 \text{ milliunit/minute}$

(continued)

Answers (Continued)

Step 4. Solve for milliliters per hour:

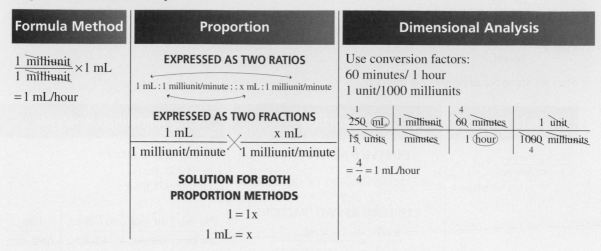

Formula Method	Proportion	Dimensional Analysis

Formula Method

$$\frac{1 \text{ milliunit}}{1 \text{ milliunit}} \times 1 \text{ mL}$$

$$= 1 \text{ mL/hour}$$

Proportion

EXPRESSED AS TWO RATIOS

1 mL : 1 milliunit/minute : : x mL : 1 milliunit/minute

EXPRESSED AS TWO FRACTIONS

$$\frac{1 \text{ mL}}{1 \text{ milliunit/minute}} \times \frac{x \text{ mL}}{1 \text{ milliunit/minute}}$$

SOLUTION FOR BOTH PROPORTION METHODS

$$1 = 1x$$
$$1 \text{ mL} = x$$

Dimensional Analysis

Use conversion factors:
60 minutes/ 1 hour
1 unit/1000 milliunits

$$\frac{250 \text{ mL}}{15 \text{ units}} \Big| \frac{1 \text{ milliunit}}{\text{minute}} \Big| \frac{60 \text{ minutes}}{1 \text{ hour}} \Big| \frac{1 \text{ unit}}{1000 \text{ milliunits}}$$

$$= \frac{4}{4} = 1 \text{ mL/hour}$$

Set the pump: total number of milliliters = 250; milliliters per hour = 1.

7. Order: 4 mcg/minute

Solution: 2 mg in 250 mL

Step 1. $\dfrac{2 \text{ mg}}{250 \text{ mL}} = 0.008 \text{ mg/mL}$

Step 2. $0.008 \times 1000 = 8 \text{ mcg/mL}$

Step 3. $\dfrac{8 \text{ mcg}}{60 \text{ mL}} = 0.133 \text{ mcg/minute}$

Step 4. Solve for milliliters per hour:

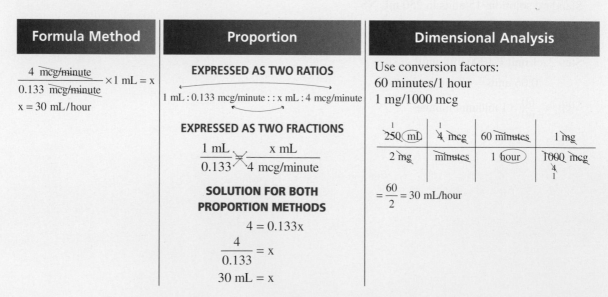

Formula Method	Proportion	Dimensional Analysis

Formula Method

$$\frac{4 \text{ mcg/minute}}{0.133 \text{ mcg/minute}} \times 1 \text{ mL} = x$$

$$x = 30 \text{ mL/hour}$$

Proportion

EXPRESSED AS TWO RATIOS

1 mL : 0.133 mcg/minute : : x mL : 4 mcg/minute

EXPRESSED AS TWO FRACTIONS

$$\frac{1 \text{ mL}}{0.133} \times \frac{x \text{ mL}}{4 \text{ mcg/minute}}$$

SOLUTION FOR BOTH PROPORTION METHODS

$$4 = 0.133x$$
$$\frac{4}{0.133} = x$$
$$30 \text{ mL} = x$$

Dimensional Analysis

Use conversion factors:
60 minutes/1 hour
1 mg/1000 mcg

$$\frac{250 \text{ mL}}{2 \text{ mg}} \Big| \frac{4 \text{ mcg}}{\text{minute}} \Big| \frac{60 \text{ minutes}}{1 \text{ hour}} \Big| \frac{1 \text{ mg}}{1000 \text{ mcg}}$$

$$= \frac{60}{2} = 30 \text{ mL/hour}$$

Set the pump: total number of milliliters = 250; milliliters per hour = 30.

8. Order: 50 mcg/kg/minute

   Solution: 2.5 g in 250 mL

   Weight: 58 kg

   58 kg × 50 mcg = 2900 mcg (order)

   Step 1. 2.5 g = 2500 mg

   $$\frac{2500 \text{ mg}}{250 \text{ mL}} = 10 \text{ mg/mL}$$

   Step 2. 10 × 1000 = 10,000 mcg/mL

   Step 3. $\dfrac{10,000}{60} = 166.67$ mcg/minute

   Step 4. Solve for milliliters per hour:

Formula Method	Proportion	Dimensional Analysis
$\dfrac{2900 \text{ mcg/minute}}{166.67 \text{ mcg/minute}} \times 1 \text{ mL}$ $= 17 \text{ mL/hour}$	**EXPRESSED AS TWO RATIOS** 1 mL : 166.67 mcg/minute : : x mL : 2900 mcg/minute **EXPRESSED AS TWO FRACTIONS** $\dfrac{1 \text{ mL}}{166.67} \diagup \dfrac{x \text{ mL}}{2900 \text{ mcg/minute}}$ **SOLUTION FOR BOTH PROPORTION METHODS** $2900 = 166.67x$ $\dfrac{2900}{166.67} = x$ $17 \text{ mL} = x$	Use conversion factors: 60 minutes/1 hour 1 g/1000 mg 1 mg/1000 mcg 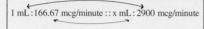 $= \dfrac{58 \times 60}{2.5 \times 4 \times 20} = \dfrac{3480}{200} = 17.4$ or 17 mL/hour

   Set the pump: total number of milliliters = 250; milliliters per hour = 17.

9. Order: 2 mcg/kg/minute

   Solution: 50 mg in 250 mL

   Weight: 80 kg

   80 kg × 2 mcg = 160 mcg (order)

   Step 1. $\dfrac{50 \text{ mg}}{250 \text{ mL}} = 0.2 \text{ mg/mL}$

   Step 2. 0.2 mg = 200 mcg

   0.2 = 200 mcg/mL

   Step 3. $\dfrac{200 \text{ mg}}{60 \text{ mL}} = 3.33$ mcg/minute

(continued)

Answers (Continued)

Step 4. Solve for milliliters per hour:

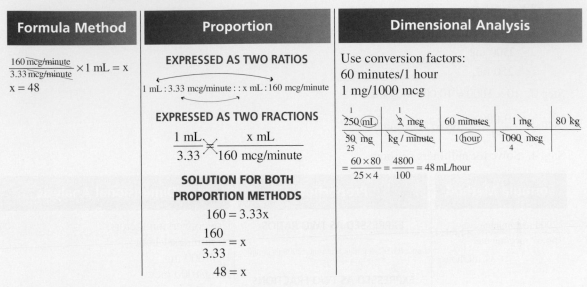

Formula Method	Proportion	Dimensional Analysis
$\dfrac{160 \overline{\text{mcg/minute}}}{3.33 \overline{\text{mcg/minute}}} \times 1 \text{ mL} = x$ $x = 48$	**EXPRESSED AS TWO RATIOS** 1 mL : 3.33 mcg/minute :: x mL : 160 mcg/minute **EXPRESSED AS TWO FRACTIONS** $\dfrac{1 \text{ mL}}{3.33} \diagup \dfrac{x \text{ mL}}{160 \text{ mcg/minute}}$ **SOLUTION FOR BOTH PROPORTION METHODS** $160 = 3.33x$ $\dfrac{160}{3.33} = x$ $48 = x$	Use conversion factors: 60 minutes/1 hour 1 mg/1000 mcg $\dfrac{250 \text{ mL}}{50 \text{ mg}} \cdot \dfrac{\overset{1}{2} \text{ mcg}}{\text{kg / minute}} \cdot \dfrac{60 \text{ minutes}}{1 \text{ hour}} \cdot \dfrac{1 \text{ mg}}{1000 \text{ mcg}} \cdot \dfrac{80 \text{ kg}}{}$ $= \dfrac{60 \times 80}{25 \times 4} = \dfrac{4800}{100} = 48 \text{ mL/hour}$

Set the pump: total number of milliliters = 250; milliliters per hour = 48.

10. Order: 200 mcg/minute

Solution: 0.1 g in 100 mL

$\qquad$ 0.1 g = 100 mg

Step 1. $\dfrac{100 \text{ mg}}{100 \text{ mL}} = 1 \text{ mg/mL}$

Step 2. 1 mg = 1000 mcg

$\qquad$ 1000 mcg/1 mL

Step 3. $\dfrac{1000 \text{ mg}}{60} = 16.67 \text{ mcg/minute}$

Step 4. Solve for milliliters per hour:

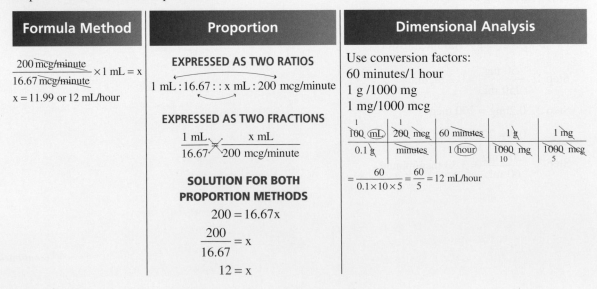

Formula Method	Proportion	Dimensional Analysis
$\dfrac{200 \overline{\text{mcg/minute}}}{16.67 \overline{\text{mcg/minute}}} \times 1 \text{ mL} = x$ $x = 11.99 \text{ or } 12 \text{ mL/hour}$	**EXPRESSED AS TWO RATIOS** 1 mL : 16.67 :: x mL : 200 mcg/minute **EXPRESSED AS TWO FRACTIONS** $\dfrac{1 \text{ mL}}{16.67} \diagup \dfrac{x \text{ mL}}{200 \text{ mcg/minute}}$ **SOLUTION FOR BOTH PROPORTION METHODS** $200 = 16.67x$ $\dfrac{200}{16.67} = x$ $12 = x$	Use conversion factors: 60 minutes/1 hour 1 g /1000 mg 1 mg/1000 mcg $\dfrac{100 \text{ mL}}{0.1 \text{ g}} \cdot \dfrac{200 \text{ mcg}}{\text{minutes}} \cdot \dfrac{60 \text{ minutes}}{1 \text{ hour}} \cdot \dfrac{1 \text{ g}}{1000 \text{ mg}} \cdot \dfrac{1 \text{ mg}}{1000 \text{ mcg}}$ $= \dfrac{60}{0.1 \times 10 \times 5} = \dfrac{60}{5} = 12 \text{ mL/hour}$

Set the pump: total number of milliliters = 100; milliliters per hour = 12.

Self-Test 4 Use of Nomogram

1. **a.** Dose is correct; $20 \text{ mg/m}^2 \times 1.96 = 39$ mg

    b. Order calls for 250 mL over ½ hour, but pump is set in milliliters per hour. Double 250 mL.

    Setting: total number of milliliters = 250; milliliters per hour = 500.

    The pump will deliver 250 mL in ½ hour.

2. **a.** Correct; $130 \text{ mg/m}^2 \times 1.77 = 230$ mg

    b. Two 100-mg tabs and three 10-mg tabs.

3. **a.** Correct; $40 \text{ mg/m}^2 \times 2 = 80$ mg

    b. Rapidly flowing IV is the primary line. Set the secondary pump: total number of milliliters = 80; milliliters per hour = 80 (see Chapter 6 for IVPB).

4. **a.** Correct; $200 \text{ mg/m}^2 \times 2 = 400$ mg

Formula Method	Proportion	Dimensional Analysis
$\dfrac{\overset{8}{\cancel{400}} \text{ mg}}{\cancel{50} \text{ mg}} \times 1 \text{ capsule}$ $= 8 \text{ capsules}$	**EXPRESSED AS TWO RATIOS** 1 capsule : 50 mg : : x capsules : 400 mg **EXPRESSED AS TWO FRACTIONS** $\dfrac{1 \text{ capsule}}{50 \text{ mg}} \bowtie \dfrac{x \text{ capsule}}{400 \text{ mg}}$ **SOLUTION FOR BOTH PROPORTION METHODS** $400 = 50x$ $\dfrac{400}{50} = x$ $8 \text{ capsules} = x$	$\dfrac{1 \text{ capsule}}{50 \text{ mg}} \Bigm| \dfrac{400 \text{ mg}}{} = \dfrac{400}{50} = 8 \text{ capsules}$

    b. Administer 8 capsules

5. **a.** Correct; $135 \text{ mg/m}^2 \times 1.6 = 216$ mg

    b. 500 mL over 3 hours; $3 \overline{)\smash{\dfrac{166.6}{500}}} = 167$

    Set the pump: total number of milliliters = 500; milliliters per hour = 167.

Self-Test 5 Heparin Protocol Calculations

1. **a.** Bolus with 40 units/kg:
    $40 \times 70 = 2800$ units

(continued)

Answers (Continued)

b. Increase rate by 2 units/kg/hour:
$2 \times 70 = 140$ units

Formula Method	Proportion	Dimensional Analysis
$\dfrac{140 \text{ units}}{25,000 \text{ units}} \times 500 \text{ mL} = x$ $x = 2.8$ mL	**EXPRESSED AS TWO RATIOS** 500 mL : 25,000 units : : x mL : 140 units **EXPRESSED AS TWO FRACTIONS** $\dfrac{500 \text{ mL}}{25,000 \text{ units}} \times \dfrac{x \text{ mL}}{140 \text{ units}}$ **SOLUTION FOR BOTH PROPORTION METHODS** $500 \times 140 = 25,000x$ $\dfrac{500 \times 140}{25,000} = x$ $2.8 \text{ mL} = x$	$\dfrac{\overset{1}{\cancel{500}} \text{ } \cancel{\text{mL}}}{\underset{50}{\cancel{25,000}} \text{ } \cancel{\text{units}}} \left| \dfrac{2 \text{ units}}{\cancel{\text{kg}} / \cancel{\text{hour}}} \right| \dfrac{70 \text{ } \cancel{\text{kg}}}{} = \dfrac{2 \times 70}{50}$ $= 2.8 \text{ mL}$

Increase rate by 2.8 mL:

$25.2 + 2.8 = 28$ mL/hour

2. a. Bolus with 40 units/kg:
$40 \times 70 = 2800$ units

b. Increase rate by 3 units/kg/hour:
$3 \times 70 = 210$ units

Formula Method	Proportion	Dimensional Analysis
$\dfrac{210 \text{ units}}{25,000 \text{ units}} \times 500 \text{ mL} = x$ $x = 4.2$ mL	**EXPRESSED AS TWO RATIOS** 500 mL : 25,000 units : : x mL : 210 units **EXPRESSED AS TWO FRACTIONS** $\dfrac{500 \text{ mL}}{25,000 \text{ units}} \times \dfrac{x \text{ mL}}{210 \text{ units}}$ **SOLUTION FOR BOTH PROPORTION METHODS** $500 \times 210 = 25,000x$ $\dfrac{500 \times 210}{25,000} = x$ $4.2 \text{ mL} = x$	$\dfrac{\overset{1}{\cancel{500}} \text{ } \cancel{\text{mL}}}{\underset{50}{\cancel{25,000}} \text{ } \cancel{\text{units}}} \left| \dfrac{3 \text{ units}}{\cancel{\text{kg}} / \cancel{\text{hour}}} \right| \dfrac{70 \text{ } \cancel{\text{kg}}}{} = \dfrac{3 \times 70}{50}$ $= 4.2 \text{ mL/hour}$

Increase rate by 4.2 mL:

$25.2 + 4.2 = 29.4$ mL/hour

3. **a.** No bolus
   b. Decrease rate by 1 unit/kg/hour:
   $1 \times 70 = 70$ units

Formula Method	Proportion	Dimensional Analysis

Formula Method

$$\frac{70 \text{ units}}{25,000 \text{ units}} \times 500 \text{ mL} = x$$

$$x = 1.4 \text{ mL}$$

Proportion

EXPRESSED AS TWO RATIOS

500 mL : 25,000 units : : x mL : 70 units

EXPRESSED AS TWO FRACTIONS

$$\frac{500 \text{ mL}}{25,000 \text{ units}} \times \frac{x \text{ mL}}{70 \text{ units}}$$

SOLUTION FOR BOTH PROPORTION METHODS

$$70 \times 500 = 25,000x$$

$$\frac{70 \times 500}{25,000} = x$$

$$1.4 \text{ mL} = x$$

Dimensional Analysis

$$\frac{\overset{1}{\cancel{500}} \text{ mL}}{\underset{50}{\cancel{25,000}} \text{ units}} \mid \frac{1 \text{ unit}}{\text{kg /hour}} \mid \frac{70 \text{ kg}}{} = \frac{70}{50}$$

$$= 1.4 \text{ mL}$$

Decrease drip by 1.4 mL:

$25.2 - 1.4 = 23.8$ mL/hour

4. **a.** No bolus
   b. Stop infusion for 1 hour;
   decrease rate by 2 units/kg/hour:
   $2 \times 70 = 140$ units

Formula Method	Proportion	Dimensional Analysis

Formula Method

$$\frac{140 \text{ units}}{25,000 \text{ units}} \times 500 \text{ mL} = x$$

$$x = 2.8 \text{ mL}$$

Proportion

EXPRESSED AS TWO RATIOS

500 mL : 25,000 units : : x mL : 140 units

EXPRESSED AS TWO FRACTIONS

$$\frac{500 \text{ mL}}{25,000 \text{ units}} \times \frac{x \text{ mL}}{140 \text{ units}}$$

SOLUTION FOR BOTH PROPORTION METHODS

$$500 \times 140 = 25,000x$$

$$\frac{500 \times 140}{25,000} = x$$

$$2.8 \text{ mL} = x$$

Dimensional Analysis

$$\frac{\overset{1}{\cancel{500}} \text{ mL}}{\underset{50}{\cancel{25,000}} \text{ units}} \mid \frac{2 \text{ units}}{\text{kg /hour}} \mid \frac{70 \text{ kg}}{} = \frac{2 \times 70}{50}$$

$$= 2.8 \text{ mL}$$

Decrease rate by 2.8 mL:

$25.2 - 2.8 = 22.4$ mL/hour

(continued)

Answers (Continued)

Self-Test 6 Insulin Protocol Calculations

1. a. $(300 - 60) \times 0.02 = 4.8$ units

Formula Method	Proportion	Dimensional Analysis
$\dfrac{4.8 \text{ units}}{100 \text{ units}} \times 100 \text{ mL} = x$ $x = 4.8 \text{ mL/hour}$	**EXPRESSED AS TWO RATIOS** 100 units : 100 mL : : x mL : 4.8 units **EXPRESSED AS TWO FRACTIONS** $\dfrac{100 \text{ mL}}{100 \text{ units}} \times \dfrac{x \text{ mL}}{4.8 \text{ units}}$ **SOLUTION FOR BOTH PROPORTION METHODS** $4.8 \times 100 = 100x$ $\dfrac{4.8 \times 100}{100} = x$ $4.8 \text{ mL/hour} = x$	$\dfrac{\cancel{100}^{1} \text{ mL}}{\cancel{100}_{1} \text{ units}} \left| \dfrac{4.8 \text{ units}}{\text{hours}} = 4.8 \text{ mL/hour} \right.$

b. Yes; $(BG - 60) \times 0.03$

2. a. $(350 - 60) \times 0.03 = 8.7$ units

Formula Method	Proportion	Dimensional Analysis
$\dfrac{8.7 \text{ units}}{100 \text{ units}} \times 100 \text{ mL} = x$ $x = 8.7 \text{ mL}$	**EXPRESSED AS TWO RATIOS** 100 units : 100 mL : : x mL : 8.7 units **EXPRESSED AS TWO FRACTIONS** $\dfrac{100 \text{ mL}}{100 \text{ units}} \times \dfrac{x \text{ mL}}{8.7 \text{ units}}$ **SOLUTION FOR BOTH PROPORTION METHODS** $8.7 \times 100 = 100x$ $\dfrac{8.7 \times 100}{100} = x$ $8.7 \text{ mL/hour} = x$	$\dfrac{\cancel{100}^{1} \text{ mL}}{\cancel{100}_{1} \text{ units}} \left| \dfrac{8.7 \text{ units}}{\text{hours}} = 8.7 \text{ mL/hour} \right.$

b. Yes; $(BG - 60) \times 0.04$

3. a. $(140 - 60) \times 0.04 = 3.2$ units

Formula Method	Proportion	Dimensional Analysis
$\dfrac{3.2 \text{ units}}{100 \text{ units}} \times 100 \text{ mL} = x$ $x = 3.2 \text{ mL}$	**EXPRESSED AS TWO RATIOS** $100 \text{ units} : 100 \text{ mL} :: x \text{ mL} : 3.2 \text{ units}$ **EXPRESSED AS TWO FRACTIONS** $\dfrac{100 \text{ mL}}{100 \text{ units}} \times \dfrac{x \text{ mL}}{3.2 \text{ units}}$ **SOLUTION FOR BOTH PROPORTION METHODS** $3.2 \times 100 = 100x$ $\dfrac{3.2 \times 100}{100} = x$ $3.2 \text{ mL/hour} = x$	$\dfrac{100 \text{ mL}}{100 \text{ units}} \Bigg| \dfrac{3.2 \text{ units}}{\text{hours}} = 3.2 \text{ mL/hour}$

Run at 3.2 mL/hour

b. Yes; $(BG - 60) \times 0.05$

4. a. $(100 - 60) \times 0.05 = 2$ units

Formula Method	Proportion	Dimensional Analysis
$\dfrac{2 \text{ units}}{100 \text{ units}} \times 100 \text{ mL} = x$ $x = 2 \text{ mL/hour}$	**EXPRESSED AS TWO RATIOS** $100 \text{ units} : 100 \text{ mL} :: x \text{ mL} : 2 \text{ units}$ **EXPRESSED AS TWO FRACTIONS** $\dfrac{100 \text{ mL}}{100 \text{ units}} \times \dfrac{x \text{ mL}}{2 \text{ units}}$ **SOLUTION FOR BOTH PROPORTION METHODS** $2 \times 100 = 100x$ $\dfrac{2 \times 100}{100} = x$ $2 \text{ mL/hour} = x$	$\dfrac{100 \text{ mL}}{100 \text{ units}} \Bigg| \dfrac{2 \text{ units}}{\text{hours}} = 2 \text{ mL/hour}$

Run at 2 mL/hour

b. No; remains $(BG - 60) \times 0.05$

(continued)

Answers (Continued)

Self-Test 7 Infusion Problems

1. The order calls for 0.5 mg/minute. Because there are 60 minutes in an hour, multiply: $0.5 \text{ mg} \times 60 = 30$ mg/hour. The standard solution is 200 mg in 200 mL. This is a 1:1 solution, so 30 mg/hour = 30 mL/hour. You can also solve using the four methods:

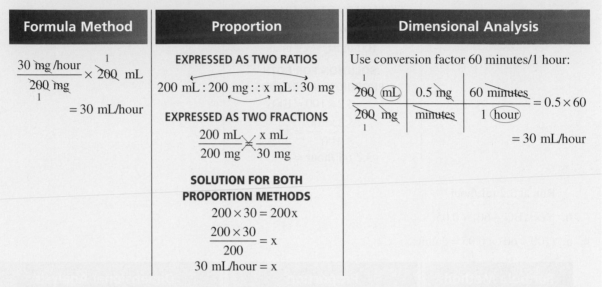

Total number of milliliters = 200; milliliters per hour = 30.

2. Order is 75 mg/hour. You have 250 mg in 250 mL (a 1:1 solution); therefore, set the pump at 75 mL/hour. You can also solve using the four methods:

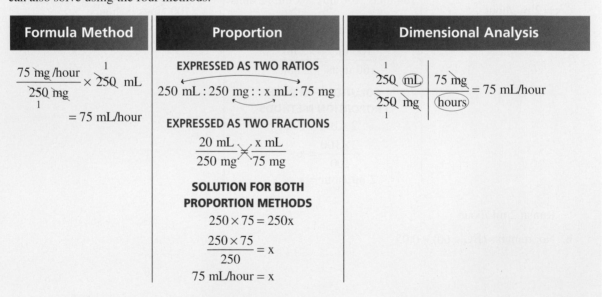

Total number of milliliters = 250; milliliters per hour = 75.

3. 2 g = 2000 mg

Order calls for 4 mg/minute. There are 60 minutes in an hour: $60 \times 4 = 240$ mg/hour.

Formula Method	Proportion	Dimensional Analysis
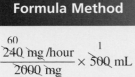 $= 60$ mL/hour	**EXPRESSED AS TWO RATIOS** 500 mL : 2000 mg : : x mL : 240 mg **EXPRESSED AS TWO FRACTIONS** $\dfrac{500 \text{ mL}}{2000 \text{ mg}} \diagup \dfrac{x \text{ mL}}{240 \text{ mg}}$ **SOLUTION FOR BOTH PROPORTION METHODS** $240 \times 500 = 2000x$ $\dfrac{240 \times 500}{2000} = x$ 60 mL/hour $= x$	Use conversion factors: 60 minutes/1 hour 1 g/1000 mg $\dfrac{\overset{1}{\cancel{500}} \; \text{mL}}{\underset{1}{\cancel{2 \text{ g}}}} \Big| \dfrac{\overset{2}{\cancel{4}} \text{ mg}}{\cancel{\text{minutes}}} \Big| \dfrac{60 \; \cancel{\text{minutes}}}{1 \; \text{hour}} \Big| \dfrac{1 \; \cancel{\text{g}}}{\underset{2}{\cancel{1000}} \; \text{mg}}$ $= \dfrac{\cancel{2} \times 60}{\cancel{2}} = 60$ mL/hour

Total number of milliliters = 500; milliliters per hour = 60.

4.

$$\dfrac{\overset{50}{\cancel{100}} \text{ mL}}{\underset{1}{\cancel{2}} \text{ hours}} = 50 \text{ mL/hour on a pump}$$

Total number of milliliters = 100; milliliters per hour = 50.

5. Calculate the milliliters per hour:

Formula Method	Proportion	Dimensional Analysis
$\dfrac{\cancel{5000 \text{ units}}/\text{hour}}{\underset{\overset{100}{1}}{\cancel{25,000 \text{ units}}}} \times \cancel{250} \text{ mL}$ $= 50$ mL/hour on a pump	**EXPRESSED AS TWO RATIOS** 250 mL : 25,000 units : : x mL : 5000 units **EXPRESSED AS TWO FRACTIONS** $\dfrac{250 \text{ mL}}{25,000 \text{ units}} \diagup \dfrac{x \text{ mL}}{5000 \text{ units}}$ **SOLUTION FOR BOTH PROPORTION METHODS** $5000 \times 250 = 25,000x$ $\dfrac{5000 \times 250}{25,000} = x$ 50 mL/hour $= x$	$\dfrac{250 \; \cancel{\text{mL}}}{\underset{5}{\cancel{25,000}} \; \cancel{\text{units}}} \Big| \dfrac{\overset{1}{\cancel{5000}} \; \cancel{\text{units}}}{\cancel{\text{hours}}} = \dfrac{250}{5}$ $= 50$ mL/hour

Total number of milliliters = 250; milliliters per hour = 50.

(continued)

Answers (Continued)

6. Calculate the milliliters per hour.

$$\frac{60 \text{ minutes}}{30 \text{ minutes}} = 2$$

Multiply: 100 mL × 2 = 200 mL/hour, or 100 mL over 30 minutes.

Total number of milliliters = 100.

7. Order: 80 mcg/minute

Supply: 50 mg in 250 mL

Step 1. $\dfrac{50 \text{ mg}}{250 \text{ mL}} = 0.2 \text{ mg/mL}$

Step 2. 0.2 × 1000 = 200 mcg/mL

Step 3. $\dfrac{200}{60} = 3.33 \text{ mcg/minute}$

Step 4. Solve for milliliters per hour:

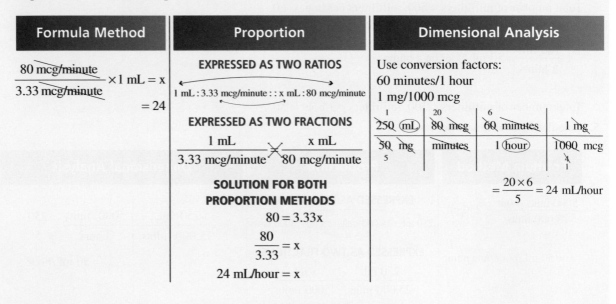

Formula Method	Proportion	Dimensional Analysis
$\dfrac{80 \text{ mcg/minute}}{3.33 \text{ mcg/minute}} \times 1 \text{ mL} = x$ $= 24$	**EXPRESSED AS TWO RATIOS** 1 mL : 3.33 mcg/minute : : x mL : 80 mcg/minute **EXPRESSED AS TWO FRACTIONS** $\dfrac{1 \text{ mL}}{3.33 \text{ mcg/minute}} \times \dfrac{x \text{ mL}}{80 \text{ mcg/minute}}$ **SOLUTION FOR BOTH PROPORTION METHODS** 80 = 3.33x $\dfrac{80}{3.33} = x$ 24 mL/hour = x	Use conversion factors: 60 minutes/1 hour 1 mg/1000 mcg $\dfrac{250 \text{ mL}}{50 \text{ mg}} \cdot \dfrac{80 \text{ mcg}}{\text{minutes}} \cdot \dfrac{60 \text{ minutes}}{1 \text{ hour}} \cdot \dfrac{1 \text{ mg}}{1000 \text{ mcg}}$ $= \dfrac{20 \times 6}{5} = 24 \text{ mL/hour}$

Set the pump: total number of milliliters = 250; milliliters per hour = 24.

8. Order: 6 mcg/kg/minute

Solution: 500 mg/250 mL

Weight: 180 lb

a. Change pounds to kilograms: $\dfrac{180 \text{ lbs}}{2.2}$

$$\begin{array}{r} 81.8 \\ 2.2 \overline{)180.00} = 82 \text{ kg} \\ \underline{176} \\ 4\,0 \\ \underline{2\,2} \\ 1\,80 \end{array}$$

b. 6 mcg/kg × 82 kg = 492 mcg

Step 1. $\dfrac{500 \text{ mg}}{250 \text{ mL}} = 2 \text{ mg/mL}$

Step 2. 2 × 1000 = 2000 mcg/mL

Step 3. $\dfrac{2000}{60} = 33.33 \text{ mcg/minute}$

Step 4. Solve for milliliters per hour:

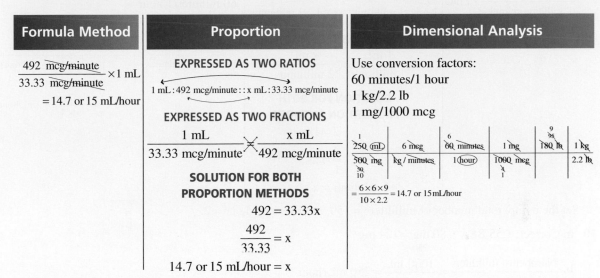

Formula Method	Proportion	Dimensional Analysis
$\dfrac{492 \cancel{\text{ mcg/minute}}}{33.33 \cancel{\text{ mcg/minute}}} \times 1 \text{ mL}$ $= 14.7 \text{ or } 15 \text{ mL/hour}$	**EXPRESSED AS TWO RATIOS** 1 mL : 492 mcg/minute : : x mL : 33.33 mcg/minute **EXPRESSED AS TWO FRACTIONS** $\dfrac{1 \text{ mL}}{33.33 \text{ mcg/minute}} \diagdown\!\!\!\!\diagup \dfrac{x \text{ mL}}{492 \text{ mcg/minute}}$ **SOLUTION FOR BOTH PROPORTION METHODS** $492 = 33.33x$ $\dfrac{492}{33.33} = x$ 14.7 or 15 mL/hour = x	Use conversion factors: 60 minutes/1 hour 1 kg/2.2 lb 1 mg/1000 mcg $= \dfrac{6 \times 6 \times 9}{10 \times 2.2} = 14.7 \text{ or } 15 \text{ mL/hour}$

Set the pump: total number of milliliters = 250; milliliters per hour = 15.

9. Order: 2 milliunits/minute

Supply: 9 units in 150 mL NS

Step 1. $\dfrac{9 \text{ units}}{150 \text{ mL}} = 0.06 \text{ units/mL}$

Step 2. 1 unit = 1000 milliunits

0.06 × 1000 = 60 milliunits/mL

Step 3. $\dfrac{60}{60} = 1 \text{ milliunit/mL}$

(continued)

Answers (Continued)

Step 4. Solve for milliliters per hour:

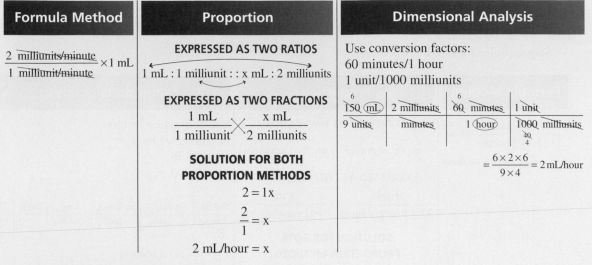

Formula Method	Proportion	Dimensional Analysis

Formula Method

$$\frac{2 \text{ milliunits/minute}}{1 \text{ milliunit/minute}} \times 1 \text{ mL}$$

Proportion

EXPRESSED AS TWO RATIOS

1 mL : 1 milliunit : : x mL : 2 milliunits

EXPRESSED AS TWO FRACTIONS

$$\frac{1 \text{ mL}}{1 \text{ milliunit}} \times \frac{x \text{ mL}}{2 \text{ milliunits}}$$

SOLUTION FOR BOTH PROPORTION METHODS

$$2 = 1x$$
$$\frac{2}{1} = x$$
$$2 \text{ mL/hour} = x$$

Dimensional Analysis

Use conversion factors:
60 minutes/1 hour
1 unit/1000 milliunits

$$\frac{\overset{6}{\cancel{150}} \text{ mL}}{9 \text{ units}} \cdot \frac{2 \text{ milliunits}}{\text{minutes}} \cdot \frac{\overset{6}{\cancel{60}} \text{ minutes}}{1 \text{ hour}} \cdot \frac{1 \text{ unit}}{\underset{4}{\overset{40}{\cancel{1000}}} \text{ milliunits}}$$

$$= \frac{6 \times 2 \times 6}{9 \times 4} = 2 \text{ mL/hour}$$

Set the pump: total number of milliliters = 150; milliliters per hour = 2.

10. a. Correct; 1.55 BSA × 80 mg = 124 mg

b. $\dfrac{\text{Number of milliliters}}{\text{Number of hours}} = \dfrac{\overset{250}{\cancel{1000}} \text{ mL}}{\underset{1}{\cancel{4}} \text{ hours}} = 250 \text{ mL/hour}$

Set the pump: total number of milliliters = 1000; milliliters per hour = 250.

1/4

50 mg/mL

Dosage Problems for Infants and Children

TOPICS COVERED

1. mg/kg body weight calculation:
   Converting ounces to pounds
   Converting pounds to kilograms
   Determining a safe dose
   mg/kg calculations
2. Body surface area calculations
3. IV medications

In previous chapters, we discussed calculations for adult medications administered orally and parenterally. This chapter considers dosage for infants and children. Wide variations in age, weight, growth, and development within this group require special care in computation. Because pediatric doses are lower than adult doses and are narrower in dosage range, a slight error can result in serious harm.

Before preparing and administering a pediatric medication, you will determine that the dose is safe for the child. Safe means that the amount ordered is neither an overdose (which can produce toxic effects) nor an underdose (which may lead to therapeutic failure). If you notice a discrepancy in the dose, consult the physician or healthcare provider who ordered the drug.

Children's medications are usually given either by mouth in a liquid form, subcutaneous, and intramuscular (IM) injections or intravenously.

- Administering liquid medications to an infant or toddler often requires gently holding the child and using a syringe or dropper (Fig. 8-1A).
- Nipples are also used to give medications to infants (this can help prevent aspiration of liquids).
- School-age children through adolescents often need to be involved in decision making when administering medication (Fig. 8-1B).
- Subcutaneous and intramuscular injections are used primarily for immunizations.
- Pediatric injections are calculated to the nearest hundredth and are often administered using a 1-mL precision (also called tuberculin) syringe.
- Pediatric IV therapy uses microdrip tubing, buretrols, other volume control sets, infusion pumps, or syringe pumps.
- In the pediatric setting, you often find infusion pumps that can be set in tenths or hundredths.

Chapter 10 gives a brief overview of pediatric medication administration. For more information related to this topic, such as needle size and injection sites, check pediatric nursing textbooks. Always follow institutional policy. Most institutions have guidelines for pediatric infusions; if no guidelines are available, consult a reliable pediatric reference. Adult guidelines are not safe for children.

Because pediatric doses must be accurate, it is advisable to use a calculator. The nurse still bears the responsibility, however, of knowing what numbers to enter into the calculator in order to calculate the correct amount. To be safe, double- or triple-check your answer.

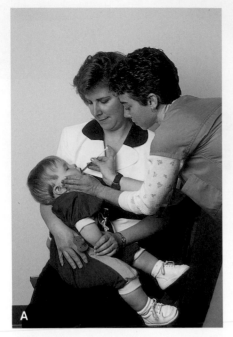

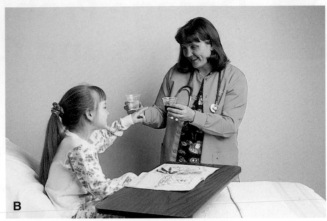

FIGURE 8-1

A. Administration of liquid medication to infants and toddlers requires gently holding the child and administering with a syringe or dropper. **B.** Administration of liquid medication to school-age children involves giving them choices—for example, what type of liquid to mix a medication that is distasteful. (Used with permission from Pillitteri, A. [2007]. *Maternal and child health nursing* [5th ed.]. Philadelphia, PA: Lippincott Williams & Wilkins, pp. 1145 and 1080.)

Recall these equivalents and abbreviations as you begin this chapter:

1 g = 1000 mg   16 oz = 1 lb

1 kg = 2.2 lb   microdrip = 60 gtt/mL

1 mg = 1000 mcg   > = greater than

1 tsp = 5 mL   < = less than

1 oz = 30 mL

Dosage Based on mg/kg

The dose of most pediatric drugs is based on milligram per kilogram of body weight or body surface area (BSA) in meters squared (m^2). This section shows you how to convert pounds to kilograms, how to estimate the safety of a dose, and, finally, how to determine the dose. To ensure accuracy, use a calculator. The next section will show how to determine dosage based on BSA.

Converting Ounces to Pounds

EXAMPLE   An infant weighs 20 lb 12 oz. Convert the ounces to pounds.

Step 1. Because there are 16 oz in 1 lb, divide the 12 oz by 16. You should get a decimal:

$$
\begin{array}{r}
0.75 \\
16\overline{)12.00} \\
\underline{11\ 2} \\
80 \\
\underline{80} \\
0
\end{array}
$$

Step 2. Add the answer to the pounds to get the total number of pounds:

$20 + 0.75 = 20.75$ lb

EXAMPLE | An infant weighs 25 lb 6 oz. Convert the ounces to pounds.

Step 1. Divide 6 by 16:

$$
\begin{array}{r}
0.375 \\
16\overline{)6.0} \\
\underline{4\ 8} \\
1\ 20 \\
\underline{1\ 12} \\
80 \\
\underline{80} \\
0
\end{array}
$$

Step 2. Add the answer to the pounds:

$25 + 0.375 = 25.375$ lb

Converting Pounds to Kilograms

EXAMPLE | A child weighs 33 lb. How many kilograms?

Step 1. Because there are 2.2 lb per 1 kg, divide the 33 lb by 2.2. Round off to the nearest hundredth (if necessary):

$$
\begin{array}{r}
15 \\
2.2\overline{)33.0} \\
\underline{22} \\
11\ 0 \\
\underline{11\ 0} \\
0
\end{array}
$$

The child weighs 15 kg.

EXAMPLE | An infant weighs 18 lb 12 oz. How many kilograms?

Step 1.   Convert ounces to pounds first:

$$\frac{12}{16} \frac{0.75}{\smash{\big)}12.0}$$
$$\underline{11\ 2}$$
$$80$$
$$\underline{80}$$
$$0$$

Step 2.   Add the answer to the pounds:

$$18 + 0.75 = 18.75 \text{ lb}$$

Step 3.   Convert to kilograms by dividing by 2.2. Round off to the nearest hundredth:

$$\frac{18.75}{2.2} \frac{8.522}{\smash{\big)}18.7\,5}$$
$$\underline{17\ 6}$$
$$1\ 15$$
$$\underline{1\ 10}$$
$$50$$
$$\underline{44}$$
$$60$$
$$\underline{44}$$

The infant weighs 8.52 kg.

SELF-TEST 1   Converting Pounds to Kilograms

Convert pounds to kilograms. Use a calculator. Round the final answer to the nearest hundredths place. Answers appear at the end of the chapter.

1. 30 lb = _____ kg
2. 15 lb 5 oz = _____ kg
3. 7¼ lb = _____ kg
4. 22 lb = _____ kg
5. 54 lb 8 oz = _____ kg

6. 4 lb 5 oz = _____ kg
7. 75 lb = _____ kg
8. 12 lb 3 oz = _____ kg
9. 66 lb = _____ kg
10. 10½ lb = _____ kg

Steps—mg/kg Body Weight

EXAMPLE   Amoxicillin (Augmentin) 150 mg po q8h is ordered for a child weighing 33 lb. Figure 8-2 shows the label for Augmentin, which comes as a dry powder. The accompanying prescribing information states that children ≤40 kg receive 6.7 to 13.3 mg/kg q8h.

We need to convert 33 lb to kg, calculate the low and high safe dose, determine whether the dose ordered is within the safe range, and prepare the dose. These are the steps:

> **STEP 1.** Convert ounces to pounds; then convert pounds to kilograms, dividing by 2.2.
>
> **STEP 2.** Determine the safe dose range in milligrams per kilograms by using a reference (such as a drug book or drug insert).
>
> **STEP 3.** Decide whether the ordered dose is safe by comparing the order with the safe dose range listed in the reference.
>
> **STEP 4.** Calculate the dose needed.

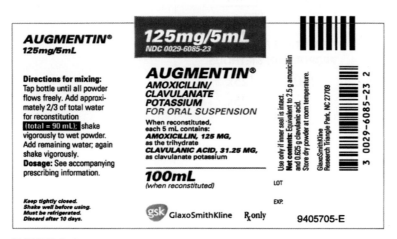

FIGURE 8-2

Label for Augmentin (amoxicillin) for oral suspension. (Courtesy of GlaxoSmithKline.)

Step 1. Convert pounds to kilograms. Divide the number of pounds by 2.2:

$$
\begin{array}{r}
15. \\
2.2\,\overline{)33.0} \\
\underline{22} \\
11\ 0 \\
\underline{11\ 0}
\end{array}
$$

The child weighs 15 kg.

Step 2. Determine the safe dose range. The literature states that the dose should range from 6.7 to 13.3 mg/kg q8h.

Low Dose	*High Dose*
6.7 mg	13.3 mg
× 15 kg	× 15 kg
100.5 mg	199.5 = 200 mg

Step 3. Is the dose safe? The safe range is 100 to 200 mg q8h. The dose ordered (150 mg q8h) is indeed safe because it falls within the 100- to 200-mg range.

Step 4.   Calculate the dose.

The label states that 90 mL water should be added gradually (see Fig. 8-2) to make a concentration of 125 mg/5 mL.

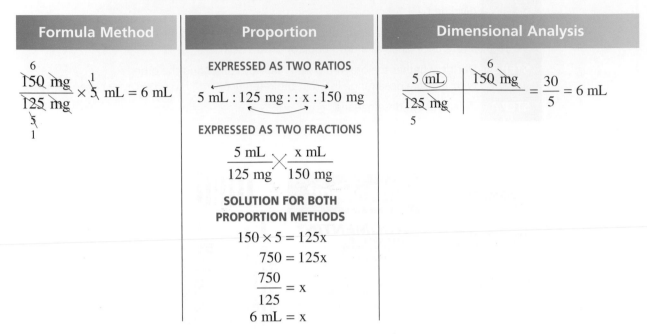

Formula Method	Proportion	Dimensional Analysis
$\dfrac{\overset{6}{\cancel{150}\ \text{mg}}}{\underset{\underset{1}{5}}{\cancel{125}\ \text{mg}}} \times \overset{1}{\cancel{5}}\ \text{mL} = 6\ \text{mL}$	**EXPRESSED AS TWO RATIOS** 5 mL : 125 mg : : x : 150 mg **EXPRESSED AS TWO FRACTIONS** $\dfrac{5\ \text{mL}}{125\ \text{mg}} \times \dfrac{\text{x mL}}{150\ \text{mg}}$ **SOLUTION FOR BOTH PROPORTION METHODS** $150 \times 5 = 125x$ $750 = 125x$ $\dfrac{750}{125} = x$ $6\ \text{mL} = x$	$\dfrac{5\ \text{(mL)}}{\underset{5}{\cancel{125}\ \text{mg}}} \left| \dfrac{\overset{6}{\cancel{150}\ \text{mg}}}{} \right. = \dfrac{30}{5} = 6\ \text{mL}$

Give 6 mL.

You can measure this dose with a calibrated safety dropper or oral syringe. For examples of this equipment, see Figure 8-3.

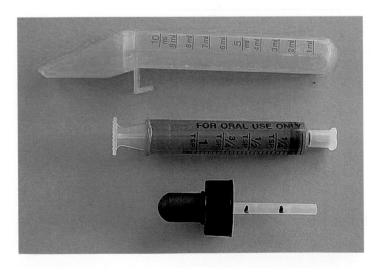

FIGURE 8-3

Examples of equipment used to obtain pediatric doses: (*top*) a medication spoon calculated in milliliters and teaspoons; (*center*) an oral syringe calculated in teaspoons; (*bottom*) a safety dropper calibrated in milliliters. (A regular syringe marked in milliliters may also be used.)

EXAMPLE   A child weighing 16 lb 10 oz is ordered furosemide (Lasix) 15 mg po bid (Fig. 8-4). Is the dose safe? What amount should you pour?

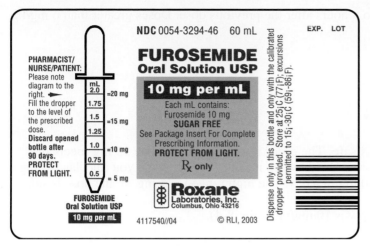

FIGURE 8-4

Label for Lasix (furosemide). (Used with permission of Roxane Laboratories, Inc.)

Step 1. Convert pounds to kilograms:

a. Change the ounces to part of a pound:

$$\frac{10}{16} \Big) \overline{\begin{matrix} 0.625 \\ 10.0 \\ 9\,6 \\ \overline{\quad 40} \\ 32 \\ \overline{\quad 80} \\ 80 \\ \overline{\quad 0} \end{matrix}}$$

The child's weight is $16 + 0.625 = 16.625$ lb.

b. Change pounds to kilograms. Round off to the nearest hundredth:

$$\frac{16.625}{2.2} \Big) \overline{\begin{matrix} 7.556 \\ 16.6\,25 \\ 15\,4 \\ \overline{\quad 1\,22} \\ 1\,10 \\ \overline{\quad 125} \\ 110 \\ \overline{\quad 150} \\ 110 \end{matrix}}$$

The child weighs 7.56 kg.

Step 2. Determine the safe dose range in milligrams per kilogram. The package insert states: The initial dose of oral furosemide (Lasix) in infants and children is 2 mg/kg body weight, given as a single dose. If the diuretic response is not satisfactory after the initial dose, dosage may be increased by 1 or 2 mg/kg no sooner than 6 to 8 hours after the previous dose. Doses greater than 6 mg/kg body weight are not recommended.

Single Dose
$$\begin{array}{r} 7.56 \text{ kg} \\ \times \quad 2 \text{ mg} \\ \hline 15.12 \text{ mg/day} \end{array}$$

High Range
$$\begin{array}{r} 7.56 \text{ kg} \\ \times \quad 6 \text{ mg} \\ \hline 45.36 \text{ mg/day} \end{array}$$

Step 3.   Decide whether the ordered dose is safe. The order is 15 mg po bid. The 15 mg meets the requirement for a single dose. The order is bid, which means twice in a day; you calculate 15 mg × 2 = 30 mg. The child will receive 30 mg in a day. The high range is 45 mg, so the dose is safe.

Step 4.   Calculate the dose needed. The supply is 10 mg/mL (Fig. 8-4).

Formula Method	Proportion	Dimensional Analysis
$\dfrac{\overset{3}{\cancel{15}} \text{ mg}}{\underset{2}{\cancel{10}} \text{ mg}} \times 1 \text{ mL} = \dfrac{3}{2}$ $= 1.5 \text{ mL}$	**EXPRESSED AS TWO RATIOS** $1 \text{ mL} : 10 \text{ mg} :: x : 15 \text{ mg}$ **EXPRESSED AS TWO FRACTIONS** $\dfrac{1 \text{ mL}}{10 \text{ mg}} \times \dfrac{x}{15 \text{ mg}}$ **SOLUTION FOR BOTH PROPORTION METHODS** $15 = 10x$ $\dfrac{15}{10} = x$ $1.5 \text{ mL} = x$	$\dfrac{1 \, \cancel{\text{mL}}}{\underset{2}{\cancel{10}} \, \cancel{\text{mg}}} \bigg| \dfrac{\overset{3}{\cancel{15}} \, \cancel{\text{mg}}}{} = \dfrac{3}{2} = 1.5 \text{ mL}$

The label states that furosemide (Lasix) comes with a calibrated safety dropper. You can use the dropper to obtain the dose of 1.5 mL.

EXAMPLE   Digoxin (Lanoxin) 37.5 mcg po × 1 is ordered for a premature infant weighing 1500 g. Is the dose safe? What amount should be given?

Step 1.   Convert grams to kilograms (1000 grams = 1 kg):

$$\frac{1500}{1000} = 1.5 \text{ kg}$$

Step 2.   Determine the safe dose range in milligrams per kilogram.

The *Nursing Drug Guide* states that the loading dose (oral) for the premature infant is 20 to 30 mcg/kg.

Low Dose	*High Dose*
1.5 kg	1.5 kg
× 20 mcg	× 30 mcg
30 mcg	45 mcg

Step 3. The ordered dose is 37.5 mcg.

The dose ordered is safe.

Step 4. Calculate the dose. Digoxin (Lanoxin) elixir (Fig. 8-5) comes in 0.125 mg/2.5 mL or 50 mcg per milliliter.

Formula Method	Proportion	Dimensional Analysis
$\dfrac{\overset{7.5}{\cancel{37.5}\ \text{mcg}}}{\underset{10}{\cancel{50}\ \text{mcg}}} \times 1\ \text{mL}$ $= 0.75\ \text{mL}$	**EXPRESSED AS TWO RATIOS** $1\ \text{mL} : 50\ \text{mcg} :: x : 37.5\ \text{mcg}$ **EXPRESSED AS TWO FRACTIONS** $\dfrac{1\ \text{mL}}{50\ \text{mcg}} \times \dfrac{x}{37.5\ \text{mcg}}$ **SOLUTION FOR BOTH PROPORTION METHODS** $37.5 = 50x$ $\dfrac{37.5}{50} = x$ $0.75\ \text{mL} = x$	$\dfrac{1\ \text{mL}}{\underset{10}{\cancel{50}\ \text{mcg}}} \left\vert\ \overset{7.5}{\cancel{37.5}\ \text{mcg}} \right. = \dfrac{7.5}{10} = 0.75\ \text{mL}$

Use a calibrated safety dropper or oral syringe (1 mL) to draw up 0.75 mL.

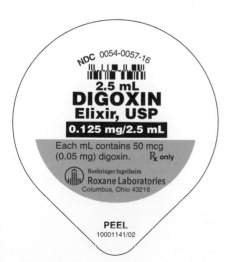

FIGURE 8-5

Label for digoxin (Lanoxin). (Courtesy of Roxane Laboratories, Inc.)

EXAMPLE   A child weighing 22 lb is prescribed acetaminophen (Tylenol) for pain. The dose prescribed is 100 mg. Is the dose safe? What amount should be given?

Step 1.   Convert pounds to kilograms

$$\frac{22}{2.2} \overline{)\begin{array}{r} 1\ 0 \\ 22\ 0 \\ \underline{22} \\ 0 \end{array}}$$

The child weighs 10 kg.

Step 2.   Determine the safe dose range in milligrams per kilogram.

The *Nursing Drug Guide* states 10–15 mg/kg/dose q4–6h. Do not exceed 5 doses in 24 hours.

Low Dose	*High Dose*
10 kg	10 kg
× 10 mg	× 15 mg
100 mg	150 mg

Step 3.   The ordered dose is 100 mg. The dose ordered is safe.

Step 4.   Calculate the dose. Tylenol (Fig. 8-6) comes 160 mg per 5 mL.

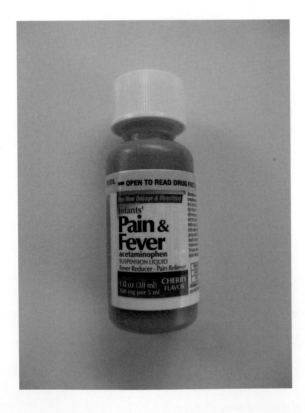

FIGURE 8-6
Label for acetaminophen (Tylenol).

Formula Method	Proportion	Dimensional Analysis
$\dfrac{100 \text{ mg}}{\underset{32}{\cancel{160} \text{ mg}}} \times \overset{1}{\cancel{5}} \text{mL}$	**EXPRESSED AS TWO RATIOS** $5 \text{ mL} : 160 \text{ mg} :: x : 100 \text{ mg}$	$\dfrac{\overset{1}{\cancel{5 \text{ mL}}} \mid 100 \cancel{\text{ mg}}}{\underset{32}{\cancel{160 \text{ mg}}}}$
$= \dfrac{100}{32} = 3.125 \text{ mL}$	**EXPRESSED AS TWO FRACTIONS** $\dfrac{5 \text{ mL}}{160 \text{ mg}} \times \dfrac{x}{100 \text{ mg}}$	$= \dfrac{100}{32} = 3.125 \text{ mL}$
	SOLUTION FOR BOTH PROPORTION METHODS $500 \text{ mg} = 160x$ $\dfrac{500}{160} = x$ $3.125 \text{ mL} = x$	

Use a calibrated safety dropper or oral syringe to draw up 3.125 mL or 3.1 mL.

EXAMPLE   A 4-year-old child is prescribed diazepam (Valium) 1.5 mg po qid. Is the dose safe? What amount should be given?

Step 1.   No weight needed.

Step 2.   Determine the safe dose range.

The *Nursing Drug Guide* states for children >6 months, 1–2.5 mg po 3–4 doses per day.

Step 3.   The ordered dose is 1.5 mg.

The dose is safe.

Step 4.   Calculate the dose. Valium (Fig. 8-7) comes 5 mg in 5 mL. So there is 1 mg in each mL. The dose will be 1.5 mL

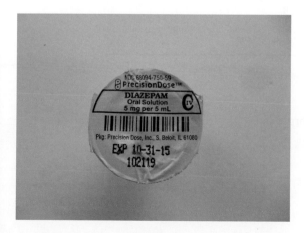

FIGURE 8-7
Label for diazepam (Valium).

EXAMPLE

A child weighing 66 lb is prescribed epinephrine subcutaneous injection for an allergic reaction. The dose prescribed is 0.3 mg. Is the dose safe? What amount should be given?

Step 1.   Convert pounds to kilograms:

$$\frac{66}{2.2} \, \overset{3 \, 0}{\big) \, \overline{66.0}}$$
$$\underline{66}$$
$$0$$

The child weighs 30 kg.

Step 2.   Determine the safe dose range in milligrams per kilogram.

The *Nursing Drug Guide* states 0.01 mg/kg subcutaneous every 20 minutes. Do not exceed 0.5 mg in a single dose.

Step 3.   The ordered dose is 0.3 mg:

$$\begin{array}{r} 30 \text{ kg} \\ \times \ 0.01 \text{ mg/kg} \\ \hline 0.3 \text{ mg} \end{array}$$

The dose is safe.

Step 4.   Calculate the dose. Figure 8-8 shows a concentration of 1 mg/mL. Therefore, 0.3 mg = 0.3 mL (no calculation needed). Use a 1-mL precision syringe for the dose.

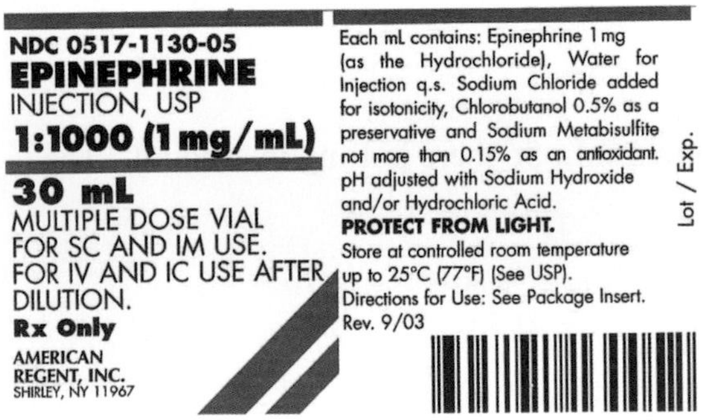

NDC 0517-1130-05
EPINEPHRINE
INJECTION, USP
1:1000 (1 mg/mL)
30 mL
MULTIPLE DOSE VIAL
FOR SC AND IM USE.
FOR IV AND IC USE AFTER
DILUTION.
Rx Only
AMERICAN
REGENT, INC.
SHIRLEY, NY 11967

Each mL contains: Epinephrine 1 mg (as the Hydrochloride), Water for Injection q.s. Sodium Chloride added for isotonicity, Chlorobutanol 0.5% as a preservative and Sodium Metabisulfite not more than 0.15% as an antioxidant. pH adjusted with Sodium Hydroxide and/or Hydrochloric Acid.
PROTECT FROM LIGHT.
Store at controlled room temperature up to 25°C (77°F) (See USP).
Directions for Use: See Package Insert.
Rev. 9/03

FIGURE 8-8

Label for subcutaneous and IM epinephrine. (Courtesy of American Regent, Inc.)

EXAMPLE

A child weighing 79 lb is prescribed morphine 1.8 mg subcutaneous stat. Is the dose safe? What amount should be given?

Step 1.   Convert pounds to kilograms

$$
\begin{array}{r}
35.9 \\
2\,2\ \overline{)79\,0} \\
\underline{66} \\
13\,0 \\
\underline{11\,0} \\
2\,00 \\
\underline{1\,98} \\
20
\end{array}
$$

The child weighs 35.9 kg.

Step 2.   Determine the safe dose range in milligrams per kilogram.

The *Nursing Drug Guide* states 0.05–0.2 mg/kg every 3–4 hours, maximum 15 mg dose.

Low Dose	*High Dose*
35.9 kg	35.9 kg
× 0.05 mg	× 0.2 mg
1.795 mg	7.18 mg

Step 3.   The ordered dose is 1.8 mg.

The dose ordered is safe.

Step 4.   Calculate the dose. Morphine (Fig. 8-9) comes 2 mg/mL.

Formula Method	Proportion	Dimensional Analysis
$\dfrac{1.8 \text{ mg}}{2 \text{ mg}} \times 1 \text{ mL}$ $= 0.9 \text{ mL}$	**EXPRESSED AS TWO RATIOS** 1 mL : 2 mg :: x mL : 1.8 mg **EXPRESSED AS TWO FRACTIONS** $\dfrac{1 \text{ mL}}{2 \text{ mg}} \times \dfrac{x \text{ mL}}{1.8 \text{ mg}}$ **SOLUTION FOR BOTH PROPORTION METHODS** 1.8 mg = 2x $\dfrac{1.8}{2} = x$ 0.9 = x	$\dfrac{1 \text{ mL}}{2 \text{ mg}} \left| \dfrac{1.8 \text{ mg}}{} \right.$ $= \dfrac{1.8}{2} = 0.9 \text{ mL}$

Use a 1 mL precision syringe for the dose.

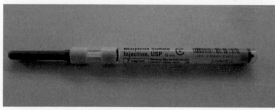

FIGURE 8-9

Morphine syringe.

SELF-TEST 2   Dosage Calculations

In these practice problems, determine whether the doses are safe and calculate the amount needed. Round the lb to kg weight conversions to the nearest hundredth. Answers appear at the end of the chapter.

1. Order: amoxicillin (Amoxil) 60 mg po q8h
   Child: Weight 20 lb
   Supply: amoxicillin (Amoxil) 125 mg/5 mL
   Literature: 20 to 40 mg/kg/day in divided doses q8h

2. Order: amoxicillin (Augmentin) 175 mg po q8h
   Child: Weight 29 lb
   Supply: Bottle of 125 mg/5 mL
   Literature: 40 mg/kg/day in divided doses q8h

3. Order: ferrous sulfate 200 mg po tid
   Child: 9 years old and weighs 30 kg
   Supply: bottle of 125 mg/5 mL
   Literature: children 6 to 12 years old, 600 mg/day, in divided doses tid

4. Order: acetaminophen (Tylenol) 80 mg po q4h prn for temp 100.9°F and above
   Child: 6 years old and weighs 20.5 kg
   Supply: chewable tablets 80 mg
   Literature: For child 6 to 8 years, give four chewable tablets. May repeat four or five times
                 daily. Not to exceed five doses in 24 hours.

5. Order: diazepam (Valium) 1 mg IM q3–4h prn
   Infant: 30 days old
   Supply: vial 5 mg/1 mL
   Literature: child <6 mo IM 1 to 2.5 mg tid or qid

6. Order: Morphine 2 mg subcutaneous q3–4h for pain
   Child: 3 years old and weighs 14 kg
   Supply: injection labeled 2 mg/mL
   Literature: starting dose 0.05 to 0.2 mg/kg; not to exceed 15 mg/dose

7. Order: metoclopramide (Reglan) 5 mg po q6h
   Child: 3 years old and weighs 30 kg
   Supply: syrup 5 mg/5 mL
   Literature: 0.1 to 0.2 mg/kg/dose up to four times a day.

8. Order: cefotaxime (Claforan) 0.5 g IM q6h
   Child: Weight 48 lb
   Supply: injection reconstituted 300 mg per 1 mL
   Literature: for children <50 kg, 100 to 200 mg/kg/day, divided q6h

9. Order: azithromycin (Zithromax) po 300 mg × 1 dose
   Child: 10 years old and weighs 30 kg
   Supply: oral suspension 100 mg/5 mL in 15-mL bottle
   Literature: children 2 to 15 years, 10 mg/kg (not more than 500 mg/dose) on day 1

10. Order: phenytoin (Dilantin) po 60 mg bid
    Infant: Weight 12 lb 8 oz
    Supply: Dilantin (phenytoin) suspension 30 mg/5 mL
    Literature: 4 to 8 mg/kg/day divided into two doses. Maximum dose is 300 mg/day.

Determining Body Surface Area in Meters Squared

A second method to determine pediatric dosage is to calculate BSA in meters squared using a chart called a nomogram (Fig. 8-10). Height is marked in the left column, weight in the right column. A line is drawn between these two marks. The point at which the line intersects the middle column indicates BSA in meters squared.

There are several mathematical formulas to calculate BSA. The following formula often is used:

$$\sqrt{\frac{weight\ (kg) \times height\ (cm)}{3600}} = \text{BSA}$$

Average BSA for children and infants:

9 year olds: 1.07 m²

10 year olds: 1.14 m²

12 to 13 year olds: 1.33 m²

Neonates: 0.25 m²

2 year olds: 0.5 m²

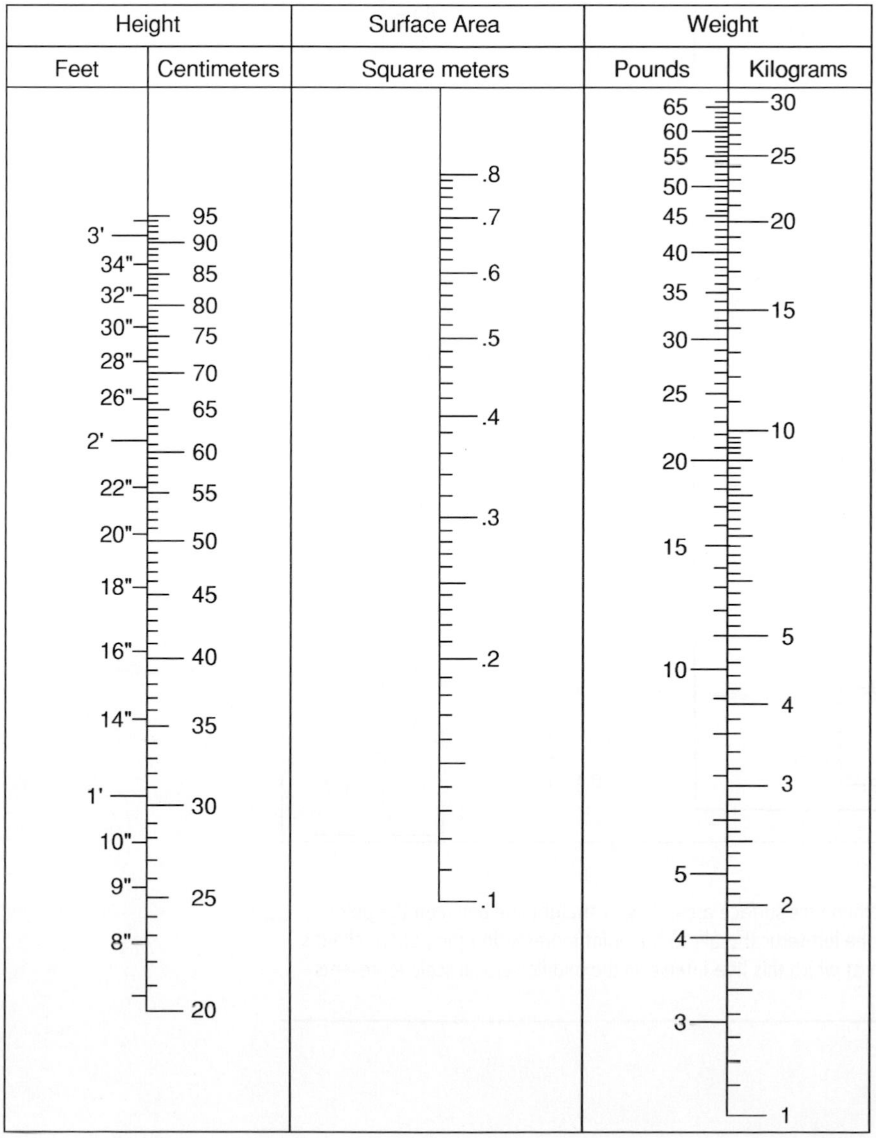

Height		Surface Area	Weight	
Feet	Centimeters	Square meters	Pounds	Kilograms

FIGURE 8-10

Nomogram for infants and toddlers.

Because of differences in growth, charts used for infants and young children are different from those for older children and adults. If a child weighs more than 65 lb or is more than 3 feet tall, use the adult nomogram (Fig. 8-11).

EXAMPLE

1. An infant with a height of 18 inches weighing 15 lb has a BSA of 0.26 m².
2. A child 4′2″ weighing 130 lb has a BSA of 1.55 m².

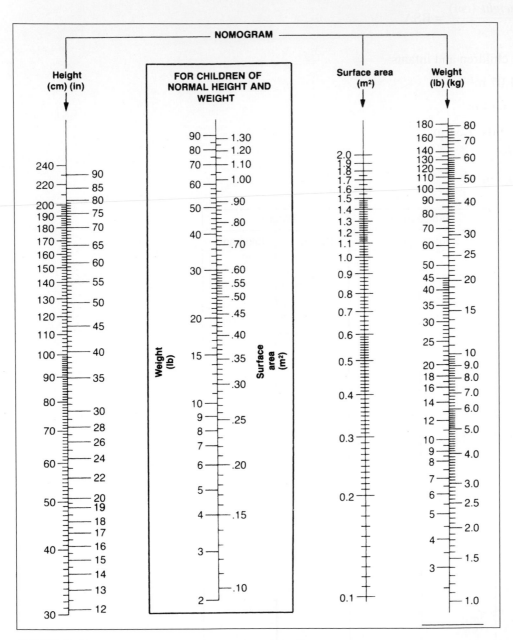

FIGURE 8-11

Nomogram for adults and children. To determine the surface area, draw a straight line between the point representing the patient/client's height on the left vertical scale to the point representing the patient/client's weight on the right vertical scale. The point at which this line intersects the middle vertical scale represents the surface area in meters squared.

BSA is used mainly in calculating chemotherapy dosages. Determining BSA can be done with a special calculator or using the Internet. One useful website for calculating BSA is *www.globalrph.com/bsa2.htm*

SELF-TEST 3   **Determining Body Surface Area**

Convert height and weight to BSA in meters squared using Figure 8-10 or 8-11. Answers appear at the end of this chapter.

Height	*Weight*	*BSA in m²*
1. 36 inches	26 lb	_____
2. 80 cm	13 kg	_____
3. 50 inches	75 lb	_____
4. 17 inches	9 lb	_____

STEPS AND RULE—m² MEDICATION ORDERS

STEP 1. Find the BSA in meters squared.

STEP 2. Determine the safe dose range by using a reference (such as a drug book or drug insert).

STEP 3. Decide whether the ordered dose is safe by comparing the order with the safe dose range listed in the reference.

STEP 4. Calculate the dose needed.

EXAMPLE

A 2-year-old child with a weight of 27 lb 12 oz and height of 35 inches is prescribed leucovorin calcium 5.5 mg po q6h × 72 hours.

Literature states dose of leucovorin for rescue after methotrexate therapy is 10 mg/m²/dose q6h × 72 hours.

Supply: 1 mg/mL reconstituted by the pharmacy

Step 1.   Use Figure 8-10.

Height, 35 inches; weight, 27 lb 12 oz (12 oz = 0.75 or ¾ lb)

Make weight 27¾ lb.

BSA = 0.55 m²

Step 2.   Safe dose is 10 mg/m²/dose q6h:

$$\begin{array}{r} 10 \text{ mg} \\ \times\, 0.55 \text{ m}^2 \\ \hline 5.5 \text{ mg} = \text{safe dose q6h} \end{array}$$

Step 3.   Order is 5.5 mg q6h. Dose is safe.

Step 4.

Formula Method	Proportion	Dimensional Analysis
$\dfrac{5.5 \text{ mg}}{1 \text{ mg}} \times 1 \text{ mL} = 5.5 \text{ mL}$	**EXPRESSED AS TWO RATIOS** $$1 \text{ mL} : 1 \text{ mg} :: x : 5.5 \text{ mg}$$ **EXPRESSED AS TWO FRACTIONS** $$\dfrac{1 \text{ mL}}{1 \text{ mg}} \times \dfrac{x}{5.5 \text{ mg}}$$ **SOLUTION FOR BOTH PROPORTION METHODS** $$5.5 = 1x$$ $$5.5 \text{ mL} = x$$	$\dfrac{1 \text{ mL}}{1 \text{ mg}} \left| \dfrac{5.5 \text{ mg}}{} \right. = 5.5 \text{ mL}$

Give 5.5 mL po q6h.

EXAMPLE   A 6-year-old child with a weight of 40 lb and height of 45 inches is prescribed methotrexate 7.5 mg po twice weekly.

Literature states methotrexate 7.5 to 30 mg/m²/dose twice weekly.

Supply: 2.5-mg tablets

Step 1.   Use Figure 8-11.

Height, 45 inches; weight, 40 lb

$BSA = 0.75$

Step 2.   Safe dose is 7.5 to 30 mg/m²/dose twice weekly:

7.5 mg	30 mg
$\times 0.75 \text{ m}^2$	$\times 0.75 \text{ m}^2$
5.625 mg	22.5 mg

Step 3.   Order is 7.5 mg po twice weekly. Dose is safe.

Step 4.

Formula Method	Proportion	Dimensional Analysis
$$\frac{\overset{3}{\cancel{7.5}} \text{ mg}}{\underset{1}{\cancel{2.5}} \text{ mg}} \times 1 \text{ tablet}$$ $$= 3 \text{ tablets}$$	**EXPRESSED AS TWO RATIOS** $$1 \text{ tablet} : 2.5 \text{ mg} :: x : 7.5 \text{ mg}$$ **EXPRESSED AS TWO FRACTIONS** $$\frac{1 \text{ tablet}}{2.5 \text{ mg}} \times \frac{x}{7.5 \text{ mg}}$$ **SOLUTION FOR BOTH PROPORTION METHODS** $$7.5 = 2.5x$$ $$\frac{7.5}{2.5} = x$$ $$3 \text{ tablets} = x$$	$$\frac{1 \text{ \textcircled{tablet}}}{\underset{1}{\cancel{2.5}} \text{ mg}} \left| \frac{\overset{3}{\cancel{7.5}} \text{ mg}}{} \right. = 3 \text{ tablets}$$

Give 3 tablets po twice weekly.

SELF-TEST 4 | Use of Nomogram

In these problems, determine whether the dose is safe, using the nomogram in Figure 8-10 or 8-11 and calculating. Answers appear at the end of the chapter.

1. Order: flecainide (Tambocor) 50 mg po q8h
   Child: 8 years; height, 50 inches; weight, 55 lb
   Supply: 50-mg tablets
   Literature: dose 100 to 200 mg/m²/24 hours in divided doses q8–12h

2. Order: methotrexate 12.5 mg po q week
   Child: 12 years; height, 59 inches; weight, 88 lb
   Supply: 2.5-mg tablets
   Literature: 10 mg/m²/dose as needed weekly to control fever and joint inflammation in rheumatoid arthritis

3. Order: prednisone (Deltasone) 5 mg po q12h
   Infant: 12 months; height, 30 inches; weight, 22 lb 8 oz
   Supply: 5 mg/5 mL syrup
   Literature: immunosuppressive dose 6 to 30 mg/m²/24 hours

4. Order: dronabinol (Marinol) po 5 mg × 1
   Child: 10 years; height, 50 inches; weight, 35 kg
   Supply: 2.5-mg capsules
   Literature: dose 5 mg/m² 1 to 3 hours before chemotherapy

5. Order: zidovudine (AZT) po 200 mg q6h
   Child: 12 years; height, 60 inches; weight, 100 lb
   Supply: 100-mg capsules
   Literature: children 3 months to 12 years, 90 to 180 mg/m² q6h, not to exceed 200 mg q6h

Administering IV Medications

IV medications are administered when a child cannot maintain an oral fluid intake, has fluid electrolyte imbalances, or requires IV medication. Dosages for IV medications are calculated in milligrams or micrograms per kilogram.

IV push (IVP) medications are calculated according to weight and are then administered, using the correct dilution and administration time. This information is in a drug handbook or administered per institutional policy. Continuous IV medications are also calculated according to weight and are then infused through an infusion pump.

IV piggyback (IVPB) medications are administered in small amounts of diluent. Consult a pediatric reference or institutional manual to determine the minimum and maximum safe amount of diluent. Drugs for IVPB must be initially diluted following the manufacturer's directions. Once you make the initial dilution, withdraw from the vial the amount of drug required to obtain the dose. IVP or IVPB drugs may also be administered with a syringe pump, which will safely deliver the medication over a specific period of time (Fig. 8-12).

Buretrols, volutrols, or other volume control units are used to administer IV fluids (Fig. 8-13). Buretrols are calibrated; they hold only 100 to 150 mL at a time, thus reducing the possibility of fluid overload. Buretrols are attached to the primary IV fluid bag. In the pediatric setting, Buretrols are usually filled with only 1 to 2 hours worth of IV fluid, so the nurse is responsible for checking the IV frequently to make sure the IV site has not infiltrated or to make sure the child is not receiving too much or too little fluid or medication. Drugs for IVPB that have been diluted can be added to a Buretrol (Fig. 8-14).

For smaller children and infants requiring IVPB medications, the medication is usually added to only 10 to 50 mL in the Buretrol, although this amount varies depending on the size and age of the child, fluid restrictions, and other factors. Always follow institutional policy regarding IV infusions.

When the Buretrol is empty of the IV medication, much of the drug will still be in the tubing. For this reason, you need to add an IV flush of 15 to 30 mL to the Buretrol after the medication is infused to ensure that the child receives the drug. This amount varies according to the length of tubing and any extension IV tubing. Follow institutional policy regarding the amount. For this text, we will use 20 mL of IV flush in the Buretrol, after the medication has infused.

Infusion pumps provide a second safeguard (Fig. 8-15). To ensure that pediatric patients/clients receive accurate dosing, you can set infusion pump rates in tenths and hundredths. In neonatal areas, syringe pumps can deliver IV fluid ranging from 1 to 60 mL. Many hospitals use premixed IVPB solutions (from the hospital pharmacy) or syringe pumps are used in place of IVPB (Fig. 8-12). The syringe pump has the medication in a large syringe, attached to a special pump, that can then deliver the medication in a specific amount of time (Figures 8-16 to 8-19).

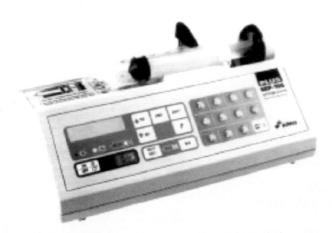

FIGURE 8-12
Syringe Pump. (Courtesy of Hospira, Inc.)

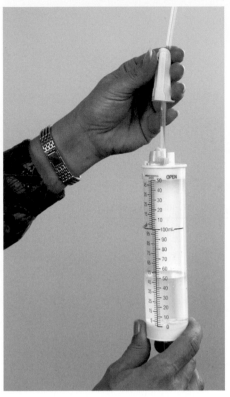

FIGURE 8-13

Volume control infusion device (Buretrol).
(Used with permission from Taylor, C. [2008].
Fundamentals of nursing [6th ed.]. Philadelphia,
PA: Lippincott Williams & Wilkins, p. 853.)

FIGURE 8-14

Adding medication to a volume control infusion device
(Buretrol). (Used with permission from Taylor, C. [2008].
Fundamentals of nursing [6th ed.]. Philadelphia, PA:
Lippincott Williams & Wilkins, p. 854.)

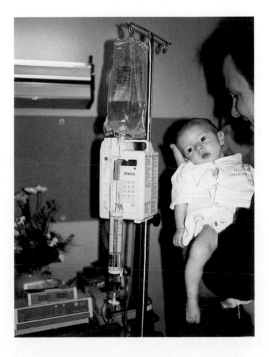

FIGURE 8-15

An infusion pump with a volume control device. (With permission
from Pillitteri, A. [2002]. *Maternal and child health nursing*
[4th ed.]. Philadelphia, PA: Lippincott Williams & Wilkins, p. 1106.)

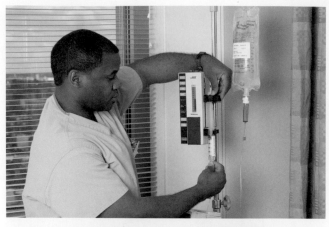

FIGURE 8-16
Inserting syringe into mini-infusion pump.

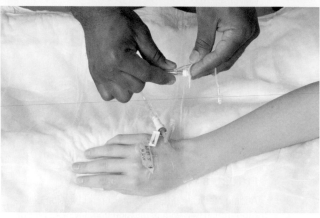

FIGURE 8-17
Cleaning access port closest to IV insertion site.

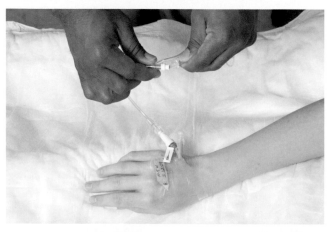

FIGURE 8-18
Connecting secondary infusion tubing to primary infusion.

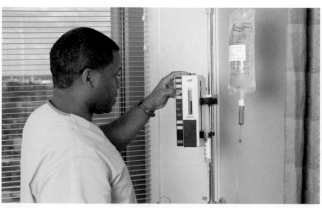

FIGURE 8-19
Programming mini-infusion pump.

This section considers the calculation of pediatric doses for IVP and IVPB administration.

> **STEPS TO SOLVING PARENTERAL PEDIATRIC MEDICATIONS IVP**
>
> **STEP 1.** Convert ounces to pounds, then convert pounds to kilograms.
>
> **STEP 2.** Determine the safe dose range in milligrams per kilogram by using a drug reference (such as a drug book or drug insert).
>
> **STEP 3.** Decide whether the ordered dose is safe by comparing the order with the safe dosage range listed in the reference.
>
> **STEP 4.** Calculate the dose needed.
>
> **STEP 5.** Check the reference for diluent and duration for administration.

Duration of Administration for IVP Drugs

To determine how fast to push the medication, you can take the volume calculated and divide by the minutes. Then take that number and divide by 4; the answer tells you approximately how much to push every 15 seconds. Or you can divide that number by 6, and the answer is approximately how much to push every 10 seconds. The important point is to push the drug slowly over the time period required and to monitor the IV infusion site. Again, a syringe pump is often used to administer IVP drugs.

EXAMPLE

> Order: cimetidine (Tagamet) 100 mg IV bid
>
> Child: 5 years; weight, 44 lb
>
> Literature: 20 to 40 mg/kg/day in divided doses q6h
>
> Dilute with 20 mL with 5% dextrose or 0.9% sodium chloride and injected over at least 2 minutes.
>
> Supply: See label (Fig. 8-20).

Step 1. Convert pounds to kilograms:

$$\begin{array}{r} 20 \\ 2.2\overline{)44.0} \\ \underline{44} \\ 0 \end{array}$$

The child weighs 20 kg.

Step 2. Determine the safe dose:

$$\begin{array}{r} 20 \text{ mg} \\ \times\ 20 \text{ kg} \\ \hline 400 \text{ mg} \end{array} \qquad \begin{array}{r} 40 \text{ mg} \\ \times\ 20 \text{ kg} \\ \hline 800 \text{ mg} \end{array}$$

Divide by 4 (since ordered q6h) to get milligrams per dose:

$$\frac{400}{4} = 100 \text{ mg} \qquad \frac{800}{4} = 200 \text{ mg}$$

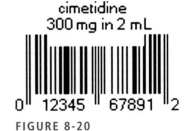

FIGURE 8-20

Cimetidine (Tagamet). (Courtesy of DeKalb Medical Center, Decatur, GA.)

Step 3.   The dose is safe. It meets the milligrams per kilogram range (100 mg).

Step 4.   Calculate the dose.

Formula Method	Proportion	Dimensional Analysis
$\dfrac{100\ mg}{300\ mg} \times 2\ mL = \dfrac{2}{3}$ or 0.67 mL	**EXPRESSED AS TWO RATIOS** 2 mL : 300 mg : : x : 100 mg **EXPRESSED AS TWO FRACTIONS** $\dfrac{2\ mL}{300\ mg} \times \dfrac{x}{100\ mg}$ **SOLUTION FOR BOTH PROPORTION METHODS** $200 = 300x$ $\dfrac{200}{300} = x$ $0.67\ mL = x$	$\dfrac{2\ \text{mL}}{300\ mg} \left| \dfrac{100\ mg}{} \right. = \dfrac{2}{3} = 0.67\ mL$

Step 5.   Dilute with 20 mL of suggested diluent. Inject over 2 minutes.

EXAMPLE

Order: furosemide (Lasix) 40 mg IV bid

Child: 10 years; weight, 40 kg.

Literature: 1 mg/kg q12h IV, no more than 6 mg/kg/day

Inject directly or into tubing of actively running IV; inject slowly over 1 to 2 minutes.

Supply: See label (Fig. 8-21).

Step 1.   Weight is in kilograms: 40 kg

Step 2.   1 mg/kg:

40 kg = 40 mg

Step 3.   40 mg bid would be a total of 80 mg:

Maximum dose: 6 mg/kg/day

40 kg × 6 = 240 mg

The dose is safe.

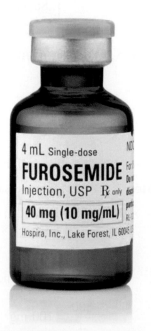

FIGURE 8-21

Furosemide (Lasix). (Courtesy of DeKalb Medical Center, Decatur, GA.)

Step 4. Calculate the dose needed.

Formula Method	Proportion	Dimensional Analysis
$\overset{4}{\dfrac{\cancel{40}\ mg}{\underset{1}{\cancel{10}\ mg}}} \times 1\ mL = 4\ mL$	**EXPRESSED AS TWO RATIOS** 1 mL : 10 mg :: x : 40 mg **EXPRESSED AS TWO FRACTIONS** $\dfrac{1\ mL}{10\ mg} \times \dfrac{x}{40\ mg}$ **SOLUTION FOR BOTH** **PROPORTION METHODS** $40 = 10x$ $\dfrac{40}{10} = x$ $4\ mL = x$	$\dfrac{1\ \cancel{mL}}{10\ \cancel{mg}}\ \bigg|\ \dfrac{40\ \cancel{mg}}{} = 4\ mL$

Step 5. Check the reference for diluent and duration for administration. To inject 4 mL over 2 minutes, you can push about ½ mL every 15 seconds. You may also use a syringe pump if available.

EXAMPLE

Order: morphine 1.5 mg IV stat

Child: 79 lb

Literature: 0.05 mg/kg/dose

Inject directly or into tubing of actively running IV; inject slowly over 1 to 2 minutes.

Supply: See label (Fig. 8-22)

Step 1. Convert pounds to kilograms.

$$\overset{35.90}{\underset{2\,2}{\overset{79}{}}\,)\,\overline{79\,0}}$$

$$\begin{array}{r} 66 \\ \hline 13\,0 \\ 11\,0 \\ \hline 2\,00 \\ 1\,98 \\ \hline 20 \end{array}$$

The child weighs 35.9 kg.

Step 2. Determine the safe dose.

$$\begin{array}{r} 35.9\ kg \\ \times\ 0.05\ mg \\ \hline 1.795\ mg\ \text{(maximum dose)} \end{array}$$

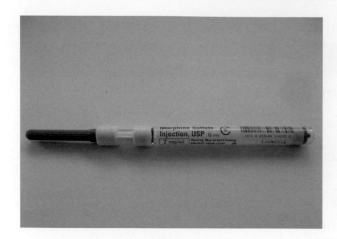

FIGURE 8-22
Morphine syringe.

Step 3. The dose is 1.5 mg.

The dose is safe.

Step 4. Calculate the dose. Morphine 2 mg in 1 mL.

Formula Method	Proportion	Dimensional Analysis
$\dfrac{1.5 \text{ mg}}{2 \text{ mg}} \times 1 \text{ mL}$ $= \dfrac{1.5}{2} = 0.75 \text{ mg}$	**EXPRESSED AS TWO RATIOS** 1 mL : 2 mg :: x mL : 1.5 mg **EXPRESSED AS TWO FRACTIONS** $\dfrac{1 \text{ mL}}{2 \text{ mg}} \times \dfrac{x \text{ mL}}{1.5 \text{ mg}}$ **SOLUTION FOR BOTH PROPORTION METHODS** 1.5 mg = 2x $\dfrac{1.5}{2} = x$ 0.75 = x	$\dfrac{1 \text{ mL}}{2 \text{ mg}} \Big| \dfrac{1.5 \text{ mg}}{}$ $= \dfrac{1.5}{2} = 0.75 \text{ mL}$

Give slowly over 1–2 minutes. Flush with normal saline. You may also use a syringe pump.

EXAMPLE

Order: atropine 0.35 mg IV × 1 for preoperative sedation.

Child: 70 lb

Literature: 0.01–0.02 mg/kg/dose

Inject directly into running IV over 1–2 minutes.

Supply: See label (Fig. 8-23)

Step 1. Convert pounds to kilograms

$$
\begin{array}{r}
31.818 \\
22 \overline{\smash{\big)}\, 70\,0} \\
\underline{66} \\
4\,0 \\
\underline{2\,2} \\
1\,80 \\
\underline{1\,76} \\
40 \\
\underline{22} \\
180
\end{array}
$$

The child weight is 31.82 kg

Step 2. Determine the safe dose.

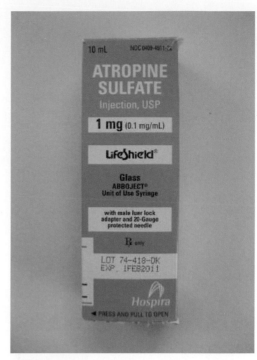

FIGURE 8-23
Atropine injection.

Low Dose	*High Dose*
31.82 kg	31.82 kg
× 0.01 mg	× 0.02 mg
0.3182 mg	0.6364 mg

Step 3. The dose 0.35 mg is safe.

Step 4. Calculate the dose.

Formula Method	Proportion	Dimensional Analysis
$\dfrac{0.35 \text{ mg}}{1 \text{ mg}} \times 10 \text{ mL}$ $= 3.5 \text{ mL}$	**EXPRESSED AS TWO RATIOS** 10 mL : 1 mg :: x : 0.35 mg **EXPRESSED AS TWO FRACTIONS** $\dfrac{10 \text{ mL}}{1 \text{ mg}} \times \dfrac{x}{0.35 \text{ mg}}$ **SOLUTION FOR BOTH PROPORTION METHODS** 0.35 × 10 mL = x 3.5 mL = x	$\dfrac{10 \text{ mL}}{1 \text{ mg}} \Bigg| \dfrac{0.35 \text{ mg}}{}$ $= 3.5 \text{ mL}$

Step 5. Inject over 1–2 minutes. Check the reference for diluent and duration of administration. You can also use a syringe pump.

When using a syringe pump (Fig. 8-12) for IVP drugs, the drugs are often pre mixed by the pharmacy. Included on the label is the patient name, medical record number, drug, dose, patient weight, and how long to administer the drug on the syringe pump (see Figs. 8-24 and 8-25). After administering the dose, there is usually a flush of normal saline of the tubing to ensure all the drug gets to the patient. Follow hospital policy for the amount of flush.

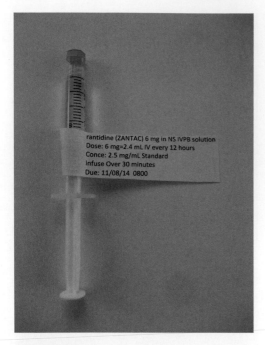

FIGURE 8-24
Ranitidine (Zantac) pre-mixed syringe.

rantidine (ZANTAC) 6 mg in NS IVPB solution
Dose: 6 mg=2.4 mL IV every 12 hours
Conce: 2.5 mg/mL Standard
Infuse Over 30 minutes
Due: 11/08/14 0800

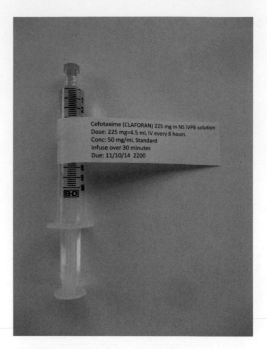

FIGURE 8-25
Cefotaxime (Claforan) pre-mixed syringe.

Cefotaxime (CLAFORAN) 225 mg in NS IVPB solution
Dose: 225 mg=4.5 mL IV every 8 hours
Conc: 50 mg/mL Standard
Infuse over 30 minutes
Due: 11/10/14 2200

STEPS TO SOLVE PARENTERAL PEDIATRIC MEDICATIONS IVPB

STEP 1. Convert ounces to pounds then convert pounds to kilograms dividing by 2.2.

STEP 2. Determine the safe dose range in milligrams per kilogram by using a reference (such as a drug book or drug insert).

STEP 3. Decide whether the ordered dose is safe by comparing the order with the safe dose range listed in the reference. Decide whether the dilution ordered meets the minimum pediatric standard by using a reference (such as a drug book or drug insert).

STEP 4. Calculate the dose needed.

STEP 5. Prepare the medication according to directions, and dilute further as needed. Add to the Buretrol (or use a syringe pump).

STEP 6. Set the pump in milliliters per hour. If the infusion time is 30 minutes, set the pump for double the amount because the pump delivers in milliliters per hour.

> **EXAMPLE** The order is 10 mL over 30 minutes. Set the pump for 20 mL/hour. It will deliver 10 mL in 30 minutes.

STEP 7. When the IV is completed, add an additional 20 mL of the IV fluid as a flush to the Buretrol to clear the tubing of the medication. Be sure to chart the flush and IVPB fluid as fluid intake. Follow institutional requirements regarding IV flush.

EXAMPLE

Order: ceftazidime (Fortaz) 280 mg IV q8h in 10 mL D5½ normal saline (NS)

Child: 4 years; weight, 17 kg

Literature: Safe dose 30 to 50 mg/kg/day
Concentration for IV use: 50 mg/mL over 30 minutes (Table 8-1)

Supply: 1 g powder. Directions: Dilute with 10 mL sterile water for injection to make 95 mg/mL; stable for 7 days if refrigerated (Fig. 8-26).

1. Weight is 17 kg.

2. Safe dose is 30 to 50 mg/kg/day.

Low Dose	*High Dose*
30 mg	50 mg
× 17 kg	× 17 kg
510 mg/day	850 mg/day

3. Order is 280 mg q8h (three doses):

280 mg × 3 = 840 mg

Dose falls within the range and is safe.

Minimum safe dilution is 50 mg/mL. Dose is 280 mg.

$$
\begin{array}{r}
5.6 \\
50\overline{)280} \\
250 \\
\hline
300 \\
300
\end{array}
$$

5.6 or 6 mL, the minimum dilution. The order of 10 mL is safe because it is more than the minimum.

TABLE 8-1 Sample of a Dilution Table for Pediatric Antibiotics

Antibiotic	Recommended Final Concentration IV	Recommended Duration of IV
Ampicillin	50 mg/mL	10–30 min
Ceftazidime (Fortaz)	50 mg/mL	10–30 min
Clindamycin (Cleocin)	6–12 mg/mL	15–30 min
Gentamicin (Garamycin)	2 mg/mL	15–30 min
Penicillin G	Infants: 50,000 units/mL Large child: 100,000 units/mL	10–30 min
Pentamidine (Nebupent)	2.5 mg/mL	1 h

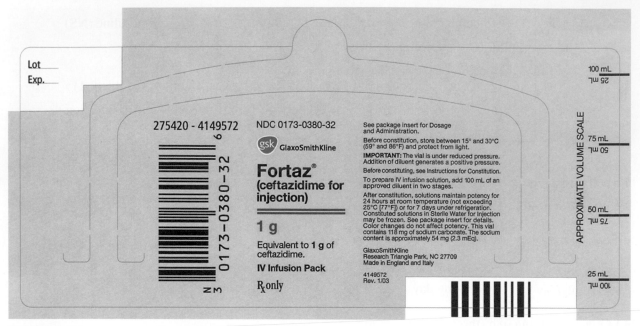

FIGURE 8-26

Label for ceftazidime (Fortaz). (Courtesy of GlaxoSmithKline.)

4. Dilute 1 g with 10 mL sterile water to make 95 mg/mL.

Formula Method	Proportion	Dimensional Analysis
$\dfrac{280 \text{ mg}}{95 \text{ mg}} \times 1 \text{ mL} = 2.9 \text{ mL}$	**EXPRESSED AS TWO RATIOS** 1 mL : 95 mg :: x : 280 mg **EXPRESSED AS TWO FRACTIONS** $\dfrac{1 \text{ mL}}{95 \text{ mg}} \times \dfrac{\text{x}}{280 \text{ mg}}$ **SOLUTION FOR BOTH PROPORTION METHODS** $280 = 95\text{x}$ $\dfrac{280}{95} = \text{x}$ $2.9 \text{ mL} = \text{x}$	$\dfrac{1 \text{ mL}}{95 \text{ mg}} \left| \dfrac{280 \text{ mg}}{} \right. = \dfrac{280}{95} = 2.9 \text{ mL}$

Withdraw 2.9 mL; label the vial and store in the refrigerator.

5. Add 10 mL from the D5½NS IV bag into the Buretrol. Add the 2.9 mL of the drug.

6. Set the pump at 20 mL/hour. The pump will deliver 10 mL in 30 minutes.

7. When the IV is completed, add an additional 20 mL of the D5½NS IV bag into the Buretrol as a flush to clear the IV tubing of medication. (Run over 5 to 10 minutes to clear the tubing.)

EXAMPLE

> Order: ampicillin 100 mg IV q6h in 10 mL D5½NS
>
> Infant: 4.3 kg
>
> Literature: The safe dose is 75 to 200 mg/kg/24 hours given q6–8h IV.
>
> Concentration for IV use: 50 mg/mL over 10 to 30 minutes (see Table 8-1).
>
> Supply: Vial of powder labeled 500 mg. Directions: Add 1.8 mL sterile water for injection to make 250 mg/mL; use within 1 hour.

1. Weight is 4.3 kg.

2. Safe dose is 75 to 200 mg/kg/24 hours given q6–8h.

Low Dose	*High Dose*
75 mg	200 mg
× 4.3 kg	× 4.3 kg
322.5 mg/24 hours	860 mg/24 hours

3. Order is 100 mg q6h (four doses):

   100 mg × 4 doses = 400 mg

   This is within the range. The dose is safe.

   Minimum safe dilution is 50 mg/mL. Dose is 100 mg.

   $$\frac{2}{50)\overline{100}} \text{ mL is the minimum dilution; 10 mL is safe.}$$

4. Add 1.8 mL sterile water for injection to 500 mg powder to make 250 mg/mL.

Formula Method	Proportion	Dimensional Analysis
$\dfrac{100 \text{ mg}}{250 \text{ mg}} \times 1 \text{ mL} = \dfrac{2}{5}$ $= 0.4 \text{ mL}$	**EXPRESSED AS TWO RATIOS** 1 mL : 250 mg :: x : 100 mg **EXPRESSED AS TWO FRACTIONS** $\dfrac{1 \text{ mL}}{250 \text{ mg}} \times \dfrac{x}{100 \text{ mg}}$ **SOLUTION FOR BOTH PROPORTION METHODS** $100 = 250x$ $\dfrac{100}{250} = x$ $0.4 \text{ mL} = x$	$\dfrac{1 \text{ mL}}{250 \text{ mg}} \left| \dfrac{100 \text{ mg}}{} \right. = \dfrac{100}{250} = 0.4 \text{ mL}$

Withdraw 0.4 mL from the vial. Discard the remainder (directions say to use within 1 hour).

5. Add 10 mL from the D5½NS IV bag into the Buretrol. Add the 0.4 mL of the drug.

6. Set the pump at 20 mL/hour. The pump will deliver 10 mL in 30 minutes.

7. When the IV is finished, add an additional 20 mL of the D5½NS bag into the Buretrol as a flush to clear the tubing of medication. (Run over 5 to 10 minutes to clear the tubing.)

EXAMPLE

Order: ceftriaxone (Rocephin) 600 mg IV q12h in 20 mL D5½NS

Child: 3 years; weight, 15 kg

Literature: safe dose up to 100 mg/kg/day in two divided doses

Concentration for IV use: 50 mg/mL over 30 minutes

Supply: 1 g powder. Directions: Dilute with 9.6 mL sterile water for injection to make 100 mg/mL; stable for 7 days if refrigerated (Fig. 8-27).

1. Weight is 15 kg.

2. Safe dose is up to 100 mg/kg/day:

$$\begin{array}{r} 100 \\ \times\ \ 15 \\ \hline 1500 \end{array}$$ mg/day or two divided doses of 750 mg each.

3. Order is 600 mg q12h (two doses).

   600 mg × 2 = 1200 mg

   The dose falls within the range and therefore is safe.

   Minimum safe dilution is 150 mg/mL. The dose is 600 mg.

   $$\frac{600}{150} = 4$$

   4 mL is the minimal dilution; 20 mL is safe.

4. Dilute 1 g with 9.6 mL sterile water to make 100 mg/mL.

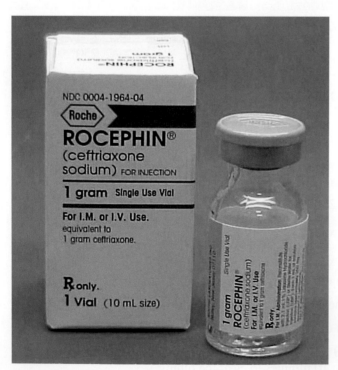

FIGURE 8-27

Ceftriaxone (Rocephin). (Reprinted with permission of Roche Laboratories, Inc. All rights reserved.)

Withdraw 6 mL; label the vial and store in the refrigerator.

Formula Method	Proportion	Dimensional Analysis
$\dfrac{600 \text{ mg}}{100 \text{ mg}} \times 1 \text{ mL} = x$ $= 6 \text{ mL}$	**EXPRESSED AS TWO RATIOS** 1 mL : 100 mg :: x : 600 mg **EXPRESSED AS TWO FRACTIONS** $\dfrac{1 \text{ mL}}{100 \text{ mg}} \times \dfrac{x}{600 \text{ mg}}$ **SOLUTION FOR BOTH PROPORTION METHODS** $600 = 100x$ $\dfrac{600}{100} = x$ $6 \text{ mL} = x$	$\dfrac{1 \text{ mL}}{100 \text{ mg}} \Big| \dfrac{600 \text{ mg}}{} = 6 \text{ mL}$

5. Add 20 mL from the D5½NS IV bag into the Buretrol. Add the 6 mL of the drug.

6. Set the pump at 40 mL/hour. The pump will deliver 20 mL in 30 minutes.

7. When the IV is completed, add an additional 20 mL of the D5½NS IV bag as a flush to clear the medication from the tubing. (Run over 5 to 10 minutes to clear the tubing.)

General Guidelines for Continuous IV Medications

1. Calculate continuous IV medications for children and infants by using the methods and formulas used in Chapter 6.

2. Continuous IV dosages are based on weight in kilograms.

3. Always use an infusion pump and/or volume control sets, or syringe pumps.

4. Use small bags of fluid to prevent fluid overload.

5. Follow institutional requirements for continuous IV infusions and IVP drugs.

6. To determine the safe dosage range, consult a pediatric text, drug reference, or drug insert.

7. Some IV medications, such as vancomycin or gentamycin, require periodic peak and trough blood levels to ensure that these drugs are not causing nephrotoxicity. Follow institutional policy.

In these practice problems, determine whether the dose is safe, calculate the amount needed, and state how the order should be administered. Round the lb to kg weight conversions to the nearest hundredth. Answers appear at the end of this chapter. Follow the steps used in the examples.

1. Order: cefuroxime (Ceftin) 200 mg IV q6h in 10 mL D5½NS
   Infant: 6 months; weight, 8 kg
   Supply: 750-mg vial of powder. Directions: Dilute with 8 mL sterile water for injection to make 90 mg/mL; stable for 3 days if refrigerated.
   Literature: The safe dose is 50 to 100 mg/kg/24 hours given q6–8h.
                Concentration for IV use: 50 mg/mL over 30 minutes

2. Order: trimethoprim/sulfamethoxazole (Bactrim) 75 mg IV q12h in 75 mL D5W over 1 hour
   Child: 3 years; weight, 15 kg
   Supply: Vial labeled 80 mg/5 mL
   Literature: Safe dose for a child is 8 to 10 mg/kg/24 hours given q12h
                Concentration for IV use: 1 mL in 15 to 25 mL (supply is a liquid)

3. Order: tobramycin (Nebcin) 100 mg IV q8h in 50 mL D5½NS
   Child: 12 years; weight, 40 kg
   Supply: vial 80 mg/2 mL
   Literature: The safe dose is 3 to 5 mg/kg/24 hours given q8h.
                Concentration for IV use: 2 mg/mL over 15 to 30 minutes

4. Order: cefotaxime (Claforan) 900 mg IV q6h in 25 mL D5½NS
   Child: 5 years; weight, 18 kg
   Supply: 1 g powder. Directions: Dilute with 10 mL sterile water for injection to make 95 mg/mL; stable in the refrigerator 10 days.
   Literature: The safe dose is 50 to 200 mg/kg/24 hours given q6h.
                Concentration for IV use: 50 mg/mL; give over 30 minutes

5. Order: nafcillin (Unipen) 150 mg IV q8h in 10 mL D5½NS
   Infant: 3 months; weight, 6 kg
   Supply: 500-mg vial of powder. Directions: Add 1.7 mL sterile water for injection to make 500 mg/2 mL; stable for 48 hours if refrigerated.
   Literature: The safe dose is 100 to 200 mg/kg/24 hours given q6h.
                Concentration for IV use: 6 mg/mL over 30 to 60 minutes

6. Order: morphine 2.5 mg IVP q4h
   Child: 8 years; weight, 30 kg
   Supply: morphine injection 1 mg/mL
   Literature: 0.05 to 0.1 mg/kg/q4h IVP. Dilute 2 to 10 mg in at least 5 mL NS. Administer over 4 to 5 minutes.

7. Order: dexamethasone (Decadron) 4 mg IVP bid
   Child: 6 years; weight, 25 kg
   Supply: Decadron 4 mg/mL injection
   Literature: 0.08 to 0.3 mg/kg/day divided q6–12h. Give undiluted IVP over 30 seconds or less.

8. Order: diphenhydramine (Benadryl) 25 mg IVP q4–6h
   Child: 12 years; weight, 45 kg
   Supply: 50 mg/mL injection
   Literature: 12.5 to 25 mg IV q4–6h; maximum dose, 300 mg/24 hours
                Give undiluted IVP over 1 minute.

| SELF-TEST 5 | Parenteral Medication Calculations (Continued) |

9. Order: digoxin (Lanoxin) maintenance dose IVP 50 mcg/day
    Infant: 15 lb
    Supply: 0.1 mg/mL injection
    Literature: 6 to 7.5 mcg/kg/day. Give undiluted or diluted in 4 mL D5W or NS over
                 5 minutes.

10. Order: methylprednisolone (Solu-Medrol) IVP 60 mg bid
    Child: 9 years; weight, 80 lb
    Supply: Solu-Medrol 40 mg/mL
    Literature: 0.5 to 1.7 mg/kg/day divided q12h. Give each 500 mg over 2 to 3 minutes.

| CRITICAL THINKING | TEST YOUR CLINICAL SAVVY |

You are working in a pediatric unit and taking care of 5-year-old Georgia Smith. Although she usually has a sweet disposition, she has her moments when she will not do anything she doesn't want to do. She is receiving IV fluids continuously and is ordered an oral medication three times a day that has an aftertaste. Each time the medication is brought to her, she refuses to take it.

A. What are techniques to help her take the medication?
B. Are there other alternatives you could use regarding the medication? How would you implement any of these alternatives?
C. Are there strategies to suggest to the family to promote easier compliance?
D. Besides reducing the possibility of fluid overload, what are some other reasons IV infusion pumps are used with children?

Another patient/client, 14-year-old Sean McBrady, is unable to swallow pills.

A. What are some alternatives to the medication?
B. Are there contraindications to any of the medication alternatives?
C. What are some ways to get children to swallow pills?
D. What would you suggest to the family to promote easier administration?

Putting it Together

Andy Bee is a 7 year old admitted to the emergency room with a 6-hour history of wheezing. The mother reports a history of "flulike" symptoms for 48 hours. He has not had any solid food for 2 days and had minimal fluid intake.

Past Medical History: Premature birth at 32 weeks. The child was on a ventilator for 1 week post-partum. Small birth weight. Asthma.

Allergies: Penicillin, causing rash and hives

Current Vital Signs: Blood pressure is 110/80, pulse 120 to 140/minute, respirations 29/minute, oxygen saturation 95%, temp 101.8, weight 30 kg

Medication Orders

methylprednisolone (Solu-Medrol) *corticosteroid, glucocorticoid* 20 mg IVP × 1, then 10 mg every 6 hours

albuterol (Proventil) *bronchodilator* 0.6 mL in 3 mL NS per nebulizer every 20 minutes × 3

acetaminophen (Tylenol) *antipyretic* liquid 400 mg po for temp >101 prn q4h

NS 10 mL/kg for 1 hour, then 100 mL/hour

ibuprofen (Motrin) *anti-inflammatory* 5 mg/kg po q6h prn for continued temp >101 if not relieved by acetaminophen (Tylenol)

ceftazidime (Fortaz) *anti-infective* 2 g IVPB q8h in 50 mL D5½NS

digoxin (Lanoxin) *cardiac glycoside* 0.72 mg/m^2 po every day

amoxicillin/clavulante (Augmentin) *anti-infective* 150 mg po q8h

ondansetron (Zofran) 0.1 mg/kg IV q8h prn nausea

Calculations

1. Calculate how many milliliters of Solu-Medrol to give. Available: Solu-Medrol vial that yields 20 mg/mL.

   a. One time dose of 20 mg

   b. Scheduled dose 10 mg every 6 hours

Putting it Together (*Continued*)

2. Calculate how many milliliters and how many teaspoons of acetaminophen (Tylenol) elixir to give.

Available: liquid acetaminophen (Tylenol) 160 mg/5 mL.

a. Conversion to milliliters

b. Conversion to teaspoons

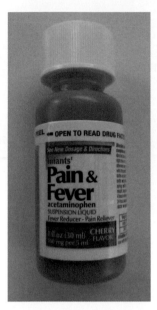

3. Calculate how many milligrams of Advil to give and how many milliliters to administer.
Available: 100 mg/5 mL.

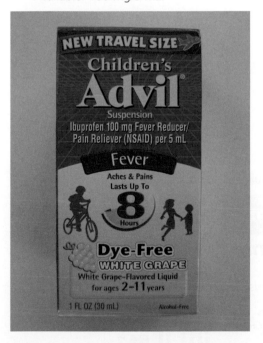

(continued)

Putting it Together (*Continued*)

4. Calculate how many milliliters of Fortaz to prepare. Calculate the infusion rate. Available: 2-g vial of powder. Dilute initially with 10 mL sterile water for injection to yield 50 mg/mL. Infuse over 30 minutes.

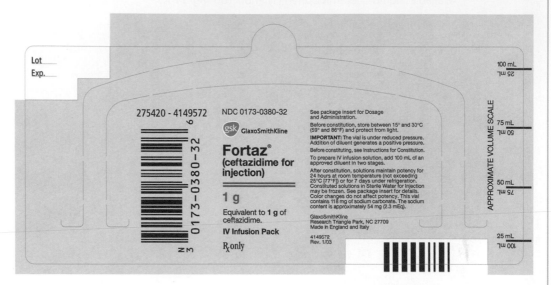

5. Calculate the dose of Digoxin. BSA is 0.9 m^2

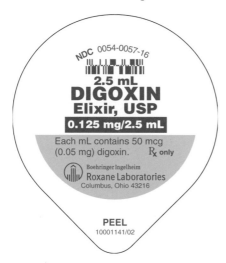

6. Calculate the dose of Augmentin. Available: 125 mg/5 mL.

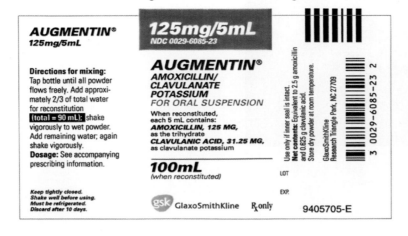

Putting it Together (*Continued*)

7. Calculate how many milligrams of Zofran. Is the dose safe? Available is 2 mg/mL. Literature states the safe dose is single dose of 0.1 mg/kg patients weighing 40 kg or less, inject over 2–5 minutes

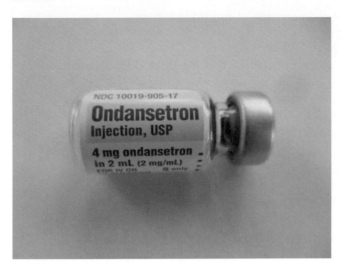

8. Calculate the amount of NS to infuse the first hour.

Critical Thinking Questions

1. Should any medication(s) be held and if so why?

2. What medication(s) should be questioned and why?

3. What route of medication may be difficult for this patient/client? What are some alternatives to medication administration for this patient/client?

4. Is the amount of NS to infuse abnormally high for this patient/client? Why or why not?

Answers in Appendix B.

PROFICIENCY TEST 1	Infants and Children Dosage Problems

*Name:*_____

Here is a mix of oral and parenteral pediatric orders. For each problem, determine the safe dose and calculate the amount to give. Round the lb to kg weight conversions to the nearest hundredth. Answers are given in Appendix A.

1. Order: vitamin K (Aquamephyton) 1 mg IM × 1 dose
   Newborn: weight, 4 kg
   Supply: vial 10 mg/mL
   Literature: Prophylaxis and treatment: 0.5 to 1 mg/dose IM, subcutaneous, IV × 1

2. Order: amoxicillin/clavulante (Augmentin) 125 mg po q8h
   Infant: 1 yr; 10 kg
   Supply: 125 mg/5 mL
   Literature: Safe dose amoxicillin/clavulanate (Augmentin): 20 to 40 mg/kg/24 hours given q8h po

3. Order: benzathine penicillin 500,000 units IM × 1 dose
   Infant: 10 months; weight, 10 kg
   Supply: vial labeled 600,000 units/mL
   Literature: Safe dose 50,000 units/kg × 1 IM. Maximum, 2.4 milliunits.

4. Order: gentamicin (Garamycin) 9 mg IV q8h in 10 mL D5½NS
   Infant: 3.6 kg
   Supply: vial 40 mg/mL
   Literature: Safe dose is 2.5 mg/kg/dose q8h.
   Concentration for IV 2 mg/mL given over 15 to 30 minutes

5. Order: docusate (Colace Syrup) 10 mg po bid
   Infant: 6.7 kg
   Supply: 20 mg/5 mL
   Literature: Infants and children under 3 years of age: 10 to 40 mg/day

6. Order: vancomycin (Vancocin) 54 mg IV q8h in 12 mL D5½NS
   Infant: 5.5 kg
   Supply: 500 mg powder
   Add 10 mL sterile water for injection to give 50 mg/mL; stable in the refrigerator 14 days.
   Literature: Safe dose is 10 mg/kg q8h IV.
   Concentration for IV 5 mg/mL; infuse over 1 hour

7. Order: chloral hydrate 350 mg po prior to electroencephalogram
   Infant: 6.7 kg
   Supply: 500 mg/5 mL
   Literature: Hypnotic for children: 25 to 50 mg/kg/dose po not to exceed 100 mg/kg

8. Order: methotrexate 10 mg po 1 to 2×/week
   Child: 12 years; height, 60 inches; weight, 40 kg; BSA, 1.32
   Supply: 2.5-mg tablet
   Literature: 7.5 to 30 mg/m^2 1 to 2×/week

9. Order: ceftazidime (Fortaz) 2 g IVPB q8h in 50 mL D5½NS
   Child: 8 years; weight, 24 kg
   Supply: 2-g vial of powder
   Dilute initially with 10 mL sterile water for injection.
   Literature: Safe dose is 2 to 6 g/24 hours given q8–12h IV
   Concentration for IV 50 mg/mL over 15 to 30 minutes

10. Order: morphine 4 mg IVP stat
    Child: weight, 35 lb
    Supply: 4 mg/mL
    Literature: Usual dose 0.05 to 0.2 mg/kg/dose q3–4h prn. Maximum dose, 15 mg.

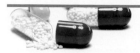

Answers

Self-Test 1 Converting Pounds to Kilograms

1. 13.64 kg

2. $\dfrac{5 \text{ oz}}{16 \text{ oz}} = 0.3125$ lb

Weight = 15.3125 lb

Change to kilograms:

$\dfrac{15.3125}{2.2} = 6.96$ kg

3. ¼ lb = 0.25 lb

Weight = 7.25 lb

Change to kilograms:

$\dfrac{7.25}{2.2} = 3.3$ kg

4. 10 kg

5. $\dfrac{8 \text{ oz}}{16 \text{ oz}} = 0.5$ lb

Weight = 54.5 lb

Change to kilograms:

$\dfrac{54.5 \text{ lb}}{2.2} = 24.77$ kg

6. $\dfrac{5 \text{ oz}}{16 \text{ oz}} = 0.3125$ lb

Weight = 4.3125 lb

$\dfrac{4.3125}{2.2} = 1.96$ kg

7. $\dfrac{75 \text{ lb}}{2.2} = 34.09$ kg

8. $\dfrac{3 \text{ oz}}{16 \text{ oz}} = 0.1875$ lb

Weight = 12.1875 lb

$\dfrac{12.1875}{2.2} = 5.54$ kg

9. $\dfrac{66 \text{ lb}}{2.2} = 30$ kg

10. ½ lb = 0.5 lb

Weight = 10.5 lb

$\dfrac{10.5}{2.2} = 4.77$ kg

Self-Test 2 Dosage Calculations

1. Step 1. $\dfrac{20}{2.2} = 9.09$ kg

Step 2. Low dose
$$\begin{array}{r} 9.09 \text{ kg} \\ \times\ 20 \text{ mg} \\ \hline 181.8 \text{ mg/day} \end{array}$$

High dose
$$\begin{array}{r} 9.09 \text{ kg} \\ \times\ 40 \text{ mg} \\ \hline 363.6 \text{ mg/day} \end{array}$$

Step 3. 60 mg × 3 doses = 180 mg/day
The order is safe, although on the low side.

(continued)

Answers (Continued)

Step 4.

Formula Method	Proportion	Dimensional Analysis
$\dfrac{60 \text{ mg}}{125 \text{ mg}} \times 5 \text{ mL} = 2.4 \text{ mL}$	**EXPRESSED AS TWO RATIOS** $5 \text{ mL} : 125 \text{ mg} :: x : 60 \text{ mg}$ **EXPRESSED AS TWO FRACTIONS** $\dfrac{5 \text{ mL}}{125 \text{ mg}} \times \dfrac{x}{60 \text{ mg}}$ **SOLUTION FOR BOTH PROPORTION METHODS** $60 \times 5 = 125x$ $\dfrac{300}{125} = x$ $2.4 \text{ mL} = x$	$\dfrac{\overset{1}{\cancel{5}} \ \text{(mL)}}{\underset{5}{\cancel{125}} \text{ mg}} \Bigg| \overset{12}{\cancel{60}} \text{ mg} = \dfrac{12}{5} = 2.4 \text{ mL}$

Give 2.4 mL po q8h.

2. Step 1. 29 lb = 13.18 kg

Step 2.
$$
\begin{array}{r}
40 \text{ mg} \\
\times\ 13.18 \text{ kg} \\
\hline
527.27 \text{ mg/day}
\end{array}
$$

Step 3. 175 mg × 3 doses = 525 mg/day. The order is safe.

$$
\begin{array}{r}
175 \text{ mg} \\
\times\quad 3 \text{ doses} \\
\hline
525 \text{ mg/day}
\end{array}
$$

Step 4.

Formula Method	Proportion	Dimensional Analysis
$\dfrac{\overset{7}{\cancel{175}} \text{ mg}}{\underset{1}{\underset{25}{\cancel{125}}} \text{ mg}} \times \overset{1}{\cancel{5}} \text{ mL} = 7 \text{ mL}$	**EXPRESSED AS TWO RATIOS** $5 \text{ mL} : 125 \text{ mg} :: x : 175 \text{ mg}$ **EXPRESSED AS TWO FRACTIONS** $\dfrac{5 \text{ mL}}{125 \text{ mg}} \times \dfrac{x}{175 \text{ mg}}$ **SOLUTION FOR BOTH PROPORTION METHODS** $5 \times 175 = 125x$ $\dfrac{875}{125} = x$ $7 \text{ mL} = x$	$\dfrac{\overset{1}{\cancel{5}} \ \text{(mL)}}{\underset{1}{\underset{25}{\cancel{125}}} \text{ mg}} \Bigg| \overset{7}{\cancel{175}} \text{ mg} = 7 \text{ mL}$

Give 7 mL po q8h.

3. It was not necessary to use Steps 1 and 2. The literature was clear. Children 6 to 12 years should receive 600 mg divided into three doses, which equals 200 mg/dose. The ordered dose is safe.

Step 4.

Formula Method	Proportion	Dimensional Analysis
$\dfrac{200}{125} \times 5 = \dfrac{1000}{125} \quad 125\overline{)1000.}\;\;8.0\text{ mL}$	**EXPRESSED AS TWO RATIOS** $5\text{ mL}:125\text{ mg}::x:200\text{ mg}$ **EXPRESSED AS TWO FRACTIONS** $\dfrac{5\text{ mL}}{125\text{ mg}} \bowtie \dfrac{x}{200\text{ mg}}$ **SOLUTION FOR BOTH PROPORTION METHODS** $5 \times 200 = 125x$ $\dfrac{1000}{125} = x$ $8\text{ mL} = x$	$\dfrac{\overset{1}{5}\;\text{(mL)}}{\underset{\underset{1}{25}}{125\text{ mg}}} \Big| \dfrac{\overset{8}{200}\text{ mg}}{} = 8\text{ mL}$

Give 8 mL po tid.

4. Tylenol 80 mg is a low dose. Literature says a child of 6 years should receive four chewable tablets. This would be 320 mg. (4×80 mg) Check with the physician or healthcare provider.

5. The literature states that children under 6 months can receive 1 to 2.5 mg IM three to four times a day. The individual dose for the infant is 1 mg. This is safe, but the physician wrote q3–4h prn for the time. This would allow six to eight doses per 24 hours. The nurse can give the first dose but should clarify the times with the physician or healthcare provider.

Step 4.

Formula Method	Proportion	Dimensional Analysis
$\dfrac{1\text{ mg}}{5\text{ mg}} \times 1\text{ mL} = 0.2\text{ mL IM}$	**EXPRESSED AS TWO RATIOS** $1\text{ mL}:5\text{ mg}::x:1\text{ mg}$ **EXPRESSED AS TWO FRACTIONS** $\dfrac{1\text{ mL}}{5\text{ mg}} \bowtie \dfrac{x}{1\text{ mg}}$ **SOLUTION FOR BOTH PROPORTION METHODS** $1 = 5x$ $\dfrac{1}{5} = x$ $0.2\text{ mL} = x$	$\dfrac{1\;\text{(mL)}}{5\text{ mg}} \Big| \dfrac{1\text{ mg}}{} = \dfrac{1}{5}\text{ or }0.2\text{ mL}$

Give 0.2 mL IM.

(continued)

Answers (Continued)

6. Step 1. Weight 14 kg

   Step 2. **Low Dose**   **High Dose**

$$\begin{array}{r} 0.05 \text{ mg} \\ \times 14 \text{ kg} \\ \hline 0.7 \text{ mg} \end{array}$$
$$\begin{array}{r} 0.2 \text{ mg} \\ \times 14 \text{ kg} \\ \hline 2.8 \text{ mg} \end{array}$$

   Step 3. The dose (2 mg) is safe and does not exceed 15 mg/dose.

   Step 4. The supply is 2 mg per 1 mL. Give 1 mL.

7. Step 1. Weight 30 kg

   Step 2. **Low Dose**   **High Dose**

$$\begin{array}{r} 0.1 \text{ mg} \\ \times 30 \text{ kg} \\ \hline 3 \text{ mg} \end{array}$$
$$\begin{array}{r} 0.2 \text{ mg} \\ \times 30 \text{ kg} \\ \hline 6 \text{ mg} \end{array}$$

   Step 3. The dose (5 mg) is safe.

   Step 4. Supply is 5 mg in 5 mL. Give 5 mL.

8. Step 1. $\dfrac{48 \text{ lb}}{2.2} = 21.82 \text{ kg}$

   Step 2. **Low Dose**   **High Dose**

$$\begin{array}{r} 100 \text{ mg} \\ \times 21.82 \text{ kg} \\ \hline 2182 \text{ mg} \end{array}$$
$$\begin{array}{r} 200 \text{ mg} \\ \times 21.82 \text{ kg} \\ \hline 4364 \text{ mg} \end{array}$$

   Step 3.

   $2182 \text{ divided q6h} = \dfrac{2182}{4} = 545.5$

   $4364 \text{ divided q6h} = \dfrac{4364}{4} = 1091$

   The dose is 0.5 g or 500 mg. The dose is too low. Contact the physician or healthcare provider.

9. Step 1. 30 kg

   Step 2.
$$\begin{array}{r} 30 \text{ kg} \\ \times 10 \text{ mg} \\ \hline 300 \text{ mg} \end{array}$$

   Step 3. The literature states not more than 500 mg/dose. The dose is safe.

Step 4.

Formula Method	Proportion	Dimensional Analysis
$\dfrac{\overset{3}{\cancel{300}} \text{ mg}}{\underset{1}{\cancel{100}} \text{ mg}} \times 5 \text{ mL} = 15 \text{ mL}$	**EXPRESSED AS TWO RATIOS** $5 \text{ mL} : 100 \text{ mg} :: x : 300 \text{ mg}$ **EXPRESSED AS TWO FRACTIONS** $\dfrac{5 \text{ mL}}{100 \text{ mg}} \bowtie \dfrac{x}{300 \text{ mg}}$ **SOLUTION FOR BOTH PROPORTION METHODS** $1500 = 100x$ $\dfrac{1500}{100} = x$ $15 \text{ mL} = x$	$\dfrac{5 \,\cancel{\text{mL}} \;\big|\; \overset{3}{\cancel{300}} \,\cancel{\text{mg}}}{\underset{1}{\cancel{100}} \,\cancel{\text{mg}}} = 15\,\text{mL}$

Give 15 mL × 1 dose.

10. Step 1. $\dfrac{8 \text{ oz}}{16} = 0.5 \text{ lb}$

$\dfrac{12.5 \text{ lb}}{2.2} = 5.68 \text{ kg}$

Step 2.
$$\begin{array}{cc} 5.68 \text{ kg} & 5.68 \text{ kg} \\ \underline{\times \quad 4 \text{ mg}} & \underline{\times \quad 8 \text{ mg}} \\ 22.72 \text{ mg} & 45.44 \text{ mg} \end{array}$$

Step 3. The dose (60 mg) is too high. Check with the physician.

Self-Test 3 Determining Body Surface Area

1. 0.54 m²   **3.** 1.1 m²

2. 0.51 m²   **4.** 0.255 m²

Self-Test 4 Use of Nomogram

1. Step 1. BSA in meters squared: 0.94.

Step 2. Determine safe dose.

Low Dose	*High Dose*
100 mg	200 mg
$\times\ 0.94$	$\times\ 0.94$
94 mg	188 mg

The safe dose is 94 to 188 mg over 24 hours.

Step 3. Is the order safe?

50 mg q8h = 50 mg × 3 = 150 mg/24 hours

The dose is safe.

Step 4. Order is 50 mg; supply is 50 mg. Give 1 tablet q8h.

(continued)

Answers (Continued)

2. Step 1. BSA in meters squared: 1.29.

   Step 2. The safe dose is:

   $$
   \begin{array}{r}
   10 \text{ mg} \\
   \times\ 1.29 \\
   \hline
   12.9 \text{ mg}
   \end{array}
   $$

   Step 3. Is the order safe? Yes; 12.5 mg is below the maximum.

   Step 4.

Formula Method	Proportion	Dimensional Analysis
$$\dfrac{\overset{5}{\cancel{12.5}} \text{ mg}}{\underset{1}{\cancel{2.5}} \text{ mg}} \times 1 \text{ tablet}$$ $$= 5 \text{ tablets}$$	**EXPRESSED AS TWO RATIOS** 1 tablet : 2.5 mg :: x : 12.5 mg **EXPRESSED AS TWO FRACTIONS** $\dfrac{1 \text{ tablet}}{2.5 \text{ mg}} \times \dfrac{x}{12.5 \text{ mg}}$ **SOLUTION FOR BOTH PROPORTION METHODS** $12.5 = 2.5x$ $\dfrac{12.5}{2.5} = x$ $5 \text{ tablets} = x$	$$\dfrac{1 \text{ tablet}}{\underset{1}{\cancel{2.5}} \text{ mg}} \Bigg|\ \dfrac{\overset{5}{\cancel{12.5}} \text{ mg}}{} = 5 \text{ tablets}$$

   Give 5 tablets po q week.

3. Step 1. BSA in meters squared: 0.46.

   Step 2. The safe dose is 6.30 mg/m²/24 hours.

Low Dose	*High Dose*
$\begin{array}{r} 6 \text{ mg} \\ \times\ 0.46 \\ \hline 2.76 \text{ mg} \end{array}$	$\begin{array}{r} 30 \text{ mg} \\ \times\ 0.46 \\ \hline 13.8 \text{ mg} \end{array}$

   The safe dose is 2.8 mg to 13.8 mg over 24 hours.

   Step 3. Order is 5 mg q12h = 5 × 2 = 10 mg q12h. The dose is safe.

   Step 4. Order is 5 mg; supply is 5 mg/5 mL. Give 5 mL po q12h.

4. Step 1. BSA in meters squared: 1.1.

   Step 2. Determine the safe dose:

   $$
   \begin{array}{r}
   5 \text{ mg} \\
   \times\ 1.1 \\
   \hline
   5.5 \text{ mg}
   \end{array}
   $$

   Step 3. Is the order safe?

   Yes. The order is 5 mg.

Step 4.

Formula Method	Proportion	Dimensional Analysis
$\dfrac{\overset{2}{\cancel{5}}\ \text{mg}}{\underset{1}{\cancel{2.5}}\ \text{mg}} \times 1\ \text{capsule}$ $= 2\ \text{capsules}$	**EXPRESSED AS TWO RATIOS** $1\ \text{capsule} : 2.5\ \text{mg} :: x : 5\ \text{mg}$ **EXPRESSED AS TWO FRACTIONS** $\dfrac{1\ \text{capsule}}{2.5\ \text{mg}} \diagup\!\!\!\!\diagdown \dfrac{x}{5\ \text{mg}}$ **SOLUTION FOR BOTH PROPORTION METHODS** $5 = 2.5x$ $\dfrac{5}{2.5} = x$ $2\ \text{capsules} = x$	$\dfrac{1\ \text{capsule}}{2.5\ \cancel{\text{mg}}}\ \Big|\ \dfrac{5\ \cancel{\text{mg}}}{} = 2\ \text{capsules}$

Give 2 capsules po × 1.

5. Step 1. BSA in meters squared: 1.4.

   Step 2.

Low Dose	*High Dose*
90 mg	180 mg
× 1.4	× 1.4
126 mg	252 mg

   Step 3. The order is 200 mg and is safe.

   It does not exceed 200 mg q6h.

   Step 4.

Formula Method	Proportion	Dimensional Analysis
$\dfrac{20\cancel{0}\ \text{mg}}{10\cancel{0}\ \text{mg}} \times 1\ \text{capsule}$ $= 2\ \text{capsules}$	**EXPRESSED AS TWO RATIOS** $1\ \text{capsule} : 100\ \text{mg} :: x : 200\ \text{mg}$ **EXPRESSED AS TWO FRACTIONS** $\dfrac{1\ \text{capsule}}{100\ \text{mg}} \diagup\!\!\!\!\diagdown \dfrac{x}{200\ \text{mg}}$ **SOLUTION FOR BOTH PROPORTION METHODS** $200 = 100x$ $\dfrac{200}{100} = x$ $2\ \text{capsules} = x$	$\dfrac{1\ \text{capsule}}{10\cancel{0}\ \cancel{\text{mg}}}\ \Big|\ \dfrac{20\cancel{0}\ \cancel{\text{mg}}}{} = 2\ \text{capsules}$

(continued)

Answers (Continued)

Self-Test 5 Parenteral Medication Calculations

1. Step 1. Weight is 8 kg.

   Step 2. The safe dose is 50 to 100 mg/kg/24 hours.

Low Dose	*High Dose*
50 mg	100 mg
× 8 kg	× 8 kg
400 mg/24 hours	800 mg/24 hours

   Step 3. Order is 200 mg q6h (4 doses).

   200 mg × 4 = 800 mg/24 hours. Dose is safe.

   Minimum safe dilution is 50 mg/mL.

   $$\frac{4 \text{ mL}}{50\overline{)200 \text{ mg}}} \text{ is the minimum dilution.}$$

   A total of 10 mL is safe.

   Step 4. Dilute 750 mg with 8 mL sterile water to make 90 mg/mL.

Formula Method	Proportion	Dimensional Analysis
$\dfrac{200 \text{ mg}}{90 \text{ mg}} \times 1 \text{ mL} = 2.2 \text{ mL}$	**EXPRESSED AS TWO RATIOS** 1 mL : 90 mg : : x : 200 mg **EXPRESSED AS TWO FRACTIONS** $\dfrac{1 \text{ mL}}{90 \text{ mg}} \diagdown \diagup \dfrac{x}{200 \text{ mg}}$ **SOLUTION FOR BOTH PROPORTION METHODS** $200 = 90x$ $\dfrac{200}{90} = x$ $2.2 \text{ mL} = x$	$\dfrac{1 \text{ } \boxed{mL}}{90 \text{ } mg} \bigg| 200 \text{ } mg = \dfrac{20}{9} = 2.2 \text{ mL}$

   Withdraw 2.2 mL of the drug into a syringe. Label the remainder and store in the refrigerator.

   Step 5. Add 10 mL from the D5½NS bag into the Buretrol.

   Add the 2.2 mL of drug.

   Step 6. Set the pump at 20 mL/hour. The pump will deliver 10 mL in 30 minutes.

   Step 7. When the IV is finished, add an additional 20 mL of the D5½NS bag into the Buretrol as a flush to clear the tubing of medication.

2. Step 1. Weight is 15 kg.

   Step 2. The safe dose is 8 to 10 mg/kg/24 hours given q12h.

Low Dose	*High Dose*
8 mg	10 mg
× 15 kg	× 15 kg
120 mg/24 hours	150 mg/24 hours

Step 3. Order is 75 mg q12h (two doses) = 150 mg/24 hours. The dose is safe.

The minimum safe dilution is 1 mL in 15 to 25 mL. The drug comes as a liquid, 80 mg/5 mL, so the dilution is safe.

Step 4. Calculate the dose.

Formula Method	Proportion	Dimensional Analysis
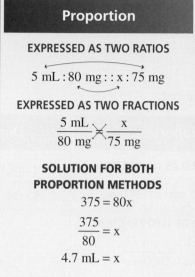	**EXPRESSED AS TWO RATIOS** 5 mL : 80 mg : : x : 75 mg **EXPRESSED AS TWO FRACTIONS** $\frac{5\ mL}{80\ mg} \times \frac{x}{75\ mg}$ **SOLUTION FOR BOTH PROPORTION METHODS** $375 = 80x$ $\frac{375}{80} = x$ $4.7\ mL = x$	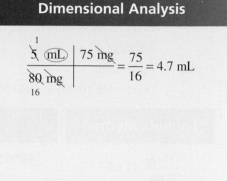

Formula Method:
$$\frac{75\ mg}{80\ mg} \times 5\ mL = 4.7\ mL$$
$$375 = 80x$$
$$4.7\ mL = x$$

Withdraw 4.7 mL of the drug into a syringe. Discard the remainder.

Step 5. Add 75 mL from the D5W bag into the Buretrol. Add the 4.7 mL of the drug.

Step 6. Order is to administer over 1 hour. Set the pump at 75.

Step 7. When the IV is completed, add an additional 20 mL of the D5W bag into the Buretrol as a flush to clear the tubing of medication.

3. Step 1. Weight is 40 kg.

Step 2. The safe dose range is 3 to 5 mg/kg/24 hours given q8h.

Low Dose	*High Dose*
3 mg	5 mg
× 40 kg	× 40 kg
120 mg/24 hours	200 mg/24 hours

Step 3. Order is 100 mg q8h (three doses):

100 mg × 3 = 300 mg

Dose is not safe. Contact the physician or healthcare provider.

4. Step 1. Weight is 18 kg.

Step 2. The safe dose is 50 to 200 mg/kg/24 hours given q6h.

Low Dose	*High Dose*
50 mg	200 mg
× 18 kg	× 18 kg
900 mg/24 hours	3600 mg/24 hours

Step 3. The order is 900 mg q6h (four doses):

900 mg × 4 = 3600 mg/24 hours

The dose is safe.

(continued)

Answers (Continued)

The minimum safe dilution is 50 mg/mL:

$$50\text{ mg}\overline{)900\text{ mg}}^{18}$$

18 mL is the minimum safe dilution.

A total of 25 mL is safe.

Step 4. 1 g powder.

Dilute with 10 mL to make 95 mg/mL.

Formula Method	Proportion	Dimensional Analysis
$\dfrac{900\text{ mg}}{95\text{ mg}} \times 1\text{ mL}$ $= 9.5\text{ mL drug}$	**EXPRESSED AS TWO RATIOS** $1\text{ mL} : 95\text{ mg} :: x : 900\text{ mg}$ **EXPRESSED AS TWO FRACTIONS** $\dfrac{1\text{ mL}}{95\text{ mg}} \bowtie \dfrac{x}{900\text{ mg}}$ **SOLUTION FOR BOTH PROPORTION METHODS** $900 = 95x$ $\dfrac{900}{95} = x$ $9.5\text{ mL} = x$	$\dfrac{1\ \text{mL}}{95\ \text{mg}} \left| \dfrac{900\ \text{mg}}{} \right. = \dfrac{900}{95} = 9.5\text{ mL}$

Withdraw 9.5 mL in a syringe.

Discard the remainder; the amount is too small to keep.

Step 5. Add 25 mL from the D5½NS bag into the Buretrol. Add the 9.5 mL of medication.

Step 6. Set the pump at 50 mL/hour. The pump will deliver 25 mL in 30 minutes.

Step 7. When the IV is finished, add an additional 20 mL of the D5½NS bag into the Buretrol as a flush to clear the tubing of medication.

5. Step 1. Weight is 6 kg.

Step 2. The safe dose is 100 to 200 mg/kg/24 hours.

Low Dose	*High Dose*
100 mg	200 mg
× 6 kg	× 6 kg
600 mg/24 hours	1200 mg/24 hours

Step 3. Order is 150 mg q8h (three doses) = 50 × 3 = 450 mg/24 hours

The dose is below range and is q8h. The literature states q6h.

The minimum safe dilution is 6 mg/mL.

The order is 150 mg:

$$6\overline{)150}^{25} = 25\text{ mL}$$

The dilution of 10 mL does not meet concentration requirements. It should be 25 mL. Consult with the physician or healthcare provider regarding the dose, times of administration, and dilution.

6. Step 1. 30 kg

Step 2. Determine the safe dose.

Low Dose	*High Dose*
0.05 mg	0.1 mg
× 30 kg	× 30 kg
1.5 mg	3 mg

Step 3. The dose is safe (2.5 mg).

Step 4. Supply: 1 mg = 1 mL

2.5 mg = 2.5 mL

Dilute in at least 5 mL NS and administer over 4 to 5 minutes.

7. Step 1. 25 kg

Step 2. Determine the safe dose.

Low Dose	*High Dose*
0.08 mg	0.3 mg
× 25 kg	× 25 kg
2 mg/day	7.5 mg/day

Step 3. The dose is slightly high. Consult the physician or healthcare provider. 4 mg bid = $4 \times 2 = 8$ mg/day.

Step 4. Supply is 4 mg/mL. Give 1 mL after notifying physician of higher dose. Administer undiluted over 30 seconds or less.

8. Step 1. 45 kg

Step 2. Determine the safe dose.

Ordered dose (25 mg) is within 12.5- to 25-mg range.

Step 3. The dose is safe.

q4h: 25 mg × 6 hours = 150 mg

q6h: 25 mg × 4 hours = 100 mg

It does not exceed 300 mg/24 hours.

Step 4.

Formula Method	Proportion	Dimensional Analysis
$\dfrac{\overset{1}{\cancel{25 \text{ mg}}}}{\underset{2}{\cancel{50 \text{ mg}}}} \times 1 \text{ mL} = 0.5 \text{ mL}$	**EXPRESSED AS TWO RATIOS** 1 mL : 50 mg : : x : 25 mg **EXPRESSED AS TWO FRACTIONS** $\dfrac{1 \text{ mL}}{50 \text{ mg}} \diagdown \dfrac{x}{25 \text{ mg}}$ **SOLUTION FOR BOTH PROPORTION METHODS** 25 = 50x $\dfrac{25}{50} = x$ 0.5 mL = x	$\dfrac{1 \text{ } \textcircled{mL}}{\underset{2}{\cancel{50 \text{ mg}}}} \left| \dfrac{\overset{1}{\cancel{25 \text{ mg}}}}{} \right. = \dfrac{1}{2}$ or 0.5 mL

Give 0.5 mL undiluted IVP over 1 minute.

(continued)

Answers (Continued)

9. Step 1. $\dfrac{15}{2.2} = 6.82$ kg

Step 2. Determine the safe dose.

Low Dose	*High Dose*
6 mcg	7.5 mcg
× 6.82 kg	× 6.82 kg
40.92 mcg/day	51.15 mcg/day

Step 3. The dose is safe (50 mcg/day).

Step 4. Calculate the dose.

Formula Method	**Proportion**	**Dimensional Analysis**
$\dfrac{\overset{1}{\cancel{50}\ \text{mcg}}}{\underset{2}{\cancel{100}\ \text{mcg}}} \times 1\ \text{mL} = 0.5\ \text{mL}$	**EXPRESSED AS TWO RATIOS** $1\ \text{mL} : 100\ \text{mcg} :: x : 50\ \text{mg}$ **EXPRESSED AS TWO FRACTIONS** $\dfrac{1\ \text{mL}}{100\ \text{mcg}} \bowtie \dfrac{x}{50\ \text{mcg}}$ **SOLUTION FOR BOTH PROPORTION METHODS** $50 = 100x$ $\dfrac{50}{100} = x$ $0.5\ \text{mL} = x$	$\dfrac{1\ \cancel{\text{mL}}}{\underset{2}{\cancel{100}\ \cancel{\text{mcg}}}} \left|\ \dfrac{\overset{1}{\cancel{50}\ \cancel{\text{mcg}}}}{}\right. = \dfrac{1}{2}\ \text{or}\ 0.5\ \text{mL}$

0.1 mg = 100 mcg/1 mL

Give 0.5 mL undiluted or diluted in 4 mL D5W or NS over 5 minutes.

10. Step 1. $\dfrac{80\ \text{lb}}{2.2} = 36.36$ kg

Step 2. Determine the safe dose.

Low Dose	*High Dose*
0.5 mg	1.7 mg
× 36.36 kg	× 36.36 kg
18.18 mg/day	61.81 mg/day

Step 3. 60 mg bid = 60 mg × 2 = 120 mg/day

The dose is too high. Contact the physician or healthcare provider.

Information Basic to Administering Drugs

In previous chapters, you learned drug forms and preparations, how to read prescriptions, and how to calculate dosages. This chapter provides the opportunity to focus on some of the nurse's responsibilities for drug therapy—drug knowledge, pharmacokinetics, and legal and ethical considerations.

 Drug Knowledge

Nursing drug handbooks are the best references for the nurse who needs a variety of information specifically designed to help assess, manage, evaluate, and teach the patient/client. The following headings represent the kind of information found in a nursing handbook.

- Generic and trade names
- Classification and category
- Side and adverse effects
- Pregnancy category
- Dosage and route
- Action

- Indications
- Contraindications and precautions
- Interactions and incompatibilities
- Nursing implications
- Signs of effectiveness
- Patient/client teaching

Two long-standing websites that include drug information are the U.S. Food and Drug Administration (http://www.fda.gov) and Rx Med (http://www.rxmed.com). Nursing publishing companies include drug information on their websites. Wolters Kluwer's site is *http://www.nursingcenter.com*. Suggestions for apps for drug information include Davis Drug Guide, Nursing Central, Lippincott's Nursing Drug Handbook, and Epocrates. The advantage of a nursing drug app is that updates can occur and therefore always have up-to-date drug information.

Generic and Trade Names

The generic name, which is not capitalized, is the name given to a drug that identifies the drug's active ingredient. In the United States, a drug can only have one generic name. The official name of the drug is the name identified in the USP (United States Pharmacopeia), and it indicates that the drug meets government standards for purity and assay.

A trade name is the brand name under which a company manufactures a generic drug. While a drug has only one generic name, it may have several trade names since the drug is produced by different manufacturers. The trade name is capitalized and is sometimes followed by the symbol®, which stands for registered trademark, or ™, which stands for trademark.

> **EXAMPLE**
>
> Acetaminophen is the generic name of several brand names: Tylenol, Paracetamol, Tempra, and others. There are 70 companies that manufacture acetaminophen.

Consumer groups have advocated that drugs be prescribed by generic name only so that the pharmacist may dispense the least expensive drug available in the market. The nurse should understand that generic drugs, because they are manufactured by different companies, are not exactly the same. Although the active ingredient in the drug meets standards of uniformity and purity, manufacturers use different fillers and dyes. These substances can cause adverse effects (e.g., severe nausea caused by the dye used in coloring).

Also, when a pharmacist dispenses the same drug with a different trade name, the patient/client may become confused and distressed about medication that appears unlike previous doses. While the active ingredient is the same, the medication size, shape, or color may vary according to trade name and manufacturer.

The nurse is responsible for knowing the generic and trade names of medications that he or she is responsible for administering.

Drug Classification and Drug Category

Drug classification is a way to categorize drugs by the way they act against diseases or disorders, especially by their effect on a particular area of the body or on a particular condition. A diuretic, for instance, acts on the kidneys; an anticonvulsant prevents seizures. Because drug classifications are a quick reference to a drug's therapeutic actions, uses, and adverse effects, they provide the administering nurse with a drug's general indications, precautions, and nursing implications.

Category (as used in this text) refers to the way a drug works at the molecular, tissue, or body system level (e.g., beta-blocker, selective serotonin reuptake inhibitor (SSRI)).

> **EXAMPLE**
>
> The classification of acetaminophen is a nonopioid analgesic and antipyretic. The category is a prostaglandin inhibitor. The drug's main action and use is to relieve mild-to-moderate pain and reduce fever.

Side Effects and Adverse Effects

Side effects are non therapeutic reactions to a drug. Because these reactions are transient, they may not require any nursing intervention. Side effects occur as a consequence of drug administration; often they are unrelated to the desired action of the drug.

Adverse effects are nontherapeutic effects that may be harmful to the patient/client and thus require lowering the dosage or discontinuing the drug. Because these effects can be life threatening, they may require medical intervention.

Idiosyncratic effects are effects from drugs that are not expected. Genetic predisposition is possibly a reason some individuals exhibit **idiosyncratic effects.** It may also be due to a hypersensitive immune reaction. Although each drug is tested extensively to determine side and adverse effects, occasionally an **idiosyncratic effect** will appear in an individual.

Drowsiness is a **side effect** that occurs with some antihistamines. A serious decrease in white blood cells (WBCs) is an **adverse effect**, resulting in lowered resistance to infection. The nurse must watch for these effects, know how to manage them, and, if necessary, teach the patient/client about them.

> **EXAMPLE**
>
> Acetaminophen has minimal side effects: it may cause a rash. Adverse effects are related to high doses and chronic use and include hepatotoxicity and renal failure.

Pregnancy Category

The U.S. Food and Drug Administration (FDA) has established the following categories for pregnant women:

A: No risk to the fetus in any trimester

B: No adverse effect demonstrated in animals; no human studies available

C: Studies with animals have shown adverse reactions; no human studies are available; given only after risks to the fetus have been considered

D: Definite fetal risk exists; may be given despite risk to the fetus if needed for a life-threatening condition

X: Absolute fetal abnormality; not to be used anytime during pregnancy

A nurse administering a drug to any woman of childbearing age should know the pregnancy categories. If the drug has a category of D or X, the nurse should inform the woman of that category's significance and determine whether there is any possibility of the woman being pregnant. If a woman has a confirmed pregnancy, the nurse should find out the pregnancy's current gestational week. The nurse also should use this circumstance as an opportunity to educate the patient/client about the risks of any current medication (whether prescribed, over the counter (OTC), herbal, or nutritional supplement) and its known or potential effects on a fetus.

EXAMPLE Acetaminophen is pregnancy category B, which indicates no adverse effect demonstrated in animals; no human studies available.

Dosage and Route

Information about the dosage and route of administration is crucial to protect against medication error. Most handbooks include, for each drug, appropriate dosage ranges for adults, the elderly, and children.

EXAMPLE Acetaminophen can be given by oral or rectal route. There is also an intravenous form. Usual dose is 325 to 650 mg every 4 to 6 hours, as needed. Children, infants, and neonates: 10 to 15 mg/kg/dose every 4 to 6 hours, as needed.

Action

Action explains how the drug works—that is, what medical experts know or believe about how the drug acts to produce a therapeutic effect. This knowledge helps the nurse understand whether a drug should be taken with food or between meals, with other drugs or alone, orally, topically, or parenterally (IM, subcutaneous, or IV).

The nurse who knows drug action can better assess, manage, and evaluate drug therapy. For example, if a particular drug is metabolized in the liver and kidney, then the nurse can apply this knowledge. Because patients/clients with liver or kidney disease may not be able to metabolize or excrete certain drugs, this particular drug could accumulate in the body and possibly cause adverse effects.

EXAMPLE Acetaminophen inhibits the synthesis of prostaglandins, which may serve as mediators of pain and fever, primarily in the central nervous system.

Indications

Indications give the reasons for using the drug. This information helps the nurse watch not only for expected effects and therapeutic response but also for any side effects and adverse effects. One of the most common questions patients/clients ask nurses is "Why am I getting this drug?" With a good understanding of indications, the nurse can answer the patient/client's question, describing the drug's expected effects.

Often a drug can be used for an indication "off label"—that is, for an indication other than the one(s) "labeled," or approved, by the FDA. The drug may be widely known to be effective in "off-label" conditions because of its side effects (e.g., diphenhydramine (Benadryl) causes sleep); or research studies may have proven the drug effective for that particular indication, but the drug hasn't yet been licensed as a treatment for it (e.g., bupropion (Wellbutrin) helps a patient/client stop smoking).

The nurse should become familiar with the typical off-label uses of particular drugs. If a medication order requests a drug for an indication other than the one for which it is labeled and approved, or other than off-label uses with which the nurse is familiar, the nurse should question the medication order.

EXAMPLE   Acetaminophen is used to relieve mild-to-moderate pain and reduce fever.

Contraindications and Precautions

The terms *contraindications* and *precautions* refer to conditions in which a drug should be either given with caution or not given at all. For instance, patients/clients who have exhibited a previous reaction to penicillin should be cautioned against taking that drug again; if a patient/client has poor kidney function, certain antibiotics must be administered with caution. Because the nurse has a responsibility to safeguard the patient/client and carry out effective nursing care, a knowledge of contraindications and precautions is important—especially in relation to patients/clients with glaucoma, renal disease, or liver disease and patients/clients who are very young or very old.

EXAMPLE   Acetaminophen is contraindicated in previous hypersensitivity and products containing alcohol. Use cautiously in clients with hepatic/renal disease, alcoholism, chronic malnutrition, severe hypovolemia, or severe renal impairment.

Interactions and Incompatibilities

When more than one drug is administered at a time, unexpected or nontherapeutic responses may occur. Some interactions are desirable: for example, naloxone (Narcan) is a narcotic antagonist that reverses the effects of a morphine overdose. Other interactions, however, are undesirable: aspirin, for instance, should avoid being taken with an oral anticoagulant because that combination may increase the possibility of an adverse effect (e.g., increased bleeding). The nurse must carefully consider some drug–herbal interactions as well.

Some drugs are incompatible and thus should not be mixed. Knowledge of incompatibilities is especially important when medications are combined for injection in IV administration. *Chemical incompatibility* usually produces a visible sign such as precipitation or color change. *Physical incompatibility,* however, may not give a visible sign, so the nurse should never combine drugs without checking a suitable reference, such as a drug compatibility chart. The nurse can also contact a pharmacist regarding incompatibilities.

A good rule of thumb: *When in doubt, do not mix.*

Interactions also may occur between drugs and certain foods. Here are some common examples. The calcium present in dairy products interferes with the absorption of tetracycline. Foods high in vitamin B_6 can decrease the effect of an antiparkinsonian drug. Foods high in tyramine, such as wine and cheese, can precipitate a hypertensive crisis in patients/clients taking MAO inhibitors. Grapefruit juice interferes with the absorption of multiple drugs.

Additionally, cigarette smoke—which can increase the liver's metabolism of drugs—may decrease drug effectiveness. People exposed even to secondhand cigarette smoke may require higher doses of medication.

> ## Common Drugs and Drug Classifications That Cause Unexpected or Nontherapeutic Responses
>
> - Monoamine oxidase (MAO) inhibitors–anticonvulsants–lithium
> - Tricyclic antidepressants–antifungals–methotrexate
> - Alcohol–barbiturates–nonsteroidal anti-inflammatory drugs (NSAIDs)
> - Aluminum–beta-blockers–oral contraceptives
> - Aminoglycosides–cimetidine–phenothiazines
> - Antacids–clonidine–phenytoin
> - Anticoagulants–cyclosporine–probenecid
> - Heparin–digoxin–rifampin
> - Coumadin–erythromycin–theophylline
> - Aspirin–isoniazid
>
> *Refer to a drug handbook for specific interactions.*

EXAMPLE

Acetaminophen may increase risk of bleeding when taking warfarin (Coumadin). Hepatotoxicity is additive with other hepatotoxic substances. Concurrent use of certain drugs may increase acetaminophen-induced liver damage. Concurrent use of other NSAIDs (nonsteroidal anti-inflammatory drugs) may increase the risk of adverse renal effects. See a drug guide for more detailed information.

Nursing Implications

To administer a drug safely and to assess, manage, and teach the patient/client, the nurse needs a knowledge of implications: whether the drug should be taken with or without food, what specific vital signs to monitor, and what lab values may be affected by the drug or may need to be ordered to check the drug's effectiveness or toxicity.

EXAMPLE

Some nursing implications with acetaminophen: Assess overall health status and alcohol usage before administering. Assess type and location of pain. Assess fever. Evaluate renal and liver functions periodically during high-dose administration. See a drug guide for detailed nursing implications.

Signs of Effectiveness

Few drug references actually list this heading, yet the nurse is expected to evaluate the drug regimen and to record and report observations. Knowledge of the drug's class, its action, and its use helps the nurse understand the expected therapeutic outcomes.

Ampicillin sodium, for instance, is a broad-spectrum antibiotic that is used for urinary, respiratory, and other infections. Signs of effectiveness might include normal temperature; the laboratory report of the WBC count, indicating a normal result; clear urine, no pain on urination, and no WBCs in urine; decreased pus in an infected wound; wound healing; a patient/client showing alertness, interest in surroundings, and improved appetite.

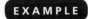 **EXAMPLE** | For acetaminophen, signs of effectiveness are relief of pain and reduction of fever.

Teaching the Patient/Client

The patient/client has a right to know the drug's name and dose, why the drug is ordered, and what effects to expect or watch for. A patient/client who will be taking a drug at home also needs specific information. Making sure that patients/clients are knowledgeable about their drugs is a professional responsibility shared by three people: the physician or healthcare provider, the nurse, and the pharmacist.

 # Pharmacokinetics

When a drug is taken *orally*, the villi of the small intestine absorb it, and the bloodstream distributes it to the cells. The body metabolizes the drug to a greater or lesser extent and then excretes it. When a drug is given *parenterally*, it bypasses the gastrointestinal system, entering the circulation more quickly—or, in the case of the IV route, immediately. The general term **pharmacokinetics** includes these drug activities: absorption, distribution, metabolism or biotransformation, and excretion.

Absorption

Effective absorption of an oral drug depends on several conditions:

- The degree of stomach acidity
- Time required for the stomach to empty
- The amount of contact with the villi in the small intestine
- The flow of blood to the villi

Other situations, too, may affect a drug's absorption:

- Enteric-coated (EC) tablets, for instance, are not meant to dissolve in the acidic stomach; they ordinarily pass through the stomach to the duodenum.
- When a patient/client receives an antacid along with an EC tablet, the pH of the stomach rises, perhaps causing the tablet to dissolve prematurely—which either can make the drug less potent or can irritate the gastric lining.
- Timed-release EC capsules that dissolve prematurely can deliver a huge dose of the drug, producing adverse effects.
- Laxatives increase gastrointestinal movement and decrease the time a drug is in contact with the villi of the small intestine, where most absorption occurs.
- Food in the stomach, however, can impair absorption.
- In particular, foods that contain calcium, such as milk and cheese, form a complex with some drugs and inhibit absorption.
- Penicillin is a good example of a drug that should be taken on an empty stomach.

Distribution

Distribution describes the drug's movement through body fluids—chiefly the bloodstream—to the cells. Drugs do not travel freely in the blood; instead, most travel attached to plasma proteins, especially albumin.

- If a drug is not attached to a plasma protein, it can attach to other cells and affect them in various ways.

- When the bloodstream contains more than one drug, the drugs may compete for binding with protein sites.

- One drug may displace another, leaving the displaced drug free to interact with the cells, and its effect on the cells will be more pronounced.

One example of this is aspirin:

- Aspirin is a common drug that displaces others; it should not be given with oral anticoagulants, which are 99% bound to albumin. Because aspirin displaces the anticoagulant, it leaves the anticoagulant free to act at the cellular level, sometimes causing the toxic effect of bleeding.

Metabolism or Biotransformation

Metabolism or biotransformation refers to the chemical change of a drug into a form that can be excreted. Most metabolism or biotransformation occurs in the liver.

- First-pass effect occurs with medications taken by mouth (enteral route).

- After ingestion, the drug is absorbed by the gastrointestinal system and then first passes through the liver, where some of the drug may be metabolized.

- Thus, the drug may not be as effective as it continues through the pharmacokinetic phases.

- The parenteral route (subcutaneous, IM, IV) bypasses the first-pass effect, so more of the drug is available to the body tissues and cells.

- One drug can interfere with the effects of another during biotransformation:

  - Barbiturates increase the liver's enzyme activity. Since this activity makes the body metabolize the drugs more rapidly, it reduces their effect.

  - Conversely, acetaminophen (Tylenol) blocks the breakdown of penicillin in the liver, thereby increasing the effect of that drug.

Excretion

The major organ of excretion—the process by which the body removes a drug—is the kidney. Drug interactions may also occur at this point. Here are two examples of this:

- The drug probenecid inhibits the excretion of penicillin and increases its length of action.

- Furosemide (Lasix), a diuretic, blocks the excretion of aspirin and can cause aspirin to produce adverse effects.

Drug interactions at the excretion stage are not necessarily harmful.

- For instance, narcotic antagonists are used intentionally to reverse the adverse effects of general anesthetics.

- This reversal action is termed *antagonism.*

- The term *synergism*, on the other hand, describes what happens when a second drug increases the intensity or prolongs the effect of a first drug.

  - A narcotic and a minor tranquilizer together, for example, produce more pain relief than the narcotic alone.

The nurse administering medications needs to be aware of possible interactions and must carefully evaluate the patient/client's response. To minimize adverse interactions, the nurse should closely review the patient/client's drug profile, administer as low a dose as possible, know the actions and the side and adverse effects of the drugs administered, and monitor the patient/client. Continued monitoring is important, because some drug interactions may take several weeks to develop.

✓ PHARMACOKINETICS: Age-Related Changes

Older Adults

Absorption

- Increased stomach acidity
- Decreased blood flow to gastrointestinal tract
- Decreased gastrointestinal motility
- Reduced body surface area

Distribution

- Decreased cardiac output/decreased heart contractility
- Decreased lean body mass
- Decreased serum albumin
- Increased body fat
- Decreased body water

Metabolism

- Decreased liver function
- Decreased hepatic blood flow

Excretion

- Decreased kidney function
- Decreased glomerular flow rate
- Decreased kidney blood flow

Medication Administration

- Decreased drug receptor sites, therefore decrease in response to drugs
- Physiologic changes increase potential for side and adverse effects
- Potential for drug interactions due to older adults taking more drugs
- Decreased cognitive function, leading to forgetfulness of drugs and dosages
- Environmental concerns: access to a pharmacy, access to medications in the living environment

Infants

Absorption

- Decreased stomach acidity
- Peripheral circulation slower
- Greater body surface area

Distribution

- Increased concentration of water
- Lower concentration of fat
- Immature liver function
- Immature blood-brain barrier

Metabolism

- Immature liver function

Elimination

- Immature renal function

Medication Administration

- Drug testing often not done on children, therefore potential side and adverse effects are not known

- Potential for more severe side and adverse effects because of immature body system
- Drug dosing varies, usually weight or body surface area based, requiring accurate dosage calculation

Cultural Considerations

- Drug metabolism and side effects can vary among different cultures, races, and ethnic groups.
- *Pharmacoanthropology* deals with differences in drug responses among racial and ethnic groups. *Ethnocultural perception* deals with various cultural perceptions and beliefs related to illness, disease, and drug therapy.
- Assessing the personal beliefs of the patient/client and the family is an essential step in drug administration.
- The nurse's communication about drugs must meet the cultural needs of the patient/client and family and must respect their culture and cultural practices.

Herbs, Herbs, Herbs

- Herbal therapy is one of the oldest forms of medication. Today, its use is worldwide, with more and more people taking herbal remedies.
- Herbal therapies and other alternative medications, however, *are not subject to FDA regulations.*
- Patients/clients should consult with their healthcare provider before beginning herbal therapy, while taking herbal therapy, whenever they experience any side effects from the products, and before discontinuing herbal medications.
- The National Center for Complementary and Alternative Medicine, under the auspices of the National Institutes of Health, studies alternative medicine and therapies (see *http://www.nccam.nih.gov*).
- The Dietary Supplement Health and Education Act of 1994 clarified regulations for herbal remedies (see *http://www.fda.gov/food/dietarysupplements/default.htm*).
- Healthcare providers need to be aware of potential drug interactions between herbal therapy and conventional drugs (both prescription and over the counter).

Tolerance

When a medication for pain or sleeping is administered frequently, the liver enzymes become skilled at rapid biotransformation.

- Thus, less of the drug is available, and the drug is less effective in relieving pain or aiding sleep.
- This reaction may be labeled "addiction" because the patient/client complains that the drug is not working and asks for more; but in fact, it is a physiologic response rather than an addictive one.
- The patient/client simply requires more of the drug or a drug with a different molecular structure.

Cumulation

When a condition—such as liver or kidney disease—inhibits biotransformation or excretion, the drug accumulates in the body. The same thing can happen when a patient/client receives too much of a drug or takes a drug too frequently. This activity, called cumulation, can produce an adverse effect.

Other factors that affect drug action include the following:

- Weight: Larger individuals need a higher dose.
- Age: People at either extreme of life respond more strongly. The liver and kidneys of infants are not well developed; in the elderly, systems are less efficient.

- Pathologic conditions, especially of liver and kidneys.

- Hypersensitivity to a drug, which causes an allergic reaction.

- Psychological and emotional state: Depression or anxiety can decrease or increase body metabolism and thus affect drug action.

Side effects and adverse reactions can occur in any system or organ. Drug knowledge will enhance the nurse's skill in observation and will lead to responsible and appropriate intervention.

Half-Life

The half-life of a drug, which correlates roughly with its duration of action, indicates how often the drug may be given to continue its therapeutic effect.

- The half-life is the time required for half of the drug to be excreted and therefore no longer available for therapeutic use.

  - For example, penicillin's half-life is 30 minutes: after 30 minutes, only half of the dose is still therapeutic.

  - After 30 more minutes, only half of *that* dose is therapeutic, and so on, until most of the drug is eliminated. Then the patient/client needs another dose.

  - In this case, the patient/client receives oral penicillin every 6 to 8 hours.

- Another example is piroxicam (Feldene):

  - It has a half-life of 48 to 72 hours and is given by mouth as a single dose once a day.

- Carisoprodol (Soma) has a half-life of 4 to 6 hours and is administered three to four times daily.

Therapeutic Range

To evaluate the effects of drug therapy, the nurse can monitor the drug concentration in the patient/client's blood or serum through the use of laboratory tests that measure the therapeutic level.

- The International System of Units (Système International d'Unités—SI) is a standard measurement system adopted by most countries.

- One of the units in SI is used to quantify the amount of drug in the blood or serum. (More details on SI can be found at *http://www.bipm.org/en/si/*.)

- Some drugs, such as theophylline (Theo-Dur), phenytoin (Dilantin), digoxin (Lanoxin), and others, require periodic measurements in order to ensure that the patient/client is receiving the right amount or not receiving too much of the drug.

- Antibiotics often are measured with peak and trough therapeutic levels:

  - The trough level is drawn from the blood before the next dose of antibiotic is due to see if there is too much drug left in the body.

  - The peak level is drawn from the blood after a dose of antibiotic to see if there is enough drug in the body to have a therapeutic effect.

  - A random drug level is done at any time to determine how much of the drug remains in the body.

Legal Considerations

Nurses must know the scope of nursing practice in the state in which they function. They should be familiar not only with government regulations—federal, state, and local—that affect nursing but also with the policies and procedures of the agency where they practice, which also have legal status. Failure to follow guidelines, or even just a lack of knowledge, can lead to liability. The website for the National Council of State Boards of Nursing (*http://www.ncsbn.org*) gives information on nurse regulation and licensure in each state; up-to-date information on legal issues is available from the website of the American Nurses Association (*http://nursingworld.org*).

In Canada, the Health Protection Branch of the Department of National Health and Welfare (*http://www.hc-sc.gc.ca/index-eng.php*) maintains the quality and safety of drug development. (Details regarding the Canadian Food and Drugs Act appear on the same site.) For information about narcotics control, see the Web page for the Controlled Drugs and Substances Act (*http://laws.justice.gc.ca/en/C-38.8/*).

Nursing practice is also affected by two other types of law: criminal and civil.

Criminal Law

Criminal law relates to offenses against the general public that are detrimental to society as a whole. Actions considered criminal are prosecuted by governmental authorities. If the defendant is judged guilty, the penalty may be a fine, imprisonment, or both.

Criminal charges include unlawful use, possession, or administration of a controlled substance. The Comprehensive Drug Abuse, Prevention and Control Act of 1970 classified drugs that are subject to abuse into one of five schedules, according to their medical usefulness and abuse potential.

* *Schedule I drugs* have no valid use and are not available for prescription use (e.g., LSD).

* *Schedule II drugs,* such as narcotics, have a valid medical use and are available for prescriptions, but they exhibit a high potential for abuse, and their misuse can lead to physical and psychological dependence. Labels for these drugs are marked with the symbol II.

  * In a hospital setting, an order for a narcotic might be valid for 3 days; once the 3 days have elapsed, however, a new order is required. A nurse who administers a controlled drug after its order has expired commits a medication error.

* *Schedule III, IV, and V drugs* are classified as having less abuse potential than schedule II drugs, but they can cause some physical and psychological dependence.

  * The labels III, IV, and V identify these drugs.

  * Examples include oxycodone (Percodan), butalbital, aspirin, and caffeine (Fiorinal) Fiorinal, diazepam (Valium), and acetaminophen with codeine (Tylenol #3).

* *Schedule II, III, IV, and V drugs* are stored in a locked cabinet or cart on nursing units, and a record is kept for each narcotic administered.

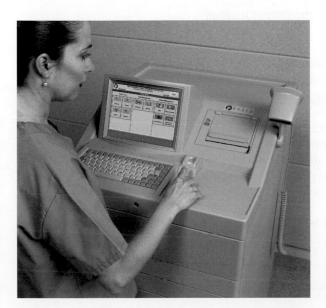

FIGURE 9-1

Pyxis Controlled Medication System. (With permission from Roach, S. [2004]. Introductory clinical pharmacology [7th ed.]. Philadelphia, PA: Lippincott Williams & Wilkins, p. 18.)

Many hospitals use the Pyxis system, a computerized locked cabinet that dispenses controlled substances (Fig. 9-1). Controlled drugs are counted for each shift, and discrepancies are reported. Government and institutional policies specify how these drugs are stored and protected.

Nurses who become impaired (unable to function) because of alcohol or drug abuse leave themselves open to criminal action, as well as to disciplinary action by the state board of nursing. Many states have laws requiring mandatory reporting of impaired nurses.

Civil Law

Civil law is concerned with the legal rights and duties of private persons. When an individual believes that a wrong was committed against him or her personally, he or she can sue for damages in the form of money.

The legal wrong is called a tort.

Malpractice, or negligence on the part of the nurse, involves four elements:

1. A claim that the nurse owed the patient/client a special duty of care—that is, that a nurse–patient/client relationship existed.

2. A claim that the nurse failed to meet the required standard. To prove or disprove this element, both sides bring in expert witnesses to testify.

3. A claim that harm or injury resulted because the nurse did not meet the required standard.

4. A claim of damages for which compensation is sought.

The nurse–patient/client relationship is a legal status that begins the moment a nurse actually provides nursing care to another person.

For administration of medications, a nurse is required by law to exercise the degree of skill and care that a reasonably prudent nurse with similar training and experience, practicing in the same community, would exercise under the same or similar circumstances.

When a nursing student performs duties that are customarily performed by a registered nurse, the courts have held the nursing student to the higher standard of care, that of the registered nurse.

Mistakes in administering medications are among the most common causes of liability, which may result from the following:

- administering the wrong dose

- giving a medication to the wrong patient/client

- giving a drug at the wrong time

- failing to administer a drug at the right time or in the proper manner

- failing to withhold a medication when indicated

A frequent cause of medication errors is either misreading the medication order of the physician or health care provider or failing to check with the physician or health care provider when the medication order is questionable. Faulty technique in administering medications, especially injections that result in injury to the patient/client, is another common medication error.

Not all malpractice is a result of negligence. Malpractice claims are also founded on the daily interaction between the nurse and the patient/client; consequently, the nurse's personality plays a major role in fostering or preventing malpractice claims. All nurses should be familiar with the principles of psychology and therapeutic communication. The surest way to prevent claims is to recognize the patient/client as a human being who has emotional as well as physical needs and to respond to these needs in a humane and competent manner.

If an error does occur, primary consideration must be given to the patient/client. These steps are followed:

- Assessment of the patient/client is done first.

- The nurse notifies the physician and the immediate nursing supervisor; students notify the instructor.

How can a nurse avoid liability claims? First and foremost are the three checks and six rights (see pp. 391–392). Accurate dosage calculation is also a safeguard against medication errors and potential liability claims.

Other Safeguards Include

- Know and follow institutional policies and procedures.
- Look up what you do not know.
- Do not leave medicines at the bedside.
- Chart carefully.
- Listen to the patient/client: "I never took that before," and the like.
- Check and double-check when a dose seems high. Most oral tablet doses range from 1/2 to 2 tablets. Most IM, intradermal, and subcutaneous injections are less than 3 mL.
- Label any powder you dilute. Label any IV bag you use.
- When necessary, seek advice from competent professionals.
- Do not administer drugs prepared by another nurse.
- Keep drug knowledge up-to-date. Attend continuing education programs and update your nursing skills.
- Label syringes after medications are drawn into the syringe.

CLINICAL POINT

✓ Medication Errors

- Prevent them.
- Don't make them.
- Don't be in a hurry.
- If you do make them, learn from your mistakes and don't make them again.
- ALWAYS give primary concern to the patient/client.

Facts

- Medication errors can cause unnecessary side effects, adverse effects, illnesses, and sometimes death.
- Medication errors are among the most common medical errors. The FDA states that there is at least one death per day and 1.3 million people are injured each year due to medication errors.
- The three most common errors are administering an improper dose, administering the wrong drug, and using the wrong route of administration.
- Medication errors are preventable. As a nurse, you can prevent medication errors by following the six rights of medication administration and three checks of medication identification (see Chapter 10). For information on medication errors, visit the FDA website (*http://www.fda.gov/Drugs/DrugSafety/ MedicationErrors/default.htm*).

Reporting

- The nurse has a legal and ethical responsibility to report medication errors immediately and to the nursing supervisor or charge nurse and physician.
- Follow institutional policy in reporting and documenting medication errors.
- The FDA maintains a confidential database for medication errors: 1-800-332-1088. The FDA medication error website is *http://www.fda.gov/Safety/MedWatch/ HowToReport/default.htm*.
- The National Coordinating Council for Medication Error Reporting and Prevention (NCCMERP) provides assistance on medication errors and promoting medication safety: 301-816-8216; the website is *http://www.nccmerp.org*.

- Error-in-medication forms or incident reports (depending on the institution) are filled out.

- Appropriate action is taken under the direction of the physician or health care provider.

To prevent malpractice claims, the nurse must render, as consistently as possible, the best possible care to patients/clients. Every nurse involved in direct care should regard prevention of malpractice claims as an integral part of daily nursing responsibilities for two fundamental reasons:

1. Such measures result in higher-quality care.

2. All affirmative measures taken to minimize malpractice will minimize the nurse's exposure to personal liability.

It is possible to render high-quality nursing care and never commit a medication error. Safe effective drug therapy is a combination of knowledge, skill, carefulness, and caring.

 # Ethical Principles in Drug Administration

Both moral and legal dimensions are involved in the administration of medications. Nurses are responsible for their actions. Here are two helpful websites that relate to ethics: Nursing Ethics Resources (*http://www.nursing ethics.ca*) and Lippincott Nursing Center's site (*http://www.nursingcenter.com/home/NursingCenterEthics.asp*).

The American Nurses Association Code of Ethics contains several statements that apply to drug therapy. Briefly stated, they are as follows:

1. The nurse provides services with respect for the patient/client's human dignity and uniqueness.

2. The nurse safeguards the patient/client's right to privacy.

3. The nurse acts to safeguard the patient/client from incompetent, unethical, or illegal practice.

4. The nurse assumes responsibility and accountability for nursing judgments and actions.

5. The nurse maintains competence in nursing.

When a nurse faces an ethical decision, several principles can serve as guides: autonomy, truthfulness, beneficence, nonmaleficence, confidentiality, justice, and fidelity.

Autonomy

Autonomy is self-determination.

- A person has the freedom to decide; knows the facts and understands them; and acts without outside force, deceit, or constraints.

- For the patient/client, this implies a right to be informed about drug therapy and a right to refuse medication.

- For the nurse, autonomy brings a responsibility to discuss drug information with the patient/client and to accept the patient/client's right to refuse.

- Autonomy also gives the nurse the right to refuse to participate in any drug therapy deemed to be unethical or unsafe for the patient/client.

Truthfulness

The nurse has an obligation not to lie.

- Telling the truth, however, is not the same as telling the whole truth.

- Ethically, it is sometimes difficult to decide what may be concealed and what must be revealed.

- In drug research, the patient/client has a right to informed consent—to be told the truth before signing as a participant.

- In double-blind studies, used to determine effectiveness, patients/clients are randomly assigned to an experimental group that receives the drug or to a control group that receives a placebo (a preparation devoid of pharmacologic effect).

- Neither the patient/client nor the nurse knows to which group he or she is assigned.

- To participate freely, the patient/client must receive full disclosure of risks and benefits and must understand the research design.

Beneficence

The principle of beneficence holds that the nurse should act in the patient/client's best interests. In fact, the respect due to the patient/client's freedom and right to self-determination can sometimes limit the nurse's actions. If the nurse overrides a patient/client's wishes, deciding himself or herself what is best for the patient/client, the nurse is violating the patient/client's rights. A conflict can arise. Forcing a patient/client to take medications or participate in a procedure can be considered battery, and a criminal charge.

Nonmaleficence

Nonmaleficence holds that the nurse must not inflict harm on the patient/client and must prevent harm whenever possible. In drug therapy, every medication administered risks inducing some undesirable side effect and/or adverse effect.

- Chemotherapy, for example, may reduce the size of a tumor but may cause nausea, vomiting, decreased white cell count, and so forth.

- The nurse anticipates the untoward effects of drugs that may occur and acts to minimize them.

Confidentiality

Confidentiality is respect for the information that a nurse learns from professional involvement with patients/clients.

- A patient/client's drug therapy and responses should be discussed only with people who have a right to know—that is, other professionals caring for the patient/client.

- The extent to which the family or significant others have a right to know depends on the specific situation and on the patient/client's wishes.

- These varying interests can cause conflict.

Justice

Justice refers to the patient/client's right to receive:

- the right drug
- the right dose
- by the right route
- at the right time.

In addition, the patient/client has a right to:

- the nurse's careful assessment, management, and evaluation of drug therapy
- use nursing actions that promote the patient/client's safety and well-being.
- the nurse's obligation is to maintain a high standard of care.

Fidelity

A nurse should keep promises made to the patient/client.

- Statements such as
  - "I'll be right back."
  - "I'll check the chart and let you know"
  - "I'll be back in 5 minutes"

create a covenant that should be respected.

Knowledge Base

Nurses should know the following:

- generic and trade names of drugs to be administered
- class and category
- average dose
- routes of administration
- use
- side effects and adverse effects
- contraindications
- nursing implications in administration
- signs of effectiveness to look for
- what drug interactions are possible.

New or unfamiliar drugs require research.

The nurse should be aware of the patient/client's diagnosis and medical history, especially relative to drugs taken.

- Be especially alert to OTC (over-the-counter) drugs, which patients/clients often do not consider important.
- Check for allergies.
- Assess the patient/client's need for drug information.
- Be prepared to implement and evaluate a nursing care plan in drug therapy.

CLINICAL POINT

✓ **Age-Specific Considerations**

- Neonatal patients/clients—The nurse needs to consider the immaturity of organ function, the importance of weight, and the precision of dosage calculation (rounding to the nearest hundredth).
- Pediatric patients/clients—The nurse needs to remember the principles of atraumatic care and to consider developmental stages.
- Geriatric patients/clients—The nurse needs to take into account decreasing organ function (especially liver and kidney), circulatory changes leading to decreased perfusion, and physical limitations (poor eyesight, decreased coordination, decreased ability to chew and/or swallow).

CRITICAL THINKING | TEST YOUR CLINICAL SAVVY

Mr. T is a patient/client receiving a drug that is in a drug study.

A. As a nurse administering this drug, what is your ethical responsibility?

B. If the patient/client asks "Is it safe to take this drug?" what is an appropriate response? If the patient/client refuses to take the drug, what should you do?

C. You agree with the patient/client that he should not take the experimental drug. What are your ethical responsibilities? What are your legal responsibilities?

Mr. T discovers from the Internet that the drug he is taking is an experimental drug and that another drug with similar actions has been released by the FDA and is available by prescription.

D. How do you respond to the information that he has acquired? What are some questions that the patient/client should ask regarding information acquired over the Internet?

E. If the patient/client asks you whether he should continue to take the experimental drug, or whether he should discontinue his participation in the drug study and obtain a prescription for the similar drug, what is an appropriate response?

F. What reasons can you give Mr. T regarding the benefits of participating in a drug study?

SELF-TEST 1 | Basic Information

Give the information requested and answer the multiple choice questions. Answers appear at the end of the chapter.

1. List at least 10 kinds of information the nurse needs to know in order to administer drugs safely.

_____   _____

_____   _____

_____   _____

_____   _____

_____   _____

2. List the five pregnancy categories used to identify the safety of drugs for the fetus and briefly define each.

_____

_____

_____

_____

_____

3. Name the major organ for the following drug activities:

a. Absorption _____   **c.** Biotransformation _____

b. Distribution _____   **d.** Excretion _____

(continued)

4. List the four elements of negligence.

_____ ,

_____ ,

_____ , and

_____

5. List at least five positive actions to avoid liability.

_____

_____

_____

_____

_____

6. List and briefly describe five ethical principles in drug therapy.

_____

_____

_____

_____

_____

7. Which term is used by the drug company to name drugs?

   a. Generic   **c.** Official

   b. Trade   **d.** Chemical

8. The term *USP* after a drug name indicates that the drug

   a. is made only in the United States

   b. meets official standards in the United States

   c. cannot be made by any other pharmaceutical company

   d. is registered by the U.S. Public Health Service

9. A patient/client is concerned about taking a cough medicine with codeine, classified as a schedule V drug. The nurse explains to the patient/client that a schedule V drug has

   a. the potential for severe drug dependencies

   b. no accepted medical use

   c. limited abuse potential

   d. no therapeutic effect

10. An adverse effect can be defined as

   a. changes that occur to the drug inside the body

   b. desired effect of the drug

   c. unintended and undesired effects of the drug

   d. mild allergic effects of a drug

Name: _____

Choose the correct answer. Answers are given in Appendix A.

1. Two drugs are given for different reasons, but drug Y interferes with the excretion of drug X. The effect of drug X would be

   a. increased
   b. decreased
   c. unchanged
   d. stopped

2. Toxicity to a drug is more likely to occur when

   a. elimination of the drug is rapid
   b. the drug is bound to the plasma protein albumin
   c. the drug will not dissolve in the lipid layer of the cell
   d. the drug is free in the blood circulation

3. Signs of effectiveness of a drug are based on what information?

   a. Action and use
   b. Untoward effects
   c. Generic and trade names
   d. Drug interaction

4. Drug classification is an aid in understanding

   a. use of the drug
   b. drug idiosyncrasy
   c. the trade name
   d. the generic name

5. Most oral drugs are absorbed in the

   a. mouth
   b. esophagus
   c. small intestine
   d. large intestine

6. Nursing legal responsibilities associated with controlled substances include

   a. storage in a locked place
   b. assessing vital signs
   c. evaluating psychological response
   d. establishing automatic 24-hour stop orders

7. Characteristics of a schedule II drug include

   a. accepted medical use with a high abuse potential
   b. medically accepted drug with low dependence possibility
   c. no accepted use in patient/client care
   d. unlimited renewals

8. The responsibilities of the nurse regarding medication in the hospital include all except

   a. prescribing drugs
   b. teaching patients/clients
   c. regulating automatic expiration times of drugs
   d. preparing solutions

(continued)

9. Which of the following illustrates a medication error?

    a. Administering a 10 AM dose at 10:20 AM
    b. Giving 2 tablets of sufisoxazole (Gantrisin) 500 mg when 1 g is ordered
    c. Pouring 5 mL of cough syrup when 1 tsp is ordered
    d. Giving digoxin (Lanoxin) IM when digoxin (Lanoxin) PO 0.25 mg is ordered

10. A nurse notices that a patient/client has an unpredictable response to a medication that is not mentioned as a potential side effect. This response can be classified as

    a. an idiosyncratic response
    b. tolerance
    c. hypersensitivity
    d. hepatotoxicity

11. The patient/client asks the nurse why two different types of antihypertensives are being administered. The nurse responds that the result is an increase of one or both of the drugs and is referred to as

    a. synergism
    b. displacement
    c. antagonism
    d. adverse effects

12. What term refers to the way the body inactivates medications?

    a. First-pass effect
    b. Biotransformation
    c. Absorption
    d. Displacement

13. A 90-year-old patient/client needs to have a lower dosage of medication than a middle-aged patient/client because of

    a. increased body fat in the elderly
    b. decreased gastrointestinal acidity
    c. decreased kidney function
    d. increased metabolism

14. A 9-month-old infant has immature liver function and a decreased capacity for biotransformation. The nurse, prior to administering medication, knows that this will

    a. reduce blood levels of certain drugs
    b. slow the metabolism of certain drugs
    c. limit the medications administered
    d. decrease drug toxicity

15. A patient/client has just eaten a large holiday celebration meal (alcohol not served). What pharmacokinetic principle would be of most concern when administering medications?

    a. Absorption
    b. Excretion
    c. Metabolism
    d. Distribution

16. A pregnant patient/client asks the nurse about taking a medication that is in pregnancy category C. The nurse states that this category

    a. fails to show risk in the first trimester
    b. should be given only if benefit justifies risk to the fetus
    c. demonstrates no risk in second or third trimesters
    d. is contraindicated in pregnant women

17. Which health practice can the nurse suggest to the patient/client which will have the least chance of causing a drug interaction?

    a. Taking a herbal remedy for depression
    b. Smoking half a pack of cigarettes per week
    c. Drinking four glasses of water a day
    d. Taking an over-the-counter medication for pain

18. A nurse monitors for a cumulative effect during a patient/client's hospital stay. A cumulative drug effect can occur when

    a. an overdose of the drug is given accidentally
    b. a drug is excreted too quickly
    c. a drug is given on an empty stomach
    d. the patient/client is unable to metabolize and/or excrete a drug

19. Adverse reactions in drugs

    a. occur only when large doses are administered
    b. are mild and not serious
    c. are not seen in healthy individuals
    d. are often sudden and may be fatal

20. Names of many drugs include

    a. several generic and several trade names
    b. several generic and one trade name
    c. one generic and one trade name
    d. one generic and several trade names

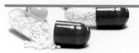

Answers

Self-Test 1 Basic Information

1. Generic/trade name, drug class and drug classification, pregnancy category, dose and route, action, use, side/adverse effects, contraindications/precautions, interactions/incompatibilities, nursing implications, evaluation of effectiveness, patient/client teaching

2. **A.** No risk to fetus
   B. No adverse effects in animals, but no human studies
   C. Animals show adverse effects; calculated risk to fetus
   D. Fetal risk exists
   X. Absolute fetal abnormality

3. **a.** Small intestines or stomach
   b. Blood
   c. Liver
   d. Kidney

4. A claim that a nurse–patient/client relationship existed

   The nurse was required to meet a standard of care

   A claim that harm or injury occurred because the standard was not met

   A claim of damages for which compensation is sought

5. Know policies and practices of the institution.
   Research unfamiliar drugs.
   Do not leave medicines at the bedside.
   Chart carefully.
   Listen to the patient/client's complaints.
   Check yourself (e.g., read labels three times).
   Label anything you dilute.
   Keep up-to-date.

6. Autonomy: freedom to decide based on knowledge with no constraint
   Truthfulness: truth telling that can create a dilemma. Is it absolute, or is there a beneficent deceit?
   Beneficence: obligation to help others
   Nonmaleficence: do no harm
   Confidentiality: keep secrets
   Justice: rights of an individual
   Fidelity: keep promises

7. b

8. b

9. c

10. c

10

Administration Procedures

TOPICS COVERED

1. Basic medication administration
2. Medication order guidelines
3. Systems of administration
4. Standard precautions
5. Guidelines for administration of drugs:
   Oral Parenteral—intramuscular, subcutaneous, IV, IV piggyback, intradermal
   Topical—ear, eye, nose drops; mucous membranes: skin, sublingual, buccal tablets;
   rectal, vaginal suppositories
6. Special considerations:
   neonatal, pediatric, geriatric

Throughout this text, we have calculated dosages and studied information related to drug therapy. This chapter is the "how to" chapter—describing the actual methods of administering drugs orally, parenterally, and topically. The adages "practice makes perfect" and "one picture is worth a thousand words" apply. Administering medications is a skilled activity that requires practice—with supervision—to ensure correct technique. As this chapter covers only the basics, you will want to work with a medication administration skill book and a pharmacology textbook as well.

Every institution has a standard procedure for administering medications, which depends on the way its drugs are dispensed: by unit-dose, in multidose containers, or a combination of the two. Institutional procedure may call for the use of a mobile cart or a locked dispensing system, or a locked cabinet at the patient's bedside. Documentation occurs with medication administration records (MARs), computerized medication administration records (CMARs), and/or the use of a bar code device.

Whatever the procedure's specifications, follow them carefully. Step-by-step attention to detail is the best safeguard to ensure the patient/client's six rights.

Three Checks and Six Rights

The nurse observes the three checks and six rights of medication administration.

Three Checks When Preparing Medications

Read the label:

1. Check the drug label with the MAR (medication administration record) when removing the container or unit-dose package.

2. Check the drug label again and compare with the MAR or CMAR immediately before pouring or opening the medication, or preparing the unit-dose.

3. Check the drug label once more when replacing the container and/or before giving the unit-dose to the patient/client.

Six Rights Before Administering Medications

1. Right medication
2. Right patient/client
3. Right dosage
4. Right route
5. Right time
6. Right documentation.

Other rights that are important: the right reason, the right drug preparation, right expiration date, right assessment, right evaluation, the right drug education, the right to refuse a drug.

Medication Orders

A correct medication order or prescription bears the patient/client's name, room number, date, name of drug (generic or trade), dose of the drug, route of administration, and times to administer the drug.

It ends with the signature of the physician or healthcare provider ordering the drug.

Types of Orders

1. Standing order with termination

> **EXAMPLE** cephalexin (Keflex) 500 mg PO every 6 hours × 7 days

2. Standing order without termination

> **EXAMPLE** digoxin (Lanoxin) 0.5 mg PO every day

3. A prn order

> **EXAMPLE** morphine 2 to 4 mg IV q 4 h prn pain

4. Single-dose order

> **EXAMPLE** atropine 0.3 mg subcutaneous 7:30 AM on call to OR

5. Stat order

> **EXAMPLE** morphine 4 mg IV stat

6. Protocols

> **EXAMPLE** for K <3.5, K 20 mEq PO q 4 hour × 2 days

Hospital guidelines provide for an automatic stop time on some classes of drugs; narcotic orders may be valid for only 3 days, antibiotics for 10 days. When first reading the order and transferring or transcribing the order, the nurse must take care to note the expiration time, thus alerting all staff who administer medications. It is still the prescriber's responsibility to rewrite the order. State laws and hospital policies vary.

Order Entry

In hospitals and other institutions, the medication orders are written by a physician or licensed healthcare provider. These orders may be written on a paper form that is in the patient/client's chart or, more often nowadays, on a computer (often called computerized order entry or COE or computerized physician order entry or CPOE).

An example of a paper form is shown in Figure 10-1.

Patient/Client Name
Medical Record Number
Date of Birth

Admitting Orders for CHF

Date/Time

       Admit to CCU
       Diagnosis: CHF
       Condition: Stable
       Allergies: Penicillin
       Activity: Bedrest x24 hours
       Vital Signs: every 2 hours, O2 sat and cardiac monitor
       Diet: AHA, low sodium
       IV: saline lock
       O2:   2L n/c

       EKG: on arrival and prn chest pain
       Troponin, CPK x3 q 8 hours
       CBC, BMP

       Medications:
       Digoxin 0.25 mg PO every day, hold if HR <60
       Aspirin 325 mg PO daily
       Protonix 40 mg PO daily
       Ampicillin 250 mg PO q 6h
       Lopressor 50 mg PO bid hold if SBP<100
       Coumadin 5 mg PO once a day
       Morphine sulfate 4–6 mg IV every 2–3 hours prn pain
       Tylenol gr X q 4h prn temp >101

Physician's Signature:

FIGURE 10-1

Sample paper medication order.

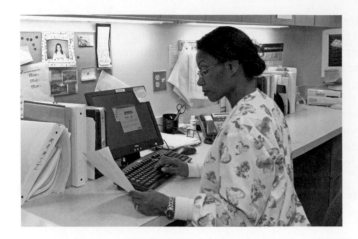

FIGURE 10-2

Checking computerized orders. (From Taylor, C. [2008]. *Fundamentals of nursing* [6th ed.]. Philadelphia, PA: Lippincott Williams & Wilkins, p. 160.)

Although other personnel, such as a unit secretary or ward clerk, may transcribe the medication orders, ultimately the nurse is responsible for transcribing the medication orders and administering the medications. Transcribing orders involves transferring the order, usually to an MAR; again, this usually is done on a paper form or the computer.

COE/CPOE allows doctors or prescribing healthcare providers to input medication orders directly onto the computer. The pharmacy receives the order and adds it to the patient/client's drug profile; subsequently, the nursing unit receives the MAR, which lists the medications and times of administration (the frequency of updates varies according to the hospital or institution). This system presents several advantages: Neither the nurse nor the pharmacist has to interpret the handwriting of the doctor or healthcare provider. The nurse does not have to transfer the written orders to an MAR, lessening the chance for error while also saving time. Moreover, a computer check identifies possible interactions among the patient/client's medications and alerts the nurse and the pharmacist. The nurse will check the medication orders on the computer (Fig. 10-2).

Medication Orders Guidelines

- Only licensed physicians or healthcare providers can write orders/prescriptions. Nurse practitioners are licensed in all states to write orders, although some restrictions apply and vary state to state.

- Medical students may write orders on charts, but orders must be countersigned by a house physician before they are legal. Medical students are not licensed.

- In states that allow nurses or paramedical personnel to prescribe drugs, these caregivers must follow hospital guidelines when carrying out orders.

- Do not carry out an order that is not clear or is illegible. Check with the physician or healthcare provider who wrote the order—do not assume anything.

- Do not carry out an order if a conflict exists with nursing knowledge. For example, meperidine (Demerol) 500 mg IM is above the average dose. Check with the physician or healthcare provider who wrote the order.

- Nursing students should not accept oral or telephone orders. The student should refer the physician to the instructor or staff nurse.

- Professional nurses may take oral or telephone orders in accord with institutional policy. The nurse must write these orders on the chart, and the physician or healthcare provider must sign them within 24 hours. Verbal orders are discouraged, and the physician should write the order if physically present in the nursing unit or has access to a computer.

Medication Administration Record (MAR)

The MAR, a daily (24-hour) record of what medications are ordered for the patient/client, also documents the medications given by the nurse. Most MARs consist of a computerized printout (Fig. 10-3), with key identifying information—the patient/client's name, identification (ID) number, room, date of admission, age, diagnosis, gender, and attending physician—printed at the top. Orders written during the shift have to be added to the printout by hand—a procedure that can lead to medication errors. Therefore, hospitals require that every shift or every 24 hours (policy varies according to institution), the nurse must check the

MCFARLAND MEDICAL CENTER
Medication Administration Record

Patient/Client Name	Room Number	Hospital Number	Diagnosis	
Curtis, Chelsea	1401	204452896	CHF	

| Allergies PCN | Admitted 5/28/14 | Age 50 | Sex F | Physician Smith, V.G. |

DOSAGE ADMINISTRATION PERIOD: 6/26/15 0600 to 6/27/15 0600

	0700–1900	1900–0700
Digoxin 0.25 mg PO every day Hold if HR <60	0900	
Aspirin 325 mg PO daily	0900	
Protonix 40 mg PO every day	0900	
Ampicillin 250 mg PO q 6h	1200 1800	2400 0600
Lopressor 50 mg PO BID Hold if SBP <100	0900	2100
Coumadin 5 mg PO once a day	1700	
Morphine sulfate 4–6 mg IV every 2–3 h prn pain		
Tylenol 650 mg q4h prn temp >101		

Signature _____ Initials ( ) Signature _____ Initials ( ) Signature _____ Initials ( )

FIGURE 10-3

A sample 24-hour computerized medication record. Scheduled drugs are listed at the top of the sheet and prn orders at the bottom. Military time is used. The nurse draws a line through the time administered and initials to indicate that the drug was administered, then signs at the bottom of the sheet.

MAR against the original orders in the chart to make sure that the orders are correct. As hospitals move to complete computerized charting, the MAR will be on the computer and charting done directly on the computer MAR.

Each healthcare setting will have different guidelines on charting medications. Generally, routine medications are assigned a scheduled time on the MAR. After the nurse gives the medication, a line is drawn through the time and initialed. If the medication is refused or held, the time is circled and initialed and then a reason given why the medication was not given. Medications prescribed on an as-needed basis (prn) are not assigned a scheduled time on the MAR; rather, after the medication is given, the time is then written on the MAR, a line crossed through that time, and then initialed. Different medications may be given at different scheduled times throughout the day. For example, warfarin (Coumadin) is given at 5 or 6 pm (1700 or 1800), so that the therapeutic effect is maximized. Follow institutional guidelines for medication administration times.

Systems of Administration

Institutions establish their own systems for administering medication. You might need to use the mobile cart, a locked medication cabinet at the central nursing station or near the patient/client's bedside, and/or computer printouts.

Unit-dose packaging is the most widely used system. Drugs are dispensed by the pharmacy and placed in individual patient/client drawers, either on a mobile cart or in a locked cabinet at the patient/client's bedside. The mobile cart can be wheeled into the patient/client's room so that you can prepare medications at the bedside for administration.

A newer system uses a scanner device, scanning the patient/client's ID band, the nurse's ID, the MAR, and the medication in unit-dose packaging. If the scan reveals any discrepancy, the device alerts the nurse.

Mobile Cart System/Locked Cabinet Near or in Patient's Room

In the mobile cart system, the pharmacy dispenses unit-dose medications directly to the patient/client's drawer in the mobile cart or locked cabinet, which is labeled with the patient/client's name. The cart/cabinet contains all of the equipment the nurse might require to administer medications.

Here's the appropriate procedure:

- When it's time to administer medications, wash your hands and roll the cart to the bedside of the first patient/client.

- Identify the patient/client using two patient/client identifiers (see p. 366).

- Unlock the cart.

- Open the medication book to that patient/client's medication sheet.

Before giving the medication, check the sheet for special nursing actions required, such as obtaining a blood pressure or heart rate. Carry out the orders, record the results, and decide whether to withhold the medication or to administer it.

First check: Place the patient/client's drawer on the top of the cart. Read each medication order, starting with the first medication listed. If you're giving a dose, choose the unit-dose from the drawer and compare the label with the order (Fig. 10-4). Check the label.

Second check: After comparing the order with the unit measure, compute the dose. Check the MAR, check the drug label, then open or prepare the unit-dose, or pour the amount of a liquid medication.

Third check: After preparing all of the patient/client's medications, check the drug label again, open the unit-dose packaging (if not done in the second check), identify the patient/client using two identifiers (see p. 366), and administer the drugs. Offer patient/client teaching. Remain with the patient/client until he or she has taken the medications, then provide any comfort measures, wash your hands, and return to the cart to chart the drugs administered. Replace the patient/client's drawer, and roll the cart to the next patient/client. When all of the medications have been administered, return the mobile cart to its designated area. (Ideally, take the MAR to the patient/client's bedside for the third check).

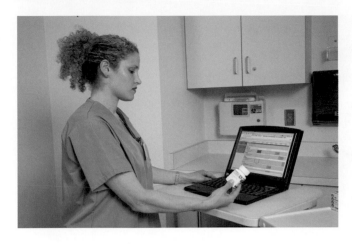

FIGURE 10-4

The nurse compares the medication with the medication order. (From Lynn, P. [2011]. *Taylor's clinical nursing skills: A nursing process approach* [3rd ed.]. Philadelphia, PA: Lippincott Williams & Wilkins, p. 158.)

This system has several advantages. Two professionals—the pharmacist and the nurse—check the medication in the drawer. All of the MARs are together on the cart, which saves time. The nurse can carry out assessment and can chart the results before pouring any medication. Immediately after administering the drugs, the nurse can sign for them.

Note that with the mobile cart systems, you must *check the label three times:* when choosing the drug, when pouring the dose or opening the medication, and before replacing the container or giving the unit-dose to the patient/client.

In a variation of the mobile cart system, the medications are locked in a cabinet at or near the patient/client's bedside. As with the original mobile cart system, the pharmacy fills the cabinet with the unit-dose medications. MARs are in the chart, which is in the cabinet, and the nurse prepares the medications in the same manner, using the three checks and the six rights. Having the medications and the patient/client's chart closer to the bedside saves time for both the patient/client and the nurse.

Many hospitals are using the computerized narcotic cart or cabinet (Pyxis system) (Fig. 10-5) to dispense all medications (controlled substances and noncontrolled medications). The computer in the cart or cabinet stores a record of each medication, when it is due, and lists this information for each patient/client. The nurse simply goes to the Pyxis with the MAR and removes the unit-doses for each patient/client by accessing the computer. The Pyxis system uses a password and often a fingerprint identifier to identify each nurse accessing this system. This system provides yet another check to make sure that the right patient/client receives the right medication, the right dose, at the right time.

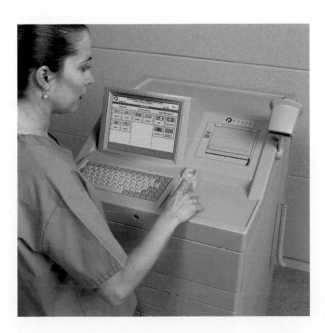

FIGURE 10-5

Pyxis Controlled Medication System. (With permission from Roach, S. [2004]. *Introductory clinical pharmacology* [7th ed.]. Philadelphia, PA: Lippincott Williams & Wilkins, p. 18.)

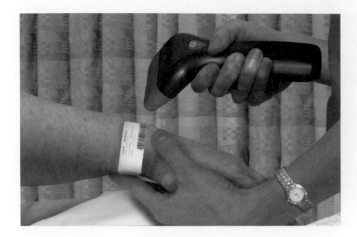

FIGURE 10-6

Scanner

Computer Scanning System

The computer scanning system uses a portable computer scanning device, which stores information about the patient/client and the medication (Fig. 10-6). The unit-dose packaging used with this system shows bar codes. The nurse's process is simple: Prepare the medications and check each one against the MAR. Use the scanning device to scan the patient/client's ID band, your own ID, the medication package, and the MAR (this system also ensures two patient/client identifiers). If the computer detects no discrepancy, you can continue to administer the medications as described in the previous section on the mobile cart system.

Knowledge Base in Giving Medications

- Nurses should know the following before giving medications:
  - generic and trade names of drugs to be administered
  - class, category of drugs to be administered
  - average adult or pediatric dose depending on the patient/client population
  - routes of administration
  - use
  - side effects and adverse effects
  - contraindications
  - nursing implications in administration
  - signs of effectiveness
  - possible drug interactions
- The nurse should be aware of the patient/client's diagnosis and medical history, especially relative to drugs taken. Be especially alert to over-the-counter drugs (OTC) or herbal remedies which patients/clients often do not consider important. Check for drug allergies.
- Assess the patient/client's need for drug information. Be prepared to implement and evaluate a nursing care plan in drug therapy.

Basic Guidelines in Giving Medications

- Always check the patient/client's ID band before administering medications (Fig. 10-7). The Joint Commission's 2014 National Patient Safety Goal 1 states that "two patient identifiers are used

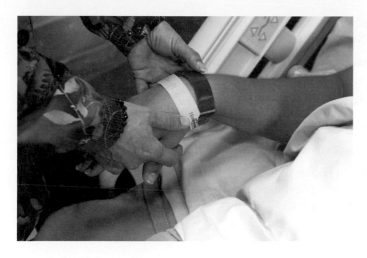

FIGURE 10-7

Checking the patient/client's armband. (From Evans-Smith, P. [2005]. *Lippincott's atlas of medication administration* [2nd ed.]. Philadelphia, PA: Lippincott Williams & Wilkins, p. 8.)

when administering medications, blood, blood components; collecting blood and other specimens for clinical testing, and providing other treatments or procedures" (see the Joint Commission website for updated information: *http://www.jointcommission.org/PatientSafety/NationalPatientSafetyGoals/*).

- Acceptable identifiers include the following:

  - The individual's name

  - An assigned ID number

  - Telephone number

  - Date of birth

  - Social security number

  - Address

  - Photograph

  - Other person-specific identifiers

- Checking a patient/client's armband and the MAR usually satisfies this requirement. Check institutional policy.

- Listen to the patient/client's comments and act on them. If a patient/client says something like "That's not mine" or "I never took this before," check carefully, then return to the patient/client with results of your investigation. Failure to do this will cause you to lose the patient/client's trust and confidence and may result in a medication error.

- If a patient/client refuses a drug, find out why. First check the chart to see if the drug was in fact ordered, then talk to the patient/client to understand his or her reasons. After charting the reason for refusal, notify the physician or healthcare provider who wrote the order.

- Watch to make sure the patient/client takes the drugs. Stay until oral drugs are swallowed.

- Keep drugs within view at all times.

- Never leave any drug at the bedside unless hospital policy permits this. If a medication is left with the patient/client, inform why the drug is ordered, how to take it, and what to expect. Later, check to determine whether the drug was taken, and record the findings.

- It is a fallacy that the nurse is no longer required to calculate or prepare drugs dispensed as unit-dose. In some instances, the pharmacy may not have the exact dose on hand or the nurse may need to administer a partial dose. The label still must be read three times.

- Labels on medication must be clear. If not, return them to the pharmacy.

- If any doubt about a drug exists, do not administer it. Check further with the physician, the healthcare provider, the pharmacist, or a supervising nurse.

- Orders issued as "stat" take precedence and must be carried out immediately.

- Perform indicated nursing actions before administering certain medications. For example, digoxin requires an apical heart rate; antihypertensives require a blood pressure reading.

- Administer medications within 30 minutes of the time scheduled.

- Keep medications within sight at all times. Never leave medications unattended.

- Do not administer a medication if assessment shows that the drug is contraindicated or that an adverse effect may have occurred as a result of a previous dose. If you withhold a drug, notify the physician or healthcare provider who wrote the order.

Documentation

Documentation is the "sixth right" of medication administration. The always-quoted axiom is still true: "If it's not charted, it's not done."

- Chart all medications after administration.

- Chart single doses, stat doses, and prn medications immediately, and note the exact time they were administered.

- Chart any nursing actions done before administering drugs (e.g., apical heart rate with digoxin or blood pressure with antihypertensives). Usually, this can be done on the MAR.

- If the drug was refused or was withheld, write the reason on the nurse's notes and/or on the MAR, notify the healthcare provider who ordered the medication, and also the time you notified the healthcare provider and any response.

Standard Precautions Applied to Administration of Medications

When you are administering drugs, there's a chance that the patient/client's blood, body fluids, or tissues can come into contact with your skin or mucous membranes. Therefore, you always risk potential exposure to serious bacterial infections, fungal infections, tuberculosis, or a long list of viruses, including these: hepatitis A virus (HAV), hepatitis B virus (HBV), hepatitis C virus (HCV), hepatitis D virus (HDV), hepatitis E virus (HEV), and the human immunodeficiency virus (HIV).

The Centers for Disease Control and Prevention (CDC) in Atlanta recommends standard precautions in caring for all patients/clients and when handling equipment contaminated with blood or blood-streaked body fluids. In 1996, the term standard precautions replaced "universal precautions." Transmission-based precautions are those used with patients/clients who have a suspected infection. For more information on these procedures, see the CDC website (http://www.cdc.gov or http://www.cdc.gov/hai/).

The following points, based on CDC guidelines, can help you determine appropriate safeguards in giving medications. Follow your institutional requirements. The safeguards you need to follow depend on the type of contact you have with patients/clients.

General Safeguards in Administering Medications

1. Oral medications: Handwashing or use of an antiseptic foam or lotion is adequate. If there's a possibility of exposure to blood or body secretions, wear gloves.

2. Injections: Both handwashing and gloves are required. Do not recap needles. Carefully dispose of used sharps, either by holding the sharp away from you in a puncture-proof container or by using a needleguard device.

3. Heparin locks, saline locks, IV catheters, and IV needles: Wash your hands and wear gloves when inserting or removing IV needles and catheters. Dispose of used sharps in a puncture-proof container or use a needleguard device.

4. Secondary administration sets or IV piggyback (IVPB) sets: Before removing this equipment from the main IV tubing, wash your hands and put on gloves. Either use a needleless device or place used needles in a puncture-proof container.

5. Application of medication to mucous membranes: Wash your hands and wear gloves (see the following guidelines for using gowns, masks, and protective eyewear).

6. Applications to skin: Before applying such drug forms as transdermal patches or applying lotions, ointments, or creams, wash your hands and wear gloves.

Hands

1. With each patient/client, always wash your hands twice—before preparing medications and after administering medications. Use of an antiseptic foam or lotion is an acceptable alternative to handwashing.

2. Wash your hands after removing your gloves, gown, mask, and protective eyewear, and wash them again before leaving any patient/client's room where you have used them.

3. If your hands have come into contact with a patient/client's blood or body fluids, wash them immediately.

4. Wash your hands after handling any equipment soiled with blood or body fluids.

Gloves

1. While administering medications, wear gloves for any direct ("hands-on") contact with a patient/client's blood, bodily fluids, or secretions.

2. Wear gloves when handling materials or equipment contaminated with blood or body fluids.

3. Whenever you use gloves, you must change them after completing procedures for each patient/client and between patients/clients.

Gowns

When administering medications, you need to wear a gown if there's a risk that your clothing may become contaminated with a patient/client's blood or body fluids.

Masks, Protective Eyewear, and Face Shields

1. A mask is required when you are caring for a patient/client on strict or respiratory isolation procedures.

2. Masks and protective eyewear or face shields are required when a medication procedure may cause blood or body fluids to splash directly onto your face, eyes, or mucous membranes.

3. You must wear masks and protective eyewear during any medication procedure known to cause aerosolization of fluids that contain chemicals or body fluids.

Management of Used Needles and Sharps

1. All used needles, syringes, sharps, stylets, butterfly needles, and IV catheters must be discarded in appropriate, labeled, puncture-proof containers.

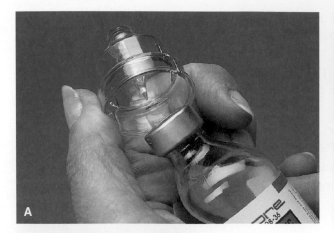
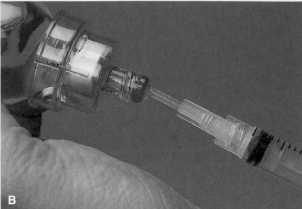
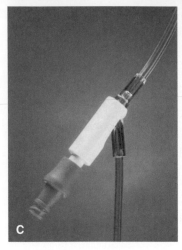

FIGURE 10-8

A. Needleless system adapter for vial. **B.** Use syringe (without needle) to withdraw medication. **C.** Needleless system for IV tubing.

2. Do not break, bend, or recap needles after using them. Immediately place needles in a puncture-proof container. If preparing the medication away from the bedside, carefully recap, if needed, to transport the medication safely.

3. Wear gloves and exercise caution when removing heparin locks, saline locks, IV catheters, and IV needles. Place them in a puncture-proof container. Never remove the IV needle from the IV tubing by hand. Instead, use either a clamp or the needle unlocking device on the sharps container. It's best to use needleless systems or needleguard devices.

4. As you dispose of a sharp, keep your eyes on the sharps (puncture-proof) container.

Needleless Systems and Needleguard Devices

Needleless systems, used to reduce the risk of needlesticks and blood-borne pathogens, work in several ways. Some syringes have a needleguard device that retracts the needle into the syringe or a cap after it is used. Needleless adapters for syringes withdraw medication from vials (Fig. 10-8). Needleless systems are also available for IV tubing and for use at the patient/client's IV site. All needleless equipment must be discarded into sharps containers.

Management of Materials Other Than Needles and Sharps

Paper cups, plastic cups, and other equipment not contaminated with blood or body fluids may be discarded according to routine hospital procedures. In situations that require strict or respiratory isolation precautions, follow the institution's established protocol.

Management of Nurse Exposed to Blood or Body Fluids

If a personal needlestick, an injury, or a skin laceration causes contact with the blood or blood-streaked body fluids of any patient/client, *act immediately*: Squeeze the area of contact if appropriate, wash the area with soap and copious amounts of water, and apply an acceptable antiseptic. If mucous membrane exposure occurs, flush the exposed areas with copious amounts of warm water. Follow the protocol established by the healthcare institution for management of needlestick injury or accidental exposure to blood or body fluids.

Routes of Administration

Oral Route

Regardless of which system you use to prepare the medications, the procedure for administering drugs requires specific steps. The oral route is the least expensive, the safest, and also the easiest to administer. For oral administration, patients/clients should have an intact gag reflex, be alert, and have a functioning gastrointestinal system.

Handwashing is required; wear gloves if there is any chance of touching mucous membranes.

1. Follow the six rights and three checks.

2. Use two patient/client identifiers to identify the patient/client.

3. Ask the patient/client if he or she has allergies to any drugs, or check the MAR or patient/client chart.

4. Before administering the medications, perform any necessary assessment (e.g., checking vital signs, apical rate, or site integrity).

5. Explain the procedure to the patient/client.

6. Assist the patient/client to a sitting position.

7. Give oral solids first, along with a full glass of water whenever possible (unless contraindicated). Then give oral liquid medications.

8. Watch to be sure the patient/client has swallowed all of the drugs.

9. Discard paper/plastic cups according to hospital procedure.

10. Make the patient/client comfortable, wash your hands, and chart the medications given.

Special Considerations for Oral Administration

SOLIDS

- Some drugs are best taken on an empty stomach; others may be taken with food. Check a drug guide to see which is needed.

- Administer irritating oral drugs along with meals or a snack (unless contraindicated) to decrease gastric irritation.

- If the patient/client is nauseated or vomiting, withhold oral medications and notify the physician/healthcare provider.

- Even if the patient/client is NPO (nothing by mouth), the patient/client may need to receive certain drugs (e.g., an anticonvulsant for a patient/client with epilepsy). Check with the doctor or healthcare provider to determine whether you can administer oral medication with a small amount of water.

- Scored tablets can be broken and have a line across the center of the tablet.

  - To break a scored tablet, use clean technique. One method is to place the tablet in a paper towel, fold the towel over, and, with your thumbs and index fingers, break the tablet along the score line. You can also use commercial pill splitters.

- Do not break unscored tablets, because you can't be certain that the drug is evenly distributed.

- Coated tablets have a coating that makes the tablets smooth and easy to swallow. Avoid crushing coated tablets unless the drug is one that can be crushed. Check a drug guide or check with a pharmacist.

  - Enteric-coated tablets are meant to dissolve in the more alkaline secretions of the intestine rather than in the highly acidic stomach juices. However, enteric-coated tablets may dissolve prematurely if a patient/client is on antacids or has a disorder that decreases stomach acidity.

  - Do not crush enteric-coated tablets.

- Prolonged-release or extended-release tablets dissolve more slowly and have a longer duration of action.

  - Do not crush prolonged-release tablets.

- Capsules are gelatin containers that hold a drug. Usually, the capsule holds the drug because the drug could irritate the stomach lining or the stomach acidity would decrease the drug's potency.

  - Avoid opening capsules. Occasionally, a capsule may be opened and combined with a semisolid such as applesauce or custard and administered to the patient/client. Always check with the physician or healthcare provider if another form may be available.

  - Do not open spansule, timespan, time release, or sustained-release capsules. These drugs are long-acting and designed to be released over time.

- If the patient/client has difficulty swallowing solids, check with the physician or healthcare provider for an order for the liquid form of the medication (if available) or crush the medications (if applicable).

- If crushing a pill won't compromise its medication, you can crush it, preferably using a commercial pill crusher. You can also crush a pill using a mortar and pestle; just make sure to clean both implements before and after crushing so no residue remains. To help a patient/client swallow the medication, you can mix a crushed drug with water or a small amount of semisolids, such as applesauce or custard.

- If the oral route is not possible, a physician or healthcare provider can order the drug parenterally (e.g., Lasix IV instead of Lasix PO).

- Lozenges are solid tablets with medication that dissolve slowly in the mouth. These may contain sugar or syrup and may be inappropriate for patients/clients with diabetes.

- Be knowledgeable about food–drug, drug–drug, and herb–drug interactions.

- When administering solid stock medications, pour them first into the container lid and then into a paper cup, using medical asepsis. Do not touch the medication. After pouring each medication into a separate cup, you can combine several solid medications into one cup. Check all unit-dose medications three times before you discard the package container.

LIQUIDS

- Shake liquid medications thoroughly before pouring; otherwise, the drug in the liquid may settle to the bottom.

- Aqueous or water-based solutions do not need to be shaken before pouring.

- Some liquid medications require dilution. Check references for directions.

- Some liquids may have to be administered through a straw. Liquid iron preparations, for example, cause discoloring and should not come in contact with teeth.

- Pour liquids at eye level, using a medicine cup. Then place them on a flat surface to accurately measure the dose. Measure at the center of the meniscus, which is the lower curve of the liquid in the cup. To keep from spilling the medication onto the label (which could make it unreadable), pour with the label up (Fig. 10-9).

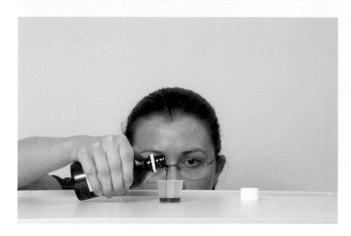

FIGURE 10-9
Eye level

- Never return any poured drug to a stock bottle once the drug has been taken from the preparation room.
- Never combine medications from two stock bottles. It is the responsibility of the pharmacist to combine drugs.
- Check drug references to determine how to disguise liquids that are distasteful or irritating. Mixing them in other liquids, such as juice, is often done unless contraindicated.
- After the patient/client has taken a liquid antacid, add 5 to 10 mL water to the cup, mix, and have the patient/client drink it as well. Because antacids are thick, some medication often remains in the cup.
- The nurse who pours medications is responsible for administering and charting. Do not give drugs that another nurse has poured.
- Syrups are solutions of sugar in water, which may disguise the medication's unpleasant taste. Because of the sugar, syrups may be contraindicated for patients/clients with diabetes.
- Elixirs are hydroalcoholic liquids that are sweetened. These may be contraindicated for patients/ clients with diabetes or a history of alcoholism.
- Fluid extracts and tinctures are alcoholic, liquid concentrations of a drug. Because these are very potent, they are ordered in small amounts. Tinctures are ordered in drops. Fluid extracts are the most concentrated of all liquids. The average dose of a fluid extract is 2 tsp or less.
- Solutions are clear liquids that contain a drug dissolved in water.
- A suspension consists of solid particles of a drug dispersed in a liquid. Be sure to shake the bottle before pouring.
- Magmas—for example, milk of magnesia—contain large, bulky particles.
- Gels—for example, magnesium hydroxide gel—contain small particles.
- Emulsions are creamy, white suspensions of fats or oils in an agent that reduces surface tension and thus makes the oil easier to swallow—for example, emulsified castor oil.
- Powders are dry, finely ground drugs, reconstituted according to directions. In liquid form, powders become oral suspensions.
- When you reconstitute a powder, write these four facts on the label: the date, the time, your initials, and the solution you made.

Nasogastric Route

When possible, obtain the medication in liquid form. Before opening capsules or crushing tablets, check with the pharmacist for alternatives. If crushing medications, crush finely so as not to clog the tube. Use either a bulb syringe or a 60-mL syringe.

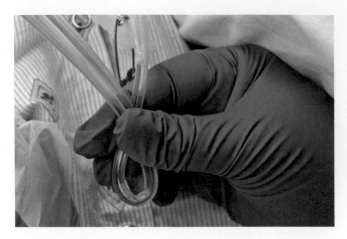

FIGURE 10-10

Bend the tube back on itself to close the tube. (From Taylor, C. [2008]. *Fundamentals of nursing* [6th ed.]. Philadelphia, PA: Lippincott Williams & Wilkins, p. 1473.)

First, dilute the medication with water. The fluid mixture should be at room temperature.

1. Follow the six rights and three checks.

2. Use two patient/client identifiers to identify the patient/client.

3. Ask the patient/client if he or she has allergies to any drugs, or check the MAR or patient/client chart.

4. Before administering the injection, perform any necessary assessment (e.g., checking vital signs, apical rate, or site integrity).

5. Explain the procedure to the patient/client.

6. Elevate the head of the bed to 30 degrees.

7. Put on your gloves and insert the syringe into the tube.

8. To check the position of the tube in the stomach, place a stethoscope on the stomach and insert about 15 mL of air. If you hear a swishing sound, the tube is in the proper place.

9. Aspirate the stomach's contents. If the patient/client has been receiving tube feedings, check institutional policy regarding residual aspirate.

10. You can also test the stomach contents for acidity by using pH paper, if available. The reasoning is that the pH paper will test more acidic, confirming placement in the stomach's acidic environment. Research supports this method, although many institutions do not have pH paper readily available on the nursing unit. One good website supporting this method is http://enw.org/Research-NGT.htm

11. Close off the tube by bending it back on itself (Fig. 10-10). Holding the syringe and bent tube in your nondominant hand, remove the bulb or plunger and leave the syringe in place.

12. Flush the tube with at least 30 mL of water (or follow institutional policy for flushing nasogastric tubes) to ensure patency (Fig. 10-11). Release the closing off of the tube; gravity will cause the water to flow in.

13. Pour the medication into the syringe (Fig. 10-12). As in step 12, gravity will cause the medication to flow in. Occasionally, you may apply slight pressure with the plunger of the syringe.

14. If the patient/client shows discomfort, stop the procedure and wait until he or she appears relaxed.

15. Before all of the medication flows in, flush the tube by adding at least 30 mL of water (or follow institutional policy for flushing nasogastric tubes) to the syringe (see Fig. 10-11).

16. Shut the tube by bending it back on itself before the syringe completely empties.

17. Remove the syringe and either clamp the tube or restart tube feedings.

18. If possible, leave the head of the bed elevated at least 30 minutes to 1 hour.

19. Make the patient/client comfortable, wash your hands, and chart the medications given.

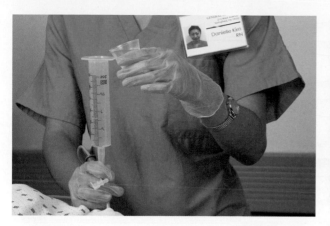

FIGURE 10-11

Flush the tube with 30 mL of water before and after giving the medication.

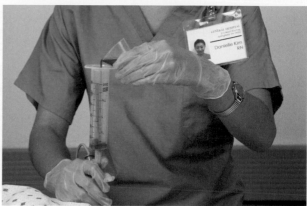

FIGURE 10-12

Pour the medication into the syringe.

Parenteral Route

General Guidelines

You can give medications by IM (intramuscular), subcutaneous, IV, IVPB, IVP (IV push), or intradermal routes. Use the parenteral route when a patient/client cannot take the drug orally, when you want to obtain a rapid systemic effect, or when the oral route would destroy a drug or render it ineffective. With parenteral routes, use aseptic technique.

Syringes for Injection

The most common syringe used for injections is a standard 3-mL size, marked in milliliters to the nearest tenth. The precision (tuberculin) syringe is marked in milliliters to the nearest hundredth. There are two insulin syringes (insulin is only given in an insulin syringe): a regular 1-mL size marked to 100 units and a 0.5-mL size (low dose) marked to 50 units.

Needles for Injections

Each of the four syringes described above has a different injection needle.

Syringe	*Gauge*	*Length (in inches)*
3 mL	20–23	1½–3
1 mL	20–28	⅝–⅞
1 mL insulin	25–26	½–⅝
½ mL low-dose insulin	25–28	½–⅝

The term *gauge* (G) indicates the needle's diameter or width. The higher the gauge number, the finer or smaller the needle's diameter. In the gauges directly above, the low-dose insulin syringe needle has the smallest diameter (28 gauge), which makes it the finest needle in this group.

The length of the needle you use depends on the route of injection. For deep IM injections, you use a long needle. For subcutaneous injections, you use a short needle. Gauge numbers 23, 25, 26, and 28 in ⅝ inch length are used in subcutaneous injections for adults and in IM injections for children and emaciated patients/clients. Numbers 20, 22, and 23 in 1 and 1½ inch lengths are used for IM injections; 20 and 21 in 1 to 2 inch lengths are for IV therapy and very viscous liquids in IM injections; and 14, 16, and 18 in 1 to 2 inch lengths are for blood transfusions.

Choosing which type of needle to use for an adult or a child depends on three factors: the route of administration, the size and condition of the patient/client, and the amount of adipose tissue present at the site (Fig. 10-13). Most hospitals use needleless systems to draw up parenteral medications and for IV therapy. This helps to prevent accidental needle sticks. IM, subcutaneous, and intradermal injections are given with the technique illustrated in Figure 10-14.

Needles usually used for **intradermal** injections are ⅜" to ⅝" (1 to 1.5 cm) long and are 25G. Such needles usually have short bevels.

Needles for **subcutaneous** injections are ⅝" to ⅞" (1.5 to 2 cm) long, have medium bevels, and are 28G to 23G.

Needles for **IM** use are 1" to 3" (2.5 to 7.5 cm) long, have medium bevels, and are 23G to 20G.

Needles for **IV** use are 1" to 3" long, have long bevels, and are 25G to 14G.

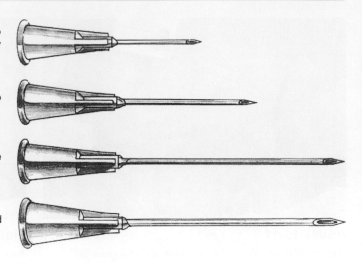

FIGURE 10-13

When choosing a needle, the nurse must consider the needle gauge, bevel, and length. Gauge refers to the inside diameter of the needle; the smaller the gauge, the larger the diameter. Bevel refers to the angle at which the needle tip is opened, and length is the distance from the tip to the hub of the needle.

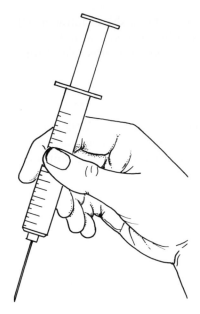

FIGURE 10-14

An injection is administered with a quick, dartlike motion into taut skin that has been spread or bunched together.

Angle of Insertion

INTRAMUSCULAR. For an IM injection, hold the syringe at a right angle to the skin. Give the injection at a 90-degree angle (Fig. 10-15). IM sites have a good blood supply, and absorption is rapid.

SUBCUTANEOUS. For subcutaneous injections, hold the syringe at a 45-degree angle, with the opening or beveled edge up, when you insert the needle. You can administer some subcutaneous injections at a 90-degree angle if the subcutaneous layer of fat is thick and the needle is short. Be careful to reach the correct site. When in doubt, use the 45-degree angle. Subcutaneous sites have a poor blood supply, and absorption is prolonged (see Fig. 10-15).

INTRADERMAL. If you're doing skin testing for allergies and tuberculosis, use a 25G or other fine needle. Hold the syringe at a 15-degree angle with the opening or beveled edge up (see Fig. 10-15).

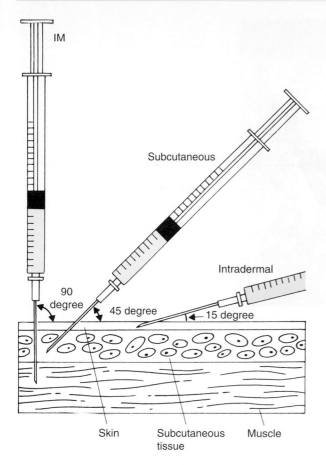

FIGURE 10-15

Comparison of angles of intersection for IM, subcutaneous, and intradermal injections.

Preparing Parenteral Medications

Handwashing is required.

DRUGS THAT ARE LIQUIDS IN VIALS

1. Clean the top of the vial with an alcohol pad.

2. Draw up into the syringe an amount of air equivalent to the desired amount of solution.

3. Inject the needle (or needleless device) through the rubber diaphragm into the vial. Some institutions require use of a filter needle, which prevents large particles from entering the syringe.

4. Expel air from the syringe into the vial (Fig. 10-16A). This increases the pressure in the vial and makes it easier to withdraw medication.

5. Invert the vial, hold it at eye level, and draw up the desired amount of medication into the syringe (Fig. 10-16B).

6. Withdraw the needle or needleless device quickly from the vial. Remove the device or needle, and attach the appropriate needle to the syringe for administration.

DRUGS THAT ARE POWDERS IN VIALS

1. Clean the top of the vial with an alcohol pad.

2. Draw up the amount of calculated diluent from a vial of distilled water or normal saline for injection. If a different diluent is indicated, follow pharmaceutical directions.

3. Add the diluent to the powder, and roll the vial between your hands to make the powder dissolve. Then, label the vial with the solution made, your initials, and the date and time.

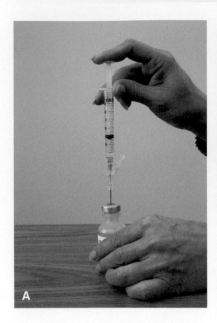
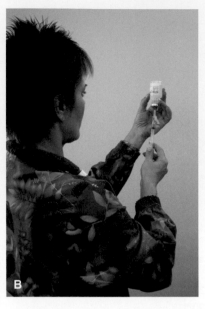

FIGURE 10-16

A. Inject air into the vial. **B.** Invert the vial, hold it at eye level, and draw up the desired amount of medication into the syringe. (From Lynn, P. [2011]. *Taylor's clinical nursing skills: A nursing process approach* [3rd ed.]. Philadelphia, PA: Lippincott Williams & Wilkins, p. 173.)

4. Clean the top of the vial again.

5. Draw up into the syringe an amount of air equivalent to the amount of solution desired.

6. Inject the needle or needleless device through the rubber diaphragm into the vial. Some institutions require use of a filter needle, which prevents large particles from entering the syringe.

7. Expel the air into the vial. This increases pressure in the vial and makes it easier to remove medication.

8. Invert the vial, hold it at eye level, and draw up the desired amount of medication into the syringe.

9. Withdraw the needle or needleless device quickly from the vial. Remove the device or needle, and attach the appropriate needle to the syringe for administration.

10. Check the directions for storing any remaining drug.

Note: When the whole amount of powder contained in a vial is needed for an IVPB medication, you can use a reconstitution device as a way of diluting the powder without a syringe.

DRUGS IN GLASS AMPULES

1. Tap the top of the ampule with your finger to clear out any drug.

2. Place an unopened alcohol pad or small gauze pad around the neck of the ampule.

3. Hold the ampule sideways.

4. Place your thumbs above the ampule neck and your index fingers below it.

5. Press down with your thumbs to break the ampule, snapping the tip away from one's self.

6. Place the ampule on a flat surface, insert the tip of the needle into the ampule, and withdraw fluid (Fig. 10-17A) *or* invert the ampule, hold it at eye level, insert the syringe needle or needleless device, and withdraw the dose (Fig. 10-17B). Some institutions require use of a filter needle, which prevents large particles from entering the syringe. *Important:* Do not add air before removing the dose, because if you do, medication will spray from the ampule.

7. Withdraw the needle or needleless device from the ampule. Remove the device or needle, and attach the appropriate needle to the syringe for administration.

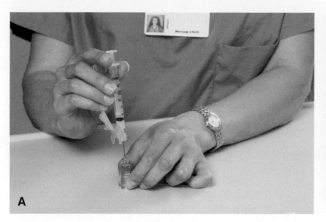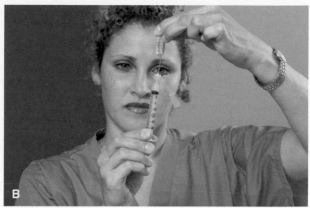

FIGURE 10-17
A. Withdrawing medication from an upright ampule. **B.** Withdrawing medication from an inverted ampule. (From Lynn, P. [2011]. *Taylor's clinical nursing skills: A nursing process approach* [3rd ed.]. Philadelphia, PA: Lippincott Williams & Wilkins, p. 170.)

UNIT-DOSE CARTRIDGE AND HOLDER

1. Insert the cartridge into the metal or plastic holder, and screw it into place (see Fig. 3-10, Chapter 3).

2. Move the plunger forward until it engages the shaft of the cartridge.

3. Twist the plunger until it is locked into the cartridge.

4. The holder is reusable, but the cartridge is not. Place the cartridge in a sharps container after use. (See *http://www.hospira.com/products/CarpujectSyringeSystem.aspx* for animation of preparing an unit-dose cartridge.)

UNIT-DOSE PREFILLED SYRINGES

1. The medication is already in the syringe (see Fig. 3-9, Chapter 3).

2. Some prefilled syringes are simple and require no action other than removing the needle cover; others are packaged for compactness and include directions for preparing the syringe for use.

3. These prefilled syringes are disposable.

MIXING TWO MEDICATIONS IN ONE SYRINGE

General Principles

1. Consult a standard reference to determine that the drugs are compatible.

2. When in doubt about compatibility, prepare medications separately and administer them into different injection sites.

3. When medications are in both a vial and an ampule, draw up the medication from the vial first.

4. When you're preparing two types of insulin in one syringe, first draw into the syringe the vial containing regular insulin. (Regular insulin has not been adulterated with protein as have other insulins such as protamine zinc insulin.)

Method

1. Clean both vials with an alcohol pad.

2. Choose one vial as the primary. *Example:* With vials of a narcotic and a nonnarcotic, the narcotic is the primary. With two insulins, regular insulin is the primary.

3. Inject air into the second vial in an amount equaling the medication to be withdrawn. Do not let the needle touch the medication.

4. Inject air into the primary vial in an amount equaling the medication to be withdrawn, then withdraw the medication in the usual way. Some institutions require use of a filter needle, which prevents large particles from entering the syringe. Make sure there are no air bubbles.

5. Insert the needle or needleless device into the second vial. Don't touch the plunger, because if you do, you might push the primary medication into the second vial.

6. Slowly withdraw the needed amount of drug from the second vial. The two medications are now combined.

7. Remove the needle or needleless device from the second vial. Remove the device or needle, and attach the appropriate needle to the syringe for administration. *Note:* Some authorities suggest changing the needle after withdrawing medication from the primary vial. Such a change may result in air bubbles, so to obtain an accurate dose, be careful when you withdraw the second medication.

Choosing the Site for Intradermal, Intramuscular, or Subcutaneous Injections

Avoid the following areas for injections: bony prominences, large blood vessels, nerves, sensitive areas, bruises, hardened areas, abrasions, and inflamed areas; areas contraindicated from previous medical procedures, such as mastectomies, renal shunts, and grafts; and areas with recent medical procedures (i.e., scars and incision lines). The site for IM injections should be able to accept 2 mL; if you're giving repeated injections, rotate sites.

Identifying the Injection Site—Adults

INTRAMUSCULAR. Common sites are the dorsogluteal, the ventrogluteal, the vastus lateralis, and the deltoid muscles.

Dorsogluteal Site. The thick gluteal muscles of the buttocks (the dorsogluteal site has been associated with possible injury due to the proximity of the sciatic nerve. Also *extensive* subcutaneous tissue at this site may cause the IM injection to actually be in the subcutaneous tissue. Follow your institutional policy regarding this injection site for IM injections).

Patient/Client's Position. Either prone or lying on the side, with both buttocks fully exposed.

Method:

- Choose the area very carefully to avoid striking the sciatic nerve, major blood vessels, or bone.
- The landmarks of the buttocks are the crest of the posterior ilium as the superior boundary and the inferior gluteal fold as the lower boundary.
- You can identify the exact site in either of these two ways:

  1. *Diagonal landmark* (Fig. 10-18):
     - Find the posterior superior iliac spine and the greater trochanter of the femur.
     - Draw an imaginary diagonal line between these two points, and give the injection lateral and superior to that line, 1 to 2 inches below the iliac crest (to avoid hitting the iliac bone).
     - If you hit the bone, withdraw the needle slightly and continue the procedure.
     - This is the preferred method because all of the landmarks are bony prominences.

  2. *Quadrant landmark* (Fig. 10-19):
     - Divide the buttocks into imaginary quadrants.
     - Your vertical line extends from the crest of the ilium to the gluteal fold.

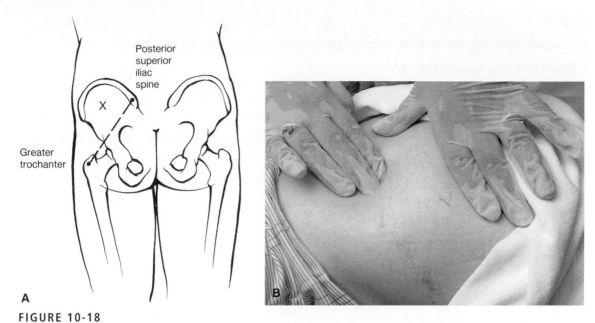

FIGURE 10-18

A. Identification of the dorsogluteal site using a diagonal between the bony prominences. **B.** Locating the exact site.

- Your horizontal line extends from the medial fold of the buttock to the lateral aspect of the buttock.
- Next, locate the upper aspect of the upper outer quadrant.
- Give the injection in this area, 1 to 2 inches below the crest of the ilium (to avoid hitting bone). To select the precise site, palpate the crest of the ilium.
- If you hit the bone when injecting, withdraw the needle slightly and continue the procedure.

Ventrogluteal Site. The ventral part of the gluteal muscle, which has no large nerves or blood vessels and less fat. This site is the safest because of those reasons.

Patient/Client's Position. Either supine, lying on the side, sitting, or standing

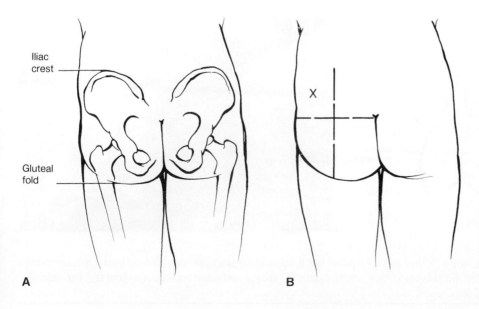

FIGURE 10-19

A. Identification of the dorsogluteal injection site using quadrants. Draw an imaginary line from the iliac crest to the gluteal fold and from the medial to the lateral buttock. **B.** The "x" indicates the injection area.

Method:

- Find the greater trochanter, the anterior superior iliac spine, and the iliac crest.
- Stand by the patient/client's knee.
- Use the hand opposite to the patient/client's leg (i.e., left leg, right hand).
- Then place the palm of your hand on the greater trochanter.
- Point your index finger toward the anterior superior iliac spine, and point your middle finger toward the iliac crest.
- The injection site lies in the center of the triangle, between your middle finger and index finger (Fig. 10-20).

Vastus Lateralis Site. The lateral thigh

Patient/Client's Position. Either supine, lying on the side, or standing

Method:

- Measure one hand's width below the greater trochanter and one hand's width above the knee (Fig. 10-21).
- Ask the patient/client to point the big toe to the center of his or her body, an action that relaxes the vastus muscle.
- Give the injection in the lateral thigh.

Deltoid Site. The upper arm, at the deltoid, a small muscle close to the radial and brachial arteries. Use this site for IM injections only if specifically ordered, and inject no more than 2 mL of medication.

Patient/Client's Position. Either sitting or lying down

Method:

- The boundaries are the lower edge of the acromion process (shoulder bone) and the axilla (armpit) (Fig. 10-22).
- Give the injection into the lateral arm between these two points, about 2 inches below the acromion process.

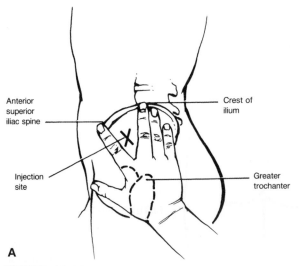

Anterior superior iliac spine

Crest of ilium

Injection site

Greater trochanter

A

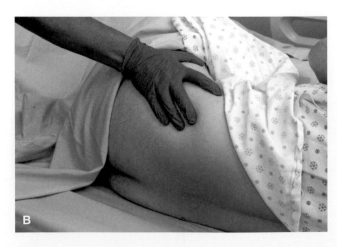

B

FIGURE 10-20

A. The ventrogluteal site for IM injections; the "x" indicates the injection site. **B.** Locating the exact site. Note the hand used is opposite to the patient/client's leg: right hand on left leg. (From Evans-Smith, P. [2005]. *Lippincott's atlas of medication administration* [2nd ed.]. Philadelphia, PA: Lippincott Williams & Wilkins, p. 31.)

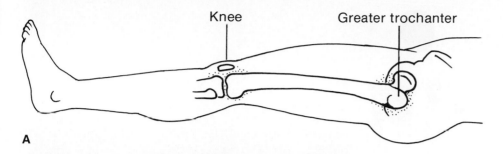

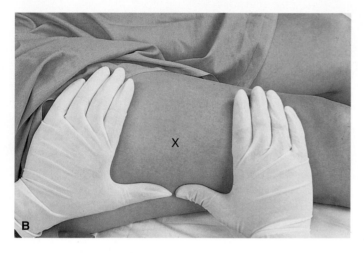

FIGURE 10-21

A. Vastus lateralis injection site. **B.** Locating the site. The "x" indicates the injection site.

SUBCUTANEOUS SITES. Commonly, the upper arms, anterior thighs, lower abdomen, and upper back (Fig. 10-23). Insulin subcutaneous is administered in the arm, lower abdomen, and thigh. Heparin subcutaneous is given in the lower abdomen.

Method:

- To avoid reaching muscle, give the injection at a 45-degree angle.

- You can give subcutaneous injections at a 90-degree angle if the subcutaneous layer of fat is thick. Diabetic patients/clients usually give their insulin only at the 90-degree angle.

- Inject no more than 1 mL of medication.

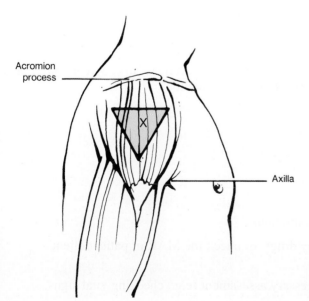

FIGURE 10-22

The deltoid muscle site for IM injections. The "x" indicates the injection site.

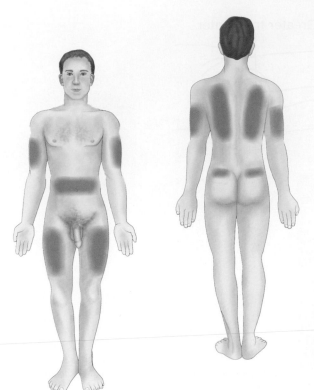

FIGURE 10-23

Sites for subcutaneous injection. The deltoid muscle may be used for subcutaneous injections, or, when ordered, for small IM injections. (From Lynn, P. [2011]. *Taylor's clinical nursing skills: A nursing process approach* [3rd ed.]. Philadelphia, PA: Lippincott Williams & Wilkins, p. 184.)

INTRADERMAL (INTRACUTANEOUS) SITE. Typically, the inner aspect of the forearm. The intradermal site is used for skin testing for allergies and diseases such as tuberculosis. Intradermal skin testing requires follow-up evaluations to determine if the skin test is positive. Injecting an antigen causes an antigen–antibody sensitivity reaction if the individual is susceptible. If the test is positive, the area will become raised, warm, and reddened.

Identifying the Injection Site—Children

The site for the IM injection in a child depends on the child's age, the child's size, and the volume and density of medication being administered. Infants cannot tolerate volumes greater than 0.5 mL in a single site. Older infants or small children can tolerate 1 mL in a single site. Needle gauges range from 21G to 25G; 27G is often used with newborns and premature infants.

The preferred site for infants is the vastus lateralis muscle (Fig. 10-24). Give the medication on the lateral aspect of the anterior thigh. After the child has been walking for more than a year, you can use the dorsogluteal site; usually, however, that site is not recommended for children less than 5 years old. For the older child and adolescent, you can use the same injection sites as for adults.

Administering Injections

Basic Guidelines for All Injections

Handwashing and gloves are required.

1. Follow the six rights and three checks.

2. Use two patient/client identifiers to identify the patient/client.

3. Ask the patient/client if he or she has allergies to any drugs, or check the MAR or patient/client chart.

4. Before administering the injection, perform any necessary assessment (e.g., checking vital signs, apical rate, or site integrity).

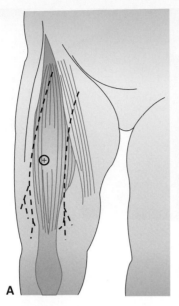
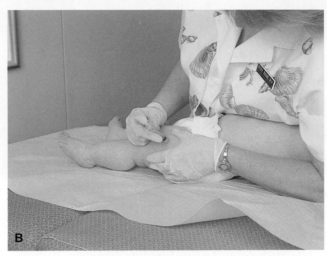

FIGURE 10-24

A. For infants under walking age, use the vastus lateralis muscle for IM injections. **B.** Technique for administering an IM injection to an infant. Note the way the nurse uses their body to restrain and stabilize the infant.
(From Pillitteri, A. [2002]. *Maternal and child health nursing* [4th ed.]. Philadelphia, PA: Lippincott Williams & Wilkins, p. 1102.)

5. Explain the procedure to the patient/client.

6. Ask the patient/client where the last injection was given. Choose a different site, because the sites should be rotated.

7. Clean the area with an alcohol pad, using a circular motion from the center out. Allow to dry.

8. Place the alcohol pad between your fingers or lay it on the patient/client's skin above the site.

INTRAMUSCULAR INJECTIONS

Follow steps 1–8 above, then:

9. After drawing up the dose, remove the needle cover.

10. Make the skin taut by mounding the tissue between your thumb and index finger or by spreading the tissue firmly.

11. Dart the needle in quickly (Fig. 10-25A).

12. Hold the barrel with your nondominant hand, and with your dominant hand pull the plunger back. This action, called aspiration, makes sure the needle is not in a blood vessel (Fig. 10-25B).

13. If blood enters the syringe, withdraw the needle, discard both the needle and the syringe into a sharps container, and prepare another injection.

14. If no blood is aspirated, inject the medication slowly (Fig. 10-25C).

15. Remove the needle quickly.

16. To inhibit bleeding, press down on the area with the alcohol pad or a dry gauze pad.

17. Do not recap the needle. Dispose of the needle and syringe in a sharps container. Make the patient/client comfortable, wash your hands, and chart the medication, documenting the site of injection.

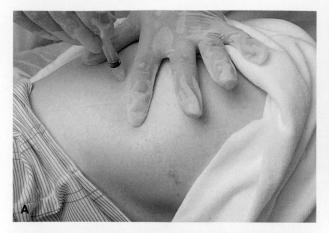

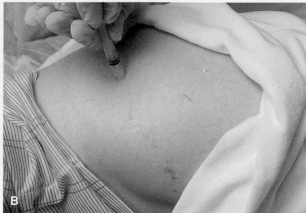

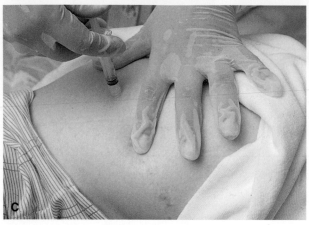

FIGURE 10-25

A. Dart the needle into the skin. **B.** Aspirate slowly. **C.** Injvect medication slowly.

Subcutaneous Heparin (or Low Molecular Weight Heparin Such as Lovenox)

A heparin injection indicates several changes in routine injection technique. Because heparin and enoxaparin (Lovenox) are anticoagulants, you must take care to minimize tissue trauma; slow bleeding at the site of the injection can cause bruising. Give the injection with a fine (25G) ½-inch needle into the lower abdominal fold, at least 2 inches from the umbilicus. Administer enoxaparin (Lovenox) in an area on the abdomen between the left or right anterolateral and left or right posterolateral abdominal wall (see Fig. 10-26).

Follow steps 1–8 above, then:

9. After drawing up the dose, change the needle to prevent leakage along the tract. (For Lovenox injections, the dose comes premixed with an air bubble in the prefilled syringe. Do not expel the air bubble before administration.)

10. With your nondominant hand, bunch (pinch) the tissue to a depth of at least 1/2 inch. If the area is obese, you can spread the skin rather than pinching it together.

11. Inject the needle at a 90-degree angle.

12. To minimize tissue damage, do not aspirate.

13. Inject the medication slowly.

14. Remove the needle quickly.

15. Do not massage the area. If the site bleeds, apply pressure with a dry gauze pad or alcohol pad for 1 to 2 minutes.

16. Do not recap the needle. Dispose of the needle and syringe in a sharps container. Make the patient/client comfortable, wash your hands, and chart the medication, documenting the site of injection.

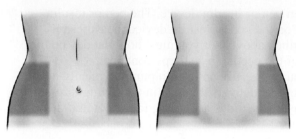

Anterior view   Posterior view

FIGURE 10-26

Sites for administration of Lovenox.

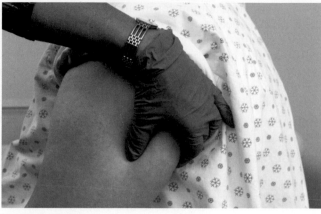

FIGURE 10-27

Pinch the tissue to a depth of at least 1/2 inch.

Subcutaneous Insulin

Insulin is administered with a special insulin syringe, measured in 100 units or 50 units (low-dose insulin syringe). Figure 10-23 shows the sites for insulin injection.

Follow steps 1–8 above, then:

9. Draw up the ordered dose in the correct insulin syringe. If you're mixing two insulins, follow the correct procedure (see pp. 146–147).

10. With another nurse, double-check the dose in the insulin syringe.

11. With your nondominant hand, bunch (pinch) the tissue to a depth of at least $\frac{1}{2}$ inch. If the area is obese, you can spread the skin rather than pinching it together (Fig. 10-27).

12. Inject the needle at a 45- or 90-degree angle (Fig. 10-28).

13. To minimize tissue damage, do not aspirate.

14. Inject the medication slowly.

15. Remove the needle quickly.

16. Do not massage the area. If the site bleeds, apply pressure with a dry gauze pad or alcohol pad for 1 to 2 minutes (Fig. 10-29).

17. Do not recap the needle. Dispose of the needle and syringe in a sharps container. Make the patient/ client comfortable, wash your hands, and chart the medication, documenting the site of injection.

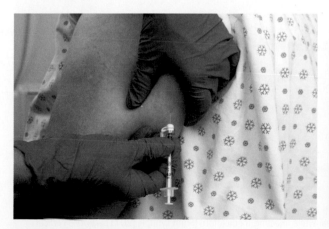

FIGURE 10-28

Inject the needle at a 45- or 90-degree angle.

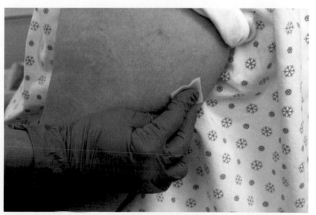

FIGURE 10-29

Applying pressure to the injection site.

You can also administer insulin with a prefilled insulin pen or insulin device. The pen or insulin device has a needle attached for each injection, and a dial on the pen or insulin device measures the correct insulin dose. The technique matches the one described above, but you must hold the device for 6 to 10 seconds before removing it from the skin. Dispose of the needle in a sharps container.

To administer insulin continuously by the subcutaneous route, use an insulin pump, typically near the abdominal area of the patient/client. The pump's preset rate delivers the insulin via tubing through a needle inserted in the subcutaneous tissue. You can adjust the settings according to the patient/client's insulin needs. Change the sites every 2 to 3 days or as needed.

Intradermal Skin Testing

Follow steps 1–8 above, then:

9. Draw up the ordered dose in a 1-mL syringe.

10. Place your nondominant hand around the arm from below, and pull the skin tightly to make the forearm tissue taut. Hold the syringe in your four fingers and thumb, with the bevel (opening) of the needle up.

11. Then insert the needle about 1/8 inch, almost parallel to the skin (Fig. 10-30A). You will be able to see the needle under the skin. Inject the solution so that it raises a small wheal (a raised bump or a blister) (Fig. 10-30B).

12. Afterward, remove the needle and allow the injection site to dry.

13. Do not massage the skin.

14. Do not recap the needle. Dispose of the needle and syringe in a sharps container. Make the patient/client comfortable, wash your hands, and chart the medication, documenting the site of injection.

Z-Track Technique for Intramuscular Injections

Some medications, such as iron dextran (Imferon) and hydroxyzine (Vistaril), are irritating to the tissues and can stain the skin. The Z-track method, used at the dorsogluteal or ventrogluteal site, can prevent medication from leaking from the tissue onto the skin.

Follow steps 1–8 above, then:

9. After preparing the medication, change the needle to prevent leakage along the tract.

10. Add 0.2 mL of air to the syringe. As the medication is injected, the air will rise to the top of the syringe and will be administered last—thus sealing off the medication and preventing it from leaking onto the skin.

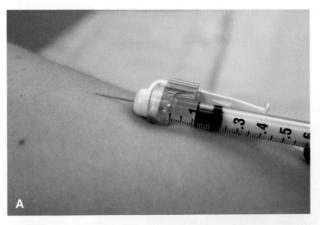
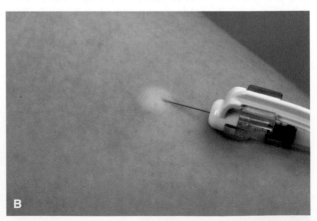

FIGURE 10-30

A. Inserting the needle almost level with the skin. **B.** Observing for wheal while injecting medication. (From Lynn, P. [2011]. *Taylor's clinical nursing skills: A nursing process approach* [3rd ed.]. Philadelphia, PA: Lippincott Williams & Wilkins, p. 182.)

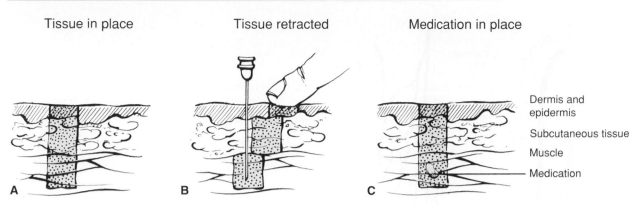

Tissue in place   Tissue retracted   Medication in place

Dermis and epidermis

Subcutaneous tissue

Muscle

Medication

A   B   C

FIGURE 10-31

Z-track technique—dorsogluteal site. The tissue is retracted to one side and held there until the injection is given. When the hand is removed, the tissue closes over the injection tract, preventing medication from rising to the surface.

11. Clean the area with an alcohol pad, using a circular motion from the center out. Allow to dry.

12. Place the alcohol pad between your fingers or lay it on the patient/client's skin above the site.

13. Use the fingers on your nondominant hand to retract the tissue to the side. Hold this position during the injection (Fig. 10-31).

14. Inject at a 90-degree angle, as usual. Before giving this injection, be sure to aspirate (Fig. 10-32).

15. After giving the injection, count 10 seconds.

16. Then remove the needle quickly.

17. Remove the hand that has been retracting the tissue.

18. Do not massage the site.

19. Using an alcohol pad or dry gauze pad, press down on the site to inhibit bleeding.

20. Do not recap the needle. Dispose of the needle and syringe in a sharps container. Make the patient/client comfortable, wash your hands, and chart the medication, documenting the site of injection.

IV Administration

Handwashing and gloves are required.
IV drugs may be given in a number of ways: continuous IV infusion, secondary or piggyback IV infusion (IVPB), IVP (IV push) (slow or fast), and flushing of an IV saline lock (sometimes called *heplock* or

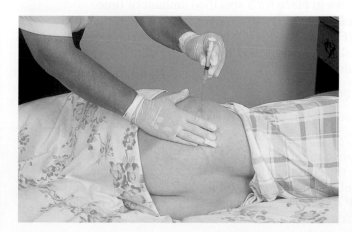

FIGURE 10-32

Displacing tissue in a Z-track manner and darting needle into tissue.

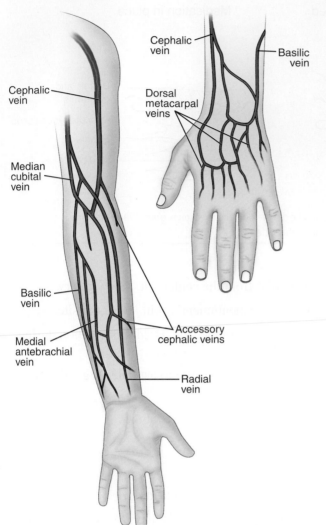

FIGURE 10-33

Infusion sites available in the hand or forearm. (From Taylor, C. [2008]. *Fundamentals of nursing* [6th ed.]. Philadelphia, PA: Lippincott Williams & Wilkins, p. 1709.)

heparin lock, although heparin is not used to flush peripheral IVs) or INT (intermittent needle therapy). Because IV medications introduce the drug directly into the bloodstream—thus having an immediate effect—you must follow strict asepsis technique.

Several types of IV needles are appropriate for inserting into a vein. The most common is the cathlon or "over the needle," in which a plastic catheter covers the needle. After inserting the needle in the vein, you withdraw the needle and the plastic catheter stays in place for a specified amount of time.

Usually, IV needles are inserted in the hand or forearm (Fig. 10-33). For long-term IV therapy, however, you can insert a central venous catheter (Fig. 10-34) or use a peripherally inserted central catheter (PICC) (Fig. 10-35). Information on IV calculations is found in Chapters 6 and 7.

Basic guidelines regarding peripheral IV therapy:

1. Use aseptic technique for insertion of the IV needle.

2. Use an occlusive dressing to secure the IV needle. Most healthcare settings use a clear plastic dressing over the IV needle site so that constant monitoring of the site can occur.

3. Verify IV fluid and IV medication orders before administration. Calculate the correct dose. Check an approved compatibility guide to determine the compatibility of IV fluids and IV medications. Flush the IV tubing between administrations of incompatible solutions. IVP drugs may or may not need to be diluted prior to administration. IVP drugs also vary as to how "fast" to push the drug. Consult institutional policy and drug handbooks.

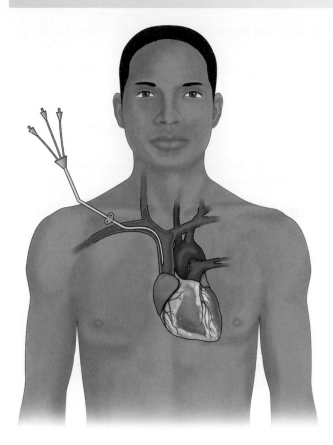

FIGURE 10-34

Triple lumen central venous catheter (TLC or CVC). (From Taylor, C. [2008]. *Fundamentals of nursing* [6th ed.]. Philadelphia, PA: Lippincott Williams & Wilkins, p. 1708.)

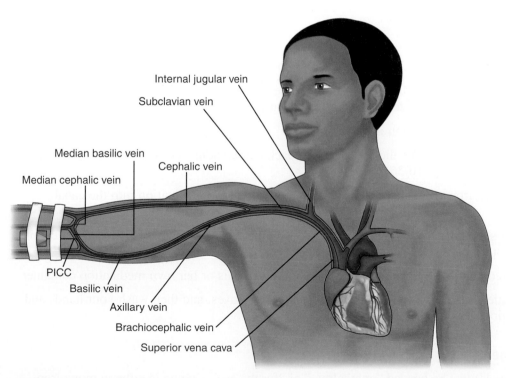

FIGURE 10-35

Peripherally inserted central catheter (PICC). (From Taylor, C. [2008]. *Fundamentals of nursing* [6th ed.]. Philadelphia, PA: Lippincott Williams & Wilkins, p. 1706.)

4. Infuse IV fluids and IV medications according to policy and procedures of the institution. Use an infusion pump if available.

5. Monitor and assess the IV site frequently and according to institutional guidelines. Monitor the IV site for swelling, color, temperature, and pain.

6. Follow institutional guidelines for changing the IV site, changing the IV fluids, and changing the IV tubing. Generally, a peripheral IV site is changed every 72 hours, IV fluids every 24 hours, and IV tubing every 72 to 96 hours.

For further information about IV insertion and IV medication administration, consult a nursing pharmacology textbook, IV therapy textbook, or nursing fundamentals textbook.

Application to Skin and Mucous Membranes

Topical drug preparations have two purposes: to cause a local effect or to act systematically. To create a systemic effect, the drug must be absorbed into the circulation.

Follow these steps for all medications:

Handwashing and gloves are required.

1. Follow the six rights and three checks.

2. Use two patient/client identifiers to identify the patient/client.

3. Ask the patient/client if he or she has allergies to any drugs, or check the MAR or patient/client chart.

4. Before administering the injection, perform any necessary assessment (e.g., checking vital signs, apical rate, or site integrity).

5. Explain the procedure to the patient/client.

Ear Drops

Follow steps 1–5 above, then:

6. The ear drops, labeled either "otic" or "auric," should be warmed to body temperature.

7. Help the patient/client into a comfortable position: either sitting upright, head tilted toward the unaffected side, or lying on the side with the affected ear up.

8. With a dropper, draw the medication into the dropper.

9. Straighten the ear canal by pulling the pinna up and back (for an adult) or down and back (for a child 3 years or younger (Fig. 10-36).

10. Placing the tip of the dropper at the opening of the canal, instill the medication into the canal (Fig. 10-37).

11. The patient/client should then rest on the unaffected side for 10 to 15 minutes. If the patient/client wishes, place a cotton ball in the canal.

12. To prevent cross-contamination, the patient/client should have his or her own medication container.

13. Make sure the patient/client is comfortable, dispose of your gloves, and then wash your hands and chart the medication.

Eye Drops or Ointment

Eye medications—which must be labeled "ophthalmic" or "for the eye"—come in either a monodrop container (a container with a droplike lid), in a bottle with a dropper; or as an ophthalmic ointment. The container is kept aseptic.

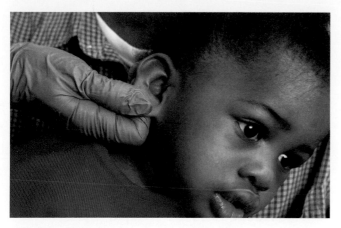

FIGURE 10-36

Technique for administering eardrops in children under 3 years old. (From Lynn, P. [2011]. *Taylor's clinical nursing skills: A nursing process approach* [3rd ed.]. Philadelphia, PA: Lippincott Williams & Wilkins, p. 244.)

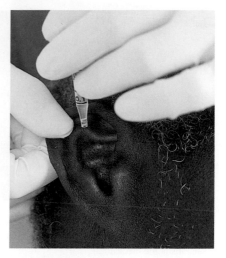

FIGURE 10-37

Straighten the ear canal and instill the medication.

CLINICAL POINT

✓ **Ear Drop Administration—Which Way?**

- Should the ear pinna be pulled up or down with adults?
- Should the ear pinna be pulled up or down with children?
- Adults are usually taller than children, so the ear pinna is pulled "up" and back for ear drops.
- Children younger than 3 years are smaller than adults, so the ear pinna is pulled "down" and back for ear drops.

Follow steps 1–5 above, then:

6. Hand the patient/client a tissue. The patient/client may sit or lie down. If exudate is present, you may need to cleanse the eyelid with cotton or gauze and either normal saline or distilled water for the eye.

7. Gently draw the patient/client's lower eyelid down to create a sac (Fig. 10-38). Instruct the patient/client to look up.

8. Then instill the liquid medication into the lower conjunctival sac, taking care not to touch the membrane.

9. If you're administering ophthalmic ointment, spread a small amount from the inner to the outer canthus of the eye.

10. After either of these procedures, instruct the patient/client to close his or her eyelids gently and rotate the eyes. The patient/client may use a tissue to wipe away excess medication.

11. Have the patient/client apply gentle pressure with the index finger to the inner canthus for a minute. This action keeps the medication from entering the tear duct (Fig. 10-39).

12. To prevent cross-contamination, each patient/client should have individual medication containers. If the medication impairs the patient/client's vision, provide a safe environment.

13. Make the patient/client comfortable. Dispose of the gloves, wash your hands, and chart the medication.

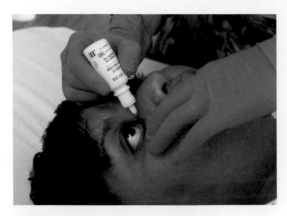

FIGURE 10-38

Gently draw the patient/client's lower eyelid down to create a sac. Instill the medication.

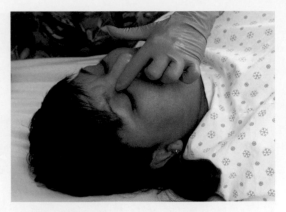

FIGURE 10-39

Apply gentle pressure with the index finger to the inner canthus for a minute.

CLINICAL POINT

✓ **Eye and Ear Abbreviations**

- The Joint Commission has identified abbreviations—including those for eye and ear medications—that can cause confusion. Although the Joint Commission does not prohibit the following abbreviations, *it's best to avoid using them:*

  - AS (left ear), AD (right ear), AU (both ears). These are often confused with the terms for eyes: OS (left eye), OD (right eye), OU (both eyes).

- Recommendations: Write out the phrases "left ear," "right ear," or "both ears," as appropriate. Write out the phrases: "left eye," "right eye," "both eyes." Be sure to write out "every day" or "daily" rather than using the abbreviation "qd," which is easily confused with "OD."

Nose Drops

Follow steps 1–5 above, then:

6. The patient/client, either sitting or lying down, may have to blow his or her nose gently to clear the nasal passageway.

7. Have the patient/client tilt his or her head back. If the patient/client is lying in bed, place a pillow under the shoulders to hyperextend the neck (unless contraindicated).

8. Insert the dropper about one third of the way into one nostril. Do not touch the nostril.

9. Instill the nose drops (Fig. 10-40) and then instruct the patient/client to maintain the position for 1 to 2 minutes. If the patient/client feels the medication flowing down the throat, he or she may sit up and bend the head down so that the medication will flow into the sinuses instead. Repeat into the other nostril if ordered.

10. To prevent cross-contamination, the patient/client should have his or her own medication container.

11. If a nasal spray is ordered, push the tip of patient/client's nose up and then place the nozzle tip just inside the nares so that when you give the medication, the spray is aiming toward the back of the nose.

12. After making the patient/client comfortable, dispose of your gloves, wash your hands, and chart the medication.

Respiratory Inhaler

An inhaler is a small, pressurized metal container that holds medication. Inhalers come in these forms: a metered-dose (MDI) inhaler, accompanied by a mouthpiece; an MDI with an extender; or a dry powder inhaler (DPI) (Fig. 10-41).

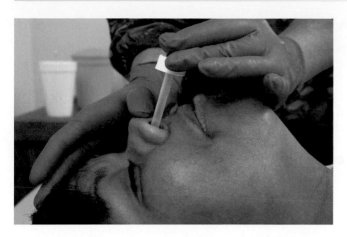

FIGURE 10-40

Administering nose drops. (From Lynn, P. [2011]. *Taylor's clinical nursing skills: A nursing process approach* [3rd ed.]. Philadelphia, PA: Lippincott Williams & Wilkins, p. 250.)

Follow steps 1–5 above, then:

6. Shake the inhaler well immediately before you use it.

7. Remove the cap from the mouthpiece.

8. Instruct the patient/client to do the following:

   • Breathe out fully, expel as much air as possible, and hold your breath.

   • Place the mouthpiece in your mouth, and close your lips around it. Keep the metal inhaler upright.

   • While breathing in deeply and slowly, use your index finger to fully depress the metal inhaler (Fig. 10-42).

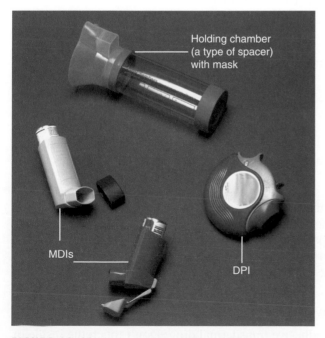

FIGURE 10-41

Examples of MDIs and spacers. (From Taylor, C. [2008]. *Fundamentals of nursing* [6th ed.]. Philadelphia, PA: Lippincott Williams & Wilkins, p. 810.)

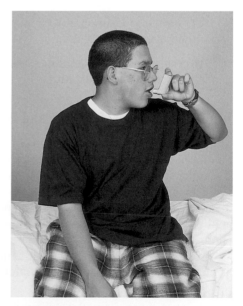

FIGURE 10-42

Many children with asthma use an MDI to administer a bronchodilator. (From Pillitteri, A. [2002]. *Maternal and child health nursing* [4th ed.]. Philadelphia, PA: Lippincott Williams & Wilkins, p. 1210.)

- Remove the inhaler from your mouth, and release your finger. Hold your breath for several seconds.

- Wait 1 minute. Then shake the inhaler again, and repeat the steps for each prescribed inhalation. (An order might read "Proventil inhaler 2 puffs qid.")

9. At least once a day, clean the mouthpiece and cap by rinsing them in warm running water. After they have dried, replace the mouthpiece and cap on the inhaler.

10. You can leave the inhaler at the patient/client's bedside stand if the institution's policy permits.

11. Make the patient/client comfortable, dispose of your gloves wash your hands, and chart the medication.

Skin Applications

Avoid personal contact with the medication so that you don't absorb any of the drug. Apply the medication with either a tongue blade, a glove, a gauze pad, or a cotton-tipped applicator. Cleanse the area as appropriate before beginning a new application.

Many kinds of medications are applied topically. Before you proceed, obtain the following information:

- How to prepare the skin

- How to apply the medication

- Whether to cover or uncover the skin

Follow steps 1–5 above, then, follow the steps for these drug preparations:

- *Powders:* The patient/client's skin should be dry. Sprinkle the medication on your gloved hands, then apply it. Use sparingly to avoid caking.

- *Lotions:* Using a gloved hand or gauze pad, pat the medication on lightly.

- *Creams:* Using gloves, rub the medication into the patient/client's skin.

- *Ointments:* Using a gloved hand or an applicator, apply an even coat and then place a dressing on the patient/client's skin.

After any of these procedures, make the patient/client comfortable, dispose of your gloves, wash your hands, and chart the medication.

Transdermal Disks, Patches, and Pads

Transdermal disks, patches, and pads are unit-dose adhesive bandages consisting of a semipermeable membrane that allows medication to be released continuously over time. Some patches are effective for 24 hours, some for 72 hours, and some last as long as 1 week.

The skin at the site should be free of hair and not subject to excessive movement; therefore, avoid distal extremities. Some patches are applied to a certain area of the body (e.g., nitroglycerin is often applied to the chest wall area). Old transdermal patches must be removed prior to the application of a new patch. At each administration, change the site. If the patch loosens with bathing, apply a new pad.

Medications appropriate for this route include hormones, nitroglycerin, antihypertensive drugs such as clonidine (Catapres), and antimotion sickness drugs such as scopolamine.

Follow steps 1–5 above, then:

6. Select a site where the skin is clear and dry, with no signs of irritation.

7. Open the packet and remove the cover from the adhesive transdermal drug. Don't touch the inside of the pad.

8. Apply the pad to the skin, pressing firmly to be certain all edges adhere.

9. Chart on the pad the date, time, and your initials.

10. Then make the patient/client comfortable, dispose of your gloves, wash your hands, and chart the medication.

Nitroglycerin Ointment

Follow steps 1–5 above, then:

6. Take a baseline blood pressure and record it. (Note that because nitroglycerin is a potent vasodilator, it may cause a drop in the blood pressure after application.)

7. To protect yourself from contact with the drug, put on gloves.

8. Then remove the previous dose and cleanse the skin.

9. Measure the prescribed dose in inches on the ruled paper that comes with the ointment.

10. Select a nonhairy site on the patient/client's trunk—chest, upper arm, abdomen, or upper back. If necessary, shave the area. (*Note:* Seek advice before shaving.)

11. Spread the measured ointment on the ruled paper, and apply the ointment in a thin layer. Do not rub it in.

12. Place the ruled paper with the ointment on the skin and then apply tape; some sources recommend covering the area with plastic wrap and taping the plastic in place.

13. Within 30 minutes, check the patient/client's blood pressure.

14. If the patient/client gets a headache (a common side effect of nitroglycerin) or if his blood pressure lowers, have him stay in bed until the blood pressure returns to normal. Treat the headaches with an ordered pain medication.

15. After making the patient/client comfortable, dispose of your gloves, wash your hands, and chart the medication.

Sublingual Tablets

The most common sublingual medication is nitroglycerin, which is prescribed to alleviate symptoms of angina pectoris. If a patient/client does not feel relief within 5 minutes, you can administer a second and then a third tablet at 5-minute intervals. If the pain continues after 15 minutes, notify the physician.
  Follow steps 1–5 above, then:

6. Instruct the patient/client to sit down and to place the tablet under the tongue.

7. If the patient/client is unable to place the tablet under the tongue, the nurse should do it, wearing a glove.

8. The patient/client should not swallow or chew the tablet but should allow it to dissolve.

9. Make sure the patient/client does not eat or drink anything with the tablet since that will interfere with the effectiveness of the medication.

10. Stay with the patient/client until the pain has stopped. For more information, consult an appropriate text.

11. After making the patient/client comfortable, dispose of your gloves, wash your hands, and chart the medication.

Buccal Tablets

Follow steps 1–5 above, then:

6. The patient/client should place the tablet between the gum and cheek.

7. Withhold food and liquids until the tablet is dissolved, and warn the patient/client not to disturb the tablet. Medication applied across mucous membranes causes rapid systemic absorption.

8. To minimize irritation, alternate doses between cheeks.

9. After making the patient/client comfortable, dispose of your gloves, wash your hands, and chart the medication.

Suppositories

Suppositories are medications molded into a base such as cocoa butter that melts at body temperature. They are shaped for insertion into the rectum, the vagina, and less commonly, the urethra. A water-soluble lubricant is used for insertion, and depth of insertion is determined by the size of the patient/client.

Rectal Suppository

Follow steps 1–5 above, then:

6. Encourage the patient/client to defecate (unless the suppository is ordered for this purpose).

7. Position the patient/client in the left lateral recumbent position.

8. After moistening the suppository with a water-soluble lubricant, instruct the patient/client to breathe slowly and deeply through the mouth. To open the anal sphincter, ask the patient/client to "bear down" as if having a bowel movement.

9. Using a gloved finger, insert the suppository past the sphincter. You will feel the suppository move into the canal (Fig. 10-43).

10. Wipe away excess lubricant, and encourage the patient/client to retain the suppository as long as possible.

11. After making the patient/client comfortable. Dispose of your gloves, wash your hands, and chart the medication.

The patient/client may insert his or her own suppository if he or she is able and wishes to do so. Provide a glove, lubricant, and suppository. After insertion, check to make sure that the suppository is in place and is not in the bed.

Vaginal Suppository or Tablet

Follow steps 1–5 above, then:

6. Ask the patient/client to void in a bedpan. (If the perineal area has excessive secretions, you may need to perform perineal care after the patient/client voids.)

7. Insert the suppository or tablet into the applicator.

8. Then assist the patient/client into a lithotomy position (lying on her back, with knees flexed and legs apart) and drape her, leaving the perineal area exposed.

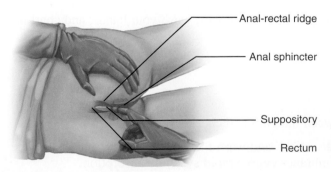

Anal-rectal ridge

Anal sphincter

Suppository

Rectum

FIGURE 10-43

Left lateral recumbent position for administration of rectal suppository.

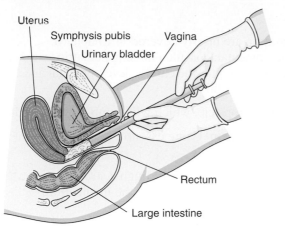

FIGURE 10-44

Vaginal applicator should be inserted down and back. (From Lynn, P. [2011]. *Taylor's clinical nursing skills: A nursing process approach* [3rd ed.]. Philadelphia, PA: Lippincott Williams & Wilkins, p. 255.)

9. Separate the labia majora and identify the vaginal opening. Then insert the applicator down and back, and eject the suppository or tablet into the vagina. (If the patient/client wishes, she can do this procedure herself.)

10. You may also insert the suppository—using gloved fingers—into the vagina.

11. Place a pad at the vaginal opening to collect secretions, and make the patient/client comfortable before you leave.

12. Wash the applicator with soap and water, wrap it in a paper towel, and leave it at the bedside.

13. Dispose of your gloves, wash your hands, and chart the medication.

Vaginal Cream

Vaginal cream is packaged either in a prefilled disposable syringe or in a tube with its own applicator. To fill the applicator, remove the cap from the tube and screw the top of the tube into the applicator's barrel. Squeeze the tube and fill the barrel to the prescribed dose. Then unscrew the tube from the applicator and cap it.

Follow steps 1–5 above, then:

6. Prepare the patient/client as described in the previous section.

7. Insert the applicator down and back, and press the plunger to empty the barrel of medication (Fig. 10-44).

8. The patient/client may do this herself if she wishes. After removing the applicator, place a pad at the vaginal opening to collect secretions.

9. Before you leave, make sure the patient/client is comfortable. She should remain in bed for a minimum of 20 minutes.

10. If the applicator is a prefilled unit-dose, dispose of it according to institutional policy. If it is reusable, wash it with soap and water, and place it in a clean paper towel on the bedside stand.

11. Dispose of your gloves, wash your hands, and chart the medication.

 Special Considerations

The basics of medication administration apply to all age groups. However, administering drugs to pediatric and geriatric patients/clients requires special considerations.

Neonatal and Pediatric Considerations

Dosages of medications for neonatal and pediatric administration are briefly covered in Chapter 8.
    Differences in medication administration are mainly developmental; consult a nursing pediatric textbook for specifics and special skills needed. The most important consideration is the child's developmental age.
    Here are some suggestions for administering oral medication to children:

- Before you administer an oral medication, offer the child a popsicle, which will numb the taste buds.

- Mix the drug with a teaspoon of puréed fruit, ice cream, or syrup. Using essential foodstuffs is not a good idea, because the child may refuse those foods later.

- Have older children pinch their nostrils closed and drink the medication through a straw. Because this technique interferes with their ability to smell, it keeps them from tasting the medication.

- For infants, use a specially manufactured medication nipple or pacifier.

IM administration in children:

- Explain the procedure to the child, using terms that he or she can easily understand.

- Predetermine the injection site to make sure the muscle is large enough to accommodate the amount and type of medication.

- To reduce the pain of deep needle administration, you can apply a topical anesthetic. An alternative method is to subcutaneously inject a local anesthetic such as lidocaine.

- A child's behavior and movements are unpredictable, so have someone help you hold the child.

- Distract the child with conversation or a toy.

- Insert the needle quickly, and inject the medication slowly.

- Use a decorative adhesive bandage to cover the injection site.

Geriatric Considerations

Before administering medications to geriatric clients, consider these changes in the geriatric client: decreased memory, decreased cognition, and decreasing organ function (especially of liver and kidney); circulatory changes leading to decreased perfusion; and physical limitations (poor eyesight, decreased coordination, decreased ability to chew and/or swallow).
    Here are some suggestions for administering oral tablets and liquids to geriatric patients/clients:

- Before administering a liquid medication, offer the patient/client a popsicle, which will numb the taste buds.

- If crushing a tablet won't compromise its medication, you can crush it and mix the fragments with a teaspoon of puréed fruit, ice cream, or syrup.

- Patients/clients who are post cardiovascular accident (CVA) often have problems with tongue mobility and/or a decreased gag reflex. To promote swallowing, you may have to place the tablet or capsule in the patient/client's mouth, toward the pharynx and on the unaffected side. Afterward, thoroughly check the patient/client's mouth to determine whether he or she has swallowed the tablet or capsule. CVA patients/clients with a feeding tube (nasogastric, oral gastric, or percutaneous endoscopic gastrostomy (PEG) tube) can receive their medications through the tube.

Subcutaneous and/or IM administration in geriatric patients/clients:

- Explain the procedure to the patient/client.

- Predetermine the injection site to make sure there is sufficient subcuticular tissue or the muscle is large enough to accommodate the amount and type of medication.

- Distract the patient/client with conversation.

- Insert the needle quickly, and inject the medication slowly.

CRITICAL THINKING **TEST YOUR CLINICAL SAVVY**

A patient/client in your outpatient clinic is to receive an IM injection. The drug literature states that the preferred site is the dorsogluteal or vastus lateralis.

A. When would the deltoid muscle be preferable over either of these sites? What are the contraindications for using the deltoid muscle?

B. The client requests the injection in the deltoid. What is your response in light of the recommended site in the drug literature?

C. If a patient/client is bedridden, which site would you choose for an IM injection and why?

D. Even though you are not actually touching the injection site, why are gloves necessary when giving IM injections?

SELF-TEST 1 **Administration Procedures**

Complete the statements about standard precautions in medication administration. Choose the correct answers for questions 11 through 20. Answers appear at the end of the chapter.

1. Name the six rights and three checks:

Six Rights

1. _____
2. _____
3. _____
4. _____
5. _____
6. _____

Three Checks

1. _____
2. _____
3. _____

2. Standard precautions should be applied when administering medications:

a. to all patients/clients
b. only to patients/clients with HIV or HBV

3. After the nurse administers an injection, the syringe and needle should be placed _____ _____ _____.

4. Five precautions stressed by the CDC include _____, _____, _____, _____, and _____.

5. Standard precautions while administering ear drop or eye drop medications include _____ _____.

(continued)

6. **a.** A nurse should wear a gown to protect his or her uniform whenever

_____

_____

   b. The nurse should wear protective eyewear whenever _____

_____

_____.

7. The primary reason patients/clients should have individual eye medication is to _____
_____.

8. Two methods of checking the positioning of a nasogastric tube are _____
_____

   and _____.

9. Identify these administration procedures as parenteral or nonparenteral.

   a. Subcutaneous injection _____   **f.** Nitroglycerin ointment _____

   b. Sublingual tablet _____   **g.** Respiratory inhaler _____

   c. Vaginal suppository _____   **h.** Nasogastric route _____

   d. Nose drops _____   **i.** Intradermal _____

   e. IM injection _____   **j.** Rectal suppository _____

10. What is the difference in administering ear drops to an adult and to a 2-year-old child? _____
_____

_____

11. Under what condition does a nurse have a right to refuse to administer a drug?

   a. The pharmacist ordered the drug.
   b. The drug is manufactured by two different companies.
   c. The drug is prescribed by a licensed physician.
   d. The dose is within the range given in the rxmed.com website.

12. When administering medication in the hospital, the nurse should:

   a. chart medications before administering them
   b. chart only those drugs that she or he personally gave the patient/client
   c. chart all medications given for the day at one time
   d. determine the best method for giving the drugs

13. A nurse reads a medication order that is not clear. What action is indicated?

   a. Ask the charge nurse to explain the order.
   b. Ask a doctor at the nurses' station for help.
   c. Check the drug reference on the unit.
   d. Check with the doctor who wrote the order.

14. When an order is written to be administered "as needed" it is called a:

   a. standing order
   b. prn order
   c. single order
   d. stat order

15. The nurse practitioner orders lorazepam (Ativan) 1 mg IV stat. The medication is given:

    a. immediately and only once
    b. once and at a specified time
    c. on an indefinite basis
    d. when the nurse determines the medication is needed

16. The nurse is to give the patient/client an IM injection. The dorsogluteal site is chosen. As the patient/client turns to expose the site, there are multiple injections that have been given in this site and the area is scarred. What should the nurse do?

    a. Give the medication at this site.
    b. Give the medication at this site, but avoid the scarred areas.
    c. Hold the medication.
    d. Select another site for administration.

17. The nurse is to give several medications via nasogastric tube. Which type of oral medication drug form may not be crushed for administration?

    a. Enteric-coated tablet
    b. Sublingual tablet
    c. Buccal tablet
    d. Liquid syrup

18. The pediatric nurse is to give an IM injection to a child that is under age 3 years. The preferred site is the:

    a. deltoid
    b. dorsogluteal
    c. vastus lateralis
    d. ventrogluteal

19. Which nursing action is most likely to increase an older patient/client's compliance and reduce medication errors? (*Hint:* Think of the changes in an older adult.)

    a. Devise a simple medication schedule.
    b. Have the family administer the drugs.
    c. Instruct the patient/client to only take over-the-counter medications.
    d. Suggest administration times when the patient/client remembers to take the medications.

You will administer the medications appropriately based on the following data. Document on the MAR. Use the guidelines on page 394-395. Answers appear at the end of the chapter.

Date: June 26, 2015
Time: 0900
Vital Signs: Temperature 101.5 oral. Respiratory rate: 32 breaths/minute. Apical heart rate: 75/minute. Blood pressure: 98/50. Drug allergies: Penicillin. No complaints of pain.

MCFARLAND MEDICAL CENTER
Medication Administration Record

Patient/Client Name	Room Number	Hospital Number		Diagnosis
Curtis, Chelsea	1401	204452896		CHF
Allergies PCN	Admitted 5/28/14	Age 50	Sex F	Physician Smith, V.G.

DOSAGE ADMINISTRATION PERIOD: 4/27/15 0600-4/28/15 0600

	0700–1900	1900–0700
Digoxin 0.25 mg PO every day Hold if HR <60	0900	
Aspirin 325 mg PO daily	0900	
Protonix 40 mg PO every day	0900	
Ampicillin 250 mg PO q 6h	1200 1800	2400 0600
Lopressor 50 mg PO BID Hold if SBP <100	0900	2100
Coumadin 5 mg PO once a day	1700	
Morphine sulfate 4–6 mg IV every 2–3 h prn pain		
Tylenol 650 mg q4h prn temp >101		

Signature _____ Initials __( )__   Signature _____ Initials __( )__   Signature _____ Initials __( )__

PROFICIENCY TEST 1—PART A	Administration Procedures

Name: _____

Choose the correct answer for each of these questions. Answers appear in Appendix A.

1. A nurse enters a patient/client room to administer the morning medications. The patient/client is in the bathroom. The nurse should:

   a. leave the medications at the bedside
   b. leave the medication after telling the family member to administer it
   c. leave with the medication and return shortly to administer it
   d. wait for the patient/client to return to bed, then leave the medications at the bedside

2. A suppository is ordered to be administered rectally. What should the nurse do first before inserting the suppository?

   a. Remove the suppository from the refrigerator 30 minutes before administration.
   b. Apply a water-based lubricant to the suppository before insertion.
   c. Dissolve the suppository in saline and then administer it as an enema.
   d. Instruct the patient/client to void in the bathroom.

3. A tuberculin skin test is performed via intradermal injection. Which angle will the nurse insert the needle?

   a. 90 degrees
   b. 45 degrees
   c. 30 degrees
   d. 15 degrees

4. A patient/client's respiratory medication is a sustained-release tablet. The nurse should avoid:

   a. administering the drug with another medication
   b. mixing the drug with an antacid
   c. crushing the tablet before administration
   d. administering the tablet with water

5. The nurse has a responsibility in drug therapy to do all except:

   a. observing the drug effects
   b. instructing the patient/client about the drug's use
   c. checking for the correct dose of the drug
   d. changing the dosage if side effects occur

6. Before administering medications to a patient/client, the nurse will do all except:

   a. withhold medication if the pulse is 100
   b. check ID using two identifiers
   c. assess the patient/client's level of consciousness
   d. respect the patient/client's right to refuse medication

7. A nurse is administering ear drops to a 5-year-old. The nurse will:

   a. pull the ear pinna downward and back for instillation
   b. pull the pinna upward and back for instillation
   c. place cotton tightly in the ear after instillation
   d. keep the child on the affected side after instillation

(continued)

8. An 84-year-old patient/client is taking a medication that has several side effects. The nurse knows that these side effects may be increased due to the patient/client's:

   a. decreased renal function
   b. increased cardiac output
   c. increased protein intake
   d. increased liver function

9. A nurse is teaching a patient/client about the rationale for administering nitroglycerin sublingually rather than orally. The nurse knows that the patient/client understands the teaching when he or she states:

   a. "the medication is absorbed more rapidly sublingually"
   b. "the medication is absorbed more rapidly if I swallow it"
   c. "the medication is absorbed at the same rate whichever way I take it"
   d. "the medication is released at a sustained rate sublingually"

10. A 170-pound patient/client is to receive an IM injection of 2 mL. The preferred site of injection is the:

    a. deltoid
    b. dorsogluteal
    c. vastus lateralis
    d. ventrogluteal

11. A nurse aspirates an IM injection and finds blood in the syringe prior to injecting the medication. What should the nurse do next?

    a. Continue to administer the medication
    b. Withdraw the needle, and restick at another location
    c. Carefully administer the medication but at a slower rate
    d. Withdraw the needle, discard the medication, and prepare another injection

12. A nurse's first check when preparing medication is:

    a. checking the patient/client's armband before administration
    b. check the unit-dose label with the MAR
    c. checking the unit-dose label with another nurse
    d. checking the unit-dose packaging after it is disposed

13. Checking the MAR before administering medication enables the nurse to determine:

    a. the name of the pharmacist who ordered the medication
    b. the correct administration time of the medication
    c. any previous medication errors
    d. orders for intake and output

14. A major advantage in the unit-dose system of drug administration is that:

    a. the drug supply is always available
    b. no error is possible
    c. the drugs are less expensive than stock distribution
    d. the pharmacist provides a second professional check

15. When a drug is to be administered sublingually, the patient/client should be instructed to:

    a. drink a full glass of water when swallowing
    b. rinse the mouth with water after taking the drug
    c. chew the tablet and allow saliva to collect under the tongue
    d. hold the medication under the tongue until it dissolves

16. Which action is correct when giving a Z-track injection?

    a. Retract the skin and hold it to one side while giving the medication.
    b. Massage the skin after giving the injection.
    c. After the needle has been inserted, do not pull back the plunger.
    d. Inject the medication quickly.

17. Which angle of injection is correctly matched with the route of administration?

    a. Intradermal—45-degree angle
    b. IM—90-degree angle
    c. Subcutaneous—30-degree angle
    d. Z track—45-degree angle

18. A patient/client asks how to put in eye drops. The nurse instructs the patient/client to place the drops:

    a. into the lower conjunctival sac
    b. under the upper lid
    c. directly on the cornea
    d. in the inner canthus

19. When administering a vaginal suppository, which statement is false?

    a. Use standard precautions.
    b. The patient/client may insert the medication.
    c. The patient/client should be lying on her back.
    d. The applicator must be kept sterile.

20. When applying the next dose of a transdermal medication, the nurse should:

    a. shave the new area and prepare with povidone–iodine
    b. cleanse the previous area and use a different site
    c. rotate the use of arms and legs as sites
    d. allow the previous patch to remain on the skin

21. After administering an injection, the nurse should:

    a. immediately recap the needle
    b. break the needle off the syringe for safety
    c. place the used syringe and needle in a nearby sharps container
    d. put on gloves to carry the syringe to the utility room

22. The nurse teaches the patient/client learning to use an inhaler to shake the inhaler, exhale fully, inhale while pushing down on the inhaler to activate it, breathe in the puff of drug, and then:

    a. hold one's breath for 1 minute
    b. hold one's breath for several seconds
    c. exhale with force
    d. exhale gently

(continued)

23. Which route of administration allows for the fastest delivery of a medication?

   a. Subcutaneous
   b. IM
   c. IV
   d. Intradermal

24. The nurse explains to the patient/client that an enteric-coated tablet is manufactured to dissolve:

   a. between the cheek and gum
   b. under the tongue
   c. in the stomach
   d. in the small intestine

25. A medication order reads "cefuroxime (Ceftin) 1 g q12h IV." This is an example of:

   a. a prn order
   b. a single order
   c. a stat order
   d. a standing order

Decide whether the following actions are correct or incorrect according to the precautions to follow when administering medications. Explain your choice. Answers appear in Appendix A.

1. A nurse wears gloves to remove an IV saline lock from a patient/client's arm. This action is

   _____

   _____

2. A nurse who has just removed a gown and gloves puts them into the disposal container in the patient/client's room and leaves the room. This action is

   _____

   _____

3. In the medication room, a nurse puts on gloves to prepare an IV for administration. This action is

   _____

   _____

4. A nurse puts on a mask to administer an oral medication to a patient/client on respiratory isolation precautions. This action is

   _____

   _____

5. A nurse applies standard precautions in caring for all patients/clients on the unit. This action is

   _____

   _____

6. A nurse wears gloves to place a transdermal pad behind a patient/client's ear. This action is

   _____

   _____

   _____

7. A nurse puts on gloves to administer a rectal suppository to a lethargic patient/client. This action is

   _____

8. A nurse whose finger has been stuck with a contaminated IV needle carefully washes his or her hands with soap and water and applies a bandage to the site. Because the patient/client's diagnosis is a brain tumor, the nurse decides that no further action is necessary. This action is

   _____

9. A nurse giving an injection to a patient/client decides not to wear gloves. This action is

   _____

   _____

   _____

(continued)

10. A nurse puts on gloves to administer an oral tablet to an alert patient/client with a positive HIV blood count. This action is

_____

_____

11. After administering an injection, the nurse carefully caps the needle. This action is

_____

_____

_____

12. A nurse wears gloves to apply nitroglycerin ointment to a patient/client's chest, even though there is no break in the skin. This action is

_____

_____

_____

13. A nurse decides not to wear gloves when administering eye drops because they are too bulky. This action is

_____

_____

_____

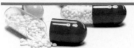

Answers

Self-Test 1 Administration Procedures

1. Right patient/client

   Right medication

   Right dosage

   Right route

   Right time

   Right documentation

   Check the drug label with the MAR when removing the container or unit-dose package.

   Check the drug label immediately before pouring or opening the medication or preparing the unit-dose.

   Check the drug label when replacing the container and/or before giving the unit-dose to the patient/client.

2. To all patients/clients. There is a risk of potential exposure to hepatitis virus and HIV that may not have been detected by standard laboratory methods.

3. In a labeled, puncture-proof sharps container

4. Handwashing, gloves, gowns, masks, and protective eyewear

5. Handwashing and gloves

6. **a.** The nurse's clothing may become contaminated with a patient/client's blood or other body fluids.

   b. A nurse is in extremely close contact with the patient/client and there is the possibility of the patient/client's blood or blood-tinged fluids being splashed or sprayed into the nurse's eyes or mucous membranes.

7. Prevent cross-contamination

8. Aspirate stomach contents and check for pH, or place a stethoscope on the stomach and insert 15 mL of air. A swishing sound indicates proper placement.

9. **a.** parenteral

   b. nonparenteral

   c. nonparenteral

   d. nonparenteral

   e. parenteral

   f. nonparenteral

   g. nonparenteral

   h. nonparenteral

   i. parenteral

   j. nonparenteral

10. In the adult, pull the ear back and up. In a 2-year-old child, pull the ear back and down.

11. a		**16.** d	
12. b		**17.** a	
13. d		**18.** c	
14. b		**19.** a	
15. a			

(continued)

Answers (Continued)

Self-Test 2 Medication Administration Record

MCFARLAND MEDICAL CENTER
Medication Administration Record

Patient/Client Name	Room Number	Hospital Number		Diagnosis
Curtis, Chelsea	1401	204452896		CHF

| Allergies
PCN | Admitted
5/28/14 | Age
50 | Sex
F | Physician
Smith, V.G. |

DOSAGE ADMINISTRATION PERIOD: 4/27/15 0600-4/28/15 0600

	0700–1900	1900–0700
Digoxin 0.25 mg PO every day Hold if HR <60	~~0900~~ AH HR: 75	
Aspirin 325 mg PO daily	~~0900~~ AH	
Protonix 40 mg PO every day	~~0900~~ AH	
Ampicillin 250 mg PO q 6h	(1200) (1800) HOLD	(2400) (0600) DUE to PATIENT/CLIENT ALLERGY
Lopressor 50 mg PO BID Hold if SBP <100	B/P 98/50 AH (0900) B/P too low	2100
Coumadin 5 mg PO once a day	1700	
Morphine sulfate 4–6 mg IV every 2–3 h prn pain		
Tylenol 650 mg q4h prn temp >101	~~900~~ AH Temp 101.5	

Signature *Andrew Hughes* Initials *(AH)*   Signature _____ Initials _____   Signature _____ Initials _____

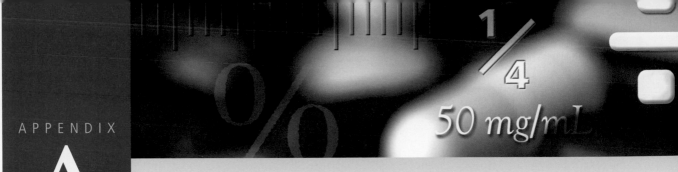

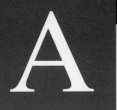

APPENDIX

A Proficiency Test Answers

Chapter 1

Test 1: Arithmetic

A. a.
$$
\begin{array}{r}
647 \\
\times\ 38 \\
\hline
5176 \\
1941\ \ \\
\hline
24586
\end{array}
$$

b.
$$\frac{\cancel{8}^{1}}{\cancel{9}_{3}} \times \frac{\cancel{12}^{\cancel{4}^{1}}}{\cancel{32}_{\cancel{4}_{1}}} = \frac{1}{3}$$

c.
$$
\begin{array}{r}
0.56 \\
\times\ 0.17 \\
\hline
392 \\
56\ \ \\
\hline
0.0952
\end{array}
$$

B. a.
$$
\begin{array}{r}
9.670 = 9.67 \\
82\overline{)793.000} \\
\underline{738}\ \ \ \ \\
55\,0\ \ \\
\underline{49\,2}\ \ \\
5\,80 \\
\underline{5\,74} \\
60
\end{array}
$$

b.
$$5\frac{1}{4} \div \frac{7}{4} = \frac{\cancel{21}^{3}}{\cancel{4}_{1}} \times \frac{\cancel{4}^{1}}{\cancel{7}_{1}} = 3$$

c.
$$
\begin{array}{r}
20. \\
0.015\,\overline{)0.300} \\
\underset{\smile}{}\ \ \underset{\smile}{}
\end{array}
$$

C. a. $\dfrac{7}{15} + \dfrac{8}{15} = \dfrac{15}{15} = 1$

b. $\dfrac{3}{8} + \dfrac{2}{5} =$

$$\frac{15}{40} + \frac{16}{40} = \frac{31}{40}$$

c. $0.825 + 0.1 = 0.925$

D. a. $\dfrac{11}{15} - \dfrac{7}{10} =$

$$\frac{44}{60} - \frac{42}{60} = \frac{2}{60} = \frac{1}{30}$$

b. $\dfrac{8}{15} - \dfrac{4}{15} = \dfrac{4}{15}$

c. $1.56 - 0.2 =$

$$
\begin{array}{r}
1.56 \\
-0.2\ \ \ = 1.36 \\
\hline
1.36
\end{array}
$$

E. a.
$$
\begin{array}{r}
0.055 = 0.06 \\
18\,\overline{)1.000} \\
\underline{90}\ \ \ \\
100 \\
\underline{90} \\
100
\end{array}
$$
$\dfrac{1}{18}$

b.
$$
\begin{array}{r}
0.375 \\
8\,\overline{)3.000} \\
\underline{24}\ \ \ \\
60 \\
\underline{56} \\
40 \\
\underline{40}
\end{array}
$$
$\dfrac{3}{8}$

F. a.
$$0.35 = \frac{\cancel{35}^{7}}{\cancel{100}_{20}} = \frac{7}{20}$$

b.
$$0.08 = \frac{\cancel{8}^{2}}{\cancel{100}_{25}} = \frac{2}{25}$$

G. a. 0.4

b. 0.8

c. 0.83

d. 0.3

H. a. $\dfrac{\cancel{20}^{5}}{\cancel{12}_{3}} = \dfrac{5}{3} \Big) \overline{5.00} 1.666 = 1.67$

$$\begin{array}{r} 3 \\ \overline{20} \\ 18 \\ \overline{20} \\ 18 \\ \overline{20} \\ 18 \end{array}$$

b. $\dfrac{\cancel{7}^{1}}{\cancel{84}_{12}} = \dfrac{1}{12} \Big) \overline{1.00} 0.083 = 0.08$

$$\begin{array}{r} 96 \\ \overline{40} \\ 36 \\ \overline{4} \end{array}$$

c. $\dfrac{6}{13} \Big) \overline{6.00} 0.461 = 0.46$

$$\begin{array}{r} 5\,2 \\ \overline{80} \\ 78 \\ \overline{20} \\ 13 \end{array}$$

I. a. 5.3   **b.** 0.63   **c.** 0.924

J. a.

decimal: $\dfrac{\frac{1}{3}}{100} = \dfrac{1}{3} \div 100 = 0.0033$

fraction: $\dfrac{1}{3} \times \dfrac{1}{100} = \dfrac{1}{300}$

ratio: $1:300$

b. decimal:

$0.8\% = \dfrac{0.8}{100} \Big) \overline{0.800} .008 = 0.008 = 0.008$

fraction: $0.8\% = \dfrac{\frac{8}{10}}{100} = \dfrac{8}{10} \div 100 = \dfrac{8}{10} \times \dfrac{1}{100} = \dfrac{\cancel{8}^{1}}{\cancel{1000}_{125}} = \dfrac{1}{125}$

ratio: $1:125$

K. a. $\dfrac{7}{100} = 00.7 = 7\%$ **b.** $1:10 = \dfrac{1}{10} = 0.10 = 10\%$ **c.** $0.008 = 0.008 \qquad 0.8\%$

L. a. $\dfrac{32}{128} = \dfrac{4}{x}$

$\dfrac{\cancel{32}^{1}x}{\cancel{32}_{1}} = \dfrac{\cancel{128}^{4} \times 4}{\cancel{32}_{1}}$

$x = 16$

b. $8:72::5:x$

$\dfrac{\cancel{8}^{1}}{\cancel{8}_{1}} x = \dfrac{\cancel{72}^{9} \times 5}{\cancel{8}_{1}}$

$x = 45$

c. $\dfrac{0.4}{0.12} = \dfrac{x}{8}$

$0.12x = 0.4 \times 8$

$\dfrac{\cancel{0.12}}{\cancel{0.12}} x = \dfrac{0.4 \times 8}{0.12}$

$x = \dfrac{3.2}{0.12} \Big) \overline{3.2000} 26.66 = 27$

$$\begin{array}{r} 2\,4 \\ \overline{80} \\ 72 \\ \overline{80} \\ 72 \\ \overline{8} \end{array}$$

$x = 27$

Chapter 2

Test 1: Exercises in Equivalents and Mixed Conversions

1. 0.1	**11.** 30	**21.** 100	**31.** 10
2. 30	**12.** ⅕	**22.** 1	**32.** 1
3. 1000	**13.** 15	**23.** 0.6	**33.** 1000 (approximate)
4. 5	**14.** 2.2	**24.** 0.01	**34.** 1
5. 15	**15.** 1000	**25.** 1	**35.** 500
6. 0.01	**16.** 0.06	**26.** 0.0005	**36.** 250
7. ½ or 0.5	**17.** 1	**27.** 0.0006	**37.** 50
8. 200	**18.** 4	**28.** 0.25	**38.** 99.32°
9. 0.03	**19.** 45	**29.** 0.001	**39.** 37.78°
10. 0.5	**20.** 40°	**30.** 125	**40.** 98.6°

Chapter 3

Test 1: Abbreviations/Military Time

1. Twice a day
2. Do not use hs. Use "at bedtime."
3. As needed
4. Do not use OU. Use "in both eyes."
5. By mouth
6. In the rectum
7. Sublingual
8. Swish and swallow
9. Do not use tiw. Use "three times weekly."
10. Milliliter
11. Every 4 hours
12. Do not use cc. Use "milliliter."
13. Do not use SC. Use "subcutaneous."
14. Do not use AU. Use "each ear."
15. Gram
16. After meals
17. Do not use qd. Use "every day."
18. Immediately
19. Every 12 hours
20. Three times a day
21. Do not use OS. Write out "in the left eye."
22. Kilogram
23. Every night
24. Every hour
25. Do not use OD. Write out "in the right eye."
26. Milliequivalent
27. Before meals
28. Four times a day
29. Milligram
30. Intramuscularly
31. 1500
32. 1715
33. 0700
34. 1045
35. 2030

Test 2: Reading Prescriptions/Interpreting Written Prescriptions

A.

1. Nembutal one hundred milligrams at the hour of sleep, as needed, by mouth (e.g., 10 PM or 2200)
2. Propranolol hydrochloride forty milligrams by mouth twice a day (e.g., 10 AM, 6 PM)
3. Ampicillin one gram intravenous piggyback every 6 hours (e.g., 6 AM, 12 noon, 6 PM, 12 midnight)
4. Tylenol three hundred twenty-five milligrams, two tablets by mouth immediately. (Give two tablets of Tylenol. Each tablet is 325 mg.)
5. Pilocarpine drops two in both eyes every 3 hours (e.g., 3 AM, 6 AM, 9 AM, 12 noon, 3 PM, 6 PM, 9 PM, 12 midnight). Do not use OU; write "in both eyes."
6. Scopolamine eight-tenths of a milligram subcutaneously immediately
7. Elixir of digoxin twenty-five hundredths of a milligram by mouth every day (e.g., 10 AM). Do not use qd; write "every day."
8. Kaochlor thirty milliequivalents by mouth twice a day (e.g., 10 AM and 6 PM)
9. Heparin six thousand units subcutaneously every 12 hours (e.g., 9 AM, 9 PM)
10. Tobramycin seventy milligrams intramuscularly every 8 hours (e.g., 6 AM, 2 PM, 10 PM or 2200)

B.

11. Colace one hundred milligrams by mouth three times a day (e.g., 10 AM, 2 PM, 6 PM)
12. Ativan one milligram intravenous push times one dose now.
13. Ten milliequivalents potassium chloride in one hundred cubic centimeters of normal saline over one hour, times one dose. Should be one hundred "milliliters."
14. Tylenol #3 two tablets by mouth every four hours as needed for pain
15. Lopressor twenty-five milligrams by mouth twice a day (e.g., 10 AM, 6 PM)

Test 3: Labels and Packaging

A. a. Individually wrapped and labeled drugs

Large stock containers of drugs

b. Glass container holding a single dose. Container must be broken to reach the drug. Any portion not used must be discarded.

Glass or plastic container with a sealed top that allows medication to be kept sterile

c. Drug applied to skin or mucous membranes to achieve a local effect. May be absorbed into the circulation and causes a systemic effect.

Drugs given by injection include subcutaneous, IM, IV, and IVPB.

d. Brand or proprietary name of manufacturer. Identified by symbol ®.

Official name of a drug as listed in the USP

e. Liquid sterile medication ready to administer

Powder or crystals diluted according to specific directions. Date and time of preparation must be written on the label and the expiration date noted.

B. a. 4   **c.** 4   **e.** 1

  b. 2   **d.** 1

C. 1. g   **4.** i   **7.** j   **9.** a

  2. e   **5.** d   **8.** c   **10.** b

  3. h   **6.** f

D. 1. Fortaz

  2. Ceftazidime

  3. Intravenous, intramuscular

  4. Varies: 3.6 mL, 10.6 mL, 100 mL

  5. 1 g

  6. Reconstitute with sterile water for injection, bacteriostatic water for injection, or 0.5% or 1% lidocaine hydrochloride injection. Dilute with 3.0 mL, approximate available volume 3.6 mL to equal 1 g (intramuscular route); 10.0 mL, approximate available volume 10.6 mL to equal 1 g (intravenous infusion); 100 mL, approximate available volume to equal 1 g (infusion pack). Shake well.

  7. Powder

  8. Protect from light. Maintains satisfactory potency for 24 hours at room temperature or for 7 days under refrigeration. Solutions in sterile water for injection that are frozen immediately after constitution in the original container are stable for 3 months when stored at −20°C. Once thawed, solutions should not be refrozen. Thawed solutions may be stored for up to 8 hours at room temperature or for 4 days in a refrigerator.

  9. Not shown

  10. 1 g (adults)

  11. Federal law prohibits dispensing without prescription. This vial is under reduced pressure. Addition of diluent generates a positive pressure. Color changes do not affect potency.

Chapter 4

Test 1: Calculation of Oral Doses

1.

Formula Method	Proportion	Dimensional Analysis
$\dfrac{\overset{10}{\cancel{20}} \text{ mEq}}{\underset{\underset{1}{\cancel{2}}}{\cancel{30}} \text{ mEq}} \times \overset{1}{\cancel{15}} \text{ mL} = 10 \text{ mL}$	**EXPRESSED AS TWO RATIOS** $15 \text{ mL} : 30 \text{ mEq} :: x : 20 \text{ mEq}$ **EXPRESSED AS TWO FRACTIONS** $\dfrac{15 \text{ mL}}{30 \text{ mEq}} \times \dfrac{x}{20 \text{ mEq}}$ **SOLUTION FOR BOTH PROPORTION METHODS** $15 \times 20 = 30x$ $\dfrac{300}{30} = x$ $10 \text{ mL} = x$	$\dfrac{\overset{1}{\cancel{15}} \text{ mL}}{\underset{2}{\cancel{30}} \text{ mEq}} \left| \dfrac{20 \text{ mEq}}{} \right. = \dfrac{20}{2} = 10 \text{ mL}$ 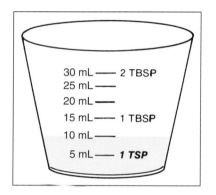

2.

Formula Method	Proportion	Dimensional Analysis
$\dfrac{\overset{2}{\cancel{150}} \text{ mg}}{\underset{1}{\cancel{75}} \text{ mg}} \times 7.5 \text{ mL} = 15 \text{ mL}$	**EXPRESSED AS TWO RATIOS** $7.5 \text{ mL} : 75 \text{ mg} :: x : 150 \text{ mg}$ **EXPRESSED AS TWO FRACTIONS** $\dfrac{7.5 \text{ mL}}{75 \text{ mg}} \times \dfrac{x}{150 \text{ mg}}$ **SOLUTION FOR BOTH PROPORTION METHODS** $7.5 \times 150 = 75x$ $\dfrac{1125}{75} = x$ $15 \text{ mL} = x$	$\dfrac{7.5 \text{ mL}}{\underset{1}{\cancel{75}} \text{ mg}} \left| \dfrac{\overset{2}{\cancel{150}} \text{ mg}}{} \right. = 7.5 \times 2 = 15 \text{ mL}$ 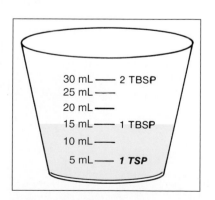

3.

Formula Method	Proportion	Dimensional Analysis

Formula Method

$$\frac{\overset{1}{\cancel{0.125}} \text{ mg}}{\underset{\underset{1}{2}}{\cancel{0.250}} \text{ mg}} \times \overset{5}{\cancel{10}} = 5 \text{ mL}$$

Proportion

EXPRESSED AS TWO RATIOS

10 mL : 0.25 mg : : x : 0.125 mg

EXPRESSED AS TWO FRACTIONS

$$\frac{10 \text{ mL}}{0.25 \text{ mg}} \times \frac{\text{x}}{0.125 \text{ mg}}$$

SOLUTION FOR BOTH PROPORTION METHODS

$$10 \times 0.125 = 0.25\text{x}$$

$$\frac{1.25}{0.25} = \text{x}$$

$$5 \text{ mL} = \text{x}$$

Dimensional Analysis

$$\frac{10 \text{ (mL)}}{\underset{2}{\cancel{0.250}} \text{ mg}} \left| \frac{\overset{1}{\cancel{0.125}} \text{ mg}}{} \right. = \frac{10}{2} = 5 \text{ mL}$$

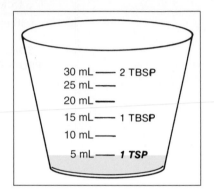

4.

Formula Method	Proportion	Dimensional Analysis

Formula Method

$$\frac{\overset{3}{\cancel{375}} \text{ mg}}{\underset{1}{\cancel{125}} \text{ mg}} \times 5 \text{ mL} = 15 \text{ mL}$$

Proportion

EXPRESSED AS TWO RATIOS

5 mL : 125 mg : : x : 375 mg

EXPRESSED AS TWO FRACTIONS

$$\frac{5 \text{ mL}}{125 \text{ mg}} \times \frac{\text{x}}{375 \text{ mg}}$$

SOLUTION FOR BOTH PROPORTION METHODS

$$5 \times 375 = 125\text{x}$$

$$\frac{1875}{125} = \text{x}$$

$$15 \text{ mL} = \text{x}$$

Dimensional Analysis

$$\frac{5 \text{ (mL)}}{\underset{1}{\cancel{125}} \text{ mg}} \left| \frac{\overset{3}{\cancel{375}} \text{ mg}}{} \right. = 5 \times 3 = 15 \text{ mL}$$

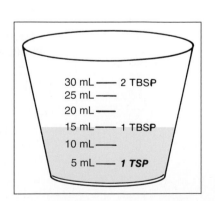

5.

Formula Method	Proportion	Dimensional Analysis
$\dfrac{\overset{2}{\cancel{40}\ \text{mg}}}{\underset{1}{\cancel{20}\ \text{mg}}} \times 2.5\ \text{mL} = 5\ \text{mL}$	**EXPRESSED AS TWO RATIOS** 2.5 mL : 20 mg :: x : 40 mg **EXPRESSED AS TWO FRACTIONS** $\dfrac{2.5\ \text{mL}}{20\ \text{mg}} \times \dfrac{\text{x}}{40\ \text{mg}}$ **SOLUTION FOR BOTH PROPORTION METHODS** $2.5 \times 40 = 20\text{x}$ $\dfrac{100}{20} = \text{x}$ $5\ \text{mL} = \text{x}$	$\dfrac{2.5\ \cancel{\text{mL}}\ \left| \overset{2}{\cancel{40}\ \cancel{\text{mg}}} \right.}{\underset{1}{\cancel{20}\ \cancel{\text{mg}}}} = 2.5 \times 2 = 5\ \text{mL}$ 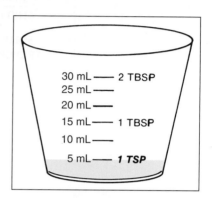

6.

Formula Method	Proportion	Dimensional Analysis
$\dfrac{0.50\ \cancel{\text{mg}}}{0.25\ \cancel{\text{mg}}} \times 1\ \text{tablet} =$ $0.25\overline{)0.50}^{\;2.} = 2\ \text{tablets}$	**EXPRESSED AS TWO RATIOS** 1 tablet : 0.25 mg :: x : 0.5 mg **EXPRESSED AS TWO FRACTIONS** $\dfrac{1\ \text{tablet}}{0.25\ \text{mg}} \times \dfrac{\text{x}}{0.50}$ **SOLUTION FOR BOTH PROPORTION METHODS** $\dfrac{0.50}{0.25} = \text{x}$ $2\ \text{tablets} = \text{x}$	$\dfrac{1\ \cancel{\text{tablet}}\ \left| \overset{2}{0.5\ \cancel{\text{mg}}} \right.}{\underset{1}{0.25\ \cancel{\text{mg}}}} = 2\ \text{tablets}$

7. Equivalent 0.1 mg = 100 mcg

Formula Method	Proportion	Dimensional Analysis
$\dfrac{100\ \cancel{\text{mcg}}}{100\ \cancel{\text{mcg}}} \times 1\ \text{capsule}$ $= 1\ \text{capsule}$	**EXPRESSED AS TWO RATIOS** 1 capsule : 100 mcg :: x : 100 mcg **EXPRESSED AS TWO FRACTIONS** $\dfrac{1\ \text{capsule}}{100\ \text{mcg}} \times \dfrac{\text{x}}{100\ \text{mcg}}$ **SOLUTION FOR BOTH PROPORTION METHODS** 100 mcg = 1 capsule	Use conversion factor 1 mg/1000 mcg: $\dfrac{1\ \cancel{\text{capsule}}\ \left| \overset{1}{\cancel{100}\ \cancel{\text{mcg}}} \right.\left| 1\ \cancel{\text{mg}} \right.}{0.1\ \cancel{\text{mg}}\ \left|\ \right.\left| \underset{10}{\cancel{1000}\ \cancel{\text{mcg}}} \right.} = \dfrac{1}{0.1 \times 10}$ $= 1\ \text{capsule}$

8.

Formula Method	Proportion	Dimensional Analysis
$\dfrac{\overset{5}{\cancel{250}}\ \text{mg}}{\underset{2}{\cancel{100}}\ \text{mg}} \times 1\ \text{tablet} = \dfrac{5}{2}$ $= 2\dfrac{1}{2}\ \text{tablets}$	**EXPRESSED AS TWO RATIOS** 1 tablet : 100 mg : : x : 250 mg **EXPRESSED AS TWO FRACTIONS** $\dfrac{1\ \text{tablet}}{100\ \text{mg}} \times \dfrac{\text{x}}{250\ \text{mg}}$ **SOLUTION FOR BOTH PROPORTION METHODS** $250 = 100\text{x}$ $\dfrac{250}{100} = \text{x}$ $2.5\ \text{tablet} = \text{x}$ or $2\dfrac{1}{2}\ \text{tablets}$	$\dfrac{1\ \text{\textcircled{tablet}}}{\cancel{100}\ \text{mg}} \;\bigg|\; \dfrac{\cancel{250}\ \text{mg}}{} = \dfrac{25}{10} = 2\dfrac{1}{2}\ \text{tablets}$

9. Equivalent 0.5 g = 500 mg

Formula Method	Proportion	Dimensional Analysis
$\dfrac{\overset{2}{\cancel{500}}\ \text{mg}}{\underset{1}{\cancel{250}}\ \text{mg}} \times 1\ \text{capsule}$ $= 2\ \text{capsules}$	**EXPRESSED AS TWO RATIOS** 1 capsule : 250 mg : : x : 500 mg **EXPRESSED AS TWO FRACTIONS** $\dfrac{1\ \text{capsule}}{250\ \text{mg}} \times \dfrac{\text{x}}{500\ \text{mg}}$ **SOLUTION FOR BOTH PROPORTION METHODS** $500 = 200\text{x}$ $\dfrac{500}{250} = \text{x}$ $2\ \text{capsules} = \text{x}$	Use conversion factor 1000 mg/1 g: $\dfrac{1\ \text{\textcircled{capsule}}}{\underset{1}{\cancel{250}}\ \text{mg}} \;\bigg|\; \dfrac{0.5\ \cancel{\text{g}}}{} \;\bigg|\; \dfrac{\overset{4}{\cancel{1000}}\ \text{mg}}{1\ \cancel{\text{g}}} = 0.5 \times 4$ $= 2\ \text{capsules}$

10. Equivalent 0.3 mg = 300 mcg

Formula Method	Proportion	Dimensional Analysis
$\dfrac{\overset{1}{\cancel{300}}\ \text{mcg}}{\underset{1}{\cancel{300}}\ \text{mcg}} \times 1\ \text{tablet} = 1\ \text{tablet}$	**EXPRESSED AS TWO RATIOS** 1 tablet : 300 mcg : : x : 300 mcg **EXPRESSED AS TWO FRACTIONS** $\dfrac{1\ \text{tablet}}{300\ \text{mcg}} \times \dfrac{\text{x}}{300\ \text{mcg}}$ **SOLUTION FOR BOTH PROPORTION METHODS** $300 = 300\text{x}$ $\dfrac{300}{300} = \text{x}$ $1\ \text{tablet} = \text{x}$	Use conversion factor 1000 mcg/1 mg: $\dfrac{1\ \text{\textcircled{tablet}}}{\cancel{300}\ \text{mcg}} \;\bigg|\; \dfrac{0.3\ \cancel{\text{mg}}}{} \;\bigg|\; \dfrac{\cancel{1000}\ \cancel{\text{mcg}}}{1\ \cancel{\text{mg}}} = \dfrac{0.3 \times 10}{3}$ $= 1\ \text{tablet}$

Test 2: Calculation of Oral Doses

1. Equivalent 0.8 g = 800 mg

Formula Method	Proportion	Dimensional Analysis
$\dfrac{\overset{2}{\cancel{800}}\ \text{mg}}{\underset{1}{\cancel{400}}\ \text{mg}} \times 1\ \text{tablet} = 2\ \text{tablets}$	**EXPRESSED AS TWO RATIOS** 1 tablet : 400 mg : : x : 800 mg **EXPRESSED AS TWO FRACTIONS** $\dfrac{1\ \text{tablet}}{400\ \text{mg}} \diagdown \dfrac{x}{800\ \text{mg}}$ **SOLUTION FOR BOTH PROPORTION METHODS** $800 = 400x$ $\dfrac{800}{400} = x$ 2 tablets = x	Use conversion factor 1000 mg/1 g: $\dfrac{1\ \text{\textcircled{tablet}}}{4\cancel{00}\ \text{mg}} \left| \dfrac{0.8\ \cancel{\text{g}}}{} \right| \dfrac{10\cancel{00}\ \text{mg}}{1\ \cancel{\text{g}}} = \dfrac{0.8 \times 10}{4}$ $= 2\ \text{tablets}$

2. Equivalent 0.3 g = 300 mg

Formula Method	Proportion	Dimensional Analysis
$\dfrac{\overset{1}{\cancel{300}}\ \text{mg}}{\underset{1}{\cancel{300}}\ \text{mg}} \times 1\ \text{tablet} = 1\ \text{tablet}$	**EXPRESSED AS TWO RATIOS** 1 tablet : 300 mg : : x : 300 mg **EXPRESSED AS TWO FRACTIONS** $\dfrac{1\ \text{tablet}}{300\ \text{mg}} \diagdown \dfrac{x}{300\ \text{mg}}$ **SOLUTION FOR BOTH PROPORTION METHODS** $300 = 300x$ $\dfrac{300}{300} = x$ 1 tablet = x	Use conversion factor 1000 mg/1 g: $\dfrac{1\ \text{\textcircled{tablet}}}{3\cancel{00}\ \text{mg}} \left| \dfrac{0.3\ \cancel{\text{g}}}{} \right| \dfrac{10\cancel{00}\ \text{mg}}{1\ \cancel{\text{g}}} = \dfrac{0.3 \times 10}{3}$ $= 1\ \text{tablet}$

3.

Formula Method	Proportion	Dimensional Analysis
$\dfrac{75\ \text{mg}}{50\ \text{mg}} \times 1\ \text{tablet} = 1\tfrac{1}{2}\ \text{tablets}$	**EXPRESSED AS TWO RATIOS** 1 tablet : 50 mg : : x : 75 mg **EXPRESSED AS TWO FRACTIONS** $\dfrac{1\ \text{tablet}}{50\ \text{mg}} \diagdown \dfrac{x}{75\ \text{mg}}$ **SOLUTION FOR BOTH PROPORTION METHODS** $75 = 50x$ $\dfrac{75}{50} = x$ $1\tfrac{1}{2}$ tablets = x	$\dfrac{1\ \text{\textcircled{tablet}}}{\underset{2}{\cancel{50}}\ \text{mg}} \left| \dfrac{\overset{3}{\cancel{75}}\ \text{mg}}{} \right. = \dfrac{3}{2} = 1\tfrac{1}{2}\ \text{tablets}$

4. $0.65 \text{ g} = 650 \text{ mg}$

Formula Method	Proportion	Dimensional Analysis
$\dfrac{\overset{2}{\cancel{650}} \text{ mg}}{\underset{1}{\cancel{325}} \text{ mg}} \times 1 \text{ tablet} = 2 \text{ tablets}$	**EXPRESSED AS TWO RATIOS** $1 \text{ tablet} : 325 \text{ mg} :: x : 650 \text{ mg}$ **EXPRESSED AS TWO FRACTIONS** $\dfrac{1 \text{ tablet}}{325 \text{ mg}} \diagdown \dfrac{x}{650 \text{ mg}}$ **SOLUTION FOR BOTH PROPORTION METHODS** $650 = 325x$ $\dfrac{650}{325} = x$ $2 \text{ tablets} = x$	Use conversion factor 1000 mg/1 g: $\dfrac{1 \text{ \textcircled{tablet}}}{325 \text{ \cancel{mg}}} \left\| \dfrac{0.65 \text{ \cancel{g}}}{} \right\| \dfrac{1000 \text{ \cancel{mg}}}{1 \text{ \cancel{g}}} = \dfrac{0.65 \times 1000}{325}$ $= 2 \text{ tablets}$

5.

Formula Method	Proportion	Dimensional Analysis
$\dfrac{10 \text{ mg}}{2.5 \text{ mg}} \times 1 \text{ tablet} = 4 \text{ tablets}$	**EXPRESSED AS TWO RATIOS** $1 \text{ tablet} : 2.5 \text{ mg} :: x : 10 \text{ mg}$ **EXPRESSED AS TWO FRACTIONS** $\dfrac{1 \text{ tablet}}{2.5 \text{ mg}} \diagdown \dfrac{x}{10 \text{ mg}}$ **SOLUTION FOR BOTH PROPORTION METHODS** $10 = 2.5x$ $\dfrac{10}{2.5} = x$ $4 \text{ tablets} = x$	$\dfrac{1 \text{ \textcircled{tablet}}}{2.5 \text{ \cancel{mg}}} \left\| \dfrac{10 \text{ \cancel{mg}}}{} \right. = \dfrac{10}{2.5} = 4 \text{ tablets}$

6.

Formula Method	Proportion	Dimensional Analysis
$\dfrac{750,000 \text{ \cancel{units}}}{100,000 \text{ \cancel{units}}} \times 1 \text{ mL} = \dfrac{75}{10}$ $= 7.5 \text{ mL}$	**EXPRESSED AS TWO RATIOS** $1 \text{ mL} : 100,000 \text{ units} :: x : 750,000 \text{ units}$ **EXPRESSED AS TWO FRACTIONS** $\dfrac{1 \text{ mL}}{100,000 \text{ units}} \diagdown \dfrac{x}{750,000 \text{ units}}$ **SOLUTION FOR BOTH PROPORTION METHODS** $750,000 = 100,000x$ $\dfrac{750,000}{100,000} = x$ $7.5 \text{ mL} = x$	$\dfrac{1 \text{ \textcircled{mL}}}{100{,}000 \text{ \cancel{units}}} \left\| \dfrac{750{,}000 \text{ \cancel{units}}}{} \right. = \dfrac{75}{10} = 7.5 \text{ mL}$ 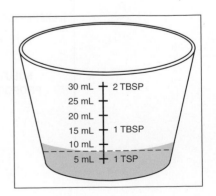

7. Equivalent 0.75 g = 750 mg

Formula Method	Proportion	Dimensional Analysis

Formula Method

$$\frac{\overset{3}{\cancel{750}} \text{ mg}}{\underset{1}{\cancel{250}} \text{ mg}} \times 5 \text{ mL} = 15 \text{ mL}$$

Proportion

EXPRESSED AS TWO RATIOS

5 mL : 250 mg : : x : 750 mg

EXPRESSED AS TWO FRACTIONS

$$\frac{5 \text{ mL}}{250 \text{ mg}} \times \frac{\text{x}}{750}$$

SOLUTION FOR BOTH PROPORTION METHODS

$$5 \times 750 = 250\text{x}$$

$$\frac{3750}{250} = \text{x}$$

$$15 \text{ mL} = \text{x}$$

Dimensional Analysis

Use conversion factor 1000 mg/1 g:

$$\frac{5 \cancel{\text{mL}}}{\underset{1}{\cancel{250} \text{ mg}}} \bigg| \frac{0.75 \cancel{\text{g}}}{} \bigg| \frac{\overset{4}{\cancel{1000}} \cancel{\text{mg}}}{1 \cancel{\text{g}}} = 5 \times 0.75 \times 4$$

$$= 15 \text{ mL}$$

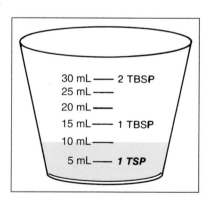

8.

Formula Method	Proportion	Dimensional Analysis

Formula Method

$$\frac{\overset{2}{\cancel{500}} \text{ mg}}{\underset{1}{\cancel{250}} \text{ mg}} \times 5 \text{ mL} = 10 \text{ mL}$$

Proportion

EXPRESSED AS TWO RATIOS

5 mL : 250 mg : : x : 500 mg

EXPRESSED AS TWO FRACTIONS

$$\frac{5 \text{ mL}}{250 \text{ mg}} \times \frac{\text{x}}{500 \text{ mg}}$$

SOLUTION FOR BOTH PROPORTION METHODS

$$5 \times 500 = 250\text{x}$$

$$\frac{2500}{250} = \text{x}$$

$$10 \text{ mL} = \text{x}$$

Dimensional Analysis

$$\frac{5 \cancel{\text{mL}}}{\underset{1}{\cancel{250} \cancel{\text{mg}}}} \bigg| \frac{\overset{2}{\cancel{500} \cancel{\text{mg}}}}{} = 5 \times 2 = 10 \text{ mL}$$

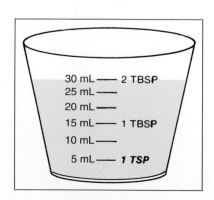

9. No arithmetic necessary. Pour 30 mL.

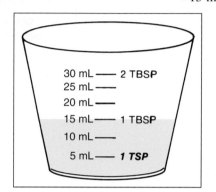

10.

Formula Method	Proportion	Dimensional Analysis
$\dfrac{\overset{2}{\cancel{160}} \text{ mg}}{\underset{1}{\cancel{80}} \text{ mg}} \times 15 \text{ mL} = 30 \text{ mL}$	**EXPRESSED AS TWO RATIOS** 15 mL : 80 mg : : x : 160 mg **EXPRESSED AS TWO FRACTIONS** $\dfrac{15 \text{ mL}}{80 \text{ mg}} \times \dfrac{\text{x}}{160 \text{ mg}}$ **SOLUTION FOR BOTH PROPORTION METHODS** $15 \times 160 = 80\text{x}$ $\dfrac{2400}{80} = \text{x}$ $30 \text{ mL} = \text{x}$	$\dfrac{15 \text{ } \textcircled{mL}}{\underset{1}{\cancel{80}} \text{ mg}} \Bigg| \overset{2}{\cancel{160}} \text{ mg} = 15 \times 2 = 30 \text{ mL}$ 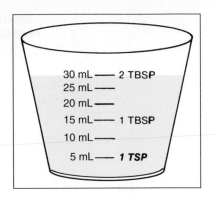

Test 3: Calculation of Oral Doses

1.

Formula Method	Proportion	Dimensional Analysis
$\dfrac{\overset{10}{\cancel{20}} \text{ mEq}}{\underset{\underset{1}{2}}{\cancel{30}} \text{ mEq}} \times \overset{1}{\cancel{15}} \text{ mL} = 10 \text{ mL}$	**EXPRESSED AS TWO RATIOS** 15 mL : 30 mEq : : x : 20 mEq **EXPRESSED AS TWO FRACTIONS** $\dfrac{15 \text{ mL}}{30 \text{ mEq}} \times \dfrac{\text{x}}{20 \text{ mEq}}$ **SOLUTION FOR BOTH PROPORTION METHODS** $15 \times 20 = 30\text{x}$ $\dfrac{300}{30} = \text{x}$ $10 \text{ mL} = \text{x}$	$\dfrac{15 \text{ } \textcircled{mL}}{\underset{6}{\cancel{30}} \text{ mEq}} \Bigg| \overset{4}{\cancel{20}} \text{ mEq} = \dfrac{15 \times 4}{6} = 10 \text{ mL}$

2.

Formula Method	Proportion	Dimensional Analysis
$$\frac{80 \text{ mcg}}{125 \text{ mcg}} \times 5 \text{ mL} = \frac{80}{25}$$ $$= \frac{16}{5} \overline{)16.0}^{\,3.2} = 3.2 \text{ mL}$$	**EXPRESSED AS TWO RATIOS** $$5 \text{ mL} : 125 \text{ mg} :: x : 80 \text{ mg}$$ **EXPRESSED AS TWO FRACTIONS** $$\frac{5 \text{ mL}}{125 \text{ mg}} \times \frac{x}{80 \text{ mg}}$$ **SOLUTION FOR BOTH PROPORTION METHODS** $$5 \times 80 = 125x$$ $$\frac{40}{125} = x$$ $$3.2 \text{ mL} = x$$	$$\frac{5 \text{ mL}}{125 \text{ mg}} \,\bigg|\, \frac{80 \text{ mg}}{} = \frac{80}{25} = 3.2 \text{ mL}$$

If you do not have a dropper bottle, you could use a syringe without the needle to obtain the dose or an oral syringe.

3. 0.02 g = 20 mg

Formula Method	Proportion	Dimensional Analysis
$$\frac{20 \text{ mg}}{10 \text{ mg}} \times 1 \text{ tablet} = 2 \text{ tablets}$$	**EXPRESSED AS TWO RATIOS** $$1 \text{ tablet} : 10 \text{ mg} :: x : 20 \text{ mg}$$ **EXPRESSED AS TWO FRACTIONS** $$\frac{1 \text{ tablet}}{10 \text{ mg}} \times \frac{x}{20 \text{ mg}}$$ **SOLUTION FOR BOTH PROPORTION METHODS** $$20 = 10x$$ $$\frac{20}{10} = x$$ $$2 \text{ tablets} = x$$	Use conversion factor 1000 mg/1 g: $$\frac{1 \text{ tablet}}{10 \text{ mg}} \,\bigg|\, 0.02 \text{ g} \,\bigg|\, \frac{1000 \text{ mg}}{1 \text{ g}} = 0.02 \times 100$$ $$= 2 \text{ tablets}$$

4. 0.5 g = 500 mg

Formula Method	Proportion	Dimensional Analysis
$$\frac{500 \text{ mg}}{250 \text{ mg}} \times 1 \text{ capsule}$$ $$= 2 \text{ capsules}$$	**EXPRESSED AS TWO RATIOS** $$1 \text{ capsule} : 250 \text{ mg} :: x : 500 \text{ mg}$$ **EXPRESSED AS TWO FRACTIONS** $$\frac{1 \text{ capsule}}{250 \text{ mg}} \times \frac{x}{500 \text{ mg}}$$ **SOLUTION FOR BOTH PROPORTION METHODS** $$500 = 250x$$ $$\frac{500}{250} = x$$ $$2 \text{ capsules} = x$$	Use conversion factor 1000 mg/1 g: $$\frac{1 \text{ capsule}}{250 \text{ mg}} \,\bigg|\, 0.5 \text{ g} \,\bigg|\, \frac{1000 \text{ mg}}{1 \text{ g}} = 0.5 \times 4$$ $$= 2 \text{ capsules}$$

5.

Formula Method	Proportion	Dimensional Analysis
$\dfrac{\overset{2}{0.\cancel{50}} \text{ mg}}{\underset{1}{0.\cancel{25}} \text{ mg}} \times 1 \text{ tablet} = 2 \text{ tablets}$	**EXPRESSED AS TWO RATIOS** 1 tablet : 0.25 mg : : x : 0.5 mg **EXPRESSED AS TWO FRACTIONS** $\dfrac{1 \text{ tablet}}{0.25 \text{ mg}} \times \dfrac{x}{0.5 \text{ mg}}$ **SOLUTION FOR BOTH PROPORTION METHODS** $0.5 = 0.25x$ $\dfrac{0.5}{0.25} = x$ 2 tablets = x	$\dfrac{1 \text{ ⃝tablet}}{0.\underset{1}{\cancel{250}} \text{ mg}} \left| \dfrac{0.\overset{2}{\cancel{500}} \text{ mg}}{} \right. = 2 \text{ tablets}$

6.

Formula Method	Proportion	Dimensional Analysis
$\dfrac{40 \text{ mg}}{\underset{1}{\cancel{5}} \text{ mg}} \times \overset{1}{\cancel{5}} \text{ mL} = 40 \text{ mL}$	**EXPRESSED AS TWO RATIOS** 5 mL : 5 mg : : x : 40 mg **EXPRESSED AS TWO FRACTIONS** $\dfrac{5 \text{ mL}}{5 \text{ mg}} \times \dfrac{x}{40 \text{ mg}}$ **SOLUTION FOR BOTH PROPORTION METHODS** $5 \times 40 = 5x$ $\dfrac{200}{5} = x$ 40 mL = x	$\dfrac{5 \text{ ⃝mL}}{\underset{1}{\cancel{5}} \text{ mg}} \left| \dfrac{\overset{8}{\cancel{40}} \text{ mg}}{} \right. = 5 \times 8 = 40 \text{ mL}$

7.

Formula Method	Proportion	Dimensional Analysis
$\dfrac{\overset{3}{\cancel{75}} \text{ mg}}{\underset{2}{\cancel{50}} \text{ mg}} \times 1 \text{ tablet} = \dfrac{3}{2} \begin{array}{r} 1.5 \\ \overline{)3.0} \end{array}$ $= 1\dfrac{1}{2} \text{ tablets}$	**EXPRESSED AS TWO RATIOS** 1 tablet : 50 mg : : x : 75 mg **EXPRESSED AS TWO FRACTIONS** $\dfrac{1 \text{ tablet}}{50 \text{ mg}} \times \dfrac{x}{75 \text{ mg}}$ **SOLUTION FOR BOTH PROPORTION METHODS** $75 = 50x$ $\dfrac{75}{50} = x$ 1.5 tablets = x or $1\dfrac{1}{2}$ tablets	$\dfrac{1 \text{ ⃝tablet}}{\underset{2}{\cancel{50}} \text{ mg}} \left| \dfrac{\overset{3}{\cancel{75}} \text{ mg}}{} \right. = \dfrac{3}{2} = 1\dfrac{1}{2} \text{ tablets}$

8.

Formula Method	Proportion	Dimensional Analysis
$\dfrac{\overset{1}{\cancel{40}} \text{ mg}}{\underset{2}{\cancel{80}} \text{ mg}} \times 1 \text{ tablet} = \dfrac{1}{2} \text{ tablet}$	**EXPRESSED AS TWO RATIOS** 1 tablet : 80 mg : : x : 40 mg **EXPRESSED AS TWO FRACTIONS** $\dfrac{1 \text{ tablet}}{80 \text{ mg}} \diagup \dfrac{x}{40 \text{ mg}}$ **SOLUTION FOR BOTH PROPORTION METHODS** $40 = 80x$ $\dfrac{40}{80} = x$ $0.5 \text{ tablet} = x$ or $\dfrac{1}{2}$ tablet	$\dfrac{1 \,\text{(tablet)}}{\underset{2}{\cancel{80}} \text{ mg}} \left| \dfrac{\overset{1}{\cancel{40}} \text{ mg}}{} \right. = \dfrac{1}{2} \text{ tablet}$

9. 0.125 mg = 125 mcg

Formula Method	Proportion	Dimensional Analysis
$\dfrac{\overset{1}{\cancel{125}} \text{ mcg}}{\underset{4\;2}{\cancel{500}} \text{ mcg}} \times \overset{5}{\cancel{10}} \text{ mL} = \dfrac{5}{2} \begin{array}{r}2.5\\[-2pt]\overline{)5.0}\end{array}$ $= 2.5 \text{ mL}$	**EXPRESSED AS TWO RATIOS** 10 mL : 500 mcg : : x : 125 mcg **EXPRESSED AS TWO FRACTIONS** $\dfrac{10 \text{ mL}}{500 \text{ mcg}} \diagup \dfrac{x}{125 \text{ mcg}}$ **SOLUTION FOR BOTH PROPORTION METHODS** $10 \times 125 = 500x$ $\dfrac{1250}{500} = x$ $2.5 \text{ mL} = x$	Use conversion factor 1000 mcg/1 mg: $\dfrac{10 \,\text{(mL)}}{\underset{1}{\cancel{500}} \text{ mcg}} \left| \dfrac{0.125 \text{ mg}}{} \right| \dfrac{\overset{2}{\cancel{1000}} \text{ mcg}}{1 \text{ mg}} = 10 \times 0.125 \times 2$ $= 2.5 \text{ mL}$

Use a syringe without a needle to measure the dose or an oral syringe.

10.

Formula Method	Proportion	Dimensional Analysis
$\dfrac{\overset{3}{\cancel{75}} \text{ mg}}{\underset{2\;1}{\cancel{50}} \text{ mg}} \times \overset{5}{\cancel{10}} \text{ mL} = 15 \text{ mL}$	**EXPRESSED AS TWO RATIOS** 10 mL : 50 mg : : x : 75 mg **EXPRESSED AS TWO FRACTIONS** $\dfrac{10 \text{ mL}}{50 \text{ mg}} \diagup \dfrac{x}{75 \text{ mg}}$ **SOLUTION FOR BOTH PROPORTION METHODS** $10 \times 75 = 50x$ $\dfrac{750}{50} = x$ $15 \text{ mL} = x$	$\dfrac{10 \,\text{(mL)}}{\underset{1}{\cancel{50}} \text{ mg}} \left| \dfrac{\overset{15}{\cancel{75}} \text{ mg}}{} \right. = 15 \text{ mL}$

11.

Formula Method	Proportion	Dimensional Analysis
$\dfrac{5\ \text{mg}}{2\ \text{mg}} \times 1\ \text{tablet} = \dfrac{5}{2} \overset{2.5}{)5.0}$ $= 2\dfrac{1}{2}\ \text{tablets}$	**EXPRESSED AS TWO RATIOS** $1\ \text{tablet} : 2\ \text{mg} :: x : 5\ \text{mg}$ **EXPRESSED AS TWO FRACTIONS** $\dfrac{1\ \text{tablet}}{2\ \text{mg}} \times \dfrac{x}{5\ \text{mg}}$ **SOLUTION FOR BOTH PROPORTION METHODS** $5 = 2x$ $\dfrac{5}{2} = x$ $2.5\ \text{tablets} = x$ or $2\dfrac{1}{2}\ \text{tablets}$	$\dfrac{1\ \text{tablet}}{2\ \text{mg}} \bigg| \dfrac{5\ \text{mg}}{} = \dfrac{5}{2} = 2\dfrac{1}{2}\ \text{tablets}$

12. 0.15 mg = 150 mcg

Formula Method	Proportion	Dimensional Analysis
$\dfrac{\overset{1}{150\ \text{mcg}}}{\underset{2}{300\ \text{mcg}}} \times 1\ \text{tablet} = \dfrac{1}{2}\ \text{tablet}$	**EXPRESSED AS TWO RATIOS** $1\ \text{tablet} : 300\ \text{mcg} :: x : 150\ \text{mcg}$ **EXPRESSED AS TWO FRACTIONS** $\dfrac{1\ \text{tablet}}{300\ \text{mcg}} \times \dfrac{x}{150\ \text{mcg}}$ **SOLUTION FOR BOTH PROPORTION METHODS** $150 = 300x$ $\dfrac{150}{300} = x$ $0.5\ \text{tablet} = x$ or $\dfrac{1}{2}\ \text{tablet}$	Use conversion factor 1000 mcg/1 mg: $\dfrac{1\ \text{tablet}}{\underset{1}{300\ \text{mcg}}} \bigg| \dfrac{\overset{0.05}{0.15\ \text{mg}}}{} \bigg| \dfrac{1000\ \text{mcg}}{1\ \text{mg}} = 0.05 \times 10$ $= 0.5\ \text{or}\ \dfrac{1}{2}\ \text{tablet}$

13.

Formula Method	Proportion	Dimensional Analysis
$\dfrac{\overset{3}{375\ \text{mg}}}{\underset{2}{250\ \text{mg}}} \times 1\ \text{tablet} = \dfrac{3}{2} \overset{1.5}{)3.0}$ $= 1\dfrac{1}{2}\ \text{tablets}$	**EXPRESSED AS TWO RATIOS** $1\ \text{tablet} : 250\ \text{mg} :: x : 375\ \text{mg}$ **EXPRESSED AS TWO FRACTIONS** $\dfrac{1\ \text{tablet}}{250\ \text{mg}} \times \dfrac{x}{375\ \text{mg}}$ **SOLUTION FOR BOTH PROPORTION METHODS** $375 = 250x$ $\dfrac{375}{250} = x$ $1.5\ \text{tablets} = x$ or $1\dfrac{1}{2}\ \text{tablets}$	$\dfrac{1\ \text{tablet}}{\underset{10}{250\ \text{mg}}} \bigg| \dfrac{\overset{15}{375\ \text{mg}}}{} = \dfrac{15}{10} = 1\dfrac{1}{2}\ \text{tablets}$

14. 0.6 g = 600 mg

Formula Method	Proportion	Dimensional Analysis
$\dfrac{\overset{2}{\cancel{600}}\text{ mg}}{\underset{1}{\cancel{300}}\text{ mg}} \times 1 \text{ tablet} = 2 \text{ tablets}$	**EXPRESSED AS TWO RATIOS** 1 tablet : 300 mg : : x : 600 mg **EXPRESSED AS TWO FRACTIONS** $\dfrac{1 \text{ tablet}}{300 \text{ mg}} \diagup \dfrac{x}{600 \text{ mg}}$ **SOLUTION FOR BOTH PROPORTION METHODS** $600 = 300x$ $\dfrac{600}{300} = x$ $2 \text{ tablets} = x$	Use conversion factor 1000 mg/1 g: $\dfrac{1 \text{ tablet}}{\underset{1}{\cancel{300}}\text{ mg}} \left\| \dfrac{\overset{0.2}{\cancel{0.6}}\text{ g}}{} \right\| \dfrac{\overset{}{\cancel{1000}}\text{ mg}}{1 \cancel{g}} = 0.2 \times 10$ $= 2 \text{ tablets}$

15.

Formula Method	Proportion	Dimensional Analysis
$\dfrac{\overset{3}{\cancel{1.5}}\text{ mg}}{\underset{\underset{1}{2}}{\cancel{1.0}}\text{ mg}} \times \overset{4}{\cancel{8}} \text{ mL} = 12 \text{ mL}$	**EXPRESSED AS TWO RATIOS** 8 mL : 1 mg : : x : 1.5 mg **EXPRESSED AS TWO FRACTIONS** $\dfrac{8 \text{ mL}}{1 \text{ mg}} \diagup \dfrac{x}{1.5 \text{ mg}}$ **SOLUTION FOR BOTH PROPORTION METHODS** $8 \times 1.5 = 1x$ $\dfrac{12}{1} = x$ $12 \text{ mL} = x$	$\dfrac{8 \cancel{\text{ mL}}}{1 \cancel{\text{ mg}}} \left\| \dfrac{1.5 \cancel{\text{ mg}}}{} \right. = 8 \times 1.5 = 12 \text{ mL}$

Use a syringe without the needle to measure the dose or an oral syringe.

16.

Formula Method	Proportion	Dimensional Analysis
$\dfrac{\overset{2}{\cancel{25.0}}\text{ mg}}{\underset{1}{\cancel{12.5}}\text{ mg}} \times 5 \text{ mL} = 10 \text{ mL}$	**EXPRESSED AS TWO RATIOS** 5 mL : 12.5 mg : : x : 25 mg **EXPRESSED AS TWO FRACTIONS** $\dfrac{5 \text{ mL}}{12.5 \text{ mg}} \diagup \dfrac{x}{25 \text{ mg}}$ **SOLUTION FOR BOTH PROPORTION METHODS** $5 \times 25 = 12.5x$ $\dfrac{125}{12.5} = x$ $10 \text{ mL} = x$	$\dfrac{5 \cancel{\text{ mL}}}{\underset{1}{\cancel{12.5}}\text{ mg}} \left\| \dfrac{\overset{2}{\cancel{25}}\text{ mg}}{} \right. = 5 \times 2 = 10 \text{ mL}$

17.

Formula Method	Proportion	Dimensional Analysis
$\dfrac{\overset{3}{\cancel{60}} \text{ mg}}{\underset{2}{\cancel{40}} \text{ mg}} \times 0.6 \text{ mL} = \dfrac{1.8}{2}$ $= 0.9 \text{ mL}$	**EXPRESSED AS TWO RATIOS** $0.6 \text{ mL} : 40 \text{ mg} :: x : 60 \text{ mg}$ **EXPRESSED AS TWO FRACTIONS** $\dfrac{0.6 \text{ mL}}{40 \text{ mg}} \times \dfrac{x}{60 \text{ mg}}$ **SOLUTION FOR BOTH PROPORTION METHODS** $0.6 \times 60 = 40x$ $\dfrac{36}{40} = x$ $0.9 \text{ mL} = x$	$\dfrac{0.6 \text{ } \textcircled{mL}}{\underset{2}{\cancel{40}} \text{ mg}} \Bigg| \dfrac{\overset{3}{\cancel{60}} \text{ mg}}{} = 0.6 \times \dfrac{3}{2} = \dfrac{1.8 \text{ mL}}{2} = 0.9 \text{ mL}$

18. $0.5 \text{ g} = 500 \text{ mg}$

Formula Method	Proportion	Dimensional Analysis
$\dfrac{\overset{2}{\cancel{500}} \text{ mg}}{\underset{1}{\cancel{250}} \text{ mg}} \times 5 \text{ mL} = 10 \text{ mL}$	**EXPRESSED AS TWO RATIOS** $5 \text{ mL} : 250 \text{ mg} :: x : 500 \text{ mg}$ **EXPRESSED AS TWO FRACTIONS** $\dfrac{5 \text{ mL}}{250 \text{ mg}} \times \dfrac{x}{500 \text{ mg}}$ **SOLUTION FOR BOTH PROPORTION METHODS** $500 \times 5 = 250x$ $\dfrac{2500}{250} = x$ $10 \text{ mL} = x$	Use conversion factor 1000 mg/1 g: $\dfrac{5 \text{ } \textcircled{mL}}{\underset{1}{\cancel{250}} \text{ mg}} \Bigg| 0.5 \text{ } \cancel{g} \Bigg| \dfrac{\overset{4}{\cancel{1000}} \text{ mg}}{1 \text{ } \cancel{g}} = 5 \times 0.5 \times 4$ $= 10 \text{ mL}$

19.

Formula Method	Proportion	Dimensional Analysis
$\dfrac{\overset{3}{\cancel{15}} \text{ mg}}{\underset{10}{\cancel{50}} \text{ mg}} \times 5 \text{ mL} = 1.5 \text{ mL}$	**EXPRESSED AS TWO RATIOS** $5 \text{ mL} : 50 \text{ mg} :: x : 15 \text{ mg}$ **EXPRESSED AS TWO FRACTIONS** $\dfrac{5 \text{ mL}}{50 \text{ mg}} \times \dfrac{x}{15 \text{ mg}}$ **SOLUTION FOR BOTH PROPORTION METHODS** $5 \times 15 = 50x$ $\dfrac{75}{50} = x$ $1.5 \text{ mL} = x$	$\dfrac{\overset{1}{\cancel{5}} \text{ } \textcircled{mL}}{\underset{10}{\cancel{50}} \text{ mg}} \Bigg| 15 \text{ mg} = \dfrac{15}{10} = 1.5 \text{ mL}$

Use a syringe without a needle to measure the dose or an oral syringe.

20.

Formula Method	Proportion	Dimensional Analysis
$\dfrac{\overset{2}{\cancel{50}}\ \text{mg}}{\underset{1}{\cancel{25}}\ \text{mg}} \times 5\ \text{mL} = 10\ \text{mL}$	**EXPRESSED AS TWO RATIOS** 5 mL : 25 mg : : x : 50 mg **EXPRESSED AS TWO FRACTIONS** $\dfrac{5\ \text{mL}}{25\ \text{mg}} \times \dfrac{\text{x}}{50\ \text{mg}}$ **SOLUTION FOR BOTH PROPORTION METHODS** $5 \times 50 = 25\text{x}$ $\dfrac{250}{25} = \text{x}$ $10\ \text{mL} = \text{x}$	$\dfrac{5\ \cancel{\text{mL}}}{\underset{1}{\cancel{25}}\ \cancel{\text{mg}}} \left| \dfrac{\overset{2}{\cancel{50}}\ \cancel{\text{mg}}}{} \right. = 5 \times 2 = 10\ \text{mL}$

Chapter 5

Test 1: Calculations of Liquid Injections

1. Equivalent 0.1 g = 100 mg

Formula Method	Proportion	Dimensional Analysis
$\dfrac{\overset{1}{\cancel{100}}\ \text{mg}}{\underset{2}{\cancel{200}}\ \text{mg}} \times 3\ \text{mL} = \dfrac{3}{2}\ \begin{array}{r} 1.5 \\ \overline{\smash{)}3.0} \end{array}$	**EXPRESSED AS TWO RATIOS** 3 mL : 200 mg : : x : 100 mg **EXPRESSED AS TWO FRACTIONS** $\dfrac{3\ \text{mL}}{200\ \text{mg}} \times \dfrac{\text{x}}{100\ \text{mg}}$ **SOLUTION FOR BOTH PROPORTION METHODS** $3 \times 100 = 200\text{x}$ $\dfrac{300}{200} = \text{x}$ $1.5\ \text{mL} = \text{x}$	Use conversion factor 1000 mg/1 g: $\dfrac{3\ \cancel{\text{mL}}}{\underset{2}{\cancel{200}}\ \cancel{\text{mg}}} \left| 0.1\ \cancel{\text{g}} \right| \dfrac{\overset{10}{\cancel{1000}}\ \cancel{\text{mg}}}{1\ \cancel{\text{g}}} = \dfrac{3 \times 0.1 \times 10}{2} = \dfrac{3}{2}$ $= 1.5\ \text{mL}$

Give 1.5 mL IM.

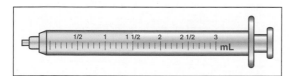

2.

Formula Method	Proportion	Dimensional Analysis

$$\frac{\overset{1}{\cancel{5}}\text{ mg}}{\underset{3}{\cancel{15}}\text{ mg}} \times 1\text{ mL} = \frac{1}{3}\overset{.333}{\overline{)1.000}}$$

$$= 0.33\text{ mL}$$

EXPRESSED AS TWO RATIOS

1 mL : 15 mg :: x : 5 mg

EXPRESSED AS TWO FRACTIONS

$$\frac{1\text{ mL}}{15\text{ mg}} \times \frac{x}{5\text{ mg}}$$

SOLUTION FOR BOTH PROPORTION METHODS

$$5 = 15x$$

$$\frac{5}{15} = x$$

$$0.33\text{ mL} = x$$

$$\frac{1\,\canc:{mL}}{\underset{3}{\cancel{15}}\text{ mg}} \;\Big|\; \frac{\overset{1}{\cancel{5}}\text{ mg}}{} = \frac{1}{3} = 0.33\text{ mL}$$

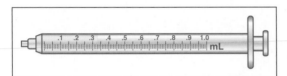

3.

Formula Method	Proportion	Dimensional Analysis

$$\frac{\overset{1}{\cancel{25}}\text{ mg}}{\underset{2}{\cancel{50}}\text{ mg}} \times \overset{1}{\cancel{2}}\text{ mL} = 1\text{ mL}$$

EXPRESSED AS TWO RATIOS

2 mL : 50 mg :: x : 25 mg

EXPRESSED AS TWO FRACTIONS

$$\frac{2\text{ mL}}{50\text{ mg}} \times \frac{x}{25\text{ mg}}$$

SOLUTION FOR BOTH PROPORTION METHODS

$$2 \times 25 = 50x$$

$$\frac{50}{50} = x$$

$$1\text{ mL} = x$$

$$\frac{2\,\cancel{mL}}{\underset{2}{\cancel{50}}\text{ mg}} \;\Big|\; \frac{\overset{1}{\cancel{25}}\text{ mg}}{} = \frac{2}{2} = 1\text{ mL}$$

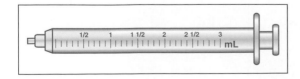

4. 20 units. Remember that Humulin insulin is a type of regular insulin and must be drawn up first into the syringe.

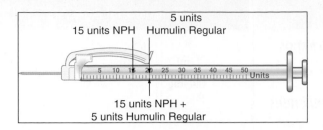

5.

Formula Method	Proportion	Dimensional Analysis

Formula Method

$$\dfrac{\overset{1}{\cancel{20}\ \text{mEq}}}{\underset{2}{\cancel{40}\ \text{mEq}}} \times \overset{10}{\cancel{20}}\ \text{mL} = 10\ \text{mL}$$

Proportion

EXPRESSED AS TWO RATIOS

20 mL : 40 mEq : : x : 20 mEq

EXPRESSED AS TWO FRACTIONS

$$\dfrac{20\ \text{mL}}{40\ \text{mEq}} \times \dfrac{x}{20\ \text{mEq}}$$

SOLUTION FOR BOTH PROPORTION METHODS

$$20 \times 20 = 40x$$

$$\dfrac{400}{40} = x$$

$$10\ \text{mL} = x$$

Dimensional Analysis

$$\dfrac{20\ \cancel{\text{mL}}}{\underset{2}{\cancel{40}\ \cancel{\text{mEq}}}} \left| \overset{1}{\cancel{20}\ \cancel{\text{mEq}}} \right. = \dfrac{20}{2} = 10\ \text{mL}$$

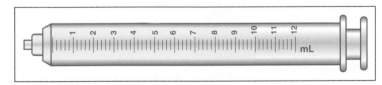

6.

Formula Method	Proportion	Dimensional Analysis

Formula Method

$$\dfrac{\overset{3}{\cancel{0.6}\ \text{mg}}}{\underset{2}{\cancel{0.4}\ \text{mg}}} \times 1\ \text{mL} = \dfrac{3}{2}\ \dfrac{1.5}{\overline{)3.0}}$$

$$= 1.5\ \text{mL}$$

Proportion

EXPRESSED AS TWO RATIOS

1 mL : 0.4 mg : : x : 0.6 mg

EXPRESSED AS TWO FRACTIONS

$$\dfrac{1\ \text{mL}}{0.4\ \text{mg}} \times \dfrac{x}{0.6\ \text{mg}}$$

SOLUTION FOR BOTH PROPORTION METHODS

$$0.6 = 0.4x$$

$$\dfrac{0.6}{0.4} = x$$

$$1.5\ \text{mL} = x$$

Dimensional Analysis

$$\dfrac{0.6\ \cancel{\text{mg}}}{} \left| \dfrac{1\ \cancel{\text{mL}}}{0.4\ \cancel{\text{mg}}} \right| \dfrac{0.6}{0.4} = 1.5\ \text{mL}$$

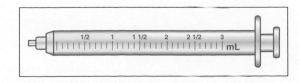

7.

Formula Method	Proportion	Dimensional Analysis
$$\dfrac{\overset{2}{\cancel{0.8}} \text{ mg}}{\underset{1}{\cancel{0.4}} \text{ mg}} \times 1 \text{ mL} = 2 \text{ mL}$$	**EXPRESSED AS TWO RATIOS** $1 \text{ mL} : 0.4 \text{ mg} :: x : 0.8 \text{ mg}$ **EXPRESSED AS TWO FRACTIONS** $\dfrac{1 \text{ mL}}{0.4 \text{ mg}} \times \dfrac{x}{0.8 \text{ mg}}$ **SOLUTION FOR BOTH PROPORTION METHODS** $0.8 = 0.4x$ $\dfrac{0.8}{0.4} = x$ $2 \text{ mL} = x$	$\dfrac{1 \;\cancel{\text{mL}}}{\underset{0.1}{\cancel{0.4}} \;\cancel{\text{mg}}} \;\Bigg|\; \dfrac{\overset{0.2}{\cancel{0.8}} \;\cancel{\text{mg}}}{} = \dfrac{0.2}{0.1} = 2 \text{ mL}$

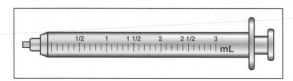

8. Equivalent 0.5 g = 500 mg

Formula Method	Proportion	Dimensional Analysis
$$\dfrac{\overset{2}{\cancel{500}} \text{ mg}}{\underset{1}{\cancel{250}} \text{ mg}} \times 1 \text{ mL} = 2 \text{ mL}$$	**EXPRESSED AS TWO RATIOS** $1 \text{ mL} : 250 \text{ mg} :: x : 500 \text{ mg}$ **EXPRESSED AS TWO FRACTIONS** $\dfrac{1 \text{ mL}}{250 \text{ mg}} \times \dfrac{x}{500 \text{ mg}}$ **SOLUTION FOR BOTH PROPORTION METHODS** $500 = 250x$ $\dfrac{500}{250} = x$ $2 \text{ mL} = x$	Use conversion factor 1000 mg/1 g: $\dfrac{1 \;\cancel{\text{mL}}}{\underset{1}{\cancel{250}} \;\cancel{\text{mg}}} \;\Bigg|\; \dfrac{0.5 \;\cancel{\text{g}}}{} \;\Bigg|\; \dfrac{\overset{4}{\cancel{1000}} \;\cancel{\text{mg}}}{1 \;\cancel{\text{g}}} = 0.5 \times 4 = 2 \text{ mL}$

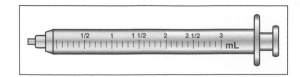

9.

Formula Method	Proportion	Dimensional Analysis
$\dfrac{200 \text{ mg}}{500 \text{ mg}} \times 2 \text{ mL} = \dfrac{4}{5} \overset{.8}{\overline{)4.0}}$ 0.8 mL	**EXPRESSED AS TWO RATIOS** 2 mL : 500 mg :: x : 200 mg **EXPRESSED AS TWO FRACTIONS** $\dfrac{2 \text{ mL}}{500 \text{ mg}} \times \dfrac{x}{200 \text{ mg}}$ **SOLUTION FOR BOTH PROPORTION METHODS** $2 \times 200 = 500x$ $\dfrac{400}{500} = x$ $0.8 \text{ mL} = x$	$\dfrac{2 \text{ mL}}{500 \text{ mg}} \bigg| \dfrac{200 \text{ mg}}{} = \dfrac{4}{5} = 0.8 \text{ mL}$

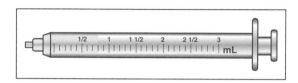

10. Equivalent 1:100 means 1 g in 100 mL

$$1 \text{ g} = 1000 \text{ mg}$$

Therefore, the solution is 1000 mg/100 mL.

Formula Method	Proportion	Dimensional Analysis
$\dfrac{7.5 \text{ mg}}{1000 \text{ mg}} \times 100 \text{ mL}$ $= \dfrac{7.5}{10} \overset{.75}{\overline{)7.50}} = 0.75$ $\quad\quad\;\; \underline{7\,0}$ $\quad\quad\;\;\; 50$ $\quad\quad\;\;\; \underline{50}$	**EXPRESSED AS TWO RATIOS** 100 mL : 1000 mg :: x : 7.5 mg **EXPRESSED AS TWO FRACTIONS** $\dfrac{100 \text{ mL}}{1000 \text{ mg}} \times \dfrac{x}{7.5 \text{ mg}}$ **SOLUTION FOR BOTH PROPORTION METHODS** $100 \times 7.5 = 1000x$ $\dfrac{7500}{1000} = x$ $0.75 \text{ mL} = x$	Use conversion factor 1 g/1000 mg: $\dfrac{\overset{1}{100} \text{ mL}}{1 \text{ g}} \bigg| \dfrac{7.5 \text{ mg}}{} \; \dfrac{1 \text{ g}}{\underset{10}{1000} \text{ mg}} = \dfrac{7.5}{10}$ $\quad\quad\quad\quad\quad\quad\quad\quad\quad = 0.75 \text{ mL}$

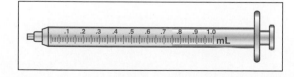

11.

Formula Method	Proportion	Dimensional Analysis

Formula Method:

$$\frac{\overset{2}{\cancel{10}\ \text{mg}}}{\underset{1}{\cancel{5}\ \text{mg}}} \times 1\ \text{mL} = 2\ \text{mL}$$

Proportion:

EXPRESSED AS TWO RATIOS

$$1\ \text{mL} : 5\ \text{mg} :: x : 10\ \text{mg}$$

EXPRESSED AS TWO FRACTIONS

$$\frac{1\ \text{mL}}{5\ \text{mg}} \times \frac{x}{10\ \text{mg}}$$

SOLUTION FOR BOTH PROPORTION METHODS

$$10 = 5x$$
$$\frac{10}{5} = x$$
$$2\ \text{mL} = x$$

Dimensional Analysis:

$$\frac{1\ \text{\textcircled{mL}}}{\underset{1}{\cancel{5}\ \text{mg}}} \left| \frac{\overset{2}{\cancel{10}\ \text{mg}}}{} \right. = 2\ \text{mL}$$

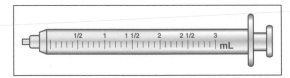

12.

Formula Method	Proportion	Dimensional Analysis

Formula Method:

$$\frac{\overset{1}{\cancel{25}\ \text{mg}}}{\underset{4}{\cancel{100}\ \text{mg}}} \times 2\ \text{mL} = x$$
$$\frac{2}{4} = x$$
$$0.5\ \text{mL} = x$$

Proportion:

EXPRESSED AS TWO RATIOS

$$2\ \text{mL} : 100\ \text{mg} :: x : 25\ \text{mg}$$

EXPRESSED AS TWO FRACTIONS

$$\frac{2\ \text{mL}}{100\ \text{mg}} \times \frac{x}{25\ \text{mg}}$$

SOLUTION FOR BOTH PROPORTION METHODS

$$25 \times 2 = 100x$$
$$\frac{50}{100} = x$$
$$0.5\ \text{mL} = x$$

Dimensional Analysis:

$$\frac{2\ \text{\textcircled{mL}}}{\underset{4}{\cancel{100}\ \text{mg}}} \left| \frac{\overset{1}{\cancel{25}\ \text{mg}}}{} \right. = \frac{2}{4} = 0.5\ \text{mL}$$

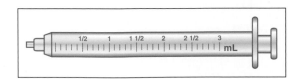

13.

Formula Method	Proportion	Dimensional Analysis
$\dfrac{50 \text{ mg}}{25 \text{ mg}} \times 1 \text{ mL} = x$ $2 \text{ mL} = x$	**EXPRESSED AS TWO RATIOS** $1 \text{ mL} : 25 \text{ mg} :: x : 50 \text{ mg}$ **EXPRESSED AS TWO FRACTIONS** $\dfrac{1 \text{ mL}}{25 \text{ mg}} \times \dfrac{x}{50 \text{ mg}}$ **SOLUTION FOR BOTH PROPORTION METHODS** $50 = 25x$ $\dfrac{50}{25} = x$ $2 \text{ mL} = x$	$\dfrac{1 \text{ mL}}{25 \text{ mg}} \left| \dfrac{\overset{2}{50 \text{ mg}}}{1} \right. = 2 \text{ mL}$

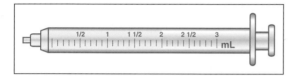

14.

Formula Method	Proportion	Dimensional Analysis
$\dfrac{0.5 \text{ mg}}{2 \text{ mg}} \times 1 \text{ mL} = x$ $\dfrac{0.5}{2} = x$ $0.25 \text{ mL} = x$	**EXPRESSED AS TWO RATIOS** $1 \text{ mL} : 2 \text{ mg} :: x : 0.5 \text{ mg}$ **EXPRESSED AS TWO FRACTIONS** $\dfrac{1 \text{ mL}}{2 \text{ mg}} \times \dfrac{x}{0.5 \text{ mg}}$ **SOLUTION FOR BOTH PROPORTION METHODS** $0.5 = 2x$ $\dfrac{0.5}{2} = x$ $0.25 \text{ mL} = x$	$\dfrac{1 \text{ mL}}{2 \text{ mg}} \left| \dfrac{0.5 \text{ mg}}{} \right. = \dfrac{0.5}{2} = 0.25 \text{ mL}$

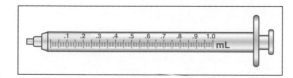

15. Equivalent 0.2 g 5 200 mg

Formula Method	Proportion	Dimensional Analysis
$\dfrac{\overset{1}{\cancel{200}} \text{ mg}}{\underset{1}{\cancel{200}} \text{ mg}} \times 2 \text{ mL} = x$ $2 \text{ mL} = x$	**EXPRESSED AS TWO RATIOS** $2 \text{ mL} : 200 \text{ mg} :: x : 200 \text{ mg}$ **EXPRESSED AS TWO FRACTIONS** $\dfrac{2 \text{ mL}}{200 \text{ mg}} \diagdown \dfrac{x}{200 \text{ mg}}$ **SOLUTION FOR BOTH PROPORTION METHODS** $2 \times 200 = 200x$ $\dfrac{400}{200} = x$ $2 \text{ mL} = x$	Use conversion factor 1000 mg/1 g: $\dfrac{\overset{1}{\cancel{2}} \text{ (mL)}}{\underset{1}{\cancel{200}} \text{ mg}} \Bigg| 0.2 \text{ g} \Bigg| \dfrac{\overset{10}{\cancel{1000}} \text{ mg}}{1 \text{ g}} = 0.2 \times 10 = 2 \text{ mL}$

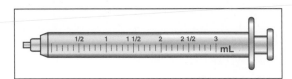

Test 2: Calculations of Liquid Injections and Injections From Powders

1.

Formula Method	Proportion	Dimensional Analysis
$\dfrac{\overset{2}{\cancel{10}} \text{ mg}}{\underset{3}{\cancel{15}} \text{ mg}} \times 1 \text{ mL} = \dfrac{2}{3} \,\overset{0.66}{\cancel{)}}\,\overline{2.00}$ $0.66 \text{ mL or } 0.7 \text{ mL}$	**EXPRESSED AS TWO RATIOS** $1 \text{ mL} : 15 \text{ mg} :: x : 10 \text{ mg}$ **EXPRESSED AS TWO FRACTIONS** $\dfrac{1 \text{ mL}}{15 \text{ mg}} \diagdown \dfrac{x}{10 \text{ mg}}$ **SOLUTION FOR BOTH PROPORTION METHODS** $10 = 15x$ $\dfrac{10}{15} = x$ $0.66 \text{ or } 0.7 \text{ mL} = x$	$\dfrac{1 \text{ (mL)}}{\underset{3}{\cancel{15}} \text{ mg}} \Bigg| \overset{2}{\cancel{10}} \text{ mg} = \dfrac{2}{3} = 0.66 \text{ or } 0.7 \text{ mL}$

Round to the nearest tenths = 0.7

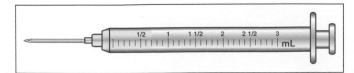

2. Equivalent 0.1 g = 100 mg

Formula Method	Proportion	Dimensional Analysis
$$\frac{\overset{1}{\cancel{100}\text{ mg}}}{\underset{2}{\cancel{200}\text{ mg}}} \times 3\text{ mL} = \frac{3}{2}\overset{1.5}{\overline{)3.0}}$$ $$= 1.5\text{ mL}$$	**EXPRESSED AS TWO RATIOS** 3 mL : 200 mg : : x : 100 mg **EXPRESSED AS TWO FRACTIONS** $$\frac{3\text{ mL}}{200\text{ mg}} \diagup \frac{x}{100\text{ mg}}$$ **SOLUTION FOR BOTH PROPORTION METHODS** $3 \times 100 = 200x$ $$\frac{300}{200} = x$$ $1.5\text{ mL} = x$	Use conversion factor 1000 mg/1 g: $$\frac{3\text{ }\textcircled{mL}}{\underset{2}{\cancel{200}\text{ mg}}} \left| \frac{0.1\text{ }\cancel{g}}{} \right| \frac{\overset{10}{\cancel{1000}}\text{ mg}}{1\text{ }\cancel{g}} = \frac{3 \times 0.1 \times 10}{2}$$ $$= 1.5\text{ mL}$$

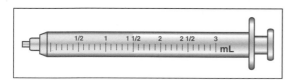

3.

Formula Method	Proportion	Dimensional Analysis
$$\frac{\overset{1}{\cancel{1000}\text{ mcg}}}{\underset{5}{\cancel{5000}\text{ mcg}}} \times 1\text{ mL} = \frac{1}{5}\overset{0.2}{\overline{)1.0}}$$	**EXPRESSED AS TWO RATIOS** 1 mL : 5000 mcg : : x : 1000 mcg **EXPRESSED AS TWO FRACTIONS** $$\frac{1\text{ mL}}{5000\text{ mcg}} \diagup \frac{x}{1000\text{ mcg}}$$ **SOLUTION FOR BOTH PROPORTION METHODS** $1000 = 5000x$ $$\frac{1000}{5000} = x$$ $0.2\text{ mL} = x$	$$\frac{1\text{ }\textcircled{mL}}{\underset{5}{\cancel{5000}\text{ mcg}}} \left| \frac{\overset{1}{\cancel{1000}}\text{ mcg}}{} \right. = \frac{1}{5} = 0.2\text{ mL}$$

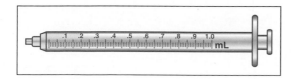

4. Equivalent 1% means 1 g in 100 mL

$$1 \text{ g} = 1000 \text{ mg}$$

Therefore, the solution is 1000 mg in 100 mL.

Formula Method	Proportion	Dimensional Analysis
$$\dfrac{\overset{5}{\cancel{25}} \text{ mg}}{\underset{\underset{2}{10}}{\cancel{1000}} \text{ mg}} \times \overset{1}{\cancel{100}} \text{ mL} = \dfrac{5}{2} \overset{2.5}{\overline{)5.0}}$$ $$= 2.5 \text{ mL}$$	**EXPRESSED AS TWO RATIOS** $$100 \text{ mL} : 1000 \text{ mg} :: x : 25 \text{ mg}$$ **EXPRESSED AS TWO FRACTIONS** $$\dfrac{100 \text{ mL}}{1000 \text{ mg}} \times \dfrac{x}{25 \text{ mg}}$$ **SOLUTION FOR BOTH PROPORTION METHODS** $$100 \times 25 = 1000x$$ $$\dfrac{2500}{1000} = x$$ $$2.5 \text{ mL} = x$$	Use conversion factor 1 g/1000 mg: $$\dfrac{\overset{1}{\cancel{100}} \text{ mL}}{1 \cancel{g}} \left| \; 25 \text{ mg} \; \right| \dfrac{1 \cancel{g}}{\underset{10}{\cancel{1000}} \text{ mg}} = \dfrac{25}{10} = 2.5 \text{ mL}$$

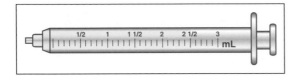

5.

Formula Method	Proportion	Dimensional Analysis
$$\dfrac{0.5 \text{ mg}}{0.4 \text{ mg}} \times 1 \text{ mL} = \dfrac{5}{4} \overset{1.25}{\overline{)5.00}}$$ $$1.25 \text{ or } 1.3 \text{ mL}$$	**EXPRESSED AS TWO RATIOS** $$1 \text{ mL} : 0.4 \text{ mg} :: x : 0.5 \text{ mg}$$ **EXPRESSED AS TWO FRACTIONS** $$\dfrac{1 \text{ mL}}{0.4 \text{ mg}} \times \dfrac{x}{0.5 \text{ mg}}$$ **SOLUTION FOR BOTH PROPORTION METHODS** $$0.5 = 0.4x$$ $$\dfrac{0.5}{0.4} = x$$ $$1.25 \text{ or } 1.3 \text{ mL} = x$$	$$\dfrac{1 \text{ mL}}{0.4 \text{ mg}} \left| \; 0.5 \text{ mg} \; \right. = \dfrac{0.5}{0.4} = 1.25 \text{ mL or } 1.3 \text{ mL}$$

Round to the nearest tenths = 1.3

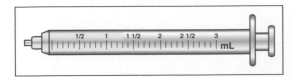

6. 13 units. Humulin insulin is a type of regular insulin and must be drawn up first into the syringe.

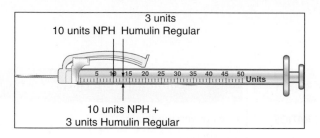

7.

Formula Method	Proportion	Dimensional Analysis
$\dfrac{1.2 \ \text{mEq}}{0.5 \ \text{mEq}} \times 1 \ \text{mL} = \dfrac{1.2}{0.5} \overline{)1.20}^{\ 2.4}$	**EXPRESSED AS TWO RATIOS** 1 mL : 0.5 mEq :: x : 1.2 mEq **EXPRESSED AS TWO FRACTIONS** $\dfrac{1 \ \text{mL}}{0.5 \ \text{mEq}} \times \dfrac{x}{1.2 \ \text{mEq}}$ **SOLUTION FOR BOTH PROPORTION METHODS** $1.2 = 0.5x$ $\dfrac{1.2}{0.5} = x$ $2.4 \ \text{mL} = x$	$\dfrac{1 \ \text{mL}}{0.5 \ \text{mEq}} \left| \ \dfrac{1.2 \ \text{mEq}}{} \right. = \dfrac{1.2}{0.5} = 2.4 \ \text{mL}$

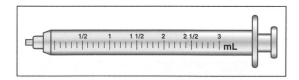

8. Equivalent 1:1000 means 1 g in 1000 mL

$$1 \text{ g} = 1000 \text{ mg}$$

Therefore, the solution is 1000 mg in 1000 mL.

$$500 \text{ mcg} = 0.5 \text{ mg}$$

Formula Method	Proportion	Dimensional Analysis
$\dfrac{0.5 \text{ mg}}{1000 \text{ mg}} \times \overset{1}{1000} \text{ mL}$ $= 0.5 \text{ mL}$	**EXPRESSED AS TWO RATIOS** $1000 \text{ mL} : 1000 \text{ mg} :: x : 0.5 \text{ mg}$ **EXPRESSED AS TWO FRACTIONS** $\dfrac{1000 \text{ mL}}{1000 \text{ mg}} \times \dfrac{x}{0.5 \text{ mg}}$ **SOLUTION FOR BOTH PROPORTION METHODS** $1000 \times 0.5 \text{ mg} = 1000x$ $\dfrac{500}{1000} = x$ $0.5 \text{ mL} = x$	Use conversion factors: 1 g/1000 mg 1 mg/1000 mcg 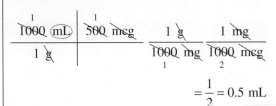 $= \dfrac{1}{2} = 0.5 \text{ mL}$

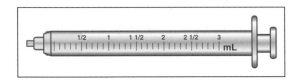

9. a. 2 mL sterile water, sodium chloride, or 1% lidocain hydrochloride for injection

   b. 1 g/2.6 mL

   c.

Formula Method	Proportion	Dimensional Analysis
$\dfrac{1 \text{ g}}{1 \text{ g}} \times 2.6 \text{ mL} = 2.6 \text{ mL}$	**EXPRESSED AS TWO RATIOS** $2.6 \text{ mL} : 1 \text{ g} :: x : 1 \text{ g}$ **EXPRESSED AS TWO FRACTIONS** $\dfrac{2.6 \text{ mL}}{1 \text{ g}} \times \dfrac{x}{1 \text{ g}}$ **SOLUTION FOR BOTH PROPORTION METHODS** $2.6 = 1x$ $\dfrac{2.6}{1} = x$ $2.6 \text{ mL} = x$	$\dfrac{2.6 \text{ mL}}{1 \text{ g}} \cdot \dfrac{1 \text{ g}}{} = 2.6 \text{ mL}$

   d. 2.6 mL

   e. Nothing is left in the vial.

   f. Discard the vial in a proper receptacle.

10. a. 1.8 mL sterile water or bacteriostatic water for injection

b. 250 mg/mL

c.

Formula Method	Proportion	Dimensional Analysis
$\dfrac{\overset{6}{\cancel{300}} \text{ mg}}{\underset{5}{\cancel{250}} \text{ mg}} \times 1 \text{ mL} = \dfrac{6}{5} \dfrac{1.2}{\overline{)6.0}}$ $= 1.2 \text{ mL}$	**EXPRESSED AS TWO RATIOS** $1 \text{ mL} : 250 \text{ mg} :: x : 300 \text{ mg}$ **EXPRESSED AS TWO FRACTIONS** $\dfrac{1 \text{ mL}}{250 \text{ mg}} \times \dfrac{x}{300 \text{ mg}}$ **SOLUTION FOR BOTH PROPORTION METHODS** $300 = 250x$ $\dfrac{300}{250} = x$ $1.2 \text{ mL} = x$	$\dfrac{1 \text{ⓜL}}{250 \text{ mg}} \ \bigg| \ \dfrac{300 \text{ mg}}{} = \dfrac{300}{250} = 1.2 \text{ mL}$

d. 1.2 mL

e. Discard the vial. Directions say solution must be used within 1 hour.

f. No. Discard the vial in an appropriate receptacle.

Test 3: Calculations of Liquid Injections

1.

Formula Method	Proportion	Dimensional Analysis
$\dfrac{\overset{1}{\cancel{0.25}} \text{ mg}}{\underset{2}{\cancel{0.50}} \text{ mg}} \times \overset{1}{\cancel{2}} \text{ mL} = 1 \text{ mL}$	**EXPRESSED AS TWO RATIOS** $2 \text{ mL} : 0.5 \text{ mg} :: x : 0.25 \text{ mg}$ **EXPRESSED AS TWO FRACTIONS** $\dfrac{2 \text{ mL}}{0.5 \text{ mg}} \times \dfrac{x}{0.25 \text{ mg}}$ **SOLUTION FOR BOTH PROPORTION METHODS** $2 \times 0.25 = 0.5x$ $\dfrac{0.50}{0.50} = x$ $1 \text{ mL} = x$	$\dfrac{2 \text{ⓜL}}{\underset{2}{\cancel{0.5}} \text{ mg}} \ \bigg| \ \dfrac{\overset{1}{\cancel{0.25}} \text{ mg}}{} = 1 \text{ mL}$

2.

Formula Method	Proportion	Dimensional Analysis
$\dfrac{40 \text{ mg}}{50 \text{ mg}} \times 2 \text{ mL} = \dfrac{8}{5}\,\overset{1.6}{)\overline{8.0}}$ $= 1.6 \text{ mL}$	**EXPRESSED AS TWO RATIOS** $2 \text{ mL} : 50 \text{ mg} :: x : 40 \text{ mg}$ **EXPRESSED AS TWO FRACTIONS** $\dfrac{2 \text{ mL}}{50 \text{ mg}} \times \dfrac{x}{40 \text{ mg}}$ **SOLUTION FOR BOTH PROPORTION METHODS** $2 \times 40 = 50x$ $\dfrac{80}{50} = x$ $1.6 \text{ mL} = x$	$\dfrac{2 \text{ mL}}{50 \text{ mg}} \left| \dfrac{40 \text{ mg}}{} \right. = \dfrac{8}{5} = 1.6 \text{ mL}$

3.

Formula Method	Proportion	Dimensional Analysis
$\dfrac{8 \text{ mg}}{15 \text{ mg}} \times 1 \text{ mL} = \dfrac{8}{15}\,\overset{0.53}{)\overline{8.00}}$ $\phantom{= \dfrac{8}{15}}\underline{7\ 5}$ $\phantom{= \dfrac{8}{15}aa}50$ $\phantom{= \dfrac{8}{15}aa}\underline{45}$ $= 0.5 \text{ mL}$	**EXPRESSED AS TWO RATIOS** $1 \text{ mL} : 15 \text{ mg} :: x : 8 \text{ mg}$ **EXPRESSED AS TWO FRACTIONS** $\dfrac{1 \text{ mL}}{15 \text{ mg}} \times \dfrac{x}{8 \text{ mg}}$ **SOLUTION FOR BOTH PROPORTION METHODS** $8 = 15x$ $\dfrac{8}{15} = x$ $0.53 \text{ or } 0.5 \text{ mL} = x$	$\dfrac{1 \text{ mL}}{15 \text{ mg}} \left| \dfrac{8 \text{ mg}}{} \right. = \dfrac{8}{15} = 0.53 \text{ mL or } 0.5 \text{ mL}$

4.

Formula Method	Proportion	Dimensional Analysis
$\dfrac{\overset{1}{50 \text{ mg}}}{\underset{2}{100 \text{ mg}}} \times 1 \text{ mL} = \dfrac{1}{2} = 0.5 \text{ mL}$	**EXPRESSED AS TWO RATIOS** $1 \text{ mL} : 100 \text{ mg} :: x : 50 \text{ mg}$ **EXPRESSED AS TWO FRACTIONS** $\dfrac{1 \text{ mL}}{100 \text{ mg}} \times \dfrac{x}{50 \text{ mg}}$ **SOLUTION FOR BOTH PROPORTION METHODS** $50 = 100x$ $\dfrac{50}{100} = x$ $0.5 \text{ mL} = x$	$\dfrac{1 \text{ mL}}{\underset{2}{100 \text{ mg}}} \left| \dfrac{\overset{1}{50 \text{ mg}}}{} \right. = \dfrac{1}{2} \text{ or } 0.5 \text{ mL}$

5.

Formula Method	Proportion	Dimensional Analysis
$\dfrac{200 \text{ mg}}{500 \text{ mg}} \times 2 \text{ mL} = \dfrac{4}{5} \overset{0.8}{\overline{)4.0}}$ $= 0.8 \text{ mL}$	**EXPRESSED AS TWO RATIOS** $2 \text{ mL} : 500 \text{ mg} :: x : 200 \text{ mg}$ **EXPRESSED AS TWO FRACTIONS** $\dfrac{2 \text{ mL}}{500 \text{ mg}} \diagup\!\!\diagdown \dfrac{x}{200 \text{ mg}}$ **SOLUTION FOR BOTH PROPORTION METHODS** $2 \times 200 = 500x$ $\dfrac{400}{500} = x$ $0.8 \text{ mL} = x$	$\dfrac{2 \text{ (mL)}}{500 \text{ mg}} \left| \dfrac{200 \text{ mg}}{} \right. = \dfrac{4}{5} = 0.8 \text{ mL}$

6.

Formula Method	Proportion	Dimensional Analysis
$\dfrac{\overset{3}{1500 \text{ mcg}}}{\underset{10}{5000 \text{ mcg}}} \times 1 \text{ mL} = \dfrac{3}{10} \overset{0.3}{\overline{)3.0}}$ $= 0.3 \text{ mL}$	**EXPRESSED AS TWO RATIOS** $1 \text{ mL} : 5000 \text{ mcg} :: x : 1500 \text{ mcg}$ **EXPRESSED AS TWO FRACTIONS** $\dfrac{1 \text{ mL}}{5000 \text{ mcg}} \diagup\!\!\diagdown \dfrac{x}{1500 \text{ mcg}}$ **SOLUTION FOR BOTH PROPORTION METHODS** $1500 = 5000x$ $\dfrac{1500}{5000} = x$ $0.3 \text{ mL} = x$	$\dfrac{1 \text{ (mL)}}{\underset{50}{5000 \text{ mcg}}} \left| \dfrac{\overset{15}{1500 \text{ mcg}}}{} \right. = \dfrac{15}{30} = 0.3 \text{ mL}$

7.

Formula Method	Proportion	Dimensional Analysis
$\dfrac{\overset{3}{0.6 \text{ mg}}}{\underset{2}{0.4 \text{ mg}}} \times 1 \text{ mL} = \dfrac{3}{2} \overset{1.5}{\overline{)3.0}}$ $= 1.5 \text{ mL}$	**EXPRESSED AS TWO RATIOS** $1 \text{ mL} : 0.4 \text{ mg} :: x : 0.6 \text{ mg}$ **EXPRESSED AS TWO FRACTIONS** $\dfrac{1 \text{ mL}}{0.4 \text{ mg}} \diagup\!\!\diagdown \dfrac{x}{0.6 \text{ mg}}$ **SOLUTION FOR BOTH PROPORTION METHODS** $0.6 = 0.4x$ $\dfrac{0.6}{0.4} = x$ $1.5 \text{ mL} = x$	$\dfrac{1 \text{ (mL)}}{\underset{2}{0.4 \text{ mg}}} \left| \dfrac{\overset{3}{0.6 \text{ mg}}}{} \right. = \dfrac{3}{2} = 1.5 \text{ mL}$

8. 0.1 g = 100 mg

Formula Method	Proportion	Dimensional Analysis
$$\frac{\overset{1}{\cancel{100}} \text{ mg}}{\underset{2}{\cancel{200}} \text{ mg}} \times 3 \text{ mL} = \frac{3}{2} \overset{1.5}{\overline{)3.0}}$$ $$= 1.5 \text{ mL}$$	**EXPRESSED AS TWO RATIOS** $$3 \text{ mL} : 200 \text{ mg} :: x : 100 \text{ mg}$$ **EXPRESSED AS TWO FRACTIONS** $$\frac{3 \text{ mL}}{200 \text{ mg}} \times \frac{x}{100 \text{ mg}}$$ **SOLUTION FOR BOTH PROPORTION METHODS** $$3 \times 100 = 200x$$ $$\frac{300}{200} = x$$ $$1.5 \text{ mL} = x$$	Use conversion factor 1000 mg/1 g: $$\frac{3 \enspace \boxed{\text{mL}}}{\underset{1}{\cancel{200}} \text{ mg}} \left| \begin{array}{c|c} 0.1 \cancel{\text{ g}} & \overset{5}{\cancel{1000}} \text{ mg} \\ \hline & 1 \cancel{\text{ g}} \end{array} \right. = 3 \times 0.1 \times 5$$ $$= 1.5 \text{ mL}$$

9.

Formula Method	Proportion	Dimensional Analysis
$$\frac{\overset{3}{\cancel{1.5}} \text{ mg}}{\underset{4}{\cancel{2.0}} \text{ mg}} \times 1 \text{ mL} = \frac{3}{4} \overset{0.75}{\overline{)3.00}}$$ $$= 0.75 \text{ mL}$$	**EXPRESSED AS TWO RATIOS** $$1 \text{ mL} : 2 \text{ mg} :: x : 1.5 \text{ mg}$$ **EXPRESSED AS TWO FRACTIONS** $$\frac{1 \text{ mL}}{2 \text{ mg}} \times \frac{x}{1.5 \text{ mg}}$$ **SOLUTION FOR BOTH PROPORTION METHODS** $$1.5 = 2x$$ $$\frac{1.5}{2} = x$$ $$0.75 = x$$	$$\frac{1 \enspace \boxed{\text{mL}}}{2 \text{ mg}} \left| \begin{array}{c} 1.5 \text{ mg} \\ \hline \end{array} \right. = \frac{1.5}{2} = 0.75 \text{ mL}$$

10.

Formula Method	Proportion	Dimensional Analysis
$$\frac{600,000 \text{ units}}{500,000 \text{ units}} \times 1 \text{ mL} = \frac{6}{5} \overset{1.2}{\overline{)6.0}}$$ $$= 1.2 \text{ mL}$$	**EXPRESSED AS TWO RATIOS** $$1 \text{ mL} : 500,000 \text{ units} :: x : 600,000 \text{ units}$$ **EXPRESSED AS TWO FRACTIONS** $$\frac{1 \text{ mL}}{500,000 \text{ units}} \times \frac{x}{600,000 \text{ units}}$$ **SOLUTION FOR BOTH PROPORTION METHODS** $$600,000 = 500,000x$$ $$\frac{600,000}{500,000} = x$$ $$1.2 \text{ mL} = x$$	$$\frac{1 \enspace \boxed{\text{mL}}}{500,000 \text{ units}} \left| \begin{array}{c} 600,000 \text{ units} \\ \hline \end{array} \right. = \frac{6}{5} = 1.2 \text{ mL}$$

11. 200 mcg = 0.2 mg

Formula Method	Proportion	Dimensional Analysis
$$\frac{0.\overset{1}{2}\ \text{mg}}{0.\underset{4}{8}\ \text{mg}} \times 1\ \text{mL} = \frac{1}{4}\overset{0.25}{\overline{\smash{)}1.00}}$$ $$= 0.25\ \text{mL}$$	**EXPRESSED AS TWO RATIOS** 1 mL : 0.8 mg : : x : 0.2 mg **EXPRESSED AS TWO FRACTIONS** $$\frac{1\ \text{mL}}{0.8\ \text{mg}} \times \frac{\text{x}}{0.2\ \text{mg}}$$ **SOLUTION FOR BOTH PROPORTION METHODS** $$0.2 = 0.8\text{x}$$ $$\frac{0.2}{0.8} = \text{x}$$ $$0.25\ \text{mL} = \text{x}$$	Use conversion factor 1 mg/1000 mg: $$\frac{1\,\text{mL}}{0.8\ \text{mg}} \left| \frac{\overset{1}{200\ \text{mcg}}}{} \right| \frac{1\ \text{mg}}{\underset{5}{1000\ \text{mcg}}} = \frac{1}{0.8 \times 5}$$ $$= 0.25\ \text{mL}$$

12. 1:4000 means   1 g in 4000 mL

                   1 g = 1000 mg, therefore, 1000 mg in 4000 mL

                   500 mcg = 0.5 mg

Formula Method	Proportion	Dimensional Analysis
$$\frac{0.5\ \text{mg}}{\underset{1}{1000\ \text{mg}}} \times \overset{4}{4000}\ \text{mL}$$ $$= \frac{0.5}{\times 4}$$ $$\overline{2\ \text{mL}}$$	**EXPRESSED AS TWO RATIOS** 4000 mL : 1000 mg : : x : 0.5 mg **EXPRESSED AS TWO FRACTIONS** $$\frac{4000\ \text{mL}}{1000\ \text{mg}} \times \frac{\text{x}}{0.5\ \text{mg}}$$ **SOLUTION FOR BOTH PROPORTION METHODS** $$4000 \times 0.5 = 1000\text{x}$$ $$\frac{2000}{1000} = \text{x}$$ $$2\ \text{mL} = \text{x}$$	Use conversion factors: 1 g/1000 mg 1 mg/1000 mcg $$\frac{4000\ \text{mL}}{1\ \text{g}} \left| \frac{\overset{1}{500\ \text{mcg}}}{} \right| \frac{1\ \text{g}}{\underset{2}{1000\ \text{mg}}} \left| \frac{1\ \text{mg}}{1000\ \text{mcg}} \right.$$ $$= \frac{4}{2} = 2\ \text{mL}$$

13.

Formula Method	Proportion	Dimensional Analysis
$$\frac{3\ \text{mg}}{2\ \text{mg}} \times 1\ \text{mL} = \frac{3}{2}\overset{1.5}{\overline{\smash{)}3.0}}$$ $$= 1.5\ \text{mL}$$	**EXPRESSED AS TWO RATIOS** 1 mL : 2 mg : : x : 3 mg **EXPRESSED AS TWO FRACTIONS** $$\frac{1\ \text{mL}}{2\ \text{mg}} \times \frac{\text{x}}{3\ \text{mg}}$$ **SOLUTION FOR BOTH PROPORTION METHODS** $$3 = 2\text{x}$$ $$\frac{3}{2} = \text{x}$$ $$1.5\ \text{mL} = \text{x}$$	$$\frac{1\ \text{mL}}{2\ \text{mg}} \left| \frac{3\ \text{mg}}{} \right. = \frac{3}{2} = 1.5\ \text{mL}$$

14. 1:1000 means   1 g = 1000 mL

1 g = 1000 mg, therefore, 1000 mg in 1000 mL

Formula Method	Proportion	Dimensional Analysis
$\dfrac{0.4 \text{ mg}}{1000 \text{ mg}} \times \overset{1}{1000} \text{ mL}$ $= 0.4 \text{ mL}$	**EXPRESSED AS TWO RATIOS** 1000 mL : 1000 mg : : x : 0.4 mg **EXPRESSED AS TWO FRACTIONS** $\dfrac{1000 \text{ mL}}{1000 \text{ mg}} \diagdown \dfrac{x}{0.4 \text{ mg}}$ **SOLUTION FOR BOTH PROPORTION METHODS** $1000 \times 0.4 = 1000x$ $\dfrac{400}{1000} = x$ $0.4 \text{ mL} = x$	Use conversion factor 1 g/1000 mg: $\dfrac{\overset{1}{1000} \text{ mL}}{1 \text{ g}} \left| \dfrac{0.4 \text{ mg}}{} \right| \dfrac{1 \text{ g}}{\underset{1}{1000} \text{ mg}} = 0.4 \text{ mL}$

15. 50% means   50 g in 100 mL

500 mg = 0.5 g

Formula Method	Proportion	Dimensional Analysis
$\dfrac{0.5 \text{ g}}{\underset{1}{50} \text{ g}} \times \overset{2}{100} \text{ mL} = 1 \text{ mL}$	**EXPRESSED AS TWO RATIOS** 100 mL : 50 g : : x : 0.5 g **EXPRESSED AS TWO FRACTIONS** $\dfrac{100 \text{ mL}}{50 \text{ g}} \diagdown \dfrac{x}{0.5 \text{ g}}$ **SOLUTION FOR BOTH PROPORTION METHODS** $100 \times 0.5 = 50x$ $\dfrac{50}{50} = x$ $1 \text{ mL} = x$	Use conversion factor 1 g/1000 mg: $\dfrac{\overset{2}{100} \text{ mL}}{\underset{1}{50} \text{ g}} \left| \dfrac{\overset{1}{500} \text{ mg}}{} \right| \dfrac{1 \text{ g}}{\underset{2}{1000} \text{ mg}} = \dfrac{2}{2} = 1 \text{ mL}$

16.

Formula Method	Proportion	Dimensional Analysis
$$\dfrac{\overset{1}{\cancel{0.75}} \text{ mg}}{\underset{2}{\cancel{1.50}} \text{ mg}} \times 1 \text{ mL} = \dfrac{1}{2} \text{ mL}$$ or 0.5 mL	**EXPRESSED AS TWO RATIOS** $1 \text{ mL} : 1.5 \text{ mg} : : x : 0.75 \text{ mg}$ **EXPRESSED AS TWO FRACTIONS** $$\dfrac{1 \text{ mL}}{1.5 \text{ mg}} \times \dfrac{x}{0.75 \text{ mg}}$$ **SOLUTION FOR BOTH PROPORTION METHODS** $0.75 = 1.5x$ $\dfrac{0.75}{1.5} = x$ $0.5 \text{ mL} = x$	$$\dfrac{1\ \cancel{\text{mL}}}{1.5\ \cancel{\text{mg}}} \ \bigg|\ \dfrac{0.75\ \cancel{\text{mg}}}{} = \dfrac{0.75}{1.5} = 0.5 \text{ mL}$$

17. 20% means 20 g in 100 mL

100 mg = 0.1 g

Formula Method	Proportion	Dimensional Analysis
$$\dfrac{\overset{}{\cancel{0.1} \ \cancel{\text{g}}}}{\underset{1}{\cancel{20} \ \cancel{\text{g}}}} \times \overset{5}{\cancel{100}} \text{ mL} = 0.5 \text{ mL}$$	**EXPRESSED AS TWO RATIOS** $100 \text{ mL} : 20 \text{ g} : : x : 0.1 \text{ g}$ **EXPRESSED AS TWO FRACTIONS** $$\dfrac{100 \text{ mL}}{20 \text{ g}} \times \dfrac{x}{0.1 \text{ g}}$$ **SOLUTION FOR BOTH PROPORTION METHODS** $100 \times 0.1 = 20x$ $\dfrac{10}{20} = x$ $0.5 \text{ mL} = x$	Use conversion factor 1 g/1000 mg: $$\dfrac{\overset{10}{\cancel{100}}\ \cancel{\text{mL}}}{20\ \cancel{\text{g}}} \ \bigg|\ \dfrac{\overset{1}{\cancel{100}}\ \cancel{\text{mg}}}{} \ \bigg|\ \dfrac{1\ \cancel{\text{g}}}{\underset{\underset{1}{10}}{\cancel{1000}}\ \cancel{\text{mg}}} = \dfrac{10}{20}$$ $$= \dfrac{1}{2} \text{ or } 0.5 \text{ mL}$$

Use a 1-mL precision syringe.

18.

Formula Method	Proportion	Dimensional Analysis
$\dfrac{\overset{1}{\cancel{0.125\ \text{mg}}}}{\underset{2}{\cancel{0.250\ \text{mg}}}} \times \overset{1}{\cancel{2}}\ \text{mL} = 1\ \text{mL}$ $\underset{1}{}$	**EXPRESSED AS TWO RATIOS** $2\ \text{mL} : 0.25\ \text{mg} :: x : 0.125\ \text{mg}$ **EXPRESSED AS TWO FRACTIONS** $\dfrac{2\ \text{mL}}{0.25\ \text{mg}} \diagdown \dfrac{x}{0.125\ \text{mg}}$ **SOLUTION FOR BOTH PROPORTION METHODS** $2 \times 0.125 = 0.25x$ $\dfrac{0.25}{0.25} = x$ $1\ \text{mL} = x$	$\dfrac{2\ \cancel{\text{(mL)}}}{0.25\ \cancel{\text{mg}}}\ \bigg|\ 0.125\ \cancel{\text{mg}} = \dfrac{0.25}{0.25} = 1\ \text{mL}$

19.

Formula Method	Proportion	Dimensional Analysis
$\dfrac{\overset{6}{\cancel{12\ \text{mg}}}}{\underset{5}{\cancel{10\ \text{mg}}}} \times 1\ \text{mL} = \dfrac{\overset{6}{\cancel{\ }}}{5} \overline{)6.0}\ 1.2$ $= 1.2\ \text{mL}$	**EXPRESSED AS TWO RATIOS** $1\ \text{mL} : 10\ \text{mg} :: x : 12\ \text{mg}$ **EXPRESSED AS TWO FRACTIONS** $\dfrac{1\ \text{mL}}{10\ \text{mg}} \diagdown \dfrac{x}{12\ \text{mg}}$ **SOLUTION FOR BOTH PROPORTION METHODS** $12 = 10x$ $\dfrac{12}{10} = x$ $1.2\ \text{mL} = x$	$\dfrac{1\ \cancel{\text{(mL)}}}{10\ \cancel{\text{mg}}}\ \bigg|\ 12\ \cancel{\text{mg}} = \dfrac{12}{10} = 1.2\ \text{mL}$

20.

Formula Method	Proportion	Dimensional Analysis
$\dfrac{\overset{5}{\cancel{10\ \text{mEq}}}}{\underset{2}{\cancel{40\ \text{mEq}}}} \times \overset{1}{\cancel{20}}\ \text{mL} = 5\ \text{mL}$ $\underset{1}{}$	**EXPRESSED AS TWO RATIOS** $20\ \text{mL} : 40\ \text{mEq} :: x : 10\ \text{mEq}$ **EXPRESSED AS TWO FRACTIONS** $\dfrac{20\ \text{mL}}{40\ \text{mEq}} \diagdown \dfrac{x}{10\ \text{mEq}}$ **SOLUTION FOR BOTH PROPORTION METHODS** $20 \times 10 = 40x$ $\dfrac{200}{40} = x$ $5\ \text{mL} = x$	$\dfrac{20\ \cancel{\text{(mL)}}}{\underset{4}{\cancel{40\ \text{mEq}}}}\ \bigg|\ \overset{1}{\cancel{10\ \text{mEq}}} = \dfrac{20}{4} = 5\ \text{mL}$

Test 4: Mental Drill in Liquids-for-Injection Problems

1. 2 mL IM

2. 5 mL IV

3. 2 mL IM

4. 1 mL IM

5. 0.5 mL IM

6. 1 mL IM

7. 0.75 mL or 0.8 mL subcutaneous

8. 1 mL subcutaneous

9. 20 mL IV

10. 2.5 mL IM

11. 0.8 mL IM

12. 2 mL IM

13. 2 mL IV

14. 1.5 mL IM

15. 1.5 mL IM

16. 0.35 mL or 0.4 mL IM

17. 1.5 mL subcutaneous

18. 1.5 mL IM

Chapter 6

Test 1: Basic IV Problems

1. a. You have 1000 mL running at 150 mL/hour, therefore

$$\frac{\overset{20}{\cancel{1000}}}{\underset{3}{\cancel{150}}} = \frac{20}{3} = 3\overline{)20.0}^{6.6} = \text{approximately 6.6 hours or 6 hours 36 minutes}$$

$$\begin{array}{r} 18 \\ \hline 2\,0 \\ 18 \\ \hline \end{array}$$

b. $\dfrac{150 \times 10}{60} = 25$ gtt/minute macrodrip

$\dfrac{150 \times 60}{60} = 150$ gtt/minute microdrip

Choose macrotubing. You could choose microtubing; however, the drip rate is hard to count.

Dimensional Analysis

$$\frac{\overset{1}{\cancel{10}}\,\text{gtt}}{1\,\cancel{mL}} \left| \frac{150\,\cancel{mL}}{1\,\cancel{hour}} \right| \frac{1\,\cancel{hour}}{\underset{6}{\cancel{60}}\,\text{minutes}} = \frac{150}{6} = 25 \text{ gtt/minute macrodrip}$$

$$\frac{\overset{1}{\cancel{60}}\,\text{gtt}}{1\,\cancel{mL}} \left| \frac{150\,\cancel{mL}}{1\,\cancel{hour}} \right| \frac{1\,\cancel{hour}}{\underset{1}{\cancel{60}}\,\text{minutes}} = 150 \text{ gtt/minute microdrip}$$

c. 25 gtt/minute macrodrip

2. a. Because the amount is small and will run over 6 hours, choose *microdrip tubing.*

b. 6 hour = 360 minutes

$$\frac{100 \times \overset{1}{\cancel{60}}}{\underset{6}{\cancel{360}}} = \frac{100}{6} = 16.6 \text{ or } 17\,\text{gtt/minute}$$

Dimensional Analysis

$$\frac{\cancel{60}\,\text{gtt}}{1\,\cancel{mL}} \left| \frac{100\,\cancel{mL}}{6\,\cancel{hours}} \right| \frac{1\,\cancel{hour}}{\cancel{60}\,\text{minutes}} = \frac{100}{6} = 16.6 \text{ or } 17 \text{ gtt/minute}$$

3. **a.** Because the stock bag is 250 mL NS, you would aseptically allow 100 mL to run off. This would leave 150 mL NS. If using an infusion pump, you could set the volume to be infused at 150 mL.

b. 3 hours = 180 minutes

Macrodrip: $\dfrac{150 \times \overset{1}{\cancel{15}}}{\underset{12}{\cancel{180}}} = \dfrac{150}{12} = 12.5$ or 13 gtt/minute

Microdrip: $\dfrac{150 \times \overset{1}{\cancel{60}}}{\underset{3}{\cancel{180}}} = \dfrac{150}{3} = 50$ gtt/minute

Microdrip because 50 gtt/minute provides a better flow. It would not be incorrect however to choose the macrodrip.

c. 50 gtt/minute (microdrip)

Dimensional Analysis

$$\frac{\overset{1}{\cancel{15}}\,\text{gtt}}{1\,\text{mL}} \cdot \frac{150\,\text{mL}}{3\,\text{hours}} \cdot \frac{1\,\text{hour}}{\underset{4}{\cancel{60}}\,\text{minutes}} = \frac{150}{12} = 12.5 \text{ or } 13 \text{ gtt/minute}$$

$$\frac{\overset{1}{\cancel{60}}\,\text{gtt}}{1\,\text{mL}} \cdot \frac{150\,\text{mL}}{3\,\text{hours}} \cdot \frac{1\,\text{hour}}{\underset{1}{\cancel{60}}\,\text{minutes}} = \frac{150}{3} = 50 \text{ gtt/minute}$$

4. 21 mL/hour

Step 1. $\dfrac{\text{Number of milliliters}}{\text{Number of hours}} = \text{mL/hour}$

$\dfrac{500\text{ mL}}{24\text{ hours}}$ $\begin{array}{r} 20.8 \\ 24\overline{)500.0} \\ \underline{48} \\ 20\,0 \\ \underline{19\,2} \end{array}$ = 21 mL/hour

Step 2 is not necessary because you have an infusion pump that delivers milliliters per hour.

5. **a.** Use a reconstitution device to add 100 mg powder to 250 mL D5W and give IVPB over 1 hour (60 minutes);
TF 5 10 gtt/mL.

$\dfrac{250 \times \cancel{10}}{\cancel{60}} = \dfrac{250}{6}$ $\begin{array}{r} 41.6 \\ 6\overline{)250.0} \end{array}$ = 42 gtt/minute

Label the IVPB.

b. Set the rate at 42 gtt/minute.

Dimensional Analysis

$$\frac{\overset{1}{\cancel{10}}\ \cancel{\text{gtt}}}{1\ \cancel{\text{mL}}}\ \bigg|\ \frac{250\ \cancel{\text{mL}}}{1\ \cancel{\text{hour}}}\ \bigg|\ \frac{1\ \cancel{\text{hour}}}{\underset{6}{\cancel{60}}\ \cancel{\text{minutes}}} = \frac{250}{6}\ \text{or 41.6 or 42 gtt/minute}$$

6. a. Order is 500 mg. Stock is 1 g in 10 mL.

        1 g 5 1000 mg, therefore 1000 mg is in 10 mL

Add 5 mL aminophylline to make 500 mg in 250 mL D5W.

Formula Method	Proportion	Dimensional Analysis
$\dfrac{500\ \text{mg}}{1000\ \text{mg}} \times 10\ \text{mL} = 5\ \text{mL}$	**EXPRESSED AS TWO RATIOS** $10\ \text{mL} : 1000\ \text{mg} :: x : 500\ \text{mg}$ **EXPRESSED AS TWO FRACTIONS** $\dfrac{10\ \text{mL}}{1000\ \text{mg}} \times \dfrac{x}{500}$ **SOLUTION FOR BOTH PROPORTION METHODS** $10 \times 500 = 1000x$ $\dfrac{5000}{1000} = x$ $5\ \text{mL} = x$	Use conversion factor 1 g/1000 mg: $\dfrac{10\ \cancel{\text{mL}}}{1\ \cancel{\text{g}}}\ \bigg|\ \dfrac{\overset{1}{\cancel{500}}\ \cancel{\text{mg}}}{}\ \bigg|\ \dfrac{1\ \cancel{\text{g}}}{\underset{2}{\cancel{1000}}\ \cancel{\text{mg}}} = \dfrac{10}{2}\ \text{or 5 mL}$

b. $\dfrac{\text{Number of milliliters}}{\text{Number of hours}} = \text{mL/hour}$

    $\dfrac{250\ \text{mL}}{8\ \text{hours}} = 31.2 = 31\ \text{mL/hour}$

Microdip: 31 mL/hour = 31 gtt/minute (no math necessary)

Label IV.

Set the rate at 31 gtt/minute.

7. 2800 mL

The patient/client gets 125 mL/hour, and there are 24 hours in a day; four times a day, the patient/client receives cefoxitin. That leaves 20 hours (24 − 4) times 125 mL/hour:

$$\begin{array}{r} 125 \\ \times\ 20 \\ \hline 2500\ \text{mL} \end{array}$$

The patient/client gets 75 mL q6h and therefore is receiving 75 mL four times in 24 hours.

So $\begin{array}{r} 75 \\ \times\ \ 4 \\ \hline 300 \end{array}$

add the 300 mL to 2500 mL = 2800 mL

8. a. 90 mL/hour—no math necessary—using an infusion pump

b.

$$\frac{\text{Total number of milliliters}}{\text{Milliliters per hour}} = \text{Hours}$$

$$90 \overline{)\begin{array}{r} 11.1 \\ 1000.0 \\ \underline{90} \\ 100 \\ \underline{90} \\ 10\,0 \end{array}}$$

Approximately 11 hours or 11 hours 6 minutes

9. 50 mg

You have 0.5 g in 500 mL. 0.5 g = 500 mg. The solution is 500 mg in 500 mL. Reducing this amount would equal 1 mg in 1 mL. Because the patient/client is receiving 50 mL/hour, the patient/client is receiving 50 mg aminophylline per hour.

10. a. You need 75 mL D5W. Take a 100-mL bag of D5W and aseptically remove 25 mL. Add 5 mL Bactrim to the 75 mL. Time is 60 minutes. The order is 75 mL/hour. No math is necessary. You have a pump in milliliters per hour (You could also use a Buretrol and add 75 mL of D5W to the Buretrol, then add the 5 mL of Bactrim).

Label the IVPB.

b. Set the pump:

For 60 minutes,

Secondary volume (mL): 75

Secondary rate (mL/hour): 75

For 90 minutes, $\dfrac{75 \times 60}{90} = 50$ mL/hour

Secondary volume (mL): 75

Secondary rate (mL/hour): 50

11. $\dfrac{3}{4} \times 150$ mL = 112.5 mL Isocal

150 mL − 112.5 mL = 37.5 mL water

12. $\dfrac{1}{2} \times 500$ mL = 250 mL Vivonex

500 mL − 250 mL = 250 mL water

13. $25\% = 0.25 = \dfrac{1}{4}$ (use any of these)

$\dfrac{1}{4} \times 400$ mL = 100 mL Osmolite

400 mL − 100 mL = 300 mL water

14. 500 mL Isocal

0 mL water

Chapter 7

Test 1: Special IV Calculations

1.

Formula Method	Proportion	Dimensional Analysis
$\dfrac{15 \text{ units/hour}}{\underset{1}{125 \text{ units}}} \times \overset{2}{250} \text{ mL} = x$ $15 \times 2 = 30$ mL/hour	**EXPRESSED AS TWO RATIOS** 250 mL : 125 units : : x : 15 units **EXPRESSED AS TWO FRACTIONS** $\dfrac{250 \text{ mL}}{125 \text{ units}} \diagdown \dfrac{x \text{ mL}}{15 \text{ units}}$ **SOLUTION FOR BOTH PROPORTION METHODS** $15 \times 250 = 125x$ $\dfrac{3750}{125} = x$ 30 mL/hour	$\dfrac{\overset{2}{250} \text{ mL}}{\underset{1}{125 \text{ units}}} \left| \dfrac{15 \text{ units}}{\text{hours}} \right. = 2 \times 15 = 30$ mL/hour

Set the pump.

Total number of milliliters: 250

Milliliters per hour: 30

2.

Formula Method	Proportion	Dimensional Analysis
$\dfrac{\overset{3}{1500} \text{ units/hour}}{\underset{\underset{1}{50}}{25,000 \text{ units}}} \times \overset{10}{500}$ $= 30$ mL/hour	**EXPRESSED AS TWO RATIOS** 500 mL : 25,000 units : : x : 1500 units **EXPRESSED AS TWO FRACTIONS** $\dfrac{500 \text{ mL}}{25,000 \text{ units}} \diagdown \dfrac{x \text{ mL}}{1500 \text{ units}}$ **SOLUTION FOR BOTH PROPORTION METHODS** $1500 \times 500 = 25,000x$ $\dfrac{750,000}{25,000} = x$ 30 mL/hour = x	$\dfrac{\overset{1}{500} \text{ mL}}{\underset{\underset{1}{50}}{25,000 \text{ units}}} \left| \dfrac{\overset{30}{1500} \text{ units}}{\text{hours}} \right. = 30$ mL/hour

Set the pump.

Total number of milliliters: 500

Milliliters per hour: 30

3. 2 mg/minute × 60 minutes = 120 mg/hour

2 g = 2000 mg

Formula Method	Proportion	Dimensional Analysis
$$\dfrac{\overset{}{\cancel{120}}\ \text{mg/hour}}{\underset{4}{\cancel{2000}}\ \text{mg}} \times \overset{1}{\cancel{500}}\ \text{mL}$$ $$= 30\ \text{mL/hour}$$	**EXPRESSED AS TWO RATIOS** 500 mL : 2000 mg : : x : 120 mg **EXPRESSED AS TWO FRACTIONS** $$\dfrac{500\ \text{mL}}{2000\ \text{mg}} \times \dfrac{x}{120\ \text{mg}}$$ **SOLUTION FOR BOTH PROPORTION METHODS** $$500 \times 120 = 2000x$$ $$\dfrac{60,000}{2000} = x$$ $$\dfrac{120}{4} = x$$ $$30\ \text{mL/hour} = x$$	Use conversion factors: 60 minutes/1 hour 1 g/1000 mg $$\dfrac{\overset{1}{\cancel{500}}\ \cancel{\text{mL}}}{\cancel{2\ \text{g}}} \left| \dfrac{\overset{1}{\cancel{2}}\ \text{mg}}{\cancel{\text{minutes}}} \right| \dfrac{60\ \text{minutes}}{1\ \cancel{\text{hour}}} \left| \dfrac{1\ \cancel{\text{g}}}{\underset{\underset{1}{2}}{\cancel{1000}}\ \text{mg}} \right.$$ $$= \dfrac{60}{2} = 30\ \text{mL/hour}$$

Set the pump.

Total number of milliliters: 500

Milliliters per hour: 30

4. Add diltiazem to the IV.

Formula Method	Proportion	Dimensional Analysis
$$\dfrac{\overset{1}{\cancel{5}}\ \text{mg}}{\underset{\underset{1}{25}}{\cancel{125}}\ \text{mg}} \times \overset{4}{\cancel{100}}\ \text{mL} = 4\ \text{mL/hour}$$	**EXPRESSED AS TWO RATIOS** 100 mL : 125 mg : : x : 5 mg **EXPRESSED AS TWO FRACTIONS** $$\dfrac{100\ \text{mL}}{125\ \text{mg}} \times \dfrac{x}{5\ \text{mg}}$$ **SOLUTION FOR BOTH PROPORTION METHODS** $$100 \times 5 = 125x$$ $$\dfrac{500}{125} = x$$ $$4\ \text{mL/hour} = x$$	$$\dfrac{100\ \cancel{\text{mL}}}{\underset{25}{\cancel{125}}\ \cancel{\text{mg}}} \left| \dfrac{\overset{1}{\cancel{5}}\ \cancel{\text{mg}}}{\cancel{\text{hours}}} \right. = \dfrac{100}{25} = 4\ \text{mL/hour}$$

Set the pump.

Total number of milliliters: 100

Milliliters per hour: 4

5. 2 g = 2000 mg

Multiply: 4 mg/minute × 60 minutes = 240 mg/hour.

Formula Method	Proportion	Dimensional Analysis
$$\frac{\overset{60}{\cancel{240}}\ \text{mg/hour}}{\underset{4\ 1}{\cancel{2000}}\ \text{mg}} \times \overset{1}{\cancel{500}}\ \text{mL}$$ $$= 60\ \text{mL/hour}$$	**EXPRESSED AS TWO RATIOS** 500 mL : 2000 mg : : x : 240 mg **EXPRESSED AS TWO FRACTIONS** $$\frac{500\ \text{mL}}{2000\ \text{mg}} \times \frac{x}{240\ \text{mg}}$$ **SOLUTION FOR BOTH PROPORTION METHODS** $500 \times 240 = 2000x$ $$\frac{120,000}{2000} = x$$ $$\frac{240}{4} = x$$ 60 mL/hour = x	Use conversion factors: 60 minutes/1 hour 1 g/1000 mg $$\frac{\overset{1}{\cancel{500}}\ \text{mL}}{\underset{1}{\cancel{2}\ \text{g}}} \left| \frac{4\ \text{mg}}{\text{minutes}} \right| \frac{\overset{30}{\cancel{60}}\ \text{minutes}}{1\ \text{hour}} \left| \frac{1\ \text{g}}{\underset{2}{\cancel{1000}}\ \text{mg}} \right.$$ $$= \frac{4 \times 30}{2} = 60\ \text{mL/hour}$$

Set the pump.

Total number of milliliters: 500

Milliliters per hour: 60

6. a. Add KCl to the IV.

Formula Method	Proportion	Dimensional Analysis
$$\frac{\overset{2}{\cancel{40}}\ \text{mEq}}{\underset{1}{\cancel{20}}\ \text{mEq}} \times 10\ \text{mL} = 20\ \text{mL}$$	**EXPRESSED AS TWO RATIOS** 10 mL : 20 mEq : : x : 40 mEq **EXPRESSED AS TWO FRACTIONS** $$\frac{10\ \text{mL}}{20\ \text{mEq}} \times \frac{x}{40\ \text{mEq}}$$ **SOLUTION FOR BOTH PROPORTION METHODS** $10 \times 40 = 20x$ $$\frac{400}{20} = x$$ 20 mL = x	$$\frac{10\ \text{mL}}{\underset{1}{\cancel{20}}\ \text{mEq}} \left| \frac{\overset{2}{\cancel{40}}\ \text{mEq}}{} \right. = 2 \times 10 = 20\ \text{mL}$$

b. Remove 20 mL IV fluid and add 20 mL of KCl to make 1000 mL.

$1 \text{ L} = 1000 \text{ mL}$

Formula Method	Proportion	Dimensional Analysis
$\dfrac{\overset{1}{\cancel{10}} \text{ mEq/hour}}{\underset{1}{\overset{4}{\cancel{40}}} \text{ mEq}} \times \overset{250}{\cancel{1000}} \text{ mL}$ $= 250 \text{ mL/hour}$	**EXPRESSED AS TWO RATIOS** $1000 \text{ mL} : 40 \text{ mEq} :: x : 10 \text{ mEq}$ **EXPRESSED AS TWO FRACTIONS** $\dfrac{1000 \text{ mL}}{40 \text{ mEq}} \times \dfrac{x}{10 \text{ mEq}}$ **SOLUTION FOR BOTH PROPORTION METHODS** $1000 \times 10 = 40x$ $\dfrac{10{,}000}{40} = x$ $250 \text{ mL/hour} = x$	Use conversion factor 1000 mL/1 L: $\dfrac{\cancel{1 \text{ L}} \;\Big|\; \overset{1}{\cancel{10}} \text{ mEq} \;\Big|\; 1000 \;\widehat{\text{mL}}}{\underset{4}{\cancel{40}} \text{ mEq} \;\Big|\; \widehat{\text{hours}} \;\Big|\; \cancel{1 \text{ L}}} = 250 \text{ mL/hour}$

Set pump at 250 mL/hour. This is a large volume, high infusion rate and KCl is a potent electrolyte; therefore, the patient/client must be on a cardiac monitor for safety. Check the order with the doctor or healthcare provider.

Total number of milliliters: 1000

Milliliters per hour: 250

7. $2 \text{ g} = 2000 \text{ mg}$

Multiply: 2 mg/minute ¥ 60 minutes/hour = 120 mg/hour

Formula Method	Proportion	Dimensional Analysis
$\dfrac{120 \text{ mg/hour}}{\underset{4}{\overset{}{\cancel{2000}}} \text{ mg}} \times \overset{1}{\cancel{500}} \text{ mL}$ $= \dfrac{120}{4} = 30 \text{ mL/hour}$	**EXPRESSED AS TWO RATIOS** $500 \text{ mL} : 2000 \text{ mg} :: x : 120 \text{ mg}$ **EXPRESSED AS TWO FRACTIONS** $\dfrac{500 \text{ mL}}{2000 \text{ mg}} \times \dfrac{x}{120 \text{ mg}}$ **SOLUTION FOR BOTH PROPORTION METHODS** $500 \times 120 = 2000x$ $\dfrac{60{,}000}{2000} = x$ $30 \text{ mL/hour} = x$	Use conversion factors: 60 minutes/1 hour 1 g/1000 mg $\dfrac{\overset{1}{\cancel{500}} \;\widehat{\text{mL}} \;\Big|\; \cancel{2} \text{ mg} \;\Big|\; 60 \;\cancel{\text{minutes}} \;\Big|\; 1 \;\cancel{\text{g}}}{\cancel{2} \;\cancel{\text{g}} \;\Big|\; \cancel{\text{minutes}} \;\Big|\; 1 \;\widehat{\text{hour}} \;\Big|\; \underset{2}{\cancel{1000}} \text{ mg}}$ $= \dfrac{60}{2} = 30 \text{ mL/hour}$

8. $\dfrac{\text{Number of milliliters}}{\text{Number of hours}} = \text{Milliliters per hour}$

$$\dfrac{500\ \text{mL}}{6\ \text{hours}}$$

$$6\ \text{hours} \overline{)\begin{array}{l} 83.0 \\ 500.0 \end{array}} = 83\ \text{mL/hour}$$

$$\begin{array}{r} 48 \\ \hline 20 \\ 18 \\ \hline 2\ 0 \\ 1\ 8 \\ \hline \end{array}$$

Dimensional Analysis

$$\dfrac{500\ \text{mL}}{6\ \text{hours}} \bigg| \dfrac{500}{6} = 83.33\ \text{or}\ 83\ \text{mL/hour}$$

Set the pump.

Total number of milliliters: 500

Milliliters per hour: 83

9.

Formula Method	Proportion	Dimensional Analysis
$\dfrac{\overset{9}{18}\ \text{units/hour}}{\underset{1}{200}\ \text{units}} \times 500\ \text{mL}$ $= 45\ \text{mL/hour}$	**EXPRESSED AS TWO RATIOS** 500 mL : 200 units : : x : 18 units **EXPRESSED AS TWO FRACTIONS** $\dfrac{500\ \text{mL}}{200\ \text{units}} \times \dfrac{x}{18\ \text{units}}$ **SOLUTION FOR BOTH PROPORTION METHODS** $500 \times 18 = 200x$ $\dfrac{900}{20} = x$ $45\ \text{mL/hour} = x$	$\dfrac{500\ \text{mL}}{200\ \text{units}} \bigg| \dfrac{18\ \text{units}}{\text{hours}} = \dfrac{5 \times 18}{2} = 45\ \text{mL/hour}$

Set the pump.

Total number of milliliters: 500

Milliliters per hour: 45

10. Order: 250 mcg/minute

Solution: 500 mg in 500 mL D5W

Step 1. $\dfrac{500\ \text{mg}}{500\ \text{mL}} = 1\ \text{mg/mL}$

Step 2. 1 mg = 1000 mcg/mL

Step 3. Divide by 60 to get micrograms per minute. $\dfrac{1000}{60} = 16.67\ \text{mcg/minute.}$

Step 4.

Formula Method	Proportion	Dimensional Analysis
$\dfrac{250 \text{ mcg/minute}}{16.67 \text{ mcg/minute}} \times 1 \text{ mL} = x$ 14.99 or 15 mL/hour	**EXPRESSED AS TWO RATIOS** 1 mL : 16.67 mcg/minute : : x : 250 mcg/minute **EXPRESSED AS TWO FRACTIONS** $\dfrac{1 \text{ mL}}{16.67 \text{ mcg/minute}} \diagup \dfrac{x}{250 \text{ mcg/minute}}$ **SOLUTION FOR BOTH PROPORTION METHODS** $250 = 16.67x$ $\dfrac{250}{16.67} = x$ 14.99 or 15 mL/hour = x	Use conversion factors: 60 minutes/1 hour 1 mg/1000 mcg $\dfrac{\overset{1}{\cancel{500}} \ \cancel{mL}}{\underset{1}{\cancel{500}} \ \cancel{mg}} \ \Bigg| \ \dfrac{\overset{1}{\cancel{250}} \ \cancel{mcg}}{\cancel{minutes}} \ \Bigg| \ \dfrac{60 \ minutes}{1 \ \cancel{hour}} \ \Bigg| \ \dfrac{1 \ \cancel{mg}}{\underset{4}{\cancel{1000}} \ \cancel{mcg}}$ $= \dfrac{60}{4} = 15 \text{ mL/hour}$

Set the pump.

Total number of milliliters: 500

Milliliters per hour: 15

11. Order: 2.5 mcg/kg/minute

   Solution: 400 mg in 250 mL

   Weight: 60 kg

   Multiply: 60 kg × 2.5 mcg = 150 mcg

   Step 1. $\dfrac{400 \text{ mg}}{250 \text{ mL}} = 1.6 \text{ mg/mL}$

   Step 2. $1.6 \times 1000 = 1600 \text{ mcg/mL}$

   Step 3. Divide by 60 $\dfrac{1600}{60} = 26.67 \text{ mcg/minute}$

   Step 4.

Formula Method	Proportion	Dimensional Analysis
$\dfrac{150 \text{ mcg/minute}}{26.67 \text{ mcg/minute}} \times 1 \text{ mL}$ = 5.6 or 6 mL/hour	**EXPRESSED AS TWO RATIOS** 1 mL : 26.67 mcg/minute : : x : 150 mcg/minute **EXPRESSED AS TWO FRACTIONS** $\dfrac{1 \text{ mL}}{26.67 \text{ mcg/minute}} \diagup \dfrac{x}{150 \text{ mcg/minute}}$ **SOLUTION FOR BOTH PROPORTION METHODS** $150 = 26.67x$ $\dfrac{150}{26.67} = x$ 5.6 or 6 mL/hour = x	Use conversion factors: 60 minutes/1 hour 1 mg/1000 mcg $\dfrac{\overset{1}{\cancel{250}} \ \cancel{mL}}{\underset{40}{\cancel{400}} \ \cancel{mg}} \Bigg| \dfrac{2.5 \ \cancel{mcg}}{\cancel{kg/minute}} \Bigg| \dfrac{\overset{15}{\cancel{60}} \ minutes}{1 \ \cancel{hour}} \Bigg| \dfrac{1 \ \cancel{mg}}{\underset{1}{\cancel{1000}} \ \cancel{mcg}} \Bigg| \overset{6}{\cancel{60}} \ kg$ $= \dfrac{2.5 \times 15 \times 6}{40} = 5.625 \text{ or } 6 \text{ mL/hour}$

Set the pump.

Total number of milliliters: 250

Milliliters per hour: 6

12. Order: 2 milliunits/minute

Solution: 9 units in 150 mL NS

Step 1. $\dfrac{9 \text{ units}}{150 \text{ mL}} = 0.06$ units/mL

Step 2. 1 unit = 1000 milliunits $0.06 \times 1000 = 60$ milliunits/mL

Step 3. Divide by 60 $\dfrac{60}{60} = 1$ milliunit/minute

Step 4.

Formula Method	Proportion	Dimensional Analysis
$\dfrac{2 \text{ milliunits/minute}}{1 \text{ milliunit/minute}} \times 1 \text{ mL} = x$ $2 \text{ mL/hour} = x$	**EXPRESSED AS TWO RATIOS** 1 mL : 1 milliunit/minute : : x : 2 milliunits/minute **EXPRESSED AS TWO FRACTIONS** $\dfrac{1 \text{ mL}}{1 \text{ milliunit/minute}} \times \dfrac{x}{2 \text{ milliunits/minute}}$ **SOLUTION FOR BOTH PROPORTION METHODS** $2 = x$ $2 \text{ mL/hour} = x$	Use conversion factors: 60 minutes/1 hour 1 unit/1000 milliunits $\dfrac{150 \text{ mL}}{9 \text{ units}} \bigg\vert \dfrac{2 \text{ milliunits}}{\text{minutes}} \bigg\vert \dfrac{60 \text{ minutes}}{1 \text{ hour}} \bigg\vert \dfrac{1 \text{ unit}}{1000 \text{ milliunits}}$ $= \dfrac{15 \times 2 \times 6}{9 \times 10} = 2$ mL/hour

Set the pump.

Total number of milliliters: 150 mL

Milliliters per hour: 2

13. a.   Correct; $100 \text{ mg/m}^2 \times 1.7 = 170$ mg

b.   1 L = 1000 mL

$\dfrac{\text{Number of milliliters}}{\text{Number of hours}} =$ Milliliters per hour

$24 \overline{)1000.0} = 42$ mL/hour, quotient 41.6
$\underline{96}$
40
$\underline{24}$
160
$\underline{144}$

Dimensional Analysis

$\dfrac{1 \text{ L}}{24 \text{ hours}} \bigg\vert \dfrac{1000 \text{ mL}}{1 \text{ L}} \bigg\vert \dfrac{1000}{24} = 41.66$ or 42 mL/hour

Set the pump.

Total number of milliliters: 1000

Milliliters per hour: 42

14. Order: 5 mcg/kg/minute

Solution: 50 mg in 250 mL

Weight: 90 kg

5 mcg × 90 kg = 450 mcg/minute

Step 1. $\dfrac{50 \text{ mg}}{250 \text{ mL}} = 0.2$ mg/mL

Step 2. $0.2 \times 1000 = 200$ mcg/mL

Step 3. Divide by 60 $\qquad \dfrac{200}{60} = 3.33$ mcg/minute

Step 4.

Formula Method	Proportion	Dimensional Analysis
$\dfrac{450 \text{ mcg/minute}}{3.33 \text{ mcg/minute}} \times 1 \text{ mL}$ $= 135$ mL/hour	**EXPRESSED AS TWO RATIOS** $1 \text{ mL} : 3.33 \text{ mcg/minute} :: x : 450 \text{ mcg/minute}$ **EXPRESSED AS TWO FRACTIONS** $\dfrac{1 \text{ mL}}{3.33 \text{ mcg}} \times \dfrac{x}{450 \text{ mcg}}$ **SOLUTION FOR BOTH PROPORTION METHODS** $450 = 3.33x$ $\dfrac{450}{3.33} = x$ $135 \text{ mL/hour} = x$	Use conversion factors: 60 minutes/1 hour 1 mg/1000 mcg $\dfrac{250 \text{ mL}}{50 \text{ mg}} \Big\vert \dfrac{5 \text{ mcg}}{\text{kg/minute}} \Big\vert \dfrac{60 \text{ minutes}}{1 \text{ hour}} \Big\vert \dfrac{1 \text{ mg}}{1000 \text{ mcg}} \Big\vert 90 \text{ kg}$ $= \dfrac{6 \times 90}{4} = 135$ mL/hour

Set the pump.

Total number of milliliters: 250

Milliliters per hour: 135

15. Order: 2 mcg/minute

Solution: 4 mg in 250 mL

Step 1. $\dfrac{4 \text{ mg}}{250 \text{ mL}} = 0.016$ mg/mL

Step 2. $0.016 \text{ mg} \times 1000 = 16$ mcg

Step 3. Divide by 60 $\qquad \dfrac{16}{60} = 0.27$ mcg/minute

Step 4.

Formula Method	Proportion	Dimensional Analysis
$\dfrac{2 \text{ mcg/minute}}{0.267 \text{ mcg/minute}} \times 1 \text{ mL}$ $= 7.4 \text{ or } 7 \text{ mL/hour}$	**EXPRESSED AS TWO RATIOS** 1 mL : 0.267 mcg/minute : : x : 2 mcg/minute **EXPRESSED AS TWO FRACTIONS** $\dfrac{1 \text{ mL}}{0.267 \text{ mcg/minute}} \times \dfrac{x}{2 \text{ mcg/minute}}$ **SOLUTION FOR BOTH PROPORTION METHODS** $2 = 0.27x$ $\dfrac{2}{0.27} = x$ 7.4 or 7 mL/hour = x	Use conversion factors: 60 minutes/1 hour 1 mg/1000 mcg 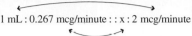 $= \dfrac{15}{2} = 7.5 \text{ or } 8 \text{ mL/hour}$ Note the difference in answers. The dimensional analysis method does not round the numbers until the final solution. The two different answers and two different pump settings could be critical in a patient/client's response to the medication. Therefore, both answers are given in this example.

Set the pump.

Total number of milliliters: 250

Milliliters per hour: 7 or 8 mL/hour (see note under dimensional analysis)

16. a. Yes. 40 units × 90 kg = 3600 units

    b. Yes. Increase rate by 2 units/kg/hour

        2 units × 90 kg = 180 units

Formula Method	Proportion	Dimensional Analysis
$\dfrac{180 \text{ units}}{25{,}000 \text{ units}} \times 500 \text{ mL}$ $= 3.6 \text{ mL/hour}$	**EXPRESSED AS TWO RATIOS** 500 mL : 25,000 units : : x : 180 units **EXPRESSED AS TWO FRACTIONS** $\dfrac{500 \text{ mL}}{25{,}000 \text{ units}} \times \dfrac{x}{180 \text{ units}}$ **SOLUTION FOR BOTH PROPORTION METHODS** $500 \times 180 = 25{,}000x$ $\dfrac{500 \times 180}{25{,}000} = x$ 3.6 mL/hour = x	$\dfrac{500 \text{ mL}}{25{,}000 \text{ units}} \Bigg| \dfrac{180 \text{ units}}{\text{hours}} = \dfrac{180}{50} = 3.6 \text{ mL/hour}$

New infusion rate: 32 + 3.6 = 35.6 mL/hour

17. **a.** Yes. 40 units × 90 kg = 3600 units

    b. Yes. Increase rate by 3 units/kg/hour:

    3 units × 90 kg = 270 units

Formula Method	Proportion	Dimensional Analysis
$\dfrac{270 \text{ units}}{\underset{50}{25{,}000 \text{ units}}} \times \overset{1}{500} \text{ mL} =$ $\dfrac{270}{50} = x$ 5.4 mL/hour	**EXPRESSED AS TWO RATIOS** 500 mL : 25,000 units : : x : 270 units **EXPRESSED AS TWO FRACTIONS** $\dfrac{500 \text{ mL}}{25{,}000 \text{ units}} \times \dfrac{x}{270 \text{ units}}$ **SOLUTION FOR BOTH PROPORTION METHODS** 500 × 270 = 25,000x $\dfrac{500 \times 270}{25{,}000} = x$ 5.4 mL/hour = x	$\dfrac{\overset{1}{500} \text{ mL}}{\underset{50}{25{,}000 \text{ units}}} \bigg| 270 \text{ units} = \dfrac{270}{50} = 5.4 \text{ mL/hour}$

New infusion rate: 32 + 5.4 = 37.4 mL/hour

18. **a.** No. Bolus.

    b. Yes. Decrease by 1 unit/kg/hour:

    1 unit × 90 kg = 90 units

Formula Method	Proportion	Dimensional Analysis
$\dfrac{90 \text{ units}}{\underset{50}{25{,}000 \text{ units}}} \times \overset{1}{500} \text{ mL} = x$ 1.8 mL/hour	**EXPRESSED AS TWO RATIOS** 500 mL : 25,000 units : : x : 90 units **EXPRESSED AS TWO FRACTIONS** $\dfrac{500 \text{ mL}}{25{,}000 \text{ units}} \times \dfrac{x}{90 \text{ units}}$ **SOLUTION FOR BOTH PROPORTION METHODS** 500 × 90 = 25,000x $\dfrac{500 \times 90}{25{,}000} = x$ 1.8 mL/hour = x	$\dfrac{\overset{1}{500} \text{ mL}}{\underset{50}{25{,}000 \text{ units}}} \bigg| \dfrac{90 \text{ units}}{\text{hours}} = \dfrac{9}{5} = 1.8 \text{ mL/hour}$

New infusion rate: 32 − 1.8 = 30.2 mL/hour

19. a. $(125 - 60) \times 0.02 = 1.3$ units/hour

Formula Method	Proportion	Dimensional Analysis
$\dfrac{1.3 \text{ units}}{100 \text{ units}} \times 100 \text{ mL}$ $= 1.3 \text{ mL/hour}$	**EXPRESSED AS TWO RATIOS** $100 \text{ mL} : 100 \text{ units} :: x : 1.3 \text{ units}$ **EXPRESSED AS TWO FRACTIONS** $\dfrac{100 \text{ mL}}{100 \text{ units}} \times \dfrac{x}{1.3 \text{ units}}$ **SOLUTION FOR BOTH PROPORTION METHODS** $100 \times 1.3 = 100x$ $\dfrac{100 \times 1.3}{100} = x$ $1.3 \text{ mL/hour} = x$	$\dfrac{100 \text{ mL}}{100 \text{ units}} \left\| \dfrac{1.3 \text{ units}}{\text{hours}} \right. = 1.3 \text{ mL/hour}$

b. Yes. $(BG - 60) \times 0.03$

20. a. $(260 - 60) \times 0.02 = 4$ units/hour

Formula Method	Proportion	Dimensional Analysis
$\dfrac{4 \text{ units}}{100 \text{ units}} \times 100 \text{ mL}$ $= 4 \text{ mL/hour}$	**EXPRESSED AS TWO RATIOS** $100 \text{ mL} : 100 \text{ units} :: x : 4 \text{ units}$ **EXPRESSED AS TWO FRACTIONS** $\dfrac{100 \text{ mL}}{100 \text{ units}} \times \dfrac{x}{4 \text{ units}}$ **SOLUTION FOR BOTH PROPORTION METHODS** $100 \times 4 = 100x$ $\dfrac{100 \times 4}{100} = x$ $4 \text{ mL/hour} = x$	$\dfrac{100 \text{ mL}}{100 \text{ units}} \left\| \dfrac{4 \text{ units}}{} \right. = 4 \text{ mL/hour}$

b. Yes. $(BG - 60) \times 0.03$

Chapter 8

Test 1: Infants and Children Dosage Problems

1. Safe dose: 0.5 mg to 1 mg/dose IM. The order is safe.

Formula Method	Proportion	Dimensional Analysis
$\dfrac{1 \text{ mg}}{10 \text{ mg}} \times 1 \text{ mL} = 0.1 \text{ mL IM}$	**EXPRESSED AS TWO RATIOS** $$1 \text{ mL} : 10 \text{ mg} :: x : 1 \text{ mg}$$ **EXPRESSED AS TWO FRACTIONS** $$\frac{1 \text{ mL}}{10 \text{ mg}} \times \frac{x}{1 \text{ mg}}$$ **SOLUTION FOR BOTH PROPORTION METHODS** $$1 = 10x$$ $$\frac{1}{10} = x$$ $$0.1 \text{ mL} = x$$	$\dfrac{1 \text{ mL}}{10 \text{ mg}} \left| \dfrac{1 \text{ mg}}{} = \dfrac{1}{10} \text{ or } 0.1 \text{ mL}$

Use a 1-mL precision syringe.

2. Safe dose: 20 to 40 mg/kg/24 hours given q8h

Low Dose	High Dose
20 mg	40 mg
× 10 kg	× 10 kg
200 mg/24 hours	400 mg/24 hours

Order is 125 mg q8h (3 doses).

125 mg × 3 doses = 375. Dose is safe.

No math necessary. Supply is 125 mg/5 mL.

Give 5 mL.

3. Safe dose: 50,000 units/kg × 1 dose

   50,000 units
  ×   10 kg
  500,000 units

The order is safe.

Formula Method	Proportion	Dimensional Analysis
$\dfrac{500,000 \text{ units}}{600,000 \text{ units}} \times 1 \text{ mL} = \dfrac{5}{6}$ $= 0.83 \text{ mL}$	**EXPRESSED AS TWO RATIOS** $1 \text{ mL} : 600,000 \text{ units} :: x : 500,000 \text{ units}$ **EXPRESSED AS TWO FRACTIONS** $\dfrac{1 \text{ mL}}{600,000 \text{ units}} \times \dfrac{x}{500,000 \text{ units}}$ **SOLUTION FOR BOTH PROPORTION METHODS** $500,000 = 600,000x$ $\dfrac{500,000}{600,000} = x$ $0.83 \text{ mL} = x$	$\dfrac{1 \text{ mL}}{600,000 \text{ units}} \left\vert \dfrac{500,000 \text{ units}}{} \right. = \dfrac{5}{6} = 0.83 \text{ mL}$

Use a 1-mL precision syringe. Give 0.83 mL IM.

4. Step 1. Weight 3.6 kg

Step 2. Safe dose: 2.5 mg/kg/dose q8h

   2.5 mg
 × 3.6 kg
   9 mg

Step 3. Order of 9 mg is safe.

Minimum safe dilution: 2 mg/mL

$\dfrac{1 \text{ mL}}{2 \text{ mg}} \times 9 \text{ mg} = \dfrac{9}{2} = 4.5 \text{ mL}$

4.5 mL is the minimum safe dilution. Therefore, 10 mL is safe.

Step 4.

Formula Method	Proportion	Dimensional Analysis
$\dfrac{9 \text{ mg}}{40 \text{ mg}} \times 1 \text{ mL} = \dfrac{9}{40} \begin{array}{r} .225 \\ \overline{)9.000} \end{array}$ $= 0.23 \text{ mL}$	**EXPRESSED AS TWO RATIOS** $1 \text{ mL} : 40 \text{ mg} :: x : 9 \text{ mg}$ **EXPRESSED AS TWO FRACTIONS** $\dfrac{1 \text{ mL}}{40 \text{ mg}} \diagdown \dfrac{x}{9 \text{ mg}}$ **SOLUTION FOR BOTH PROPORTION METHODS** $9 = 40x$ $\dfrac{9}{40} = x$ $0.23 \text{ mL} = x$	$\dfrac{1 \text{ mL}}{40 \text{ mg}} \bigg| \dfrac{9 \text{ mg}}{} = \dfrac{9}{40} = 0.23 \text{ mL}$

Use a 1 mL precision syringe to draw up 0.23 mL.

Step 5. Add about 10 mL from the D5½NS bag into the Buretrol. Add the 0.23 mL drug.

Step 6. Set the pump at 20 mL/hour because 20 mL in 1 hour will deliver the 10 mL in 30 minutes.

Step 7. When the IV is completed, add an additional 20 mL of the D51/2NS bag into the Buretrol as a flush.

5. Safe dose: infants and children younger than 3 years, 10 to 40 mg. The dose (10 mg) is safe.

Formula Method	Proportion	Dimensional Analysis
$\dfrac{10 \text{ mg}}{20 \text{ mg}} \times 5 \text{ mL} = \dfrac{5}{2}$ $= 2.5 \text{ mL po}$	**EXPRESSED AS TWO RATIOS** $5 \text{ mL} : 20 \text{ mg} :: x : 10 \text{ mg}$ **EXPRESSED AS TWO FRACTIONS** $\dfrac{5 \text{ mL}}{20 \text{ mg}} \diagdown \dfrac{x}{10 \text{ mg}}$ **SOLUTION FOR BOTH PROPORTION METHODS** $5 \times 10 = 20x$ $\dfrac{50}{20} = x$ $2.5 \text{ mL} = x$	$\dfrac{5 \text{ mL}}{20 \text{ mg}} \bigg| \dfrac{\overset{1}{10 \text{ mg}}}{\underset{2}{}} = \dfrac{5}{2} = 2.5 \text{ mL}$

6. Step 1. Weight is 5.5 kg

Step 2. Safe dose: 10 mg/kg q8h IV

10 mg
× 5.5 kg
55 mg q8h

Step 3. The dose of 54 mg is safe, although a little low on dosage.

Minimum safe dilution: 5 mg/mL; infuse over 1 hour.

$$\frac{1 \text{ mL}}{5 \text{ mg}} \times 54 \text{ mg} = \frac{54}{5} = 10.8 \text{ or } 11 \text{ mL}$$

Infuse over 1 hour

Step 4. To the 500-mg powder, add 10 mL sterile water for injection to make 50 mg/mL.

Formula Method	Proportion	Dimensional Analysis
$\frac{54 \text{ mg}}{50 \text{ mg}} \times 1 \text{ mL} = \frac{54}{50}$ $= 50\overline{)54.00}$ gives 1.08, $4\,00$ $= 1.1 \text{ mL}$	**EXPRESSED AS TWO RATIOS** $1 \text{ mL} : 50 \text{ mg} :: x : 54 \text{ mg}$ **EXPRESSED AS TWO FRACTIONS** $\frac{1 \text{ mL}}{50 \text{ mg}} \times \frac{x}{54 \text{ mg}}$ **SOLUTION FOR BOTH PROPORTION METHODS** $54 = 50x$ $\frac{54}{50} = x$ $1.08 \text{ or } 1.1 \text{ mL} = x$	$\frac{1 \text{ mL}}{50 \text{ mg}} \bigg| \frac{54 \text{ mg}}{} = \frac{54}{50} = 1.08 \text{ or } 1.1 \text{ mL}$

Withdraw 1.1 mL of the drug, label the vial, refrigerate.

Step 5. Add about 12 mL from D5½NS bag into the Buretrol. Add 1.1 mL drug.

Step 6. Set the pump for 12 mL/hour.

Step 7. When the IV is completed, add an additional 20 mL of the D5½NS bag into the Buretrol as a flush.

7. Safe dose: 25 to 50 mg/kg/dose

Low Dose
25 mg
× 6.7 kg
167.5 mg/dose

High Dose
50 mg
× 6.7 kg
335 mg/dose

Order of 350 mg is not safe. Consult the physician or healthcare provider.

8. Step 1. BSA is 1.32.

Step 2. Safe dose: 7.5 to 30 mg/m^2

Low Dose
1.32 BSA
× 7.5 mg
9.9 mg/dose

High Dose
1.32 BSA
× 30 mg
39.6 mg/dose

Step 3. Order is 10 mg. Dose is safe.

Step 4.

Formula Method	Proportion	Dimensional Analysis
$\dfrac{10 \text{ mg}}{2.5 \text{ mg}} \times 1 \text{ tablet} = 4 \text{ tablets}$	**EXPRESSED AS TWO RATIOS** $1 \text{ tablet} : 2.5 \text{ mg} :: x : 10 \text{ mg}$ **EXPRESSED AS TWO FRACTIONS** $\dfrac{1 \text{ tablet}}{2.5 \text{ mg}} \times \dfrac{x}{10 \text{ mg}}$ **SOLUTION FOR BOTH PROPORTION METHODS** $10 = 2.5x$ $\dfrac{10}{2.5} = x$ $4 \text{ tablets} = x$	$\dfrac{1 \text{ tablet}}{2.5 \text{ mg}} \left\lvert \dfrac{\overset{4}{10 \text{ mg}}}{\underset{1}{}} \right. = 4 \text{ tablets}$

9. Step 1: Weight is 24 kg

   Step 2: Safe dose is 2 to 6 g in a 24-hour period divided into either q8h or q12h.

   Step 3: The order is 2 g q8h (3 doses).

   $2 \text{ g} \times 3 \text{ doses} = 6 \text{ g}$. The order is safe.

   Minimum safe dilution is 50 mg/mL over 15 to 30 minutes (2 g = 2000 mg)

   $$\frac{1 \text{ mL}}{50 \text{ mg}} \times 2000 \text{ mg} = \frac{2000}{50} = 40 \text{ mL}$$

   40 mL is the minimum safe dilution: 50 mL is safe.

   Step 4. Order is 2 g. Stock is a 2-g powder.
   Directions say to dilute initially with 10 mL sterile water for injection. Draw the total amount into a syringe.

   Step 5. Add 40 mL from the D5⅓NS bag into the Buretrol. Add the medication from the syringe.

   Step 6. Set the pump for 100 mL/hour. It will deliver 50 mL in 30 minutes.

   Step 7. When the IV is completed, add an additional 20 mL of the D5½NS bag into the Buretrol as a flush.

10. Usual dose is 0.05 to 0.2 mg/kg/dose.

    Step 1. $\dfrac{35 \text{ lb}}{2.2} = 15.91 \text{ kg}$

    Low Dose

    $\begin{array}{r} 0.05 \text{ mg/kg} \\ \times\, 15.91 \text{ kg} \\ \hline 0.7955 \text{ mg/dose} \end{array}$

    High Dose

    $\begin{array}{r} 0.2 \text{ mg/kg} \\ \times\, 15.91 \text{ kg} \\ \hline 3.182 \text{ mg/dose} \end{array}$

    Step 2. 4 mg is too high of a dose. Contact the physician or healthcare provider.

Chapter 9

Test 1: Basic Drug Information

1. a	**5.** c	**9.** d	**13.** c	**17.** c
2. d	**6.** a	**10.** a	**14.** b	**18.** d
3. a	**7.** a	**11.** a	**15.** a	**19.** d
4. a	**8.** a	**12.** b	**16.** b	**20.** d

Chapter 10

Test 1: Administration Procedures

Part A

1. c	**6.** a	**11.** d	**16.** a	**21.** c
2. b	**7.** b	**12.** b	**17.** b	**22.** b
3. d	**8.** a	**13.** b	**18.** a	**23.** c
4. c	**9.** a	**14.** d	**19.** d	**24.** d
5. d	**10.** d	**15.** d	**20.** b	**25.** d

Part B

1. Correct. As the needle or catheter is removed, there is a possibility of bleeding at the site. In addition, the nurse should carefully carry the needle or catheter to a puncture-proof sharps container.

2. Incorrect. The nurse must wash his or her hands before leaving the room.

3. Incorrect. It is not necessary to wear gloves to prepare an IV because there is no contact at this time with the patient/client's blood or body fluids.

4. Correct. Standard precautions state that a mask must be worn when the patient/client is on strict or respiratory isolation precautions.

5. Correct. There is a potential risk of exposure to hepatitis B virus and HIV. Laboratory testing may not show the presence of the virus or antibodies to the virus immediately, so precautions should be taken with all patients/clients.

6. Correct. Although transdermal pads are applied to intact skin, standard precaution require gloves.

7. Correct. Standard precautions state wearing gloves when coming in contact with mucous membranes.

8. Incorrect. The nurse should squeeze the finger and, after washing hands with soap and water, scrub the area with povidone–iodine (Betadine) or another accepted antiseptic. In addition, the needlestick should be reported to the proper authority and the protocol for exposure to blood should be carried out. Standard precautions apply to all patients/clients regardless of the diagnosis.

9. Incorrect. There is always a possibility or risk when doing an invasive procedure such as an injection.

10. Incorrect. Because the patient/client is alert and can take the medicine cup from the nurse, handwashing is adequate. However, the nurse could wear gloves if there is possibility of contact with mucous membranes.

11. Incorrect. The CDC guidelines advise the nurse not to recap a needle, but to place it immediately in a puncture-proof container.

12. Correct. Nitroglycerin ointment is a potent vasodilator. Wearing gloves protects the nurse against the drug's effect.

13. Incorrect. The nurse's fingers may come in contact with mucous membrane when administering eye drops.

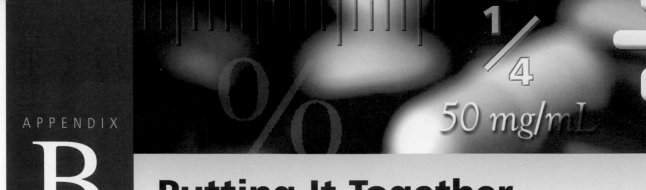

Putting It Together Answers

Chapter 4

Calculations

1.

Formula Method	Proportion	Dimensional Analysis
$\dfrac{7.5 \text{ mg}}{5 \text{ mg}} \times 1 \text{ tablet} = x$ $1\dfrac{1}{2}$ tablets $= x$	**EXPRESSED AS TWO RATIOS** 1 tablet : 5 mg : : x : 7.5 tablets **EXPRESSED AS TWO FRACTIONS** $\dfrac{1 \text{ tablet}}{5 \text{ mg}} \diagdown \dfrac{x}{7.5 \text{ tablets}}$ **SOLUTION FOR BOTH PROPORTION METHODS** $7.5 = 5x$ $\dfrac{7.5}{5} = x$ $1\dfrac{1}{2}$ tablets $= x$	$\dfrac{1 \text{ tablet}}{\cancel{5} \text{ mg}} \Bigg| \dfrac{\cancel{7.5}^{\,1.5} \text{ mg}}{} = 1\dfrac{1}{2}$ tablets

2.

Formula Method	Proportion	Dimensional Analysis
$\dfrac{\cancel{20} \text{ mg}}{\cancel{10} \text{ mg}} \times 1 \text{ tablet} = x$ 2 tablets $= x$	**EXPRESSED AS TWO RATIOS** 1 tablet : 10 mg : : x : 20 mg **EXPRESSED AS TWO FRACTIONS** $\dfrac{1 \text{ tablet}}{10 \text{ mg}} \diagdown \dfrac{x}{20 \text{ mg}}$ **SOLUTION FOR BOTH PROPORTION METHODS** $20 = 10x$ $\dfrac{20}{10} = x$ 2 tablets $= x$	$\dfrac{1 \text{ tablet}}{\cancel{10} \text{ mg}} \Bigg| \dfrac{\cancel{20}^{\,2} \text{ mg}}{} = 2$ tablets

3. 500 mcg = 0.5 mg
250 mcg = 0.25 mg

Formula Method	Proportion	Dimensional Analysis
$\dfrac{0.75 \text{ mg}}{0.5 \text{ mg}} \times 1 \text{ tablet} = x$ $1\dfrac{1}{2}$ tablets = x	**EXPRESSED AS TWO RATIOS** 1 tablet : 0.5 mg : : x : 0.75 mg **EXPRESSED AS TWO FRACTIONS** $\dfrac{1 \text{ tablet}}{0.5 \text{ mg}} \times \dfrac{x}{0.75 \text{ mg}}$ **SOLUTION FOR BOTH PROPORTION METHODS** 0.75 mg = 0.5x $\dfrac{0.75}{0.5} = x$ $1\dfrac{1}{2}$ tablets = x	Use conversion factor 1000 mcg/1 mg: $\dfrac{1 \text{ tablet}}{500 \text{ mcg}} \left\vert \dfrac{0.75 \text{ mg}}{} \right\vert \dfrac{\overset{2}{1000} \text{ mcg}}{1 \text{ mg}} = 0.75 \times 2$ $= 1\dfrac{1}{2}$ tablets

OR

Formula Method	Proportion	Dimensional Analysis
$\dfrac{0.75 \text{ mg}}{0.25 \text{ mg}} \times 1 \text{ tablet} = x$ 3 tablets = x	**EXPRESSED AS TWO RATIOS** 1 tablet : 1.25 mg : : x : 0.75 mg **EXPRESSED AS TWO FRACTIONS** $\dfrac{1 \text{ tablet}}{0.25 \text{ mg}} \times \dfrac{x}{0.75 \text{ mg}}$ **SOLUTION FOR BOTH PROPORTION METHODS** 0.75 mg = 0.25x $\dfrac{0.75}{0.25} = x$ 3 tablets = x	Use conversion factor 1000 mcg/1 mg: $\dfrac{1 \text{ tablet}}{250 \text{ mcg}} \left\vert \dfrac{0.75 \text{ mg}}{} \right\vert \dfrac{\overset{4}{1000} \text{ mcg}}{1 \text{ mg}} = 0.75 \times 4$ $= 3$ tablets

4. 500 mg = 0.5 mg
   250 mcg = 0.25 mg

Formula Method	Proportion	Dimensional Analysis

Formula Method

$$\frac{0.25 \text{ mg}}{0.5 \text{ mg}} \times 1 \text{ tablet} = x$$

$$\frac{1}{2} \text{ tablet} = x$$

Proportion

EXPRESSED AS TWO RATIOS

1 tablet : 0.5 mg : : x : 0.25 mg

EXPRESSED AS TWO FRACTIONS

$$\frac{1 \text{ tablet}}{0.5 \text{ mg}} \times \frac{x}{0.25 \text{ mg}}$$

SOLUTION FOR BOTH PROPORTION METHODS

0.25 mg = 0.5x

$$\frac{0.25}{0.5} = x$$

$$0.5 \text{ or } \frac{1}{2} \text{ tablet} = x$$

Dimensional Analysis

Use conversion factor 1000 mcg/1 mg:

$$\frac{1 \text{ tablet}}{500 \text{ mcg}} \left| 0.25 \text{ mg} \right| \frac{1000 \text{ mcg}}{1 \text{ mg}} = 0.25 \times 2$$

$$= \frac{1}{2} \text{ tablet}$$

OR

Formula Method	Proportion	Dimensional Analysis

Formula Method

$$\frac{0.25 \text{ mg}}{0.25 \text{ mg}} \times 1 \text{ tablet} = x$$

$$1 \text{ tablet} = x$$

Proportion

EXPRESSED AS TWO RATIOS

1 tablet : 0.25 mg : : x : 0.25 mg

EXPRESSED AS TWO FRACTIONS

$$\frac{1 \text{ tablet}}{0.25 \text{ mg}} \times \frac{x}{0.25 \text{ mg}}$$

SOLUTION FOR BOTH PROPORTION METHODS

$$\frac{0.25}{0.25} = x$$

$$1 \text{ tablet} = x$$

Dimensional Analysis

Use conversion factor 1000 mcg/1 mg:

$$\frac{1 \text{ tablet}}{250 \text{ mcg}} \left| 0.25 \text{ mg} \right| \frac{1000 \text{ mcg}}{1 \text{ mg}} = 0.25 \times 4$$

$$= 1 \text{ tablet}$$

5. 500 mcg = 0.5 mg
250 mcg = 0.25 mg

Formula Method	Proportion	Dimensional Analysis
$\dfrac{0.125 \text{ mg}}{0.5 \text{ mg}} \times 1 \text{ tablet} = x$ 0.25 or $\dfrac{1}{4}$ tablet $= x$ (may be unable to quarter the tablet)	**EXPRESSED AS TWO RATIOS** 1 tablet : 0.5 mg : : x : 0.125 mg **EXPRESSED AS TWO FRACTIONS** $\dfrac{1 \text{ tablet}}{0.5 \text{ mg}} \times \dfrac{x}{0.125 \text{ mg}}$ **SOLUTION FOR BOTH PROPORTION METHODS** $0.125 \text{ mg} = 0.5x$ $\dfrac{0.125 \text{ mg}}{0.5 \text{ mg}} = x$ 0.25 or $\dfrac{1}{4}$ tablet $= x$	Use conversion factor 1000 mcg/1 mg: $\dfrac{1 \text{ tablet}}{500 \text{ mcg}} \Big| 0.125 \text{ mg} \Big| \dfrac{1000 \text{ mcg}}{1 \text{ mg}} = 0.125 \times 2$ $= 0.25$ or $\dfrac{1}{4}$ tablet

OR

Formula Method	Proportion	Dimensional Analysis
$\dfrac{0.125 \text{ mg}}{0.25 \text{ mg}} \times 1 \text{ tablet} = x$ $\dfrac{1}{2}$ tablet $= x$	**EXPRESSED AS TWO RATIOS** 1 tablet : 0.25 mg : : x : 0.125 mg **EXPRESSED AS TWO FRACTIONS** $\dfrac{1 \text{ tablet}}{0.25 \text{ mg}} \times \dfrac{x}{0.125 \text{ mg}}$ **SOLUTION FOR BOTH PROPORTION METHODS** $0.125 = 0.25x$ $\dfrac{0.125}{0.25} = x$ $\dfrac{1}{2}$ tablet $= x$	Use conversion factor 1000 mcg/1 mg: $\dfrac{1 \text{ tablet}}{250 \text{ mcg}} \Big| 0.125 \text{ mg} \Big| \dfrac{1000 \text{ mcg}}{1 \text{ mg}} = 0.125 \times 4$ $= \dfrac{1}{2}$ tablet

6.

Formula Method	Proportion	Dimensional Analysis
$\dfrac{30 \text{ mEq}}{10 \text{ mEq}} \times 750 \text{ mg} = x$ $2250 \text{ mg} = x$	**EXPRESSED AS TWO RATIOS** 750 mg : 10 mEq : : x : 30 mEq **EXPRESSED AS TWO FRACTIONS** $\dfrac{750 \text{ mg}}{10 \text{ mEq}} \times \dfrac{x}{30 \text{ mEq}}$ **SOLUTION FOR BOTH PROPORTION METHODS** $750 \times 30 = 10x$ $\dfrac{22500}{10} = x$ $2250 \text{ mg} = x$	$\dfrac{750 \text{ mg}}{10 \text{ mEq}} \Big| \dfrac{30 \text{ mEq}}{} = 375 \times 6 = 2250 \text{ mg}$

7. $0.25 \text{ mg} = 250 \text{ mcg}$
$0.5 \text{ mg} = 500 \text{ mcg}$

Formula Method	Proportion	Dimensional Analysis
$\dfrac{250 \text{ mcg}}{125 \text{ mcg}} \times 1 \text{ tablet} = x$ $2 \text{ tablets} = x$	**EXPRESSED AS TWO RATIOS** $1 \text{ tablet} : 125 \text{ mg} :: x : 250 \text{ mcg}$ **EXPRESSED AS TWO FRACTIONS** $\dfrac{1 \text{ tablet}}{125 \text{ mcg}} \times \dfrac{x}{250 \text{ mg}}$ **SOLUTION FOR BOTH PROPORTION METHODS** $250 = 125x$ $\dfrac{250}{125} = x$ $2 \text{ tablets} = x$	Use conversion factor 1000 mcg/1 mg: $\dfrac{1 \text{ tablet}}{125 \text{ mcg}} \left| 0.25 \text{ mg} \right| \dfrac{1000 \text{ mcg}}{1 \text{ mg}} = 0.25 \times 8$ $= 2 \text{ tablets}$

OR

Formula Method	Proportion	Dimensional Analysis
$\dfrac{500 \text{ mcg}}{125 \text{ mcg}} \times 1 \text{ tablet} = x$ $4 \text{ tablets} = x$	**EXPRESSED AS TWO RATIOS** $1 \text{ tablet} : 125 \text{ mg} :: x : 500 \text{ mg}$ **EXPRESSED AS TWO FRACTIONS** $\dfrac{1 \text{ tablet}}{125 \text{ mg}} \times \dfrac{x}{500 \text{ mg}}$ **SOLUTION FOR BOTH PROPORTION METHODS** $500 = 125x$ $\dfrac{500}{125} = x$ $4 \text{ tablets} = x$	Use conversion factor 1000 mcg/1 mg: $\dfrac{1 \text{ tablet}}{125 \text{ mcg}} \left| 0.5 \text{ mg} \right| \dfrac{1000 \text{ mcg}}{1 \text{ mg}} = 0.5 \times 8$ $= 4 \text{ tablets}$

8.

Formula Method	Proportion	Dimensional Analysis
$\dfrac{\overset{2}{40} \text{ mg}}{\underset{1}{20} \text{ mg}} \times 1 \text{ tablet} = x$ $2 \text{ tablets} = x$	**EXPRESSED AS TWO RATIOS** $1 \text{ tablet} : 20 \text{ mg} :: x : 40 \text{ mg}$ **EXPRESSED AS TWO FRACTIONS** $\dfrac{1 \text{ tablet}}{20 \text{ mg}} \times \dfrac{x}{40 \text{ mg}}$ **SOLUTION FOR BOTH PROPORTION METHODS** $40 = 20x$ $\dfrac{40}{20} = x$ $2 \text{ tablets} = x$	$\dfrac{1 \text{ tablet}}{\underset{1}{20} \text{ mg}} \left| \overset{2}{40} \text{ mg} \right. = 2 \text{ tablets}$

9.

Formula Method	Proportion	Dimensional Analysis
$\dfrac{650 \text{ mg}}{160 \text{ mg}} \times 5 \text{ mL}$ $= \dfrac{65 \times 5}{16}$ $= 20.3 \text{ or } 20 \text{ mL}$	**EXPRESSED AS TWO RATIOS** $5 \text{ mL} : 160 \text{ mg} :: x : 650 \text{ mg}$ **EXPRESSED AS TWO FRACTIONS** $\dfrac{5 \text{ mL}}{160 \text{ mg}} \times \dfrac{x}{650 \text{ mg}}$ **SOLUTION FOR BOTH PROPORTION METHODS** $5 \times 650 = 160x$ $\dfrac{3250}{160} = x$ $20.3 \text{ or } 20 \text{ mL} = x$	$\dfrac{5 \text{ mL} \mid 650 \text{ mg}}{160 \text{ mg}}$ $= \dfrac{65 \times 5}{16}$ $= 20.3 \text{ or } 20 \text{ mL}$

10. $1 \text{ g} = 1000 \text{ mg}$

Formula Method	Proportion	Dimensional Analysis
$\dfrac{1000 \text{ mg}}{200 \text{ mg}} \times 1 \text{ tablet} = x$ $5 \text{ tablets} = x$	**EXPRESSED AS TWO RATIOS** $1 \text{ tablet} : 200 \text{ mg} :: x : 1000 \text{ mg}$ **EXPRESSED AS TWO FRACTIONS** $\dfrac{1 \text{ tablet}}{200 \text{ mg}} \times \dfrac{x}{1000 \text{ mg}}$ **SOLUTION FOR BOTH PROPORTION METHODS** $1000 = 200x$ $\dfrac{1000}{200} = x$ $5 \text{ tablets} = x$	Use conversion factor 1000 mg/1 g: $\dfrac{1 \text{ tablet} \mid 1 \text{ g} \mid \overset{5}{1000 \text{ mg}}}{\underset{1}{200 \text{ mg}} \mid 1 \text{ g}} = 5 \text{ tablets}$

Critical Thinking Questions

The "answers" are suggested, and there may be other correct comments, suggestions, and answers.

1. Any of the medications that need conversion to another measurement system increases the potential for error, since it takes knowledge of the correct conversion and calculation of that conversion. Xanax in micrograms, K-dur in milliequivalents, and digoxin in micrograms would have a higher potential for error.

2. Digoxin has the following parameter: hold if HR $<$ 60. The heart rate in the scenario is above 60, so it is safe to give. Alprazolam (Xanax) is given for anxiety and acetaminophen (Tylenol) for mild pain. There are no contraindications for these medications, but you would assess if the patient/client is having these symptoms. Since lisinopril (Prinivil) is an antihypertensive, you would hold the medication if the blood pressure was too low—without a specific parameter, it would be best to check with the healthcare provider how "low" is "too low."

3. Does the medication come in liquid form? If so, use that instead of the tablets. Does the drug come in a tablet with a higher dosage? If so, recalculate with the higher dosage.

4. Alprazolam (Xanax) does not have a route. Tylenol does not have a route although it comes in liquid form, so it could be presumed to be the po route. But the order needs to be clarified.

5. Could any of the pills be safely crushed and mixed with a food or drink? Is there a liquid form of the medication available? Is there another route available to administer the medications? For example, Famotidine (Pepcid) also can be given intravenously.

Chapter 5

Calculations

1.

Formula Method	Proportion	Dimensional Analysis
$$\frac{40 \text{ mg}}{10 \text{ mg}} \times 1 \text{ mL} = 4 \text{ mL}$$	**EXPRESSED AS TWO RATIOS** 1 mL : 10 mg : : x : 40 mg **EXPRESSED AS TWO FRACTIONS** $$\frac{1 \text{ mL}}{10 \text{ mg}} \times \frac{x}{40 \text{ mg}}$$ **SOLUTION FOR BOTH PROPORTION METHODS** $$40 = 10x$$ $$\frac{40}{10} = x$$ $$4 \text{ mL} = x$$	$$\frac{1 \text{ mL}}{10 \text{ mg}} \Bigg| \frac{\overset{4}{40} \text{ mg}}{1} = 4 \text{ mL}$$

2.

Formula Method	Proportion	Dimensional Analysis
$$\frac{2500 \text{ units}}{5000 \text{ units}} \times 1 \text{ mL} = x$$ $$0.5 \text{ mL} = x$$	**EXPRESSED AS TWO RATIOS** 1 mL : 5000 units : : x : 2500 units **EXPRESSED AS TWO FRACTIONS** $$\frac{1 \text{ mL}}{5000 \text{ units}} \times \frac{x}{2500 \text{ units}}$$ **SOLUTION FOR BOTH PROPORTION METHODS** $$2500 = 5000x$$ $$\frac{2500}{5000} = x$$ $$0.5 \text{ mL} = x$$	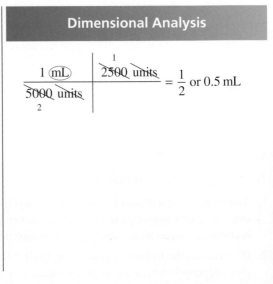

$$\frac{1 \text{ mL}}{\underset{2}{5000 \text{ units}}} \Bigg| \frac{\overset{1}{2500} \text{ units}}{} = \frac{1}{2} \text{ or } 0.5 \text{ mL}$$

3.

Formula Method	Proportion	Dimensional Analysis
$\dfrac{8000 \text{ units}}{20{,}000 \text{ units}} \times 1 \text{ mL} = x$ $0.4 \text{ mL} = x$	**EXPRESSED AS TWO RATIOS** $1 \text{ mL} : 20{,}000 \text{ units} : : x : 8000 \text{ units}$ **EXPRESSED AS TWO FRACTIONS** $\dfrac{1 \text{ mL}}{20{,}000 \text{ units}} \times \dfrac{x}{8000 \text{ units}}$ **SOLUTION FOR BOTH PROPORTION METHODS** $8000 = 20{,}000x$ $\dfrac{8000}{20{,}000} = x$ $0.4 \text{ mL} = x$	$\dfrac{1 \text{ mL}}{20{,}000 \text{ units}} \left| \dfrac{8000 \text{ units}}{} \right. = \dfrac{8}{20} = 0.4 \text{ mL}$

4. Yes, give insulin if blood glucose >150.

$$\frac{200-50}{20} = \frac{150}{20} = 7.5 \text{ units}$$

Round to 8 units.

5.

Formula Method	Proportion	Dimensional Analysis
$\dfrac{\overset{4}{\cancel{100}} \text{ mg}}{\underset{5}{\cancel{125}} \text{ mg}} \times 2 \text{ mL} = x$ $\dfrac{8}{5} = x$ $1.6 \text{ mL} = x$	**EXPRESSED AS TWO RATIOS** $2 \text{ mL} : 125 \text{ mg} : : x : 100 \text{ mg}$ **EXPRESSED AS TWO FRACTIONS** $\dfrac{2 \text{ mL}}{125 \text{ mg}} \times \dfrac{x}{100 \text{ mg}}$ **SOLUTION FOR BOTH PROPORTION METHODS** $2 \times 100 = 125x$ $\dfrac{200}{125} = x$ $1.6 \text{ mL} = x$	$\dfrac{2 \text{ mL}}{\underset{5}{\cancel{125}} \text{ mg}} \left| \dfrac{\overset{4}{\cancel{100}} \text{ mg}}{} \right. = \dfrac{8}{5} = 1.6 \text{ mL}$

6.

Formula Method	Proportion	Dimensional Analysis
$\dfrac{12.5 \text{ mg}}{25 \text{ mg}} \times 1 \text{ mL} = x$ $0.5 \text{ mL} = x$	**EXPRESSED AS TWO RATIOS** $1 \text{ mL} : 25 \text{ mg} :: x : 12.5 \text{ mg}$ **EXPRESSED AS TWO FRACTIONS** $\dfrac{1 \text{ mL}}{25 \text{ mg}} \times \dfrac{x \text{ mL}}{12.5 \text{ mg}}$ **SOLUTION FOR BOTH PROPORTION METHODS** $12.5 = 25x$ $\dfrac{12.5}{25} = x$ $0.5 \text{ mL} = x$	$\dfrac{1 \text{ mL}}{25 \text{ mg}} \mid \dfrac{12.5 \text{ mg}}{} = \dfrac{1}{2} \text{ or } 0.5 \text{ mL}$

7. Vasotec should be administered.

Formula Method	Proportion	Dimensional Analysis
$\dfrac{0.625 \text{ mg}}{1.25 \text{ mg}} \times 1 \text{ mL} = x$ $0.5 \text{ mL} = x$	**EXPRESSED AS TWO RATIOS** $1 \text{ mL} : 1.25 \text{ mg} :: x : 0.625 \text{ mg}$ **EXPRESSED AS TWO FRACTIONS** $\dfrac{1 \text{ mL}}{1.25 \text{ mg}} \times \dfrac{x}{0.625 \text{ mg}}$ **SOLUTION FOR BOTH PROPORTION METHODS** $0.625 \text{ mg} = 1.25x$ $\dfrac{0.625}{1.25} = x$ $0.5 \text{ mL} = x$	$\dfrac{1 \text{ mL}}{1.25 \text{ mg}} \mid \dfrac{0.625 \text{ mg}}{} = \dfrac{0.625}{1.25} = 0.5 \text{ mL}$

8. 1 g = 1000 mg

Formula Method	Proportion	Dimensional Analysis
$\dfrac{\overset{2}{1000} \text{ mg}}{\underset{1}{500} \text{ mg}} \times 1 \text{ mL} = x$ $2 \text{ mL} = x$	**EXPRESSED AS TWO RATIOS** $1 \text{ mL} : 500 \text{ mg} :: x : 1000 \text{ mg}$ **EXPRESSED AS TWO FRACTIONS** $\dfrac{1 \text{ mL}}{500 \text{ mg}} \times \dfrac{x}{1000 \text{ mg}}$ **SOLUTION FOR BOTH PROPORTION METHODS** $1000 = 500x$ $\dfrac{1000}{500} = x$ $2 \text{ mL} = x$	Use conversion factor 1000 mg/1 g: $\dfrac{1 \text{ mL}}{500 \text{ mg}} \mid \dfrac{1 \text{ g}}{} \mid \dfrac{\overset{2}{1000} \text{ mg}}{1 \text{ g}} = 2 \text{ mL}$

Critical Thinking Questions

The "answers" are suggested, and there may be other correct comments, suggestions, and answers.

1. IV push drugs must be reconstituted and/or diluted according to manufacturer directions and institutional guidelines. IV push drugs must be administered over a certain amount of time as specified in manufacturer directions and/or institutional guidelines. IV push drugs are given through a patent and intact IV site. During administration, if the IV site appears infiltrated, the administration is stopped and further assessment completed.

2. Insulin calculations must be checked with another licensed personnel (in most institutions). This is to ensure accuracy in calculation and preparation. Care should be taken to read the formula correctly, as often the formulas vary from institution to institution and patient/client to patient/client, and even varies with one patient/client depending on the insulin protocol.

   Administration precautions include making sure the correct route is used (only regular insulin can be given IV) and choosing a site according to insulin administration guidelines. (See Chapter 10 or any nursing pharmacology textbook.)

3. Insulin dosages can be miscalculated as with any drug. "U" must be written as "units" per the Joint Commission's "do not use" abbreviations list because the "u" can be mistaken for a number. If the sliding scale formula changes (as it often does depending on the patient/client's glucose level), then care must be taken to use the new formula and calculate the new dose correctly. Most institutions require a "double-check" with two licensed personnel.

4. Heparin dosages can be miscalculated as with any drug. "U" must be written as units per the Joint Commission's "do not use" abbreviations list because the "u" can be mistaken for a number. Heparin comes in two different strengths, 10,000 units in 1 mL and 1000 units in 1 mL, and these are often mistaken because the vials are very similar. Many institutions require two licensed personnel to double check the heparin dose.

5. Type 2 diabetics often experience higher glucose levels and more variance of their glucose level in the hospital because it is a more stressful situation physically and emotionally, increasing the glucocorticoids in their body and therefore raising their blood glucose. This patient is also on methylprednisolone (Solu-Medrol), and any exogenous steroid will raise blood glucose.

6. Phenergan should be held because it is listed under the patient's drug allergies. The patient/client has a history of renal cell carcinoma and nephrectomy—an assessment of renal function needs to be done. Medications that may need to be given in a lower dose would include furosemide (Lasix) and vancomycin. These two drugs may also need to be given at separate times because of the renal involvement. The PTT needs to be checked to determine the safe dose of heparin.

Chapter 6

Calculations

1. $$\frac{100 \text{ mL} \times 60 \text{ gtt}}{60 \text{ minutes}} = 100 \text{ gtt/minute}$$

$$\frac{100 \text{ mL} \times \overset{1}{20} \text{ gtt}}{\underset{3}{60} \text{ minutes}} = \frac{100}{3} = 33.33 \text{ or } 33 \text{ gtt/minute}$$

2. $$\frac{100 \text{ mL} \times \overset{2}{60} \text{ gtt}}{\underset{1}{30} \text{ minutes}} = 200 \text{ gtt/minute}$$

$$\frac{100 \text{ mL} \times 20 \text{ gtt}}{30 \text{ minutes}} = \frac{200}{3} = 66.66 \text{ or } 67 \text{ gtt/minute}$$

3. $\dfrac{50 \text{ mL} \times \overset{2}{\cancel{60}} \text{ gtt}}{\underset{1}{\cancel{30}} \text{ minutes}} = 100 \text{ gtt/minute}$

(*Guidelines:* Infuse 50 mL over 30 minutes if no direction is given.)

$\dfrac{50 \text{ mL} \times \overset{}{\cancel{15}} \text{ gtt}}{\underset{2}{\cancel{30}} \text{ minutes}} = \dfrac{50}{2} = 25 \text{ gtt/minute}$

4. $\dfrac{1000 \text{ mL}}{40 \text{ mL}} = 25 \text{ hours}$ (hospital policy usually requires a fluid bag change every 24 hours)

5.
Gentamicin	100 mL (daily) (over 1 hour)	
Cubicin	100 mL (daily) (over 30 minutes)	
Zosyn	50 mL (over 30 minutes)	
	$\times$ 4 (6 hours = 4 doses)	
	200 mL (30 minutes ×4 = 2 hours)	

NS   40 mL/hour × 20.5 hours
(24 hours − 3.5 hours that
antibiotics are running)

$\begin{array}{r} 40 \text{ mL/hour} \\ \times\, 20.5 \text{ hour} \\ \hline 820 \text{ mL} \end{array}$

Total intake: Total IVPB = 400 mL

820 mL primary IV fluid + 400 mL IVPB fluid = 1220 mL

Critical Thinking Questions

The "answers" are suggested, and there may be other correct comments, suggestions, and answers.

1. The patient complains of nausea and vomiting. The po medications may be held and/or another route substituted (check with physician or healthcare provider for an order). Lisinopril (Prinivil) and nifedipine (Procardia) should be held because of the low blood pressure and physician or healthcare provider notified.

2. Each antibiotic works against different organisms (note the suffixes in the names—cillin, -mycin, -micin—they are each a different category of anti-infective). The cause of the infection may not be known yet (usually dependent on the results of cultures), so the three antibiotics together would kill most bacteria. After the cause of the infection is known, then perhaps only one antibiotic would be used.

3. 40 mL × 6 hours = 240 mL. The IV solution may not be infusing at the correct rate due to miscalculation of rate (if using gtt/minute) or setting the wrong rate on the infusion pump. If the infusion is running by gravity, then the patient's position can affect the flow rate. If the patient only has one IV infusion site, then the primary fluid (NS) will be stopped when the antibiotics are infusing. The nurse should not try to "catch up" unless there is a specific order to change or increase the rate.

4. Yes, the dose is 20 mg. The order reads "For doses over 10 mg, must be IVPB." Mix in 50 mL and give over 30 minutes. (If direction is not given as to amount and rate, use 50 mL as a minimum amount over 30 minutes.)

Chapter 7

Calculations

1. 30 mg in 500 mL D5W

$\dfrac{30 \text{ mg}}{500 \text{ mL}} = 0.06 \text{ mg/mL}$

$0.06 \text{ mg} \times 1000 \text{ mcg} = 60 \text{ mcg/mL}$

2. Dose 100 mcg/minute

$100 \text{ mcg} \times 60 \text{ minute} = 6000 \text{ mcg/hour}$

Formula Method	Proportion	Dimensional Analysis
$\dfrac{\overset{100}{\cancel{6000} \text{ mcg}}}{\underset{1}{\cancel{60} \text{ mcg}}} \times 1 \text{ mL}$ $= 100 \text{ mL/hour}$	**EXPRESSED AS TWO RATIOS** $1 \text{ mL} : 60 \text{ mcg} :: x : 6000 \text{ mcg}$ **EXPRESSED AS TWO FRACTIONS** $\dfrac{1 \text{ mL}}{60 \text{ mcg}} \times \dfrac{x}{6000 \text{ mcg}}$ **SOLUTION FOR BOTH PROPORTION METHODS** $6000 = 60x$ $\dfrac{6000}{60} = x$ $100 \text{ mL/hour} = x$	Use conversion factors: 60 minutes/1 hour 1 mg/1000 mcg (combines # 1 and # 2) $\dfrac{\overset{1}{\cancel{500}} \text{ mL}}{\underset{1}{\cancel{30} \text{ mg}}} \left| \dfrac{100 \text{ mcg}}{\text{minutes}} \right| \dfrac{\overset{\overset{1}{\cancel{2}}}{\cancel{60} \text{ minutes}}}{1 \text{ hour}} \left| \dfrac{1 \text{ mg}}{\underset{\underset{1}{2}}{\cancel{1000} \text{ mcg}}} \right.$ $= 100 \text{ mL/hour}$

Set the pump at 100 mL/hour.

3. $\dfrac{4 \text{ mg}}{500 \text{ mL}} = 0.008 \text{ mg/mL}$

$0.008 \text{ mg} \times 1000 \text{ mcg} = 8 \text{ mcg/mL}$

4. Dose: 0.5 mcg/minute

$0.5 \times 60 \text{ minutes} = 30 \text{ mcg/minute}$

Formula Method	Proportion	Dimensional Analysis
$\dfrac{30 \text{ mcg}}{8 \text{ mcg}} \times 1 \text{ mL} = 3.75 \text{ mL}$ or 4 mL/hour	**EXPRESSED AS TWO RATIOS** $1 \text{ mL} : 8 \text{ mcg} :: x : 30 \text{ mcg}$ **EXPRESSED AS TWO FRACTIONS** $\dfrac{1 \text{ mL}}{8 \text{ mcg}} \times \dfrac{x}{30 \text{ mcg}}$ **SOLUTION FOR BOTH PROPORTION METHODS** $30 = 8x$ $\dfrac{30}{8} = x$ 3.75 or 4 mL/hour $= x$	Use conversion factors: 60 minutes/1 hour 1 mg/1000 mcg (combines # 1 and # 2) $\dfrac{\overset{1}{\cancel{500}} \text{ mL}}{\underset{1}{\cancel{4} \text{ mg}}} \left| \dfrac{0.5 \text{ mcg}}{\text{minutes}} \right| \dfrac{\overset{15}{\cancel{60} \text{ minutes}}}{1 \text{ hour}} \left| \dfrac{1 \text{ mg}}{\underset{2}{\cancel{1000} \text{ mcg}}} \right.$ $= \dfrac{0.5 \times 15}{2} = 3.75 \text{ or } 4 \text{ mL/hour}$

Set the pump at 3.75 or 4 mL/hour.

5. 12 units/kg/hour

$12 \text{ units} \times 90 \text{ kg} = 1080 \text{ units/hour}$

6.

Formula Method	Proportion	Dimensional Analysis
	EXPRESSED AS TWO RATIOS	(combines # 5 and # 6)

Formula Method:

$$\frac{1080 \text{ units}}{25{,}000 \text{ units}} \times 500 \text{ mL}$$

$$= 21.6 \text{ mL/hour}$$
$$\text{or } 22 \text{ mL/hour}$$

Proportion:

EXPRESSED AS TWO RATIOS

$$500 \text{ mL} : 25{,}000 \text{ units} :: x : 1080 \text{ units}$$

EXPRESSED AS TWO FRACTIONS

$$\frac{500 \text{ mL}}{25{,}000 \text{ units}} \times \frac{1 \text{ mL}}{1080 \text{ units}}$$

SOLUTION FOR BOTH PROPORTION METHODS

$$500 \times 1080 = 25{,}000x$$

$$\frac{500 \times 1080}{25{,}000} = x$$

$$21.6 \text{ or } 22 \text{ mL/hour} = x$$

Dimensional Analysis:

$$\frac{500 \text{ mL}}{25{,}000 \text{ units}} \left| \frac{12 \text{ units}}{\text{kg/hour}} \right| \frac{90 \text{ kg}}{} = \frac{12 \times 9}{5}$$

$$= 21.6 \text{ or } 22 \text{ mL/hour}$$

Set the pump at 21.6 or 22 mL/hour; next PTT is due in 6 hours.

7.

Formula Method	Proportion	Dimensional Analysis

Formula Method:

$$\frac{x}{100 \text{ mL}} \times 1 \text{ mL} = 10 \text{ mg/mL}$$

$$\frac{x}{100} \times 100 = 10 \times 100$$

$$x = 1000 \text{ mg}$$

Proportion:

EXPRESSED AS TWO RATIOS

$$x : 100 \text{ mL} :: 10 \text{ mg} : 1 \text{ mL}$$

EXPRESSED AS TWO FRACTIONS

$$\frac{10 \text{ mg}}{1 \text{ mL}} \times \frac{x \text{ mg}}{100 \text{ mL}}$$

SOLUTION FOR BOTH PROPORTION METHODS

$$10 \times 100 = 1x$$

$$1000 \text{ mg} = x$$

Dimensional Analysis:

$$\frac{10 \text{ mg}}{1 \text{ mL}} \left| \frac{100 \text{ mL}}{} \right| \frac{10 \times 100}{} = 1000 \text{ mg}$$

8a. Order: 5 mcg/kg/minute

5 mcg × 90 kg = 450 mcg/minute

Step 1: $\dfrac{1000 \text{ mg}}{100 \text{ mL}} = 10$ mg in 1 mL

Step 2: 10 mg × 1000 = 10,000 mcg in 1 mL

Step 3: Divide by 60 to get micrograms per minute:
$$\frac{10{,}000}{60} = 166.67 \text{ mcg/minute}$$

Step 4: Solve. Round to the nearest whole number.

Formula Method	Proportion	Dimensional Analysis

Formula Method

$$\frac{450 \text{ mcg/minute}}{166.67 \text{ mcg/minute}} \times 1 \text{ mL}$$
$$= 2.69 \text{ mL or 3 mL/hour}$$

Proportion

EXPRESSED AS TWO RATIOS

1 mL : 166.67 mcg/minute : : x : 450 mcg/minute

EXPRESSED AS TWO FRACTIONS

$$\frac{1 \text{ mL}}{166.67 \text{ mcg/minute}} \times \frac{x}{450 \text{ mcg/minute}}$$

SOLUTION FOR BOTH PROPORTION METHODS

$$450 = 166.67x$$

$$\frac{450}{166.67} = x$$

2.69 mL or 3 mL/hour = x

Dimensional Analysis

Use conversion factors:

60 minutes/1 hour

1 mg/1000 mcg

(combines all steps)

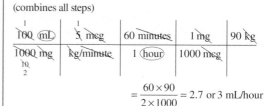

$$= \frac{60 \times 90}{2 \times 1000} = 2.7 \text{ or 3 mL/hour}$$

Set the pump at 2.69 or 3 mL/hour.

8b. Order: 50 mcg/kg/minute

50 mcg × 90 kg = 4500 mcg/minute

(Steps 1 to 4 unchanged)

Formula Method	Proportion	Dimensional Analysis

Formula Method

$$\frac{4500 \text{ mcg/minute}}{166.67 \text{ mcg/minute}} \times 1 \text{ mL}$$
$$= 26.99 \text{ or 27 mL/hour}$$

Proportion

EXPRESSED AS TWO RATIOS

1 mL : 166.67 mcg/minute : : x : 4500 mcg/minute

EXPRESSED AS TWO FRACTIONS

$$\frac{1 \text{ mL}}{166.67 \text{ mcg/minute}} \times \frac{x}{4500 \text{ mcg/minute}}$$

SOLUTION FOR BOTH PROPORTION METHODS

$$4500 = 166.67x$$

$$\frac{4500}{166.67} = x$$

26.99 or 27 mL/hour

Dimensional Analysis

Use conversion factors:

60 minutes/1 hour

1 mg/1000 mcg

(combines all steps)

$$= \frac{6 \times 9}{2} = 27 \text{ mL/hour}$$

Set the pump at 26.99 or 27 mL/hour.

Critical Thinking Questions

The "answers" are suggested, and there may be other correct comments, suggestions, and answers.

1. The medication dosages may need to be adjusted based on the patient/client's renal failure. Also, the dosages and/or administration times may be adjusted based on when the patient/client receives dialysis.

2. The two vasopressors are different medications and have different actions (Neo-Synephrine is an alpha-adrenergic agonist; Levophed is an alpha-adrenergic agonist and beta1-adrenergic agonist), but the end result is to raise the blood pressure. Different doses of different medications may work better, and different patient/clients react differently.

3. The patient/client is intubated, and there are no immediate plans to extubate her because of her serious medical condition. Diprivan will sedate and allow the patient/client to rest on the ventilator. The sedation will also help to decrease oxygen demand on the heart, thereby helping the cardiomyopathy and overall improving the medical condition.

4. A calcium channel blocker such as nifedipine may help atrial fibrillation, but the patient/client is allergic to calcium channel blockers.

5. The two vasopressors may be causing the increased heart rate because of their affect on the alpha and beta receptors.

6. IV push drugs are given slowly to infuse the amount of drug concentration given over a longer time. This may be to prevent side effects—in this case with Protonix, to prevent nausea.

Chapter 8

Calculations

1a. Dose: 20 mg

Formula Method	Proportion	Dimensional Analysis
$\dfrac{\overset{1}{\cancel{20\text{ mg}}}}{\underset{1}{\cancel{20\text{ mg}}}} \times 1\text{ mL} = 1\text{ mL}$	**EXPRESSED AS TWO RATIOS** $1\text{ mL} : 20\text{ mg} :: x : 20\text{ mg}$ **EXPRESSED AS TWO FRACTIONS** $\dfrac{1\text{ mL}}{20\text{ mg}} \times \dfrac{x}{20\text{ mg}}$ **SOLUTION FOR BOTH PROPORTION METHODS** $20 = 20x$ $\dfrac{20}{20} = x$ $1\text{ mL} = x$	$\dfrac{1\ \text{mL}}{\underset{1}{\cancel{20\text{ mg}}}} \left| \dfrac{\overset{1}{\cancel{20\text{ mg}}}}{} \right. = 1\text{ mL}$

1b. Dose: 10 mg

Formula Method	Proportion	Dimensional Analysis
$\dfrac{\overset{1}{\cancel{10\text{ mg}}}}{\underset{2}{\cancel{20\text{ mg}}}} \times 1\text{ mL} = \dfrac{1}{2}\text{ or } 0.5\text{ mL}$	**EXPRESSED AS TWO RATIOS** $1\text{ mL} : 20\text{ mg} :: x : 10\text{ mg}$ **EXPRESSED AS TWO FRACTIONS** $\dfrac{1\text{ mL}}{20\text{ mg}} \times \dfrac{x}{10\text{ mg}}$ **SOLUTION FOR BOTH PROPORTION METHODS** $10 = 20x$ $\dfrac{10}{20} = x$ $\dfrac{1}{2}\text{ or } 0.5\text{ mL} = x$	$\dfrac{1\ \text{mL}}{\underset{2}{\cancel{20\text{ mg}}}} \left| \dfrac{\overset{1}{\cancel{10\text{ mg}}}}{} \right. = \dfrac{1}{2}\text{ or } 0.5\text{ mL}$

2a. Dose: 400 mg

Formula Method	Proportion	Dimensional Analysis
$\dfrac{400 \text{ mg}}{160 \text{ mg}} \times \overset{1}{5} \text{ mL} = \dfrac{400}{32}$ $= 12.5 \text{ mL}$	**EXPRESSED AS TWO RATIOS** 5 mL : 160 mg : : x : 400 mg **EXPRESSED AS TWO FRACTIONS** $\dfrac{5 \text{ mL}}{160 \text{ mg}} \times \dfrac{x}{400 \text{ mL}}$ **SOLUTION FOR BOTH PROPORTION METHODS** $5 \times 400 = 160x$ $\dfrac{2000}{160} = x$ $12.5 \text{ mL} = x$	Use conversion factor 1 tsp/5 mL: (combines both steps) $\dfrac{1 \text{ tsp}}{5 \text{ mL}} \ \bigg| \ \dfrac{5 \text{ mL}}{160 \text{ mg}} \ \bigg| \ \dfrac{400 \text{ mg}}{} = \dfrac{40}{16} = 2.5 \text{ or } 2\frac{1}{2} \text{ tsp}$

2b. 12.5 mL = how many teaspoons

   1 tsp = 5 mL

Formula Method	Proportion	Dimensional Analysis
$\dfrac{12.5 \text{ mL}}{5 \text{ mL}} \times 1 \text{ tsp} = 2.5 \text{ tsp}$	**EXPRESSED AS TWO RATIOS** 1 tsp : 5 mL : : x : 12.5 mL **EXPRESSED AS TWO FRACTIONS** $\dfrac{1 \text{ tsp}}{5 \text{ mL}} \times \dfrac{x}{12.5 \text{ mL}}$ **SOLUTION FOR BOTH PROPORTION METHODS** $12.5 = 5x$ $\dfrac{12.5}{5} = x$ $2.5 \text{ tsp or } 2\frac{1}{2} \text{ tsp} = x$	See above for dimensional analysis method.

3. 5 mg/kg

   5 × 30 = 150 mg

Formula Method	Proportion	Dimensional Analysis
$\dfrac{150 \text{ mg}}{100 \text{ mg}} \times \overset{1}{5} \text{ mL} = 7.5 \text{ mL}$	**EXPRESSED AS TWO RATIOS** 5 mL : 100 mg : : x : 150 mg **EXPRESSED AS TWO FRACTIONS** $\dfrac{5 \text{ mL}}{100 \text{ mg}} \times \dfrac{x}{150 \text{ mg}}$ **SOLUTION FOR BOTH PROPORTION METHODS** $5 \times 150 = 100x$ $\dfrac{750}{100} = x$ $7.5 \text{ mL} = x$	(combines all steps) $\dfrac{5 \text{ mL}}{100 \text{ mg}} \ \bigg| \ \dfrac{5 \text{ mg}}{\text{kg}} \ \bigg| \ \dfrac{30 \text{ kg}}{} = \dfrac{150}{20} = 7.5 \text{ mL}$

4. Dose: 2 g = 2000 mg

Formula Method	Proportion	Dimensional Analysis
$\dfrac{\overset{40}{\cancel{2000}\text{ mg}}}{\underset{1}{\cancel{50}\text{ mg}}} \times 1\text{ mL} = 40\text{ mL}$	**EXPRESSED AS TWO RATIOS** 1 mL : 50 mg :: x : 2000 mg **EXPRESSED AS TWO FRACTIONS** $\dfrac{1\text{ mL}}{50\text{ mg}} \times \dfrac{x}{2000\text{ mg}}$ **SOLUTION FOR BOTH PROPORTION METHODS** $2000 = 50x$ $\dfrac{2000}{50} = x$ $40\text{ mL} = x$	Use conversion factor 1000 mg/1 g: $\dfrac{1\;\cancel{\text{mL}}}{\underset{1}{\cancel{50}\text{ mg}}} \left| \dfrac{2\;\cancel{\text{g}}}{} \right| \dfrac{\overset{20}{\cancel{1000}\text{ mg}}}{1\;\cancel{\text{g}}} = 20 \times 2 = 40\text{ mL}$

Infuse over 30 minutes. Set the pump at 80 mL/hour. The pump will deliver 40 mL in 30 minutes. Follow directions to infuse via Buretrol.

5. 0.72 mg × BSA

= 0.72 × 0.9 = 0.648 mg

6. Dose = 150 mg

Formula Method	Proportion	Dimensional Analysis
$\dfrac{150\;\cancel{\text{mg}}}{125\;\cancel{\text{mg}}} \times 5\text{ mL} = \dfrac{750}{125}$ $= 6\text{ mL}$	**EXPRESSED AS TWO RATIOS** 5 mL : 125 mg :: x : 150 mg **EXPRESSED AS TWO FRACTIONS** $\dfrac{5\text{ mL}}{125\text{ mg}} \times \dfrac{x}{150\text{ mg}}$ **SOLUTION FOR BOTH PROPORTION METHODS** $750 = 125x$ $\dfrac{750}{125} = x$ $6\text{ mL} = x$	$\dfrac{5\;\cancel{\text{mL}}}{\underset{5}{\cancel{125}\text{ mg}}} \left| \dfrac{\overset{6}{\cancel{150}\text{ mg}}}{} \right. = \dfrac{30}{5} = 6\text{ mL}$

7. 0.1 mg/kg = 0.1 × 30 = 3 mg. The dose is safe.

8. 10 mL/kg/hour = 10 × 30 = 300 mL for 1 hour

Critical Thinking Questions

The "answers" are suggested, and there may be other correct comments, suggestions, and answers.

1. Hold (and discontinue) the Augmentin—it contains amoxicillin and the patient/client is allergic to penicillin. Check with the physician or healthcare provider about giving ceftazidime (Fortaz)—sometimes the patient/client will have a cross-sensitivity to other antibiotics if allergic to penicillin, especially cephalosporins, which is the classification for Fortaz.

2. Digoxin is ordered, and there does not seem to be a medical condition that warrants the order. There may be a medical history of a cardiac condition that the nurse is unaware of. Check with the physician or healthcare provider. Ondansetron (Zofran) is usually not prescribed prn for children 6 months to 8 years. It is prescribed mainly for postoperative nausea/vomiting or prevention of chemotherapy-induced nausea/vomiting. Check with the physician or healthcare provider who ordered the ondansetron (Zofran) dose.

3. The po route may be difficult given the history of "flulike" symptoms and no food and minimal drink for 28 hours. Check if any of the medications can be given via another route (need to have the physician or healthcare provider order a different route). If the patient/client has decreased nausea, check to see if the medications can be given in a liquid form.

4. The amount to be infused is 300 mL for 1 hour. Although this is a large dose of fluid for a child, the child's condition (no food and minimal drink for 48 hours) may warrant the fluid in order to prevent further dehydration. The 100 mL/hour is also a higher dose but again may be needed for the child's condition. Close monitoring of the infusion is needed.

Chapter 9

Critical Thinking Questions

The "answers" are suggested, and there may be other correct comments, suggestions, and answers.

A. The nurse's responsibility is to inform the patient/client of information pertinent to the drug and the drug study. There are set guidelines provided by the FDA and the drug manufacturer that guide the nurse and other healthcare professionals in being part of a drug study. The patient/client must give informed consent. The nurse, ethically, cannot interject his or her opinion regarding the drug or drug study.

B. Again, guidelines from the FDA and drug manufacturer should be followed when patients/clients ask questions such as, "Is it safe to take this drug?" Oftentimes, there may be an assigned person (associated with the research study) to answer questions such as this or a website. The nurse should direct the patient/client to these resources. If the patient/client refuses to take the drug, the nurse should note this with accurate documentation.

C. Ethically, there are several principles that may guide a response. Beneficence, nonmaleficence, and truthfulness are some of the principles that may guide a response. The principle of autonomy may ultimately be the most important because it is the patient/client's decision whether to take the experimental drug and/or participate in the drug study. Legally, a nurse's actions are based on his or her job responsibilities and how they are defined. If a practice setting utilizes research on a regular basis, the nurse is expected to participate even if beliefs are different.

D. The nurse could ask the patient/client for more information; direct the patient/client to the physician, healthcare provider, or resource person regarding the drug study; or research the drugs involved with available resources. The patient/client needs to look at the website as to its reliability and ask questions such as Who is the author of the website? What is the site's origin? When the site was last updated? What is the purpose of the website? What is evidence that the information on the site is accurate and current?

E. Guidelines from answer C may be addressed. Autonomy is still the principle to emphasize—that it is the patient/client's decision whether to proceed in the drug study.

F. Drug studies are used to determine the effectiveness of the drug and the safety of the drug. By participation, the drug may benefit the patient/client directly (i.e., provide treatment for a disorder) or may benefit others in the long term. Although serious side and adverse effects will hopefully be avoided, the side effects experienced by participants will help to determine the safety of the drug for future use.

Chapter 10

Critical Thinking Questions

The "answers" are suggested, and there may be other correct comments, suggestions, and answers.

A. The deltoid may be used if there is any contraindication to using the other two sites. Some of the contraindications may be surgery in those areas, thereby increasing the sensitivity, or increase in scar tissue; lack of adequate muscle in those areas; and other tissue damage in those areas (i.e., pressure ulcers, bruising, and swelling). Patient/client preference can be considered. Contraindications to the deltoid muscle include the same; plus, any injection of more than 2 mL (some texts say no more than 1 mL) should not be given in the deltoid.

B. The nurse can share the information from the drug literature as to the preferred site. If there are no other contraindications, the nurse may give the shot in the deltoid.

C. Either site may be used, although using the vastus lateralis site may be easier in positioning the patient/client. Also, if the patient/client is incontinent, the vastus lateralis may be a cleaner site.

D. There is always a possibility of body fluids being introduced when administering an IM shot (blood or interstitial fluid).

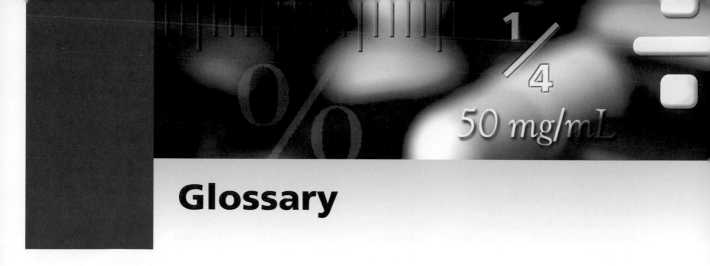

Glossary

Absorption   passing of a drug in the body across tissue into the general circulation, so that the drug becomes active in the body

ac   before meals

ad lib   as desired

ADD-Vantage system   method of reconstitution in which the powdered form of the drug is in a special container attached to the IV fluid. The nurse opens the container and mixes the IV fluid with the powder, so that the system remains closed and sterile.

Adverse effects   nontherapeutic effects that may be harmful

Aerosol   method of drug administration in which the solid drug is delivered in a liquid spray

Agonist   drug that binds with cell receptors to invoke a cellular response, usually similar to the cell's action

Allergic reaction   reaction to a drug involving the body's antibody response to a perceived antigen (in this case, the medication)

Ampule (ampoule)   sealed glass container for powdered or liquid drugs

Amt   amount

Analgesic   drug to relieve or minimize pain

Anaphylactic shock   severe allergic reaction that results in a shock state

Anaphylaxis   severe allergic reaction

Antagonism   interaction between two drugs in which the combined effect is less than the sum of the effects of the drugs acting separately

Antagonist   drug that binds with cell receptors to block the cellular response

Antibiotic   drug that inhibits or kills bacteria, fungi, or protozoans

Anticoagulant   drug that inhibits formation of blood clots

Antiemetic   drug that prevents vomiting and reduces nausea

Antihypertensive   drug that lowers blood pressure

Antitussive   drug used to suppress coughing

Anxiolytic   drug that relieves anxiety

Apothecary system   measurement system using grains and minims, introduced into the United States from England in colonial times

Aqueous suspension   medication or solution prepared with water

Arabic numbers   the numerals 1,2,3,4,5,6,7,8,9,0, as used in arithmetic

AS, AD, AU   left ear, right ear, both ears. The Joint Commission states "DO NOT USE" these abbreviations; instead, write out "left ear," "right ear," or "both ears," as appropriate.

Autonomy   self-determination. The patient/client has a right to be informed about drug therapy and to refuse it.

Avoirdupois system   measurement system using ounces and pounds; used for patient/client weight and some drugs

Bactericidal   drug action that kills an organism

Bacteriostatic   drug action that inhibits an organism's ability to grow and reproduce

Bacteriostatic water   solution used for mixing and dissolving medications; a sterile preparation of water, containing a small amount of benzyl alcohol as a preservative

Bar code   system of vertical bars of varying width on products. It can be laser scanned for information about the product and cost.

Beneficence   an ethical principle; acting in the best interests of the patient/client; "doing good"

bid   twice a day

Bioavailability   availability of a drug once it is absorbed and transported in the body to the site of its action

Biotransformation   conversion of an active drug to an inactive compound

Blister pack or **bubble pack**   drug packaging that seals the drug between clear plastic and cardboard; often used in multipackaging

Body surface area or **BSA**   calculation of meters squared, based on height and weight, as shown in a nomogram

BP   blood pressure

Bronchodilator   drug that dilates the bronchioles of the lungs

Buccal   route of administration in which a drug is placed in the pouch between the teeth and cheek

Buretrol   plastic container, usually 100 to 150 mL in volume, that can be attached to IV tubing and is used to administer medications; also known as Volutrol or Soluset

C   Centigrade, Celsius

Caplet   smooth, oval-shaped, coated tablet

Cap or **capsule**   gelatin container that holds a drug in a solid or liquid form

Cardiac glycoside   drug that increases cardiac contractility and increases cardiac output. Lanoxin (digoxin) is the most commonly used cardiac glycoside.

Carpuject   prefilled, disposable syringe cartridge; also called Tubex

Cartridge   cylindrical device (plastic or glass) containing medication

CC or **cc**   cubic centimeter; equal to 1 mL. The Joint Commission states "DO NOT USE" this abbreviation; instead, use "mL."

CDC   Centers for Disease Control and Prevention

Central or **central IV line**   IV line, introduced through the vein, with the tip ending near the superior vena cava

Chemical name   drug name derived from its chemical structure

Chemotherapy   drug treatment for cancer

Civil law   statutes concerned with the rights and duties of individuals

Clark's Rule   way to determine dosage of medications for children older than 2 years of age; based on weight

cm   centimeter

Combination drugs   drugs that contain more than one active medication

Common factor   number that is a factor of two different numbers (i.e., 3 is a factor of 6 and 9)

Common fraction   fraction with a whole number in the numerator and denominator (i.e., 7/9)

Compliance   taking a medication as prescribed or following label instructions

Computerized medication record   medication administration recording system that is accessed from the computer. Medication recording software programs often have safeguards to reduce medication errors.

Computerized system of medication administration   system of medication administration that coordinates information with a bar code system of verifying patient/client identity and the correct medication

Concentration   amount of drug in a solution, in either fraction, decimal, or percentage form

Continuous infusion   infusion that continually delivers fluids intravenously

Contraindication   situation in which a drug should be avoided

Controlled drug   a drug, controlled by federal, state, and local law, that may lead to drug abuse or dependence

Corticosteroids   hormones that help the body respond to stress; also used in immune response, anti-inflammatory. In the body, the adrenal cortex produces corticosteroids.

CR   controlled release

Cream   semisolid drug preparation applied externally to the skin or mucous membrane

Criminal law   statutes that protect the public against actions harmful to society

Cross tolerance   becoming tolerant to one drug, then acquiring tolerance to another drug; either a similar drug, a drug from a similar category, or a drug with a similar classification

CSF   cerebrospinal fluid

Cumulation or **Accumulation**   inability of the body to metabolize one dose of a drug before another dose is administered; leads to increased concentration of the drug in the body and possible toxicity

d   day

D or **Dextrose**   an IV infusion fluid that contains dextrose (sugar). Common solutions are D5W, which is a solution of 5% dextrose dissolved in water (equals 5 g of dextrose in each 100 mL of water), and D10W, which is a solution of 10% dextrose dissolved in water (equals 10 g of dextrose in each 100 mL of water).

D/C   discharge or discontinue. The Joint Commission states "DO NOT USE" this abbreviation; instead, write out "discharge" or "discontinue" as appropriate.

DEA   U.S. Drug Enforcement Administration

Delayed-release tablet   tablet given by mouth that has a delayed release of its contents and therefore a delay or slowing in drug response or drug action

Denominator   bottom number of a fraction

Dermal route   topical application of a drug to the skin

Diluent   liquid used to dissolve a solid (usually a powder) into a solution

Dilution   making a solution less concentrated or weaker

Dimensional analysis   method of problem solving that allows conversion between different units

Disch   discharge

Displacement   increase in the volume of fluid added to a powder when the powder dissolves and goes into solution

Distribution   movement of a drug through body fluids (chiefly blood) to cells

Dividend   number to be divided (e.g., in "40 divided by 5," 40 is the dividend)

Divisor   number by which the dividend is divided (e.g., in "40 divided by 5," 5 is the divisor)

dL   deciliter, 100 mL

Dose   amount of drug to be given at one time or the total amount to be given

dr   dram; an apothecary measurement rarely used. One fluid dram equals approximately 4 mL.

DR   delayed release

Drip chamber   part of the IV tubing where the IV fluid can be observed dripping. The drops are regulated by observing the drip chamber, counting the number of drops per minute, and adjusting with the roller clamp or other device.

Drip or **Drop factor**   number of drops of an IV fluid in 1 mL; listed on the IV tubing set or package

Drip rate   number of drops of an IV solution to be infused per minute

Drop   tiny sphere of liquid, abbreviated gtt. In the apothecary system (rarely used), 1 drop =1 minim.

Dropper   device to administer fluid; usually a small glass or plastic tube, with a rubber suction bulb on one end, to draw the fluid into the tube

Drug   chemical agent used in the treatment, diagnosis, or prevention of disease

Dry powder inhaler or **DPI**   inhaler that converts a solid drug into a fine powder

Elixir   clear, aromatic, sweetened alcoholic preparation

Emulsion   suspension of a fat or oil in water with the aid of an agent to reduce surface tension

Enteral   refers to the small intestine

Enteral feedings   delivery of liquid feedings through a tube

Enteral route   drugs given orally or through nasogastric (N/G) or percutaneous endoscopic gastrostomy (PEG) tubes

Enteric coating   layer placed over a tablet or capsule to prevent dissolution in the stomach; used to protect the drug from gastric acid or to protect the stomach from drug irritation

Epidural route   medication is administered into the space around the dura mater of the spinal column

ER   extended release

Ethics   system of values and morals

Excretion   physiologic elimination of substances from the body

Expectorant   drug to increase bronchial secretions

Expiration date   date after which a drug cannot be administered; the last day of the month stamped on the label

Extended-release tablet   tablet with a special coating or ingredients that allow it to dissolve in a slower time, thereby extending the drug response and drug action; often abbreviated "XL" (extended length), "LA" (long acting), or "XR" (extended release)

F   Fahrenheit

FDA   U.S. Food and Drug Administration

Fidelity   ethical principle; the nurse or healthcare provider keeps promises made to a patient/client.

Film-coated tablet   compressed, powdered drug that is smooth and easy to swallow because of its outer shell covering

First-pass effect   drugs administered orally that pass from the intestine to the liver and are partially metabolized before entering the circulation

fl. oz.   fluid ounce; equal to 30 mL

Flow rate   number of milliliters per hour of IV fluid to be infused

Fluid extract or **fluidextract**   potent alcoholic liquid concentration of a drug

Formulary reference for pharmacists and other healthcare providers with lists of drugs, drug combinations, and so forth

Fraction division of one number by another

Fried's Rule rule to calculate drug dosages for infants younger than 1 year; based on age

g gram

Gauge diameter or width of a needle; the higher the gauge number, the finer the needle

Gel aqueous suspension of small particles of an insoluble drug in a hydrated form

Gelatin-coated liquid capsule a capsule with liquid medication inside, covered with a gelatin coating to seal and make the capsule one-piece

Generic name official name of a drug as listed in the United States or other pharmacopoeia

Glucocorticoids hormones that help the body respond to stress. In the body, glucocorticoids are manufactured by the adrenal cortex.

gr grain; approximately equal to 60 or 65 mg; an apothecary measure rarely used

Gram weight of 1 mL of water at 4°C; basic unit of weight in the metric system

Gravity infusion using the flow of gravity to infuse fluid intravenously. The flow rate may change depending on how high the IV fluids are placed and the position of the patient/client

gtt drop or drops

gtt/min or **gtt per minute** drops of IV fluid infusing per minute; calculated by observing the number of drops in the drip chamber per minute

G-tube gastrostomy tube; a tube inserted into the stomach that can be used for drug administration and enteral feedings

h or **hr** hour

Half-life time that a drug is metabolized by 50% in the body

Heparin IV or subcutaneous anticoagulant. Most healthcare institutions have a protocol that directs how the heparin is calculated, administered, and monitored. Two licensed nurses must double-check the dosage, to monitor side effects.

Hepatotoxic drug or side effects of a drug that may affect the liver

Hep-Lock venous access device (IV catheter) that remains in place in the vein with a cap or port on the end. The device must be flushed periodically to maintain patency of the vein. Heparin was formerly the drug of choice to flush the device; most institutions now use a normal saline flush.

Household system measurement system based on household items of measurement; uses teaspoon, tablespoon, and cup

hs hour of sleep, at bedtime. The Joint Commission states "DO NOT USE" this abbreviation; instead, write out "at bedtime."

hypo hypodermic syringe or injection

I & O intake and output

Idiosyncratic unexplained or unusual reaction to a drug

IM intramuscular

Improper fraction fraction with the numerator larger or equal to the denominator

Incompatibility mixture of two or more drugs that results in a harmful chemical or physical interaction

Indwelling infusion port implantable port device that is placed for long-term IV therapy, placed subcutaneously, then connected to an IV cannula that is inserted in a central vein and ends in the superior vena cava. Trade names include Port-a-Cath, Infuse-a-Port, Passport.

Infusion pump electronic pump that infuses fluid and/or medication intravenously. The pump can be set to control amount, time, and volume and to measure volume infused. "Smart" pumps can also be programmed to deliver amounts of drug per hour, per minute, and per weight.

Inhalant vapors that are inhaled via the nose, lungs, or trachea

Inhaler device used to spray liquid or powder in a fine mist into the lungs during inspiration

inj injection

Insulin hormone to regulate glucose and energy metabolism; can be given exogenously and is manufactured from beef or pork or synthetically. Most healthcare institutions have a protocol that directs how the insulin is calculated, administered, and monitored. Two licensed nurses must double-check the dosage, to monitor the side effects.

INT intermittent needle device. Same as the Hep-Lock, a venous access device (IV catheter) that remains in place in the vein with a cap or port on the end. The INT must be flushed periodically to maintain patency of the vein; usually, this is with a normal saline flush.

Intake amount of liquid ingested, usually fluids by mouth, IV fluids, or tube feedings

Interaction either desirable or undesirable effects produced by giving two or more drugs together

Intra-articular medication injected into the joints

Intradermal or **ID** injection given into the upper layers of the skin

Intramuscular or **IM** injection given into the muscle

Intrathecal administration into the cerebrospinal fluid via the subarachnoid space

Intravenous or **IV** medication given by injection or infusion into a vein

Isotonic solutions that have the same osmotic pressure as physiologic body fluids

IU international unit. The Joint Commission states "DO NOT USE" this abbreviation; instead, write out "international units."

IV intravenous

IV bolus intravenous bolus of medication or fluid; usually given in a larger amount and infused more rapidly than other infusions

IVP intravenous push of medication or fluid; similar to IV bolus; many medications are given as an IV push; a specific dilution and amount of time to push the medication is given (usually per drug insert or institutional protocol).

IVPB intravenous piggyback; medication placed in an infusion set and attached to the main line IV for delivery to the patient/client

Joint Commission an organization responsible for safety in hospitals and other healthcare settings. In 2004, the Joint Commission issued a list of abbreviations "DO NOT USE" in order to decrease errors.

J-tube tube placed in the jejunum that can be used for drug administration and enteral feedings

Justice ethical principle; all patients/clients receive the same care; and it is the nurse's obligation to provide safe care.

k or **kg** kilogram

Kardex trade name for a card filing system that contains information regarding nursing care of each patient/client. Usually, Kardex is a term used for any system that contains orders and nursing interventions for a patient/client; can be a hard copy or on a computer chart.

Lactated Ringer's solution IV solution containing fluid and electrolytes; used for replacement of losses of fluid and electrolytes, commonly abbreviated "LR." Lactated Ringer's solution, mixed with 5% dextrose, is abbreviated D5LR; it contains dextrose, in addition to the LR solution.

Latex-free infusion set   infusion tubing that is manufactured free of latex, which can cause an allergic reaction in individuals with a latex allergy

lb   pound

Liter or **L**   a unit of fluid volume in the metric system; equal to one tenth of a cubic meter

Loading dose   higher dose given at the initiation of drug therapy in order to build up the therapeutic effect

Lotion   liquid suspension intended for external use

Lot number   number assigned to a drug by the manufacturer

Lowest common denominator   smallest number that is a multiple of all denominators

Lowest terms   smallest numbers possible in the numerator and denominator of a fraction. Reducing a fraction to lowest terms means that the numerator and denominator cannot be reduced further.

Lozenge   flat, round, or rectangular preparation held in the mouth until the medicine dissolves

Luer-Lok syringe   syringe with a special tip that allows a needle or needleless device to lock onto the syringe

Lumen   opening; usually refers to the opening in a needle

Macrodrip chamber, Macrodrip tubing   IV tubing with a drip chamber that has a drip factor from 10 to 20 drops per milliliter. Each manufacturer of IV tubing will specify the drip factor on the tubing or the packaging.

Magma   bulky suspension of an insoluble preparation in water that must be shaken before pouring

mcg   microgram. Previously abbreviated as µg; The Joint Commission recommends "DO NOT USE."

MDI   metered-dose inhaler; an aerosol device that consists of two parts—a canister under pressure and a mouthpiece. Finger pressure on the mouthpiece opens a valve that discharges one dose.

Measuring cup   cup to measure liquid, with markings on the side of the cup showing various measurements, usually household and/or metric markings

Medication   another word for drug; sometimes used to pertain to a drug that has been administered

Medication administration record or **MAR**   documentation of drugs

received by the patient/client or schedule of drugs to be received

Medication cup   cup used to administer medication. The cup may have markings on the side to measure a liquid dose, or it may be a small paper or plastic cup to place pills in before administering to a patient/client.

Medication error   preventable error in medication administration, usually related to one of the six rights (see Chapter 9)

Medication order   order for medication, prescribed by a physician, nurse practitioner, or licensed healthcare prescriber; elements of the order include patient/client name, name of medication, dosage, frequency, and route

Medication ticket   system of administering medication, where the medication is checked with a small ticket that has the medication order written on it. This system is rarely used because of the medication errors associated with transcription and with misplacing tickets.

Meniscus   curved surface of a liquid in a container

Metabolism   chemical biotransformation of a drug to a form that can be excreted

Meter or **m**   unit of length in the metric system; equals 39.27 inches

Metric system   measurement system that uses meters, liters, and grams; common system used worldwide except in the United States. It is a widely used system in dosages of drugs based on units of 10.

mg   milligram

MgSO4   magnesium sulfate. The Joint Commission states "DO NOT USE" this abbreviation; instead, write out "magnesium sulfate," because this abbreviation can be confused with MSO4.

Microdrip chamber, microdrop tubing   IV tubing with a drip chamber that has a drip factor of 60 drops per milliliter.

Military time   time based on a 24-hour clock rather than the traditional 12-hour clock

Milliequivalent or **mEq**   number of grams of solute in a 1-mL solution; used to measure electrolytes and some medications

min   minute

minim   apothecary measure, rarely used, that equals 1/60 of a dram; also equal to one drop

Mixed number   whole number and a fraction (e.g., $1^{11}/_{42}$)

ML or **mL**   milliliter

mm   millimeter

mo   month

MS, MSO4   morphine sulfate. The Joint Commission states "DO NOT USE" this abbreviation; instead, write out "morphine sulfate," because this abbreviation can be confused with MgSO4.

Multidose   large stock containers of medication

Narcotic   natural or synthetic drug related to morphine; or a large classification of drugs that include hallucinogens, central nervous system stimulants, and illegal drugs

Nebulizer   device to convert liquid drugs into a fine mist, to use via an inhaled route

NDC   national drug code; number used by pharmacists to identify a drug and the packaging method

Needle   sterile, stainless steel device used to inject medications into the body or to withdraw blood or other fluids

Needleless infusion system   blunt plastic cannula used on a syringe to pull fluid into the syringe and/or inject fluid through a rubber needleless connector of IV tubing or an INT device

Nephrotoxic   drug or side effects of a drug that may affect the renal system

N/G tube   tube inserted through the nasal opening into the stomach; can be used for drug administration and enteral feedings

Nomogram   tabular illustration of BSA, based on height and weight

Nonmaleficence   ethical principle; to do no harm to the patient/client

Nonparenteral drugs   drugs administered via topical, rectal, or oral route

Nonprescription drug   drug obtained without a prescription; also called over-the-counter or OTC

NPO   nothing by mouth

NS or **Normal saline**   IV infusion fluid that contains sodium chloride. Common solutions include 0.9 NS, which is a solution of 0.9% saline dissolved in water (equals 0.9 g of saline in each 100 mL of water); 0.45% NS, which is a solution of 0.45% saline dissolved in water (equals 0.45 g of saline in each 100 mL of water); and 0.33% NS, which is a solution of 0.33% saline dissolved in water (equals 0.33 g of saline in each 100 mL of water).

Numerator   top number of a fraction

OD   right eye (suggested "DO NOT USE"—write out "right eye")

Official name   drug's official name as listed in the United States Pharmacopeia and the National Formulary

O/G tube   tube inserted through the oral cavity into the stomach; can be used for drug administration and enteral feedings

Ointment semisolid preparation in a petroleum or lanolin base, for external use

Ophthalmic pertaining to the eye

Oral route drugs given through the mouth; abbreviated PO

OS left eye (suggested "DO NOT USE"—instead write out "left eye")

OTC over-the-counter

Otic pertaining to the ear

Ototoxic drug or side effects of a drug that may affect the ear

OU both eyes (suggested "DO NOT USE"—instead write out "both eyes")

Output measurement of amount of body waste, fluid, or drainage (i.e., urine output, stool, etc.)

oz ounce

Parenteral general term that means administration by injection (IV, IM, or subcutaneous)

Paste thick ointment used to protect the skin

Pastille disk-like solid that slowly dissolves in the mouth

Patch small adhesive that releases medication over an extended period of time; applied topically

pc after meals

PCA patient-controlled analgesia, controlled by a special pump that allows the patient/client to self-administer pain medication as needed

PDR *Physician's Desk Reference,* a resource book and online reference that details drug information

PEG tube special type of gastrostomy tube; the abbreviation stands for "percutaneous endoscopic gastrotomy." This tube, designed to be more permanent than other feeding tubes, can be used for drug administration and enteral feedings.

Percentage parts per hundred, designated by a percent sign (%)

Percentage solution a solid dissolved in a liquid that represents a percentage of the total weight of the solution; measured in grams per 100 mL of solution

Peripheral or **Peripheral line** IV line placed in a peripheral vein

Pharmacodynamics study of the chemical and physical effects of drugs in the body

Pharmacogenetics chemical and physical effects in the body to a drug related to a person's genetics

Pharmacokinetics science of the factors that determine how much drug reaches the site of action in the body and is excreted

Pharmacology study of the origin, nature, chemical effects, and uses of drugs

Pharmacopoeia medical reference containing information about drugs

Pharmacotherapeutics study of the use of drugs to treat, prevent, and diagnose diseases

Piggyback medication placed in an IV infusion set attached to the mainline IV, for delivery to the patient/client

Placebo inert substance used in place of a drug to determine the drug's psychological effect and the physiologic changes caused by the psychological response

PO by mouth, oral

Potency strength of a drug at a specific concentration or dose

Powder finely ground solid drug or mixture of drugs for internal or external use

PPN peripheral parenteral nutrition

PR per rectum

Precision syringe 1-mL syringe with an attached small-gauge (G) needle (23G or smaller) that is used to draw up amounts of medication less than 1 mL; also called tuberculin syringe

Prefilled cartridge small vial with an attached needle that fits into a metal or plastic holder for injection

Prefilled syringe liquid, sterile medication that is ready to administer without further preparation

Prepackaged syringe same as prefilled syringe

Prescription order for medication, written by an authorized prescriber

Prescription drug drug that requires a prescription; usually regulated by state laws

Prime number whole number divisible only by 1 and itself; a whole number that cannot be reduced any further (i.e., 3, 5, 7)

PRN as needed

Product answer in multiplication

Prolonged-release or **Slow-release tablet** powdered, compressed drug that disintegrates more slowly and has a longer duration of action

Proper fraction fraction with a numerator smaller than the denominator

Proportion set of ratios or fractions

Proprietary name brand or trade name of a generic medication

Protocol specific set of drug orders referring to certain physical conditions or lab values that must be met before drug administration; also used when titrating certain drugs (i.e., insulin and heparin)

pt patient or pint

Pyxis trade name of an automated system of dispensing medications or supplies. The system keeps track of medications/supplies used and

dispenses them in a secure way, with identification of the nurse and patient/client.

q each, every

q4h every 4 hours

q6h every 6 hours

q8h every 8 hours

q12h every 12 hours

qd every day. The Joint Commission states "DO NOT USE" this abbreviation; instead, write out "every day."

qid four times a day

qod every other day. The Joint Commission states "DO NOT USE" this abbreviation; instead, write out "every other day."

qt quart

Quotient answer in division

Ratio way to compare numbers; the numbers are separated by a colon, such as 1:5, which reads "one is to five."

Reconstitution dissolving a powder to a liquid form

Rectal route or **PR** medication administered through the rectum

Reduce to simplify

Reducing fractions simplifying a fraction so that the numerator and denominator can be divided only by 1. To do this, find the largest number that can divide into the numerator and denominator evenly.

Registration symbol registered trademark that signifies the trade name of a medication or other medical device that is registered by the manufacturing company. There are certain exclusive rights associated with a registered trademark. The symbol is "®."

Roller clamp small device with IV tubing that has a roller. When the roller is turned (usually with the thumb), the flow of the IV is regulated (increased or decreased).

Roman numerals numbering system from ancient Rome, based on certain letters (i.e., X, V, L, C, I); used with the apothecary system of measurement

Rounding reducing decimal places in a number. A number may be rounded off to the nearest tenth, hundredth, thousandth, and so forth; a number may also be reduced to the nearest whole number.

Routine order order written for a drug that will be administered on a certain schedule or regular basis

Rx prescription

Saline lock rubber needleless device that is attached to the indwelling IV catheter (plastic needle) with or without a short IV tubing attached to it. This device is flushed with saline (formerly flushed with heparin) to prevent the IV catheter from clotting and to allow access to the IV as needed.

SC or **SQ**   subcutaneous. The Joint Commission states "DO NOT USE" this abbreviation; instead, write out "subcutaneous" or "subq."

Scheduled drug   drug in one of five categories (in the United States) that is based on the drug's potential for misuse, abuse, or addiction

Scored tablet   compressed, powdered drug with a line down the center so that the tablet can be broken in half

SI units   International System of Units; a measurement adapted from the metric system that is used in most developed countries to provide a standard language

Single order   medication that is to be given once

Slide clamp   device on IV tubing with a narrow opening that increases to a wider opening. The IV tubing can be pushed into the narrow opening to reduce or stop the flow rate, or it can be pushed into the wider opening, thereby increasing the flow rate.

Sodium chloride (NS)   saline solution, either an IV solution (see Normal saline) or a flush solution used for IV catheters (needles)

Solute   substance dissolved in another substance (the solvent)

Solution or **sol**   clear liquid that contains a drug dissolved in water

Solvent   substance capable of dissolving another substance (the solute)

Spansule   long-acting capsule that contains drug particles coated to dissolve at different times

Spirits   concentrated alcoholic solutions of volatile substances

SR   sustained release

Standing order   drug order written to cover certain situations; the drug is administered only when those conditions are met

Stat   immediately

Stat order   drug to be given immediately

Subcutaneous   tissue between the skin and muscle

Sublingual tablet   powdered drug that is compressed or molded into a solid shape that dissolves quickly under the tongue

Suppository   mixture of a drug with a firm base, molded into a shape to be inserted into a body cavity

Suspension   solid particles of a drug dispersed in a liquid that must be shaken to obtain an accurate dose

Sustained-release capsule   gelatinous capsule enclosing medication that

is slowly released into the body; abbreviated "SR"

Syringe   sterile, hollow barrel, usually made of plastic (but may be glass), with graduated markings and a piston device in the barrel, that is used to pull fluid into the syringe and push the fluid into the body

Syringe pump   electronic IV pump with a syringe plunger that delivers medication at a set rate and/or volume; used with patient-controlled analgesia (PCA), ambulatory patients/clients, or pediatric/infant patients/clients.

Syrup or **syr**   solution of sugar in water to disguise the unpleasant taste of a medication

Tablet or **tab**   powdered drug that is compressed or molded into a solid shape; may contain additives that bind the powder or aid in its absorption

Tbsp or **tbsp**   tablespoon

Teratogen   drug that can cause birth defects

Ticket   medication administration system (rarely used) that uses small medication tickets, listing the medication, dose, amount, frequency, and time; use the three specified checks before administering the medication.

tid   three times a day

Timed release   small beads of drug in a capsule coated to delay absorption

Tincture   alcoholic or hydroalcoholic solution of a drug

Titration   gradually adjusting the dose of a medication to achieve a response

Tolerance   decreased responsiveness to a drug after repeated exposure

Topical   route of administration in which a drug is applied to the skin or mucous membrane

Toxicity   nontherapeutic effect that may result in damage to tissues or organs

TPN   total parenteral nutrition

Trade name   brand or proprietary name, identified by the symbol that follows the name

Transcribe   to rewrite or copy. In nursing and in hospitals, a drug order is usually transcribed usually to another form that records and documents administration of medications.

Transdermal   medicated drug molecules contained in a unique polymer patch applied to the skin for slow absorption

Troche   flat, round, or rectangular preparation held in the mouth (or placed in the vagina) until the drug dissolves

Tsp or **tsp**   teaspoon

Tube feeding   method of providing nutrition for a patient/client through a feeding tube; can also refer to the

high-calorie, high-protein nutritional solution that is used

Tuberculin syringe   1-mL syringe with a small-gauge needle attached (27G or smaller) that is used to draw up amounts of medication less than 1 mL; also called a precision syringe

U   units. The Joint Commission states "DO NOT USE" this abbreviation; instead, write out "unit."

U-50 syringe   syringe marked in units with a small-gauge needle attached (27G or smaller) that is used for insulin injections. The syringe is 0.5 mL in volume, and the markings are per unit (1,2,3,4,5, etc.).

U-100 syringe   syringe marked in units with a small-gauge needle attached (27G or smaller) that is used for insulin injections. The syringe is 1 mL in volume, and the markings are per 2 units (2,4,6,8, etc.).

Ung   ointment

Unit dose   individually wrapped and labeled dose of a drug

Unit system   measurement system using units to measure amounts of drugs. Drugs that use this system include heparin, penicillin, and insulin.

Universal precautions   procedures to protect against infection that are used while caring for all patients/clients and when handling contaminated equipment

USP   United States Pharmacopeia, a public standard-setting authority for prescription and over-the-counter medicines; see *www.usp.org*

Vaginal route   medication inserted or injected into the vagina

Vasopressor   drug that constricts blood vessels, thereby raising blood pressure

Veracity   ethical principle; tell the truth

Vial   glass container with a rubber stopper containing one or more doses of a drug

Volutrol   plastic container, usually 100 to 150 mL in volume, that can be attached to IV tubing and is used to administer medications; also known as Buretrol or Soluset

wt   weight

Young's Rule   rule used to calculate drug dosages for children ages 1 to 12 years, based on the age of the child

Y-site   location on IV tubing where medication can be administered through a rubber, needleless connector. The site looks like a "Y."

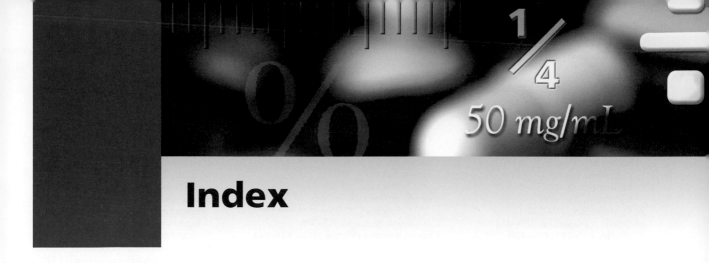

Index

Note: Locators followed by 'f' or 't' refer to figure or table, respectively.